Neuroradiology

A Study Guide

Thanks for a great year (almost!) All the best
W[illegible]

Always remember that food and bathroom breaks are a luxury enjoyed only when patients are gone —
Thanks for the great memories — call anytime — love
Michele

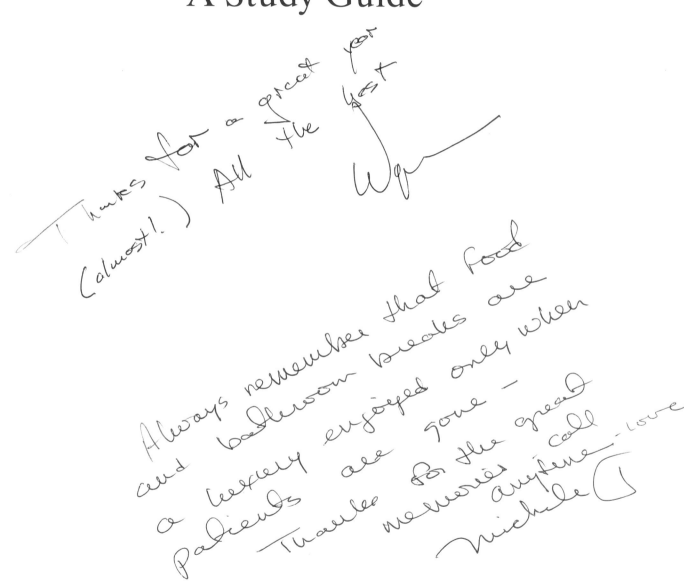

Neuroradiology
A Study Guide

Chi S. Zee, M.D.

Professor of Radiology and Neurosurgery
University of Southern California School of Medicine
Los Angeles, California

McGRAW-HILL
Health Professions Division

New York St. Louis San Francisco Auckland Bogotá
Caracas Lisbon London Madrid Mexico City Milan Montreal
New Delhi San Juan Singapore Sydney Tokyo Toronto

McGraw-Hill
A Division of The McGraw-Hill Companies

Zee: Neuroradiology: A Study Guide

1 2 3 4 5 6 7 8 9 0 KGPKGP 9 8 7 6 5

ISBN 0-07-057128-7

This book was set in Times Roman by Publication Services, Inc.
The editors were Martin J. Wonsiewicz and Susan Finn;
the production supervisor was Richard Ruzycka.
The project was managed by Hockett Editorial Service.
Quebecor Printing/Kingsport was printer and binder.

This book is printed on acid-free paper.

Library of Congress Catalog Card Number: 95-081159

To my wife, Rosa,
and our sons, Edward and Oliver

Contents

Contributors*

Scott Agran, M.D. [Appendix 2]
Clinical Assistant Professor
University of Southern California School of Medicine
Los Angeles, California

Jamshid Ahmadi, M.D. [13]
Professor of Radiology, Neurology, and Neurosurgery
LAC + USC Medical Center
Los Angeles, California

David G. Ashley, M.D. [10]
Staff Neuroradiologist
Northwest Radiology
Bellingham, Washington

William O. Bank, M.D. [17]
Professor and Director
Interventional Neuroradiology
George Washington University Medical Center
Washington, D.C.

Terry S. Becker, M.D. [6]
Associate Clinical Professor and Chief of ENT Radiology
University of Southern California School of Medicine
Sherman Oaks, California

William D. Boswell, M.D. [23]
Associate Clinical Professor of Radiology
Executive Vice-Chairman
Department of Radiology
University of Southern California School of Medicine
Kenneth Norris Cancer Hospital and Research Institute
Los Angeles, California

William G. Bradley, M.D. [16]
Director of Magnetic Resonance Imaging
Long Beach Memorial Hospital and MR Center
Long Beach, California

David P. Chason, M.D. [Appendix 3]
Assistant Professor of Radiology
University of Texas—Southwestern Medical Center
Chief of Neuroradiology
Parkland Memorial Hospital
Austin, Texas

Patrick M. Colletti, M.D. [23]
Associate Professor of Radiology
Director of Magnetic Resonance Imaging
University of Southern California School of Medicine
Imaging Science Center
Los Angeles, California

Sylvie Destian, M.D. [14]
Associate Clinical Professor of Radiology
University of Southern California School of Medicine
Los Angeles, California

Steven Epner, M.D. [4]
Clinical Instructor of Radiology
University of Southern California School of Medicine
LAC + USC Medical Center
Los Angeles, California

D.M. Forrester, M.D. [24]
Associate Professor of Radiology
Director of Resident and Fellowship Program
University of Southern California School of Medicine
LAC + USC Medical Center
Los Angeles, California

Michael I. Ginsburg, M.D. [Appendix 3]
Clinical Instructor of Radiology
University of Texas—Southwestern Medical Center
Austin, Texas

John Go, M.D. [7]
Clinical Instructor of Radiology
University of Southern California School of Medicine
LAC + USC Medical Center
Los Angeles, California

Edwin R. Hudson, M.D. [17]
Clinical Instructor of Radiology
George Washington University Medical Center
Washington, D.C.

James E. Huprich, M.D. [1]
Director of Radiology
Department of Radiology
University of Southern California University Hospital
Los Angeles, California

Benjamin C.P. Lee, M.D. [20]
Associate Professor of Radiology
Washington University Medical Center
St. Louis, Missouri

*The numbers in brackets following the contributor name refer to chapter(s) authored or coauthored by the contributor.

Michael Lefkowitz, M.D. [17]
Fellow in Neuroradiology
University of Southern California School of Medicine
Los Angeles, California

William W.M. Lo, M.D. [8]
Clinical Professor of Radiology
University of Southern California School of Medicine
St. Vincent Medical Center
Los Angeles, California

Mathew Lotysch, M.D. [2]
Staff Neuroradiologist
Mercy Hospital Department of Radiology
Bakersfield, California

George Magre, M.D. [Appendix 1]
Assistant Professor of Radiology
University of Southern California School of Medicine
Chief of MRI
University of Southern California University Hospital
Los Angeles, California

Mukul Maheshwari, M.D. [20]
Clinical Instructor of Radiology
University of Southern California School of Medicine
Los Angeles, California
Long Island Diagnostic
East Setauket, New York

Mark Mehringer, M.D. [18]
Associate Professor and Chairman
Department of Radiology
Harbor-UCLA Medical Center
Torrance, California

Marvin D. Nelson, Jr., M.D. [22]
Associate Professor of Radiology
University of Southern California School of Medicine
Department of Radiology
Children's Hospital—Los Angeles
Los Angeles, California

Charles North, M.D. [2]
Staff Neuroradiologist
Mercy Hospital Department of Radiology
Bakersfield, California

Wayne J. Olan, M.D. [17]
Assistant Professor of Radiology
George Washington University Medical Center
Washington, D.C.

Leonard Petrus, M.D. [3]
Assistant Professor of Radiology
UCLA School of Medicine
Department of Radiology
Olive View Medical Center
Sylmar, California

George Pjura, M.D. [11]
Clinical Instructor of Radiology
University of Southern California School of Medicine
Los Angeles, California

Karen Ragland, M.D. [11]
Clinical Instructor of Radiology
University of Southern California School of Medicine
Los Angeles, California

Hervey D. Segall, M.D. [22]
Professor of Radiology
Director of Neuroradiology
University of Southern California School of Medicine
LAC + USC Medical Center
Los Angeles, California

Tereasa M. Simonson, M.D. [19]
Associate Professor of Neuroradiology
Department of Radiology
University of Iowa College of Medicine
Iowa City, Iowa

Dale Sue, M.D. [5]
Staff Neuroradiologist
Director of Magnetic Resonance Imaging
Plaza Imaging Center, White Memorial Medical Center
Los Angeles, California

Lawrence N. Tanenbaum, M.D. [21]
Staff Neuroradiologist
JFK Medical Center
Edison, New Jersey

James S. Teal, M.D. [25]
Professor and Chairman
Department of Radiology
Howard University School of Medicine
Washington, D.C.

George P. Teitelbaum, M.D. [9]
Associate Professor of Neurosurgery
University of Southern California University Hospital
Los Angeles, California

Michael R. Terk, M.D. [24]
Assistant Professor of Radiology
Director of Musculoskeletal Imaging
University of Southern California School of Medicine
Imaging Science Center
Los Angeles, California

Fong Y. Tsai, M.D. [15]
Professor and Chairman
Department of Radiology
University of Missouri
Truman Medical Center
Kansas City, Missouri

Ay-Ming Wang, M.D. [19]
Co-Chief, Neuroradiology
Clinical Professor of Radiology
University of Missouri
Kansas City School of Medicine
Diagnostic Radiology
William Beaumont Hospital
Royal Oak, Michigan

Alyssa T. Watanabe, M.D. [9]
Clinical Instructor of Radiology
University of Southern California School of Medicine
Los Angeles, California

William T.C. Yuh, M.D. [19]
Professor of Radiology
Director of MRI and Neuroradiology
Department of Radiology
University of Iowa Hospital
Iowa City, Iowa

Chi S. Zee, M.D. [11, 12]
Professor of Radiology and Neurosurgery
University of Southern California School of Medicine
Director of Neuroradiology
USC University Hospital
Los Angeles, California

Foreword

Neuroradiology has been recognized as a subspecialty at the University of Southern California School of Medicine for nearly 35 years. Norman E. Leeds, coming from Juan Taveras's new Fellowship program in New York in 1961, was the ideal person to start a lineage of excellent educators in neuroradiology. Following Norm's return to the East Coast, first William Bruce Anderson, and then Calvin L. Rumbaugh and R. Thomas Bergeron, upheld the tradition which continues to the present day. Norm, Cal, and Tom all later authored excellent textbooks in their area of interest, but these were written after each had left the institution which is now known as the LAC + USC Medical Center. Thus, Chi Zee's *Neuroradiology: A Study Guide* has the distinction of being the first textbook to be edited by an incumbent USC neuroradiologist.

Since the early times when there were only one or two staff members, many outstanding neuroradiologists have trained and practiced at the various USC hospitals—the LAC + USC Medical Center, the Children's Hospital of Los Angeles, the Norris Cancer Center, and the USC University Hospital. Chi Zee, a distinguished product of our neuroradiology training program, has called on these colleagues and other accomplished friends to compile this book. Chi coordinated this effort while taking on important responsibility in neuroradiology at the USC University Hospital and he did not have the luxury of much totally free "academic time." In view of his single-mindedness during this period of time, Chi can well serve as a model for the clinical academician of the future. I congratulate him for this achievement and also acknowledge his much-appreciated contributions to our educational program in neuroradiology at USC over the years.

It is no coincidence that this text appears as the American Board of Radiology moves forward with the development of subspecialty certification in Neuroradiology. It is sincerely hoped that readers who use *Neuroradiology: A Study Guide* to prepare for examinations leading to a CAQ (Certificate of Added Qualifications) will find this book most rewarding.

Hervey D. Segall, M.D.
Los Angeles, California

Preface

This book was created as a study guide to neuroradiology. It is designed as an easily readable text for radiology and neuroscience residents and as a reference for clinicians and practicing radiologists. This book covers three major areas: brain and its coverings; spine and its contents; and head and neck as required by Certificate of Added Qualification. The book is reasonably comprehensive with a large number of statistics and data within it, but it is not an exhaustive reference book. Suggested readings categorized according to specific subjects are included at the end of each chapter for more in-depth study.

This book consists of 25 chapters and is the joint effort of multiple authors, many of whom are well published experts in their specific field. Normal anatomy, pathology, radiology, and clinical information are discussed. Discussion in radiology is focused on computed tomography and magnetic resonance imaging. Other imaging modalities, such as cerebral angiography, radionuclide scan, and skull radiograph are also discussed where necessary. Basic imaging techniques as well as recent advances are also included.

I hope that this book will be a concise, easily readable, and practical source of relevant information.

☐ ACKNOWLEDGMENTS

Special thanks go to my secretary, Mrs. Kelly Stewart, for her invaluable help; Janelle Rich and Yvonne Klausmeier for their secretarial support; Jane Pennington, senior medical editor at McGraw-Hill, who started the project with me; Martin J. Wonsiewicz, who took over the project, and his assistant Laurie Mathews; Susan Finn, the editing supervisor, and Rachel Youngman of Hockett Editorial Service; Dr. Hervey Segall for helping me get interested in the project and for his encouragement; and Drs. James Halls and William Boswell for their support.

I would like to express my sincere appreciation to all the contributors for delivering excellent chapters in such a short time frame and working it into their busy schedules.

Many thanks to Ellen Close and Rod Faccio at USC Medical Graphics and Tom Meichelbock, Orlando Ramirez, Glen Davis, Robert Travlee, and Robert Salinas at the LAC + USC Medical Center Photo Lab.

My thanks for all the technologists at LAC + USC Imaging Science Center and USC University Hospital, especially Linda Needham, Blaine Horvath, and Shellee James.

Finally, I thank my wife, Rosa, for letting me use the dining room as a study and for her moral support, and my sons, Edward and Oliver, for help in transcribing part of the manuscript.

CHAPTER 1

Skull

James E. Huprich

In this era of spiral computed tomography (CT) and echo planar imaging, is there a diagnostic role for plain films of the skull? Thirty years ago the diagnostic tools of the neuroradiologist consisted of plain films, angiography, pneumoencephalography, and Pantopaque (iophendylate) myelography. Plain tomographic images of the sella were carefully examined for clues suggesting the presence of an intrasellar tumor. Evidence of significant intracranial injury from trauma was inferred from the finding of a fracture on a skull series. Thankfully, we no longer need to rely on such indirect methods to make an accurate diagnosis. We have come a long way diagnostically, and one could argue that there is no longer place for skull films in our diagnostic armamentarium. But in order to appreciate how far we have come, we need to see where we started. What we have learned from these less technologically demanding tools forms a useful basis for understanding disease processes in the modern era. Plain films provide superb spatial resolution in examining calvarial lesions and intracranial calcifications. In this regard, plain films prove a useful adjunct to more sophisticated technologies.

The emphasis in this chapter will be on the plain-film appearance of selected disorders of the skull. Tables discussing common differential diagnoses have been included for those who want only a brief review of this subject. The findings of CT and magnetic resonance imaging (MRI) will be discussed when pertinent.

☐ BONY CALVARIUM (Tables 1–1 through 1–5)

NORMAL STRUCTURES SIMULATING DISEASE

Venous Lakes Venous or diploic lakes are normally seen in the parietal bones and near the torcular Herophili. Diploic veins are seen to communicate with these widened venous channels. Their appearance consists of irregular, somewhat oval or round areas of radiolucency rarely greater than 2 cm in longest diameter. "Parietal star" is an appropriate description of the radiographic appearance. When the appearance is more round or oval, distinction from metastatic disease or multiple myeloma may be difficult. Tangential views of the skull usually demonstrate their middle-table origin and their benign nature, leaving the inner and outer table undisturbed.

Pacchionian Granulations Arachnoid granulations project into the lumen of venous sinuses, or the venous lacunae, just lateral to the dural sinuses. Because of their association with the venous sinuses, pacchionian granulations are always located parasagittally. Large pacchionian granulations may cause smooth, focal elevations of the inner table. Occasionally, they may be large enough to produce a deformity of the outer table also. Tangential views that demonstrate their smooth, funneled edges in the inner table belie their benign origin from inside the skull. The presence of a smooth cortical margin is an important sign in distinguishing pacchionian granulations from aggressive lesions.

Parietal Foramina These structures are seldom confused with disease. Parietal foramina consist of two symmetrical lucencies on either side of the sagittal suture located in the posterior third of the parietal bone. These openings allow passage of emissary veins. They are normally very small, but—in an unusual benign familial developmental condition—they can be several centimeters in diameter.

Hyperostosis Frontalis Interna This benign condition is so common that it is included here as a normal variant even though its etiology is unknown. It occurs in 15 percent of women over 40 years of age (can be associated with mild mental retardation and obesity in menopausal women in Morgagni's syndrome). It is rare in men except those with acromegaly. Radiographically, the inner table of both halves of the frontal bone becomes irregularly thickened, resembling a "choppy sea." The areas occupied by the superior sagittal sinus and cortical veins are spared these changes, making this a valuable differential diagnostic point. Rarely, the hyperostosis can involve the whole calvarium (hyperostosis calvariae diffusa).

CONGENITAL / DEVELOPMENTAL

Cephalocele Cephaloceles are skull defects associated with herniated brain contents. The herniated structures in meningoceles consist of meninges and cerebrospinal fluid (CSF). Meningoencephaloceles include brain, meninges, and CSF. Most encephaloceles are isolated; however, occipital cephaloceles may be associated with neural tube defects such as myelomeningocele (7 percent) and diastematomyelia (3 percent). Parietal cephaloceles (10 to 15 percent), occurring between the lambda and the bregma, can be associated with midline brain defects such as absent corpus callosum, Dandy-Walker malformation, lobar holoprosencephaly, and Chiari II malformation. Head scans by CT or MRI help to sort these out.

These *midline* round defects affect both tables of the skull and have a smooth, sclerotic margin. The appearance of these lesions is sufficiently characteristic to allow an accurate diagnosis. When small, they may be confused with a congenital dermal sinus, but the absence of a scalp dimple overlying the skull defect favors a diagnosis of cephalocele. In this country, 75 percent of cephaloceles occur between the foramen magnum and the lambda in the occipital region.

Osteopetrosis This bone dysplasia is a complex disease of four different types. The autosomal recessive lethal type is apparent early in the patient's life and, as the name implies, causes death in childhood, usually from recurrent infection as a result of marrow cavity obliteration. The intermediate recessive type is less severe. Patients are of short stature, afflicted with anemia and hepatomegaly, and sustain pathologic fracture. The recessive type with tubular acidosis, also known as "marble brain," consists of osteopetrosis, renal tubular acidosis, and cerebral calcifications; these patients are frequently mentally retarded. The least severe type is the autosomal dominant type, also known as Albers-Schönberg disease. These patients may be relatively asymptomatic, and the disease is detected because of pathologic fracture. The last two types of osteopetrosis may be associated with a normal life span.

Radiographically, all four types are characterized by generalized osteosclerosis. There is failure of differentiation between the cortex and medullary cavity in the long bones. The presence of "bone within bone" is unusual but characteristic. The entire skull is affected, but the base is more severely involved. The calvarium is also sclerotic, with obliteration of the vascular and diploic markings. The mastoids and paranasal sinuses are poorly developed and the sella appears small. There may be foraminal narrowing with cranial nerve palsies. Osteomyelitis, especially of maxilla and mandible as a result of periodontal disease, is common.

Fibrous Dysplasia Fibrous dysplasia is a disease of unknown etiology in which the osteoblasts fail to mature and differentiate. The *monostotic form* (70 to 80 percent) is frequently asymptomatic and is discovered only incidentally. Skull and facial bone involvement occurs in 20 to 30 percent of these patients. The *polyostotic form* (20 to 30 percent) usually presents before the age of 10 with bone pain, pathologic fractures, skeletal deformity (especially facial), and cranial nerve palsies as a result of foraminal narrowing. Skull and facial involvement occurs in more than 50 percent of these patients. McCune-Albright syndrome includes fibrous dysplasia (almost always the polyostotic type), precocious female sexual development and cutaneous pigmentation. Café au lait spots may be seen in over 50 percent of those with the polyostotic form but can be seen with less frequency in the monostotic form.

Skull abnormalities seen in fibrous dysplasia may be sclerotic or cystic. The more common sclerotic form consists of dense, expanded bone with loss of the diploic space and of trabecular pattern. The affected areas of the skull may be localized or extensive. The sclerotic pattern is more commonly seen when both the skull base and facial bones are involved along with the calvarium. Occasionally, in the calvarium the disease may manifest itself as a "doughnut" lesion—a relatively lucent center with a thick, sclerotic peripheral zone. The cystic form usually involves the calvarium and consists of a blisterlike expansion and thinning of the outer table, with a ground-glass appearance centrally. This may resemble a hemangioma but lacks the typical pattern of trabeculation.

Malignant degeneration is rare in fibrous dysplasia (0.5 percent). However, evidence suggests that up to 37 percent of patients will show progression of their lesions as adults. Therefore it would seem reasonable to follow these patients both clinically and radiologically.

Table 1–1
DIFFERENTIAL DIAGNOSIS: SOLITARY SKULL DEFECTS

Condition	Distinguishing Features
Normal structures	
Venous lake	Involves diploic space only. More common in parietal bones ("parietal star").
Pacchionian granulation	Involves inner table > middle table > outer table. Always parasagittal. Cortical margin.
Cephalocele	Smoothly marginated midline defect in occipital bone of child. May have associated congenital malformations.
Meningioma	Rarely produces pure lytic destruction. Parasagittal. Involves inner table > middle table > outer table.
Hemangiomas	Arise from diploic space, expand to outer table. "Sunburst" or "soap bubble" trabeculation. Evidence of previous hemorrhage on MRI.
Epidermoid/dermoid	Purely lytic defect (uncalcified) most common in temporal and occipital squamosa. Sclerotic rim.
Metastasis	Single metastasis—consider renal or thyroid carcinomas. Middle table involved first. Bony invasion from scalp tumor affects outer table first.
Leptomeningeal cyst	Occur in children. Oval shape with beveled edges suggesting intracranial origin. Clinical history of trauma, neurologic deficit.
Eosinophilic granuloma	Uncalcified defect with uneven destruction of table producing "hole within a hole." Nonsclerotic margin except with healing. Button sequestrum.
Paget's disease	Begins in frontal or occipital, sparing vertex initially. Well-defined lytic lesion without sclerotic margins. Associated skeletal lesions. Basilar invagination. Progresses to healing phase ("cotton-wool").
Postsurgical	Other signs of surgery—clips, sutures, etc.
Osteomyelitis	Early-widening of diploic channels. Progress to coalescent, irregular lucency.

Table 1–2
DIFFERENTIAL DIAGNOSIS: MULTIPLE SKULL DEFECTS

Condition	Distinguishing Features
Normal structures	
Venous lake	Involves diploic space only. More common in parietal bones ("parietal star")
Pacchionian granulation	Involves inner table > middle table > outer table. Always parasagittal. Cortical margin.
Parietal foramina	Small symmetrical lucencies on either side of sagittal suture in posterior third of parietal bone.
Metastases/myeloma	Multiple, irregular lucencies of similar size involving all three tables. Evidence of bony metastases elsewhere in 90% of cases.
Histiocytosis	Round, or oval punched-out lesions with well defined margins arising from the diploic space. Occasionally, a "button sequestrum" is seen. Uneven destruction of inner and outer tables produces "hole within a hole."
Hyperparathyroidism	Mottled demineralization of "ground-glass" appearance. Indistinctness of cortical margins of vascular grooves. Focal destruction is rare (brown tumor).
Osteomyelitis	Early—vague lucencies in diploic space or widening of diploic venous channels. Later—involvement of inner and outer tables. Lucencies coalesce into wide geographic areas of destruction.
Radiation necrosis	Multiple small areas of radiolucency in a pattern corresponding to location of radiation port.

Craniosynostosis Primary craniosynostosis (Table 1–6) may be apparent at birth or during the first few years of life. Typically, the neonate presents with a deformed calvarium or misshapen face, thought to be the result of intrauterine positioning or birth trauma. When the deformity does not resolve, in utero craniosynostosis is considered. In others, the skull is normal at birth and the deformity gradually becomes apparent during the period of rapid calvarial growth. The majority of cases are without apparent cause (primary). Less commonly, craniosynostosis may occur as a result of metabolic disease (rickets, hyperthyroidism, hypervitaminosis D), hematologic disorders (sickle cell disease, thalassemia), or due to decreased intracranial pressure (shunted hydrocephalus, cerebral atrophy, dysgenesis). Craniosynostosis has been described in association with over sixty syndromes.

Table 1–3
DIFFERENTIAL DIAGNOSIS: FOCAL INCREASED SKULL DENSITY

Condition	Distinguishing Features
Osteoma	Involves inner or outer table and spares the middle table. Well-marginated, flat-based domes of dense bone. *External margin is smooth.* May involve frontal sinus.
Meningioma	Focal thickening of inner table with *poorly defined external margin.* May have associated minimal central lysis. Enlarged meningeal artery groove.
Paget's disease	"Cotton-wool" appearance. Trabecular coarsening. Vertex spared or involved after lower portion of skull. Pagetoid lesions in lumbar spine and pelvis.
Fibrous dysplasia	Thickened inner and outer tables at the expense of the diploic space. Loss of trabecular pattern. Some portions of skull may be spared. Skull base and facial bones almost always involved.

Table 1–4
DIFFERENTIAL DIAGNOSIS: DIFFUSE INCREASED SKULL DENSITY

Condition	Distinguishing Features
Osteopetrosis	"Bone within bone" appearance. Changes in skull base greater than in calvarium. Small paranasal sinuses, mastoids, and sella. Anemia, hepatosplenomegaly.
Fibrous dysplasia	Thickened inner and outer tables at the expense of the diploic space. Loss of trabecular pattern. Some portions of skull may be spared. Skull base and facial bones almost always involved.
Paget's disease	"Cotton-wool" appearance. Trabecular coarsening. Vertex spared or involved after lower portion of skull. Pagetoid lesions in lumbar spine and pelvis.
Metastases	Purely sclerotic changes are unusual. Osteoblastic metastases most common with breast and prostate cancer. Destruction frequently has geographic pattern.
Fluorosis	"Chalky" appearance of calvarium and base. Axial skeleton always more affected than skull. Exuberant osteophytes and ligamentous calcification in spine.

Table 1–5
CAUSES OF DIFFUSE CALVARIAL THICKENING

Condition	Features
Anemias	Thickening of diploic space. Thinning of the outer table with "hair-on-end" pattern. Sparing of occipital squamosa.
Myelofibrosis	Thickened inner and outer tables at the expense of the diploic space, producing diffuse osteosclerosis. Axial skeleton and proximal ends of femur and humerus affected. Anemia, hepatosplenomegaly.
Phenytoin (Dilantin)	Thickening of diploic space. History of phenytoin use since childhood.
Shunted hydrocephalus	Thickening of diploic space. History of hydrocephalus, possible neurologic deficit.
Acromegaly	Thickening of all tables. Enlarged sella (80–90%). Expanded frontal sinuses and mastoids. Enlargement and elongation of mandible.
Fibrous dysplasia	Thickened inner and outer tables at the expense of the diploic space. Loss of trabecular pattern. Some portions of skull may be spared. Skull base and facial bones almost always involved.
Paget's disease	"Cotton-wool" appearance. Trabecular coarsening. Vertex spared or involved after lower portion of skull. Pagetoid lesions in lumbar spine and pelvis.

It is commonly associated with Apert's syndrome (acrocephalosyndactyly), Carpenter's syndrome (acrocephalopolysyndactyly) and Crouzon disease (craniofacial dysostosis).

Calvarial growth occurs as a result of sutural widening and ossification of the membranous bony plates. Skull growth occurs in a plane perpendicular to the sutures. The growing brain provides the driving force for this skull enlargement. The most rapid brain growth occurs during the first 2 years of life. Premature closure of major sutures produces abnormal head shape and facial deformity. It is important to detect craniosynostosis early in a child's life. Early detection and treatment prevents more severe skull and facial deformity from occurring and also allows normal brain growth to contribute to this reshaping.

Table 1–6
CRANIOSYNOSTOSIS

Sutures Involved	Skull Deformity	Comments
Sagittal	Dolichocephaly Scaphocephaly	Accounts for 50% of cases. More common in males. Usually isolated and not associated with syndromes. Usually not associated facial deformity.
Metopic	Trigonocephaly	Usually isolated deformity. Associated facial deformities—ethmoid hypoplasia, hypotelorism, tilting of orbits inward.
Bilateral coronal	Brachycephaly	Commonly associated with other suture closure (50%). Frequently associated with syndromes. Facial deformities—"harlequin eye," shortening anterior fossa, shallow orbits, vertical sphenoid wings.
Unilateral coronal	Plagiocephaly	Produces unilateral flattening of skull.
Bilateral lambdoid	Brachycephaly	Small posterior fossa. No associated facial deformities.
Unilateral lambdoid	Plagiocephaly	Produces minimal changes in skull and no facial changes.

The major sutures include the metopic and sagittal sutures, in the midline, and the coronal, lambdoid, and squamosal sutures—the paired sutures. Significant deformity results from closure of one or more of the major sutures. Minor suture closure (frontonasal, frontoethmoid, frontosphenoid, parietomastoid, occipitomastoid, and mendosal) is frequently associated with closure of a major suture. When isolated, minor suture closure seldom results in significant deformity.

Major radiographic signs of craniosynostosis include sclerosis or bridging of the suture, beaking of the margins of the suture, or indistinctness of the suture margins. Only a short segment of the sutural abnormality may be involved, even though the deformity of the skull may be profound. Secondary changes include the reshaping of the face and skull and are the result of the early sutural closure. Prominent convolutional markings, which are normally apparent in children aged 4 to 7 years, may become apparent much earlier. The magnitude of the facial and skull deformities is dependent on the timing of premature suture closure, the distance the suture closure is from the other sutures and the face, the amount of growth normally occurring at the suture; and association with other suture closures.

Sagittal synostosis is the most common form of craniosynostosis, accounting for 50 percent of cases. It is more common in males (3:1) and may be inherited as an autosomal trait. It is seldom associated with syndromic findings. Side-to-side growth is restricted, producing narrowing of the forehead and elongation of the skull (dolichocephaly or scaphocephaly = "long-headedness"). An indentation over the convexity at the site of earliest closure of the suture may be apparent on the lateral skull film. If facial abnormalities are present, additional craniosynostosis should be suspected, since such findings are not common in isolated sagittal synostosis.

Bilateral coronal synostosis is more frequently seen in association with malformation syndromes. It is commonly associated with other sutural closures (50 percent). The facial and skull deformities in isolated bicoronal synostosis demonstrate bilateral harlequin eye deformity (elevation of the superolateral portion of the orbital roof), shortening of the anterior fossa with flattening of the frontal bone (brachycephaly = "short-headedness"), shallow orbits, and vertically slanted and anteriorly bowed sphenoid wings. *Unilateral coronal synostosis* is common and produces unilateral flattening of the skull (plagiocephaly = "oblique-headedness").

Metopic synostosis produces a classic keel-shaped deformity of the anterior skull known as trigonocephaly ("triangle-headedness"). Most secondary features are visible on the anteroposterior frontal view and include ethmoid hypoplasia, hypotelorism, and tilting of the orbits toward each other. In most cases metopic synostosis is an isolated abnormality.

Bilateral lambdoid synostosis causes a brachycephalic skull and a small, flattened posterior fossa. Since it is located far from the face, facial and orbital deformity is not seen. *Unilateral lambdoid synostosis* may produce only subtle changes on the skull films.

Computed tomography plays a valuable role in the management of these patients. It not only demonstrates the changes in the skull in planes and in detail not possible with plain films but also identifies intracranial abnormalities that may influence the decision for surgical therapy. If CT demonstrates that the underlying brain has insufficient capacity to grow, brain expansion will not provide the stimulus to remodel the skull after surgical correction of the skull abnormality. In addition, three-dimensional image reconstruction provides valuable information in preoperative planning.

Dyke-Davidoff-Mason Syndrome (Cerebral Hemiatrophy) Plain film findings indicating unilateral cerebral atrophy were first described by Dyke. The characteristic findings consist of unilateral calvarial thickening (especially of the diploic space); expansion of the ipsilateral ethmoid, frontal, and mastoid sinuses; elevation of the ipsilateral petrous ridge and sphenoid wing; tilting of the planum sphenoidale; and asymmetry of the anterior clinoids. These findings—when combined with clinical findings of hemiparesis, seizures, and mental retardation—

are usually sufficient to make the diagnosis. In questionable cases, CT or MRI findings (hemiatrophy ipsilateral to the skull changes) will confirm the diagnosis.

OSTEOMYELITIS

Osteomyelitis is rarely seen in the United States today. When present, the source of the infection is usually from infected sinuses or mastoid air cells, puncture wounds of the scalp, or infected craniotomy sites. Osteomyelitis of the bony calvarium has a different appearance from that seen elsewhere. Periosteal reaction is extremely rare. Sequestra are unusual. Rapid and widespread involvement is the rule, due to the extensive diploic venous network and the common potential spaces adjacent to the inner and outer table of the skull (epidural and subgaleal). There is no radiographic characteristic that permits diagnosis of a specific organism. The acute and chronic phases of the disease, however, have distinct radiographic appearances.

Acute osteomyelitis is always a lytic process. Roentgenographic signs of untreated osteomyelitis can appear 7 to 10 days after the clinical onset of the disease. The process begins as small, vague lucencies or widening and blurring of the margins of the diploic venous channels. As the disease progresses, these small lucencies become larger and better defined, coalescing into larger areas. All three tables of the calvarium may be involved. Clinical signs of infection are usually present. Associated radiographic signs, such as a clouded sinus or mastoid, postsurgical defect, and so on may suggest the origin of the infection. Left untreated, neurologic complications and death are inevitable.

Acute osteomyelitis of a craniotomy site tends to be more confined to the avascular bone flap. The rich vascular supply of the overlying scalp permits ingrowth of granulation tissue and rapid and sometimes complete resorption of the bone flap.

Chronic osteomyelitis appears radiographically as both a sclerotic and lytic process, with the sclerotic process predominating. It may be secondary to tuberculosis, syphilis, or fungal organisms.

NEOPLASMS

Hemangioma These lesions appear as lytic lesions of less than 4 cm with a "sunburst" or "soap bubble" pattern of trabeculation, occasionally with a sclerotic margin. This abnormal bony trabeculation within the lesion distinguishes hemangiomas from epidermoids, which contain no internal trabeculation. Hemangiomas arise from the diploic space, expand the outer table, and may produce a palpable lump. When vertical trabeculation is a prominent feature on tangential views, these lesions may infrequently be confused with osteogenic sarcoma. Atypical lesions without the classic linear trabeculated appearance may be difficult to distinguish from epidermoid, eosinophilic granuloma, or even meningioma. Magnetic resonance imaging may show evidence of previous hemorrhage.

Epidermoid and Dermoid Tumors Epidermoid and dermoid tumors both arise from inclusion of ectodermal epithelial elements at the time of neural tube closure or during formation of the secondary cerebral vesicles. Dermoids contain dermal appendages. Epidermoids contain keratohyaline material and desquamated squamous epithelium but no dermal appendages.

Epidermoids may be congenital or may also be acquired, as a result of traumatic implantation of epidermis into deeper underlying tissues, with subsequent formation of desquamated keratin-containing cyst. Only 10 percent of central nervous system epidermoids occur in the diploic space (40 to 50 percent, cerebellopontine (CP) angle; 10 to 15 percent, parasellar, middle fossa). Epidermoids, or cholesteatomas, are characterized by a purely lucent defect with a well-defined sclerotic rim most frequently occurring in the temporal or occipital squamosa. The degree of expansion of the diploic space may be great, but there usually remains a rim of sclerotic inner and outer table. Unlike dermoids, epidermoids seldom contain intralesional calcifications. A peripheral rim of calcification may be seen on CT examinations in 25 percent of cases.

Dermoid cysts are far less common than epidermoids; they occur in younger patients and tend to arise in more midline locations. A dermal sinus and external dimple may be present in the skin over the lesion, commonly the midline of the occiput. Dermoids may contain sebaceous and sweat glands as well as hair. The breakdown products of these dermal appendages result in the fatlike signal characteristics on CT and MRI. Dystrophic calcifications or the presence of dental enamel are common pathologic findings. Intradiploic dermoids are extremely rare and radiographically similar to epidermoids, but they tend to be more inhomogeneous, with areas of sclerosis and osteolysis combined with fine linear calcifications.

Meningiomas Meningiomas are the most common nonglial neoplasm of the central nervous system. Over half arise over the convexities and especially in the parasagittal regions near the middle third of the sagittal sinus. Meningiomas in these locations produce local radiographic changes in the calvarium in half or more of cases (bony changes recognizable by CT in approximately 18 percent). The calvarial changes may be osteolytic (rare), osteoblastic, or, most frequently, a mixed pattern. Earliest changes may consist of focal thickening of the inner table, visible only on tangential views of the skull or on CT sections perpendicular to the inner table using bone windows. As the tumor grows, central lysis of the inner table may occur, accompanied by sclerosis near the periphery of the lesion. Meningiomas of the planum sphenoidale may produce a characteristic "blistering" of the floor of the anterior fossa along with a sclerotic reaction.

These tumors are vascular and usually derive their blood supply from meningeal arteries. Convexity meningiomas are usually supplied by an enlarged middle meningeal artery. The arterial dilatation may produce unilateral enlargement and tortuosity of middle meningeal artery groove and enlargement of the foramen spinosum.

Extracranial meningiomas occur in less than 1 percent of cases. When these tumors arise intraosseously, they may appear purely osteoblastic and may resemble fibrous dysplasia.

Calcifications, associated with meningiomas, will be discussed later in this chapter.

Metastases and Multiple Myelomas Any tumor that metastasized to bone can metastasize to the skull. Ninety percent of patients with calvarial metastases also have extracranial metastatic disease. Because of its rich blood supply, the calvarium is more commonly involved than the skull base. Breast (48 percent) and lung carcinoma (14 percent) are the most common metastatic lesions to the calvarium, followed by prostate, renal, thyroid, and melanoma. Solitary skull metastases occur most often in patients with renal and thyroid carcinoma.

Even when extracalvarial metastases are sclerotic, the skull lesions are usually lytic. Any of the three tables of the skull may be involved, or in any combination. Lesions are usually detected when they are 5 mm or more in size. The margins of the lesions may be ill defined, ragged or show permeative destruction. Except in some cases of breast or prostate metastases, there is no sclerosis or new bone formation.

Occasionally, metastases may produce "geographic" destruction of the calvarium, which may be difficult to distinguish from osteomyelitis. Other tumors that may produce a similar appearance are neuroblastoma, melanoma, metastatic sarcoma, and leukemia.

Multiple myeloma manifests itself radiologically as an osteolytic process frequently indistinguishable from metastatic disease. It affects the axial skeleton predominantly. The skull is the third most frequently affected bony structure after the vertebral column and ribs. Classically, myeloma appears as multiple rounded, well-circumscribed lucencies a few millimeters in diameter, without reactive sclerosis. Diffuse sclerosis is seen in 3 percent of patients but seldom in the skull. Mandibular involvement in one-third of cases may help to differentiate myeloma from metastatic disease.

Osteomas Osteomas may involve either table, but more commonly they involve the inner table. Osteomas appear as flat-based, well-marginated domes of dense bone. They are sometimes separated, at least to some extent, from the underlying outer table by a thin radiolucent line. They do not involve the diploic space. If they involve the inner table, they may be difficult to distinguish from the sclerotic reaction associated with meningiomas except for their smooth internal margin. They frequently involve the frontal sinus and can occasionally produce obstruction of the sinus ostia.

HEMATOLOGIC/METABOLIC/ENDOCRINE

Anemias Congenital hemolytic anemias produce such significant bone marrow hyperplasia that characteristic radiographic changes are common. Because the diploic space is an important site of hematopoiesis, changes in the cranial vault are common. In hemolytic anemias, the diploic space expands and thins the outer table. If the stimulus to produce erythrocytes is great enough, the hyperplastic marrow breaks through the outer table and marrow proliferates in the subperiosteal space. Eventually the cortical bone in the outer table may become destroyed and replaced by vertically oriented, calcified, thin columns of bone ("hair-on-end") devoid of a cortical mantle. It is thought that normal intracranial pressure prevents diploic expansion inward, therefore the inner table is unaffected. The occipital squamosa inferior to the internal occipital protuberance contains no marrow; therefore diploic widening and radial spiculation is not seen here.

Radiographic changes range from mild widening of the diploic space to hair-on-end spiculation in the calvarium and facial bone changes. The radiographic changes, however, are an unpredictable and unreliable index of the severity of the anemia, but more severe radiographic changes tend to occur in infants and children. The most striking changes tend to occur in patients with beta-thalassemia major. In the most severe cases, the hair-on-end pattern is seen. Swelling of the marrow in the facial bones inhibits the pneumatization of the maxillary sinuses and produces malocclusion of the jaws and, as a result of overgrowth of the central incisors, a "rodent" facies results. Swelling of the upper maxilla may displace the orbits laterally and produce hypertelorism. Less severe changes consist of diploic expansion, with preservation of the outer table or mild diploic expansion with granular osteoporosis. These less severe changes are seen in 50 percent of patients with sickle cell disease and in 25 percent of those with sickle cell trait. They are also seen in hereditary spherocytosis, iron-deficiency anemia in childhood, and other hemolytic anemias.

Myelofibrosis Myelofibrosis is an uncommon disease associated with bone marrow fibrosis and extramedullary hematopoiesis. It represents the bone marrow's response to a myeloproliferative disorder (chronic granulocytic leukemia, polycythemia rubra vera, and essential thrombocythemia). When it arises without obvious primary cause, it is known as primary myelofibrosis. Pathologically, bone marrow biopsies show focal or diffuse areas of hypercellularity combined with trabecular thickening and overgrowth. The disease affects middle-aged to elderly men and women with signs of hepatosplenomegaly; anemia, with an increased number of nucleated red cells; leukocytosis or leukopenia; abnormal white cells; and increased, decreased, or normal platelet counts.

The calvarium is affected in 25 percent of cases, as usually manifest by thickening of the internal surface of the inner and outer tables, resulting in narrowing of the medullary space. The osteosclerosis is usually homogeneous and the vascular markings become dramatically visible against the thickened bone. The axial skeleton is predominantly affected in this condition, along with the proximal ends of the humerus and femur. Systemic mastocytosis has a very similar appearance and may be difficult to differentiate. The osteophytosis seen in fluorosis is not seen in myelofibrosis and is therefore a helpful distinguishing feature. Paget's disease, metastases, osteomalacia, and renal osteodystrophy are usually sufficiently different in appearance to allow distinction.

Langerhans' Cell Histiocytosis Histiocytosis is traditionally classified into three types—eosinophilic granuloma (the most common and benign form), Hand-Schüller-Christian disease (the most varied, with chronic disseminated osseous lesions), and Letterer-Siwe disease (the acute form, with rapid fatal progression). Lesions of the skull are similar in all three forms. Distinction among the types is based on differences in histology, age of onset, and extent of disease.

Eosinophilic granulomas arise from the diploic space, most commonly in the parietal and temporal petrous bone. Their appearance consists of round or ovoid punched-out lesions with well-defined margins and an occasional sclerotic center—a "button sequestrum." (Button sequestrum is also seen in radiation necrosis, osteomyelitis, fibrous dysplasia, multiple myeloma, Paget's disease, dermoid tumors, and, rarely, metastasis.) Although the full thickness of the calvarium is usually involved, uneven destruction of the inner and outer tables may produce a "hole-within-a-hole" appearance. Characteristically, no sclerosis is seen at the margin except during healing. More aggressive forms of histiocytosis X may produce more extensive involvement of the skull.

Paget's Disease Skull involvement (65 percent) in Paget's disease is second in frequency only to involvement of the lumbar spine and pelvis (76 percent). Three stages of Paget's disease are recognized. The osteolytic phase, also known as osteoporosis circumscripta, is most commonly seen in the skull. It appears as a well-defined lytic lesion, without sclerotic margins, beginning in the frontal bone or occiput. It is virtually never seen near the vertex without first being present lower in the skull. Suture lines do not provide a barrier for growth of these lesions, and the abnormality may involve a large area of the skull. When its margins are irregular or poorly defined, rather than the more usual rounded or scalloped appearance, osteoporosis circumscripta may resemble malignancy or osteomyelitis. The presence of Paget's elsewhere will aid in making this distinction.

The lytic phase is almost invariably followed by evidence of osteogenesis. Areas of both osteolysis and osteosclerosis merge imperceptibly with each other. The trabecular pattern is thickened and disorganized and the tables of the skull become thickened. These first two phases represent the active stages of the disease and are accompanied by local hyperthermia and elevations in serum alkaline phosphatase and hydroxyproline.

The third stage of Paget's disease is the inactive or healing phase. Laboratory abnormalities become normal during this stage. The lesions become more sclerotic and the thickening of the tables of the calvarium become more obvious. During the sclerotic phase this disease may be confused with other similarly appearing conditions. Hyperostosis frontalis interna affects the inner table of the frontal bones symmetrically and is seen more commonly in women. Fibrous dysplasia more commonly affects the facial bones and usually does not display the coarsened trabecular pattern seen with Paget's. Certain anemias, such as thalassemia and sickle cell disease, produce thickening of the outer table with a hair-on-end appearance usually sufficiently different in appearance to distinguish them from Paget's. Occasionally, osteoblastic metastases may resemble the "cotton-wool" lesions of healing Paget's. The presence of pagetoid lesions elsewhere helps to differentiate Paget's from other conditions.

Sarcomatous degeneration in Paget's lesions occurs in less than 5 percent of cases. The most common associated tumor is osteogenic sarcoma. Its diagnosis can be suspected by observing areas of increasing osteolysis in a pagetoid skull.

Hyperparathyroidism Among patients with primary hyperparathyroidism, calvarial changes occur in approximately 10 to 20 percent. Pathologically, there is osteoclastic resorption in all tables of the calvarium, associated with reparative fibrosis and formation of poorly calcified immature bone. Brown tumors (unusual today), representing localized accumulation of fibrous tissue and giant cells, are unusual in the calvarium and occur more commonly in the mandible. The most frequent finding in the skull is mottled demineralization. As the disease advances, the mottled granularity is replaced by a more homogeneous ground-glass appearance. The cortical margins of the vascular grooves and the margins of the inner and outer table become less distinct. Focal areas of demineralization, up to several centimeters in size, may appear. Less commonly, focal areas of sclerosis or generalized increased mineralization may be seen. With successful surgical removal of the parathyroid gland abnormality, these areas of demineralization may become sclerotic as a result of healing. The presence of calcifications in the falx and tentorium and vascular calcifications is more commonly seen in secondary rather than primary hyperparathyroidism (e.g., renal osteodystrophy).

IATROGENIC LESIONS

Leptomeningeal Cysts Leptomeningeal cysts, or "growing skull fractures," result from herniation of arachnoid membrane through a skull fracture. This accounts for the frequent oval shape of these lesions. The pulsations of the CSF cause gradual expansion of the fracture. The beveled edges and preferential erosion of the inner table belie their intracranial origin. These lesions are more common in children and generally result from diastatic parietal bone fractures. As a result of the initial trauma, there is usually underlying brain damage, which may be obvious clinically. If the herniated arachnoid is multiloculated, the margins of the cyst appear scalloped.

Radionecrosis Radiographic changes in the calvarium as a result of radiation therapy occur with absorbed doses of 3500 cGy or more. The radiographic changes generally take years to occur. The common pattern of multiple small areas of radiolucency may be difficult to distinguish from osteomyelitis, metastatic disease, and multiple myeloma. Sometimes the pattern may be that of mixed areas of osteolysis and sclerosis. The correspondence of the radiographic changes with the location of the radiation treatment ports is a valuable differential diagnostic point.

Abnormalities Caused by Medications and Other Chemical Agents Chronic use of phenytoin (Dilantin) has been associated with diffuse calvarial thickening. This phenomenon is more common in patients who have been on phenytoin therapy since childhood. The increase in calvarial thickness is attributable to widening of the diploic space.

Chronic fluorine intoxication, or fluorosis, occurs most commonly in people who live in areas where the fluoride level in drinking water exceeds 4 ppm. Ninety percent of the absorbed fluorine is excreted, mainly in the urine. The majority of the retained fluorine is deposited in the calcified tissues. Characteristically, the axial skeleton is more severely involved, with the extremities and skull usually less affected. Increasing trabecular condensation leads to a chalky appearance throughout the thorax, spine, and pelvis. These changes, along with findings of exuberant vertebral osteophyte formation and ligamentous calcification, are virtually diagnostic of this disease. Changes in the skull, although unusual, are seen in both the base and the vault. These changes consist of increased density of all the tables without significant overall thickening. Successful treatment may result in partial reversal of these changes.

☐ BASILAR INVAGINATION AND PLATYBASIA

As pointed out by Dr. Smoker in her fine article discussing the craniovertebral junction (see "Suggested Readings"), detailed discussions of the craniovertebral junction are conspicuously absent from standard texts. This is unfortunate since so much confusion exists regarding abnormalities in this area. Much of the confusion stems from misunderstanding of the terms used to define these abnormalities.

Basilar invagination and *basilar impression* both refer to an abnormally high position of the vertebral column with respect to the skull base. Radiographic diagnosis is based on alteration in one or more craniometric measurements. The most commonly used reference lines and angles are Chamberlain's line, McGregor's line, Wakenheim's clivus baseline, and Welcher's basal angle (Diagram 1–1). As pointed out by Dr. Smoker, it is far easier to apply these measurement to a sagittal MRI image than a skull film.

The term *basilar invagination* is used when the cause is developmental. Developmental anomalies responsible for basilar invagination usually involve hypoplasia of one of the components of the craniovertebral junction, such as basioccipital hypoplasia or fusion, occipital condyle hypoplasia, bifid posterior arch of the atlas, Klippel-Feil syndrome, and other anomalies that produce hypoplasia of the craniovertebral junction components. *Basilar impression*, on the other hand, is the term used when the cause is secondary or acquired. Diseases that cause softening of the skull base to produce basilar impression are Paget's disease, rheumatoid arthritis, osteomalacia, hyperparathyroidism, osteogenesis imperfecta, Hurler's

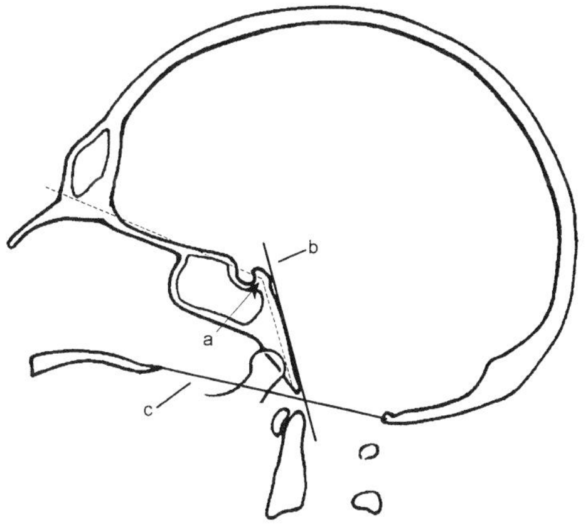

Diagram 1–1 Craniometric evaluation of basilar invagination, basilar impression, and platybasia. *a. Welcher basal angle* is formed at the intersection of the nasion-tuberculum line and the tuberculum-basion line. If greater than 140°, platybasia exists. *b. Wackenheim clivus baseline* is formed by drawing a line parallel to the posterior clival margin. The extended line should fall tangent to the posterior margin of the tip of the odontoid. The intersection of this line with the posterior spinal line should be greater than 150°. *c. Chamberlain line* is drawn from the posterior tip of the hard palate to the opisthion (posterior margin of the foramen magnum). The distance to the tip of the odontoid should be from 1 to 6 mm.

syndrome, rickets, and skull base infection. Either basilar impression or basilar invagination exists when Chamberlain's line, McGregor's line or Wakenheim's clival baseline indicates an abnormally high position of the upper cervical spine. Platybasia, on the other hand, is strictly an *anthropometric term* referring to abnormal flattening of the Welcher basal angle. Although usually associated with basilar invagination or basilar impression, it may be an isolated finding.

□ INTRACRANIAL CALCIFICATIONS

PHYSIOLOGIC CALCIFICATION

The term *physiologic calcifications* is meant to describe calcifications that occur normally. The term may, however, only reflect our lack of understanding of their etiology. The incidence of these "normal" calcifications varies, not only among different geographic regions and between the two genders but also with metabolic states. For example, the incidence of pineal calcification is higher among normocalcemic patients with urinary tract calculi. Physiologic calcifications become more prevalent as we age and may reflect a degenerative process.

Pineal calcifications are the most common intracranial calcifications. The incidence in adult North Americans, as detected on plain films, is approximately 60 percent. Pineal calcification may be seen in children but should be considered abnormal if seen in a patient less than 6 years old. The calcifications appear as an amorphous or clumped group less than 1 cm in diameter approximately 3 cm posterior and superior to the dorsum sellae. If the calcifications measure more than 1 cm in diameter, an abnormality such as a calcifying neoplasm should be suspected. Calcifications may be only faintly visible on the lateral view. When they are detected on the anteroposterior view, the center of the calcifications should not be displaced more than 2 mm from the midpoint of the biparietal line. Habenular calcifications are seen approximately 5 mm anterior to the pineal in 30 percent of adults. The appearance is that of an elongated "C" open posteriorly.

Dural calcifications tend to occur in specific areas. Calcification of the anterior portion of the falx is the most common and occurs in 7 to 9 percent of adults. It appears on the frontal view as a linear streak involving one or both leaves of the dural reflection. Calcification of the dura of the superior sagittal sinus is more common in females (falx calcification is more common in males) and appears as a V-shaped structure at the vertex on the anteroposterior skull. Calcifications of the tentorial reflection extending from the petrous pyramid to the posterior clinoid process (petroclinoid ligament) and a portion of the diaphragma sella (interclinoid ligament) are also commonly seen (approximately 10 percent). Extensive dural calcifications have been described in disorders of calcium homostasis, pseudoxanthoma elasticum, and basal cell nevus syndrome.

Calcification in the choroid plexus may occur anywhere but is commonly seen in the atria of the lateral ventricle. It is seen on skull films in 10 percent of adults and may appear amorphous, nodular, or reticulated. Significant asymmetry in calcification is common. Calcification occurring in other areas of the choroid (particularly the temporal horn) suggests the presence of neurofibromatosis type 2.

Basal ganglion calcification, commonly seen as a normal finding on CT examinations, should be considered abnormal when visible on skull films. They may be visible in the anterior part of the globus pallidus and are sometimes accompanied by calcification in the dentate nucleus. On the frontal views, the calcifications are in the characteristic location and consist of truncated V's with the limbs of the V projected toward the frontal sinuses. On the lateral view, the calcifications form an arch paralleling the squamosal suture. The causes of calcification of the basal ganglion are listed in Table 1–7.

PHAKOMATOSES

Tuberous Sclerosis Intracranial calcifications are seen in 50 percent of patients with this disease. Calcifications are multiple in 75 percent and bilateral in 50 percent of patients. The calcifications are not characteristic and consist of scattered, granular groups. In 40 to 52 percent of patients, well-circumscribed unilateral focal areas of hyperostosis are seen in the frontal or parietal regions and may be confused with intracranial calcifications. The intracranial calcifications may be located within the cortical tubers, the subependymal nodules, or in subependymal giant-cell astrocytomas and therefore may be widely scattered.

Neurofibromatosis Nonneoplastic calcifications are unusual in neurofibromatosis and generally occur only in type 2 disease. They have been described in the choroid, particularly the temporal horn and cerebellum, and are occasionally seen on the cortical surface. Their appearance is granular, similar to that of tuberous sclerosis. Calcifications may also be seen in the neoplasms associated with neurofibromatosis.

Sturge-Weber Syndrome Intracranial calcifications are seen on plain films in 50 to 60 percent of patients with Sturge-Weber syndrome. They appear as so-called "tram-track" calcifications near the cortical surface. The calcifications occur in the middle layers of the cortex and are probably degenerative in nature, secondary to ischemia as a result of venous stasis from lack of normal venous drainage. The parallel calcifications are the result of calcification in adjacent gyri separated by a sulcus. The calcifications are seldom seen before the age of two and tend to occur on the same side as the cutaneous nevus.

Table 1–7
CAUSES OF BASAL GANGLION CALCIFICATION

Condition	Features
Physiologic	Commonly seen on CT, abnormal if calcifications seen on plain films.
Hypoparathyroidism/ pseudohypoparathyroidism	Hypocalcemia and hyperphosphatemia. There may be a history of thyroidectomy or this may be familial. Calvarial thickening and hypoplastic dentition.
Wilson's disease	Extrapyramidal signs. Kayser-Fleischer rings. Cirrhosis. Hypodense putamen on CT. High signal in putamen, dentate, thalamus, and brainstem on T2-weighted MRI images.
Fahr's disease	Familial. Microcephaly, spasticity, seizures, progressive neurologic deterioration.
Cockayne's syndrome	Familial diffuse demyelinating process. Microcephaly. Abnormal facies. Kyphoscoliosis. Dwarfism.
Down's syndrome	Mental retardation. Brachycephaly. Abnormal facies. Skull-base deformities. Cervical spinal stenosis. Atlantoaxial subluxation. Hypoplastic temporal lobe and inferior frontal gyrus.
Mineralizing angiopathy	Seen in children following radiation and methotrexate therapy for leukemia. Associated with calcifications in subcortical white matter.
Hypoxic-ischemic encephalopathy	Accompanied by severe atrophy or encephalomalacia and profound neurologic deficit. History of perinatal anoxia, carbon monoxide poisoning.
Lead intoxication	Seizures, hemiparesis, optic atrophy, generalized weakness. "Lead" lines in ends of long bones.
AIDS	Children born of HIV-positive mother. Progressive spastic quadriparesis. Failure to thrive. Generalized cerebral atrophy.
Toxoplasmosis	Congenital. Hydrocephalus. Bilateral chorioretinitis. Calcifications may be scattered.

NEOPLASMS

In earlier times, before CT and MRI, it was thought that the appearance and location of calcifications seen in intracranial tumors on plain films might lead to a definitive histologic diagnosis. Unfortunately, this proved not to be true. Except in a few instances, each tumor type may be associated with a wide variety of morphologic styles of calcification, none of which is distinctive enough to allow confident diagnosis of tumor type. Location of calcification and associated skull changes greatly narrows the diagnostic possibilities and in some cases (e.g., corpus callosum lipoma, craniopharyngioma), strongly suggests a specific histologic diagnosis.

Neuroglial Tumors The incidence of calcifications associated with astrocytomas seen on plain films is 9.3 percent. As expected, calcification is more commonly seen on CT exams. The type of calcifications produced in these tumors is not sufficiently characteristic to allow specific diagnosis. Earlier literature pointed out that calcifications are more common in infratentorial astrocytomas occurring in younger patients. The explanation for this observation may be that calcification more commonly occurs in lower-grade astrocytomas, which tend to occur in younger patients who also have a higher incidence of infratentorial tumors than adults. Anaplastic astrocytomas and glioblastoma multiforme, which arise from more benign tumors, tend to have a higher incidence of calcification. Pilocytic astrocytomas (optochiasmatic-hypothalamic gliomas) are calcified on CT in 10 percent of cases. The majority of subependymal giant cell astrocytomas, seen in tuberous sclerosis, calcify.

Calcification in oligodendrogliomas is common (40 percent). The incidence of calcification is the same in all age groups. Differences do exist with respect to location of the tumor—frontal and parietal tumors tend to calcify more frequently than tumors at other locations. As with the other gliomas, the morphology of the calcifications is not distinctive.

Calcification is also commonly seen in ependymomas (20 percent) and choroid plexus neoplasms. Only a few cases of calcification in choroid plexus papillomas visible on plain films have been reported, so the exact incidence is not known. Eighty-five percent of these tumors occur in young children. Physiologic calcification of the choroid would be unusual at this age and therefore probably does not account for the high incidence seen with CT.

Calcification has also been reported in some mixed glial-neuronal and neuronal tumors (ganglioglioma, central neurocytoma).

Pineal Region Tumors Because of the frequency of physiologic calcification in the pineal gland, neoplasms that arise in this area are frequently "calcified." Calcification within pineal tumors may either be produced by the neoplasm or the physiologic calcifications may be displaced or altered by tumor. Tumor-generated calcifications are more commonly associated with pineal-cell tumors (pineocytoma and pineoblastoma) and teratomas than by the more common germ-cell tumors. Alterations in the normal appearance of the calcifications should be sought in patients suspected of having a pineal region tumor. Table 1–8 summarizes the findings on plain films which should lead to further investigation for

Table 1–8
PLAIN-FILM FINDINGS SUGGESTIVE OF PINEAL REGION NEOPLASM

Calcified pineal in child under 5 years of age
Pineal region calcifications greater than 10 mm in diameter
Displaced pineal calcification
Unusual appearance of pineal calcifications

pineal neoplasm, such as performance of a CT or MRI examination.

Parasellar Tumors Pituitary adenomas seldom calcify (less than 5 percent). Of the parasellar neoplasms, craniopharyngiomas calcify most frequently (75 to 80 percent). In nearly two-thirds of cases, the calcifications are seen above the diaphragma. The majority of calcifications are nodular or floccular in appearance. Curvilinear calcifications are also commonly seen in the walls of the cystic components.

Chordomas Calcification is seen in skull-base chordomas in 30 to 70 percent of cases. In the majority of cases, the calcifications can be distinguished from those similar appearing calcifications in craniopharyngioma by their retrosellar location and the associated destructive changes (90 percent) in the clivus, sella, and petrous bone. In some cases the calcifications may be very dense and well organized, similar to those seen in osteochondral tumors (discussed elsewhere).

Meningiomas Calcification in meningiomas is unusual (10 percent incidence on plain films; 20 to 25 percent incidence on CT scans) and far less frequent than associated bony changes (50 percent). *Psammomatous calcification* is a term borrowed from pathology and refers to the granular calcifications sometimes seen in meningiomas. Alternately, calcifications can be very dense ("brain stone"), curvilinear, or resemble a "sunburst" pattern. As is the case with most tumoral calcifications, their location (parasagittal, suprasellar, etc.) is far more important as a distinguishing feature than their appearance.

Lipomas The exact incidence is unknown, but calcification in corpus callosum lipomas usually has a characteristic appearance. The calcification that occurs in the lateral walls of the tumor and on the frontal skull films suggests a midline calcified cystic lesion. These lesions are associated with callosal dysgenesis in half the cases.

INFECTIONS

Cysticercosis Intracranial calcifications seen in cysticercosis usually appear as 1- to 2-mm nodules scattered throughout the brain (collapsed, calcified cyst) or as a 0.5-mm ringlike calcification comprising an eccentric nodule (dead scolex within a calcified cyst). Films of the extremities may demonstrate rice-sized calcification in the muscles, with the long axis of the calcification oriented parallel with the muscle bundles.

Tuberculosis Intracranial tuberculosis exists in two forms—meningeal and parenchymal. As tuberculous meningitis heals, curvilinear or branching calcific plaques or "popcorn" calcifications may be seen in the region of the basilar cisterns. This appearance differs from the calcifications seen in parenchymal infections (tuberculomas), which tend to produce nodular calcifications with a crenated margin. Both types of calcification may be seen together, since parenchymal and meningeal involvement is common (11 percent). Solitary tuberculomas are twice as common as multiple ones.

Toxoplasmosis and Cytomegalovirus These two congenital viral infections are discussed together because the appearance of the intracranial calcifications is indistinguishable. At one time it was felt that cytomegalovirus (CMV) more commonly presented with visible calcifications at birth and that the calcifications of toxoplasmosis appeared later. This proved untrue. The calcifications in both diseases may be seen at birth or soon after. Calcifications occur commonly in both diseases (CMV, 25 percent; toxoplasmosis, 32 to 59 percent). They are typically located in the periventricular region but may be widespread. Intracranial calcifications are not seen in the acquired form of these diseases in immunocompromised patients.

VASCULAR CALCIFICATION

Atherosclerotic calcification is commonly seen in the carotid siphon of older individuals and does not necessarily indicate significant associated vascular obstruction. The calcifications appear as ring shadows lateral to the floor of the sella on the frontal projection and as curvilinear shadows in one or both walls of the carotid, overlying the sella, on the lateral view. Calcification occurring with aneurysms and arteriovenous malformations is also usually curvilinear. Calcification visible on plain films in symptomatic saccular aneurysms is probably less than 5 percent. The incidence is higher for giant aneurysms (22 percent) and is rare in mycotic aneurysms. Approximately 25 percent of arteriovenous malformations contain visible calcifications. These may occur in the nidus, the feeding or draining vessel, or within associated aneurysms.

TRAUMATIC CALCIFICATION

Significant calcification in traumatic intracerebral hematoma is disputed and its incidence is rare at best. Case reports in the older literature describe "brain stones" thought to be the result of previous strokes or traumatic hemorrhage.

Calcification in chronic subdural hematomas is a rare (less than 0.5 percent) but well-accepted phenomenon. It occurs more often in the parietal or temporoparietal region and is characterized by a "tissue paper"-like sheet of calcification adjacent to the inner table. The margins of the calcification are usually well corticated. If associated with long-standing atrophy from birth trauma, there may be thickening of the calvarium.

☐ SELLAR ENLARGEMENT

PLAIN-FILM ANATOMY OF THE SELLA TURCICA

Thirty years ago, any competent neuroradiologist knew the bony anatomy of the sellar region in great detail. This was necessary, since so many intracranial processes produced changes, often subtle, in the sellar structures. In this section we are going to revisit this slice of history.

The *planum sphenoidale* represents the posterior midline portion of the floor of the anterior fossa. The posterior margin of the planum is marked by an inconstant elevation, the *limbus sphenoidale*. This structure is separated from the anterior boundary of the pituitary fossa, the *tuberculum sellae*, by a shallow groove for the optic chiasm, *the chiasmatic groove*. From the tuberculum, the sellar floor sweeps down and posteriorly to the base of the *dorsum sellae*. Some portion of the floor of the sella shares a common bony wall with the adjacent sphenoid sinus. Indeed, the architecture of the sphenoid sinus greatly influences the normal appearance of the floor of the sella and its reaction to intracranial processes. The dorsum sellae along with the floor of the sella are the most common sellar structures in which radiographic abnormalities occur in response to disease. The *posterior clinoid processes* are symmetrical bony prominences projecting upward, forward, and laterally. The *anterior clinoid processes* arise from the lesser wings of the sphenoid lateral to the tuberculum sellae and project posteriorly.

Neuroradiologists used to spend a great deal of time pondering the sella, trying to determine whether the pituitary fossa was enlarged on a lateral skull film. If you had a dime, the task became much easier because a U.S. dime is 17.5 mm in diameter and the upper limits of normal for the anteroposterior dimension of the pituitary fossa (as measured from the anterior wall below the tuberculum to the posterior wall below the tip of the dorsum), on a 40-in. lateral skull film is 17 mm. The height of the pituitary fossa is measured from the lowest point of the floor to a line drawn from the tuberculum to the tip of the dorsum and should not exceed 13 mm. The area of the sella on the lateral view should not exceed 130 mm^2.

PLAIN FILM CHANGES OF SELLAR ENLARGEMENT

Chromophobe adenomas produce archetypal radiographic findings of sellar enlargement (Table 1–9). As the tumor grows, the pituitary fossa balloons and the dorsum becomes curved. Early on, the cortical margins remain intact. Adenomas frequently produce asymmetrical expansion of the sella, manifest on the lateral view as a "double floor." Correlation with the anteroposterior view reveals this asymmetrical involvement of the sellar floor. When isolated, this sign should be interpreted cautiously, since it can be normal. As the tumor continues to grow, the cortex at the base of the dorsum may become eroded and there may be extension into the sphenoid. The competency of the diaphragma sella (the dural roof of the sella) and the character of the bone between the floor of the sella and the sphenoid sinus seem to determine whether the expanding mass grows upward or downward. The growing tumor may erode and displace the dorsum and posterior clinoids upward and posteriorly (the anterior clinoids may also be displaced upward). The direction of displacement of the anterior and posterior clinoids and

Table 1–9
CAUSES OF SELLAR ENLARGEMENT

Condition	Features
Pituitary adenoma	"Ballooned sella." Expansion into sphenoid sinus. Tip of dorsum and clinoids displaced *upward.* No intratumoral calcification.
Craniopharyngioma	Suprasellar calcifications. Sellar enlargement may be mild or sella may appear flattened. "Whittled" dorsum and anterior and posterior clinoid processes that may be displaced *downward.*
Aneurysm	"Double floor" appearance or enlarged carotid sulcus. Ipsilateral thinning of anterior clinoid process and widening of superior orbital fissure. Curvilinear calcifications.
Hydrocephalus	Demineralization or erosion of dorsum and posterior clinoid processes with displacement *downward.* Mild or absent sellar enlargement.
Intrasellar herniation of arachnoid (empty sella)	Sellar expansion may be indistinguishable from intrasellar mass. More common in women (4:1). Asymptomatic. Appearance on MRI and CT is characteristic.

tip of the dorsum is extremely useful in determining the epicenter of the mass. Eosinophilic and basophilic adenomas less commonly produce expansion of the sella. The presence of other bony changes of acromegaly (large mandible, prominent paranasal sinuses) is helpful in suggesting the presence of an eosinophilic adenoma.

Three-quarters of craniopharyngiomas are entirely suprasellar. Because of this location, sellar enlargement is less common and less dramatic than with pituitary adenomas. Instead, craniopharyngiomas tend to "whittle away" at the anterior and posterior clinoids and the tip of the dorsum, producing a flattened rather than a ballooned sella. The presence of calcification (75 to 80 percent) is a helpful differential point. Occasionally, these tumors produce a sclerotic reaction in the sella (11 percent), and this finding must be differentiated from that produced by meningiomas (which usually involves the planum or sphenoid wing, sparing the sellar floor) and, rarely, chordoma.

Intracavernous carotid aneurysms, due to their lateral position usually do not cause symmetrical enlargement of the sella. The carotid groove, on the lateral margin of the sellar floor, may become enlarged and produce a double floor. The anterior clinoid may become thinned on its undersurface, and there may be associated widening of the superior orbital fissure. The presence of curvilinear calcifications is also a helpful sign.

Dilatation of the inferior recesses of the third ventricle may cause expansion of the sella. This is usually seen in cases of posterior third ventricular or aqueductal obstruction of long standing. Because of the proximity of the recesses to these structures, the dorsum sellae and posterior clinoid processes are almost always affected to a greater extent than is the degree of expansion of the pituitary fossa. These bony structures become demineralized and eroded and fragments are displaced downward. The changes may appear similar to those seen with craniopharyngioma. The presence of calcifications in craniopharyngiomas helps to distinguish them.

Intrasellar herniation of arachnoid may produce sellar expansion, which is indistinguishable from intrasellar tumors. Intrasellar herniation of arachnoid is seen in 24 percent of autopsies. Its etiology is related to a wide opening in the diaphragma sella allowing arachnoid herniation. The sellar enlargement is thought to result from pulsations of the CSF against the sellar walls. It is more commonly seen in women by a ratio of 4:1. Fortunately, CT and MRI findings are characteristic.

SUGGESTED READING

1. DuBoulay GH: *Principles of X-Ray Diagnosis of the Skull,* 2nd ed. London, Butterworths, 1981.
2. Fernbach SK, Feinstein KA: Radiologic evaluation of the child with craniosynostosis. *Neurosurg Clin North Am* 2:569, 1991.
3. Kaplan SB et al: Radiographic manifestations of congenital anomalies of the skull. *Radiol Clin North Am* 29:195, 1991.
4. Lane B: Erosions of the skull. *Radiol Clin North Am* 12:257, 1974.
5. Moser RP: From the archives of the AFIP: Fibrous dysplasia. *Radiographics* 10:519, 1990.
6. Newton TH, Potts DG: *Radiology of the Skull and Brain,* vol 1, Books 1 and 2. St Louis, Mosby, 1971.
7. Osborn AG: *Diagnostic Neuroradiology,* St Louis, Mosby-Yearbook, 1994.
8. Resnick D: *Bone and Joint Imaging.* Philadelphia, Saunders, 1989.
9. Smoker WRK: Craniovertebral junction: Normal anatomy, craniometry, and congenital anomalies. *Radiographics* 14:255, 1994.
10. Taveras JM, Wood EH: *Diagnostic Neuroradiology,* 2d ed. Baltimore, Williams & Wilkins, 1976.
11. Weinberg PE: *Neuroradiology Test and Syllabus.* Reston, VA, American College of Radiology, 1990.

☐ QUESTIONS (True or False)

1. Fibrous dysplasia
- **a.** Skull and facial involvement is seen in 50 percent of polyostotic disease.
- **b.** Skull involvement may be sclerotic or cystic.
- **c.** Sclerotic skull lesions more commonly associated with skull base and facial involvement.
- **d.** Café au lait spots not seen in monostotic disease.
- **e.** Progresson of lesions is not seen in adulthood.

2. Craniosynostosis
- **a.** Skulls appear abnormal at birth in patients with craniosynostosis.
- **b.** Skull growth occurs independent of brain growth.
- **c.** Bilateral coronal synostosis is the most frequent type.
- **d.** Sagittal synostosis is usually not associated with syndromic findings.
- **e.** Plagiocephaly means "triangle-headedness."

3. Calvarial neoplasms
- **a.** "Sunburst" trabecular pattern is commonly seen with hemangiomas.
- **b.** Dermoids arise from ectodermal and mesodermal elements.
- **c.** Dermoids are far less common than epidermoids.
- **d.** Epidermoids never calcify.
- **e.** Epidermoids may be congenital or acquired.

4. Meningioma
- **a.** Bony changes are radiographically visible in 50 percent of convexity meningiomas.
- **b.** Osteolytic bony changes do not occur.
- **c.** Planum meningiomas may cause "blistering" of the floor of the anterior fossa.
- **d.** Calcifications are visible in plain films in 20 to 25 percent of cases.
- **e.** Calcifications associated with meningiomas are characteristic.

5. Hematologic disorders
- **a.** Skull changes in hemolytic anemia begin in the outer table.
- **b.** The occipital squamosa is usually spared in hemolytic anemia.
- **c.** Skull changes are seen with thalassemia and sickle cell disease only.
- **d.** Expansion of the middle table is seen in myelofibrosis.
- **e.** Systemic mastocytosis has a similar appearance to myelofibrosis.

6. Paget's disease
- **a.** Skull involvement is second in frequency only to pelvis and lumbar spine.
- **b.** Paget's does not cross suture lines.
- **c.** Thickening of the trabecular pattern is a characteristic finding.
- **d.** Facial involvement is a common feature used to distinguish Paget's from fibrous dysplasia.
- **e.** Sarcomatous degeneration occurs in 5 percent of cases.

7. Basilar invagination and platybasia
- **a.** Chamberlain's line is used to differentiate basilar invagination and basilar impression.
- **b.** Platybasia refers to flattening of the basal angle.
- **c.** Basilar invagination refers to acquired alterations in the craniovertebral relationships.
- **d.** Craniometric measurements are best made from plain skull films.
- **e.** Basilar impression and basilar invagination are usually asymptomatic.

8. Physiologic calcifications
- **a.** The incidence does not vary with sex or geographic region.
- **b.** Pineal calcifications are visible in adults on 70 percent of skull films.
- **c.** Pineal calcification should be considered abnormal if seen before 12 years of age.
- **d.** Calcification of the dura of the superior sagittal sinus is more common in females.
- **e.** Calcification in the choroid in the atria of the lateral ventricle suggests the presence of NF 2.

9. Abnormal intracranial calcifications
- **a.** Calcifications in the basal ganglion seen on skull films should always be considered abnormal.
- **b.** Intracranial calcifications are uncommon in NF-1.
- **c.** Intracranial calcifications are seen in 50 to 60 percent of patients with Sturge-Weber disease.
- **d.** High-grade gliomas calcify more commonly than low-grade tumors.
- **e.** Plain-film calcifications are seen in 37 percent of oligodendrogliomas.

10. Sellar enlargement
- **a.** Marked sellar enlargement is common with craniopharyngiomas.
- **b.** The height of the pituitary fossa should not exceed 17 mm.
- **c.** Dilatation of the third ventricle commonly causes changes in the anterior clinoids.
- **d.** Calcification within a pituitary adenoma helps to distinguish it from intrasellar herniation of arachnoid.
- **e.** One-half of all craniopharyngiomas are suprasellar.

☐ ANSWERS

1. **a.** T
b. T
c. T
d. F
e. F

2. **a.** F
b. F
c. F
d. T
e. F

3. **a.** T
b. F
c. T
d. F
e. T

4. **a.** T
   b. F
   c. T
   d. F
   e. F

5. **a.** F
   b. T
   c. F
   d. F
   e. T

6. **a.** T
   b. F
   c. T
   d. F
   e. T

7. **a.** F
   b. T
   c. F
   d. F
   e. F

8. **a.** F
   b. F
   c. F
   d. T
   e. F

9. **a.** T
   b. T
   c. T
   d. F
   e. F

10. **a.** F
    b. T
    c. F
    d. F
    e. F

CHAPTER

2

Skull Base and Cranial Nerves

Charles North
Mathew Lotysch

☐ NORMAL ANATOMY

FORAMINA, FISSURES, CANALS, AND THEIR IMPORTANT CONTENTS

As you begin to read this, may we suggest that you utilize a skull specimen to aid your comprehension of the structures we will be reviewing.

The skull base comprises five bones: the ethmoid, frontal, sphenoid, temporal, and occipital lobes (Diagrams 2–1 and 2–2).

Ethmoid Bone The ethmoid bone is the small bone situated in the midline anterior to the sphenoid bone and comprising the dorsal aspect of the nasal ethmoid complex. When viewed from the interior of the skull the main features of the ethmoid are the paired cribriform plates and the crista galli. The cribriform plates are very thin and have multiple perforations, which accommodate the passage of the several small branches of the first cranial nerve. With a dissected ethmoid bone, the grooves for the anterior and posterior ethmoidal arteries and nerves can be detected as they run along the frontoethmoid suture, but they are hidden by the frontal bone in the intact specimen and are rarely noted on computed tomography (CT). The major feature of either lateral aspect of the ethmoid is the laminae papyracea. The ethmoid cells are obscured by the frontal bone in the intact specimen.

Sphenoid Bone The major components of the sphenoid bone are the greater and lesser wings and the central body, with the pterygoid processes extending inferiorly. The greater wings provide the bulk of the floor of the middle cranial fossae. Several important foramina are situated medially. The foramen rotundum is located anteriorly and contains the maxillary (V_2) branch of the fifth cranial nerve as well as the small artery of the foramen rotundum. Moving dorsally, the next foramen encountered is the foramen ovale. It contains the mandibular (V_3) branch of the fifth cranial nerve as well as the accessory meningeal artery and, occasionally, the lesser petrosal nerve. Dorsolateral to the foramen ovale, you will find the foramen spinosum, which contains the middle meningeal artery. If you view the middle cranial fossa from behind in the coronal plane, these foramina, as described by Grant, form a crescent with the superior orbital fissure lying superiorly and the foramina rotundum, ovale, and spinosum following inferiorly. Also part of this crescent are two foramina that are inconstant. The foramen of Vesalius or sphenoid emissary foramen is found posterior and medial to the foramen rotundum when present. The other is the canal of Arnold or the canaliculus innominatus, which can be detected between the foramen ovale and the foramen spinosum. It transmits parasympathetic fibers to the parotid gland and a branch of the lesser superficial petrosal nerve, which structures usually pass through the foramen ovale. Posterior and medial to the foramen spinosum lies the foramen lacerum. This is a unique structure, since it is not a true foramen but rather a fibrous structure through which nothing passes. However, it is important, since the carotid artery lies along the cranial surface. The vidian canal is located along the anterior margin of the greater wing as it joins the body of the sphenoid along the lateral inferior margin of the sphenoid sinus and runs anteriorly to the pterygoid plates. It is also known as the pterygoid canal. It contains the vidian nerve and artery and is usually seen on coronal computed tomography (CT) or magnetic resonance imaging (MRI).

The lesser sphenoid wings are essentially triangular structures that abut anteriorly with the orbital roof portion of the frontal bones. The inferior aspect defines the superior margin of the superior orbital fissure as well as the dorsal aspect of the orbital roof. The anterior clinoid

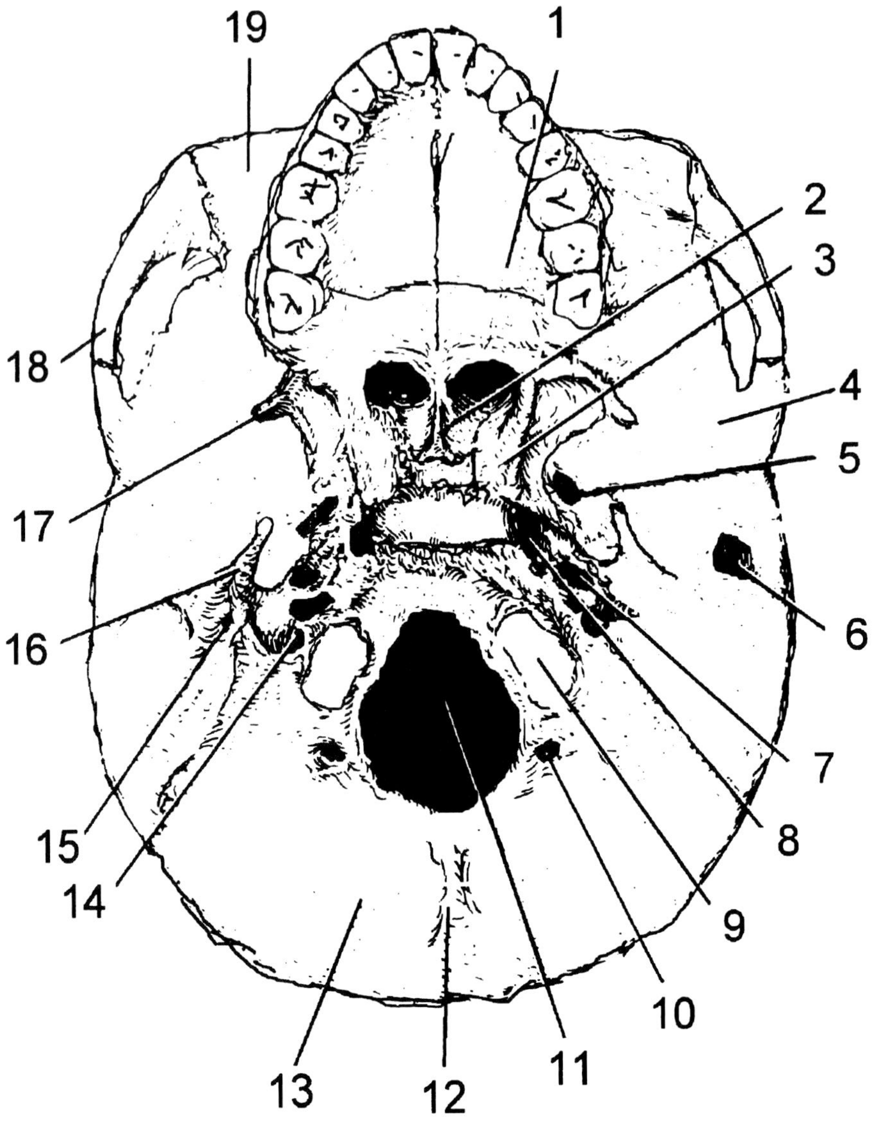

Diagram 2–1

1. Hard palate
2. Vomer
3. Medial pterygoid plate
4. Temporal bone
5. Foramen ovale
6. External acoustic meatus
7. Carotid canal
8. Foramen lacerum
9. Occipital condyle
10. Posterior condyloid canal
11. Foramen magnum
12. External occipital protuberance
13. Occipital bone
14. Jugular foramen
15. Stylomastoid foramen
16. Styloid process
17. Lateral pterygoid plate
18. Zygomatic arch
19. Maxilla

processes are located on the dorsal medial aspect of the lesser wings; they are the anterior point of attachment of the tentorium. The optic canal, which contains the optic nerve (cranial nerve II) and the ophthalmic artery, lies along the medial aspect of the lesser wing as it joins the body of the sphenoid.

The sphenoid body is the central segment of the sphenoid bone. It comprises the sphenoid sinuses inferiorly and forms the sella turcica superiorly, extending from its articulation with the cribriform plate anteriorly to the midclivus posteriorly. This latter junction is the sphenooccipital synchondrosis, which is fused to the occiput in adults. Fusion generally occurs near 16 years of age. Anteriorly, the body forms the planum sphenoidale, which flows into the lesser sphenoid wings. Look for the chiasmatic sulcus, which lies just under the optic chiasm between the planum sphenoidale and the tuberculum sellae. The chiasm is somewhat variable in its relationship to the tuberculum; in about 20 percent of cases, it will be positioned nearly vertical to the tuberculum. This is important to recognize, since the anterior (prefixed) position of the chiasm can present a major obstacle to the neurosurgical access to the pituitary gland from a frontal surgical approach.

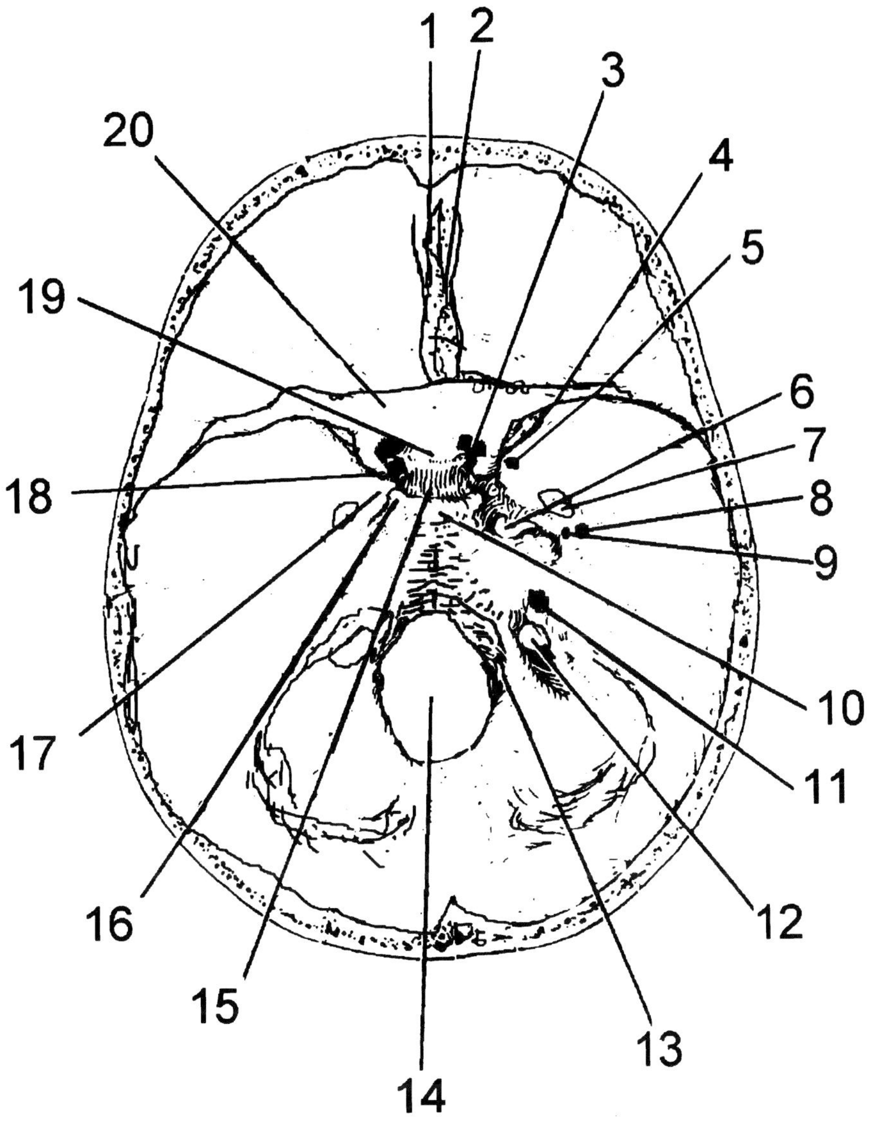

Diagram 2–2

1. Crista galli
2. Cribriform plate
3. Optic canal
4. Superior orbital fissure
5. Foramen rotundum
6. Foramen lacerum
7. Foramen ovale
8. Foramen spinosum
9. Canal of Arnold (innominate canal)
10. Dorsum sella
11. Internal acoustic meatus
12. Jugular foramen
13. Hypoglossal canal
14. Foramen magnum
15. Sella turcica
16. Posterior clinoid process
17. Carotid groove
18. Anterior clinoid process
19. Tuberculum sella
20. Sphenoid bone

The sella turcica is bounded anteriorly by the bony ridge, which includes the tuberculum sella; and posteriorly by the dorsum sella and posterior clinoids. Its floor is also the roof of the sphenoid sinuses, and it is defined superiorly by the membranous diaphragm sella. The lateral aspect may or may not have middle clinoid processes. More important, on the lateral aspect are the cavernous sinuses, which contain several important structures. These include cranial nerves (CN) III, IV, V_1, V_2, and VI as well as the cavernous carotid artery segment. Much of the remainder of the cavernous sinuses are made up of venous sinusoids, which extend from the petrous to the orbit and communicate from side to side by somewhat variable posterior and anterior sinuses.

Occipital Bone The occiput is assembled from the basiocciput, exocciput, and supraocciput. The basiocciput represents the dorsal aspect of the clivus (dorsal to the spheno-occipital synchrondosis) and the jugular tubercules and defines the anterior aspect of the foramen magnum. The paired exoccipital segments define the lateral aspects of the foramen magnum, including the occipital condyles. There are two paired canals to be noted at the condyles. These are the hypoglossal canal, which contains CN XII; a meningeal branch of the ascending pharyngeal artery; and an emissary vein. The hypoglossal canal is also referred to as the anterior condylar canal. The other pair are the posterior condylar canals, which are not consistently present; when they are, they contain a prominent vein connecting deep cervical veins to the transverse or jugular sinuses. This vein has been confused with a pathologic structure on CT and MRI. The supraoccipital bone segment extends upward from the dorsal foramen magnum to form the bulk of the floor of the posterior fossa. While sutures delineate these bones at birth, they are usually fused by the seventh year. The superior margin of the occiput is at the lambdoid suture. The groove for the transverse sinuses is oriented horizontally at the midpoint between the dorsal foramen magnum and lambdoid sutures.

The foramen magnum is, as its name implies, the largest foramen of the skull base. Important structures passing through the foramen magnum include the medulla oblongata, spinal accessory nerves (CN XI), vertebral arteries, anterior and posterior spinal arteries, communicating veins to the internal vertebral venous plexus, and meninges. The cerebellar tonsils lie adjacent to the foramen's superior margin but are known to migrate downward with posterior fossa masses and Arnold-Chiari malformations, with ensuing compression of the brainstem.

Temporal Bone The paired temporal bones are composed of five segments. The styloid and squamosal segments are of relatively minor concern. The petrous, tympanic, and mastoid areas are of considerably more interest.

The styloid process represents the dorsal terminus of the hyoid arch and is located posteriorly and laterally to the stylomastoid foramen on the inferior exocranial surface of the temporal bone.

The squamosal bone includes the zygomatic process anteriorly, which joins the zygomatic bone to form the zygomatic arch. The bulk of the squamous is a basically flat structure that, anteriorly, joins the greater wing of the sphenoid and defines the lateral margin of the middle cranial fossa.

The petrous portion of the temporal bone resembles a pyramid, with the apex oriented toward the sphenoid body and its base toward the tympanic part of the temporal bone. It abuts the petrosquamous fissure anteriorly and the foramen lacerum anteromedially. The key feature on its superior surface is the arcuate eminence, which covers the superior semicircular canal. Dorsally, the dominant structure is the jugular foramen, which lies at the junction of the petrous pyramid and the occiput. The internal auditory meatus—also known as the porus acousticus—is situated medially, whereas the smaller vestibular aqueduct is more inferior and lateral to the internal auditory meatus. Just inferior to the internal auditory meatus lies the cochlear aqueduct, which communicates between the cerebellopontine angle cistern and the inner ear via the perilymphatic duct.

The jugular fossa, by location and content, becomes an important area to master. The jugular foramen is just inferior and medial to the internal auditory meatus and travels inferiorly to exit the skull base posterior to the carotid canal and lateral to the occipital condyle. Within the petrous bone, it is separated from the carotid canal by the jugular spine. The foramen is usually divided into the pars nervosa medially and the pars vascularis laterally. The pars nervosa contains the glossopharyngeal nerve (CN IX) and its sensory branch to the middle ear, Jacobsen's nerve, and the inferior petrosal sinus. The jugular vein is the largest occupant of the pars vascularis. They are often asymmetrical with the right usually being the larger one. The vagus nerve (CN X) is located medially in the pars vascularis. The spinal accessory nerve (CN XI) traverses the pars vascularis of the jugular foramen just posterior to the vagus nerve. Also present are meningeal branches of the ascending pharyngeal artery.

The carotid canal is another important structure of the temporal bone, with its exocranial orifice identified medial to the styloid process and anterior to the jugular fossa. It ascends vertically about a centimeter into the petrous pyramid before it turns anteriorly and medially in the horizontal plane until it reaches the superior surface of the foramen lacerum. Not surprisingly, it contains the carotid artery and a few sympathetic fibers.

The internal auditory canal, which extends laterally from the porus acousticus—or internal auditory meatus—contains CN VII and VIII. Viewed in cross section, it can be conceptualized as representing a circle divided into four quadrants. The horizontal division is provided by the crista falciformis and vertically by Bill's bar. CN VII occupies only the anterior superior quadrant. The cochlear division of CN VIII occupies the anterior inferior quadrant. Posteriorly lie the superior and inferior vestibular divisions of CN VIII. Laterally, CN VII extends to the geniculate ganglion and CN VIII to the cochlea and semicircular canals.

The inner ear makes up the lateral aspect of the petrous pyramid. This area—which includes the cochlea, semicircular canals, and vestibule—is known as the otic capsule or osseous labyrinth. There is also the membranous labyrinth, which is composed of perilymph and endolymph and is contained within the osseous labyrinth. Its three components are the cochlear duct, the saccule and utricle within the vestibule, and the semicircular ducts within the semicircular canals. The cochlear duct communicates with the saccule but is blind at its other end. The three semicircular canals empty into the utricle with the superior and posterior sharing a common junction, the crus communis, medially. The utricle merges into the vestibule, which connects to the middle ear cavity via the oval window. The perilymph and endolymph are essentially the membranous lining of the bony labyrinth.

The perilymph is within the cochlea and the endolymph in the semicircular canals, vestibular aqueduct, and cochlear duct.

The cochlea is a spiral structure with 2½ turns, with the largest (basal turn) getting the half circle. The cochlea meets the middle ear cavity at the round window.

The geniculate ganglion is located just lateral to the cochlea and contains CN VII. Seventh-nerve fibers arrive from the brainstem via the internal auditory canal, and, passing across the roof of the vestibule at the ganglion, there is a right angle bend known as the genu. From here the nerve descends via the bony facial canal along the dorsal border of the middle ear cavity; it exits at the styloid foramen. The greater and lesser petrosal nerves exit anteriorly from the ganglion and travel to the pterygopalatine ganglion and otic ganglion respectively. The petrosal branch of the middle meningeal artery travels with the seventh nerve through the thin section CT.

The tympanic portion of the petrous bone is essentially the middle ear cavity. The lateral margin is the tympanic membrane and annulus. The medial margin has the oval and round windows, with the cochlear promontory between them, as well as the facial nerve canal and the bulge from the lateral semicircular canal. The anterior wall is a thin, bony separation between middle ear and carotid artery. The eustachian tube and a tympanic branch of the carotid artery pass through it. Superiorly, the tegmen provides a thin, bony roof. Posteriorly, look for the pyramidal eminence and fossa of the incus. Finally, the floor is a bony separation of the middle ear and the jugular bulb. Occasionally this is dehiscent, which results in the jugular bulb bulging into the hypotympanium. The segment of the middle ear cavity known as mesotympanium contains the stapes, long process of the incus, and manubrium of the malleus. This section also contains the stapedius muscle and the tensor tympani muscle. Above the level of the tympanic membrane is the area defined as the epitympanium. It is noted for the scutum, a bony prominence that forms the superior aspect of the tympanic annulus. Just medial to the scutum is Prusak's space, a frequent locus for cholesteatoma. The head of the malleus plus the body and short process of the incus are also found in the epitympanium. The remainder of the tympanic portion is the external auditory canal, which lies lateral to the tympanic membrane. The anterior aspect of this external segment also delineates the posterior aspect of the glenoid fossa for the temporal mandibular joint.

The mastoid area has several structures of interest, including the mastoid antrum, additus ad antrum, facial nerve canal, and Korner's septum. The antrum is a large air space in the mastoid bone that connects to the epitympanium via the additus ad antrum. There is a bony ridge, a remnant of the petrosquamosal suture separating the medial and lateral aspects of the mastoid air cells, known as Korner's septum. The seventh-nerve canal is a continuation of the neural canal, descending dorsal to the middle ear cavity, which passes through the medial mastoid area to exit at the styloid foramen.

Cranial Nerves You will undoubtedly recall that there are 12 cranial nerves, all of which have significant relationships with the skull base. The short version is summarized in Table 2–1, which outlines the significant *gozindas* (a term borrowed from my father-in-law's concept of math—e.g., 3 gozinda 6 two times).

Table 2–1
THE "GOZINDAS"

Foramen	Important Contents
Cribriform plate	Olfactory nerve and ethmoidal artery
Optic canal	Optic nerve and ophthalmic artery
Inferior orbital fissure	Infraorbital artery, veins, and nerve (V_2 branch)
Superior orbital fissure	CN III, IV, V_1, and VI, middle meningeal artery branch, and superior ophthalmic vein
Foramen rotundum	V_2 nerve, foramen rotundum arteries, emissary vein
Vidian canal	Vidian nerve and artery
Foramen ovale	CN V_3, accessory meningeal branch of maxillary artery, and emissary vein
Foramen spinosum	Middle meningeal artery and recurrent branch of V_3
Carotid canal	Internal carotid artery and sympathetic plexus
Stylomastoid foramen	CN VII
Foramen lacerum	Nothing
Jugular foramen	Pars nervosa: CN IX, Jacobsen's nerve and inferior petrosal sinus Pars vascularis: CN X and XI, jugular bulb and meningeal artery branches
Hypoglossal (anterior condylar) canal	CN XII
Internal auditory canal	CN VII and VIII
Foramen magnum	Medulla oblongata, spinal portion of CN XI, vertebral aa, and anterior and posterior spinal aa

The olfactory nerve, CN I, begins with multiple small fibers in the upper nasal cavity. These pass through the cribriform plates to join the olfactory bulbs. The olfactory nerves pass dorsally along the inferior surface of the frontal lobe in the olfactory sulcus, reaching the olfactory trigone, and then into the limbus. The course of this nerve anterior to the trigone can be visualized by MRI.

The optic nerve, CN II, extends dorsally from the globe through the optic canal, where it is accompanied by the ophthalmic artery. Continuing dorsally, the nerve reaches the optic chiasm, which is superior to the anterior aspect of the sella turcica. The optic tracts continue dorsally along the inferior thalamus to the lateral geniculate body. From here the optic radiations extend dorsally to the calcarine cortex of the occipital lobe.

The oculomotor nerve, CN III, begins with the third-nerve nucleus in the tegmentum of the dorsal midbrain and runs anteriorly through the red nucleus and substantia nigra, exiting on the medial aspect of the cerebral peduncles. It travels between the superior cerebellar artery and the posterior cerebral artery as it goes anteriorly to pass beneath the posterior communicating artery. Continuing forward, the third nerve is found in the superior and lateral cavernous sinus adjacent to the internal carotid artery. After passing through the cavernosus sinus, it traverses the superior orbital fissure into the orbit. In the orbit, it supplies all the extraocular muscles except the lateral rectus and superior oblique. It also interconnects to the parasympathetic innervation to the pupil and lens via the ciliary ganglion.

The trochlear nerve, CN IV, has its nucleus ventral to the cerebral aqueduct and slightly caudal to the third nucleus. It extends dorsally around the aqueduct, where it crosses to the opposite side and then exits the midbrain to swing anteriorly along the free edge of the tentorium. The fourth cranial nerve is unique in two respects: it is the smallest cranial nerve and the only one to decussate. In the cavernous sinus, it is found inferior to CN III and also runs through the superior orbital fissure into the orbit, where it supplies the superior oblique muscle.

The trigeminal nerve, CNV, is the motor nerve for the muscles of mastication and the sensory nerve for the face and much of the scalp. It has three divisions; ophthalmic, maxillary, and mandibular, which are often referred to as V_1, V_2, and V_3, respectively. The nucleus is located anterolateral to the fourth ventricle and is composed of four segments. They are the mesencephalic nucleus, the principal sensory nucleus, the motor nucleus, and the spinal tract nucleus. The nerve fibers run anteriorly from the nuclear complex to exit the pons anterolaterally through the prepontine cistern. They then enter Meckel's cave, where the trigeminal or Gasserian ganglion is formed; it, by the way is a sensory ganglion. The three major branches exit the ganglion and V_1 and V_2 travel through the inferior and lateral aspect of the cavernous sinus. V_1 exits the cavernous sinus through the superior orbital fissure and trifurcates into the lacrimal, frontal, and nasociliary branches. V_2 passes anteriorly through the foramen rotundum into the superior aspect of the pterygopalatine fossa. The infraorbital nerve is the anterior continuation, which traverses the infraorbital fissure. V_3 is different in two ways: it is both motor and sensory and it does not travel through the cavernous sinus. In fact, V_3 extends inferiorly from the trigeminal ganglion through the foramen ovale into the masticator space, where it innervates the muscles of mastication and receives sensation from the lower face and jaw.

The abducens nerve, CN VI, arises from its nucleus in the paramedian pons near the craniad aspect of the floor of the fourth ventricle. The fibers descend ventrally through the pons to exit medially, at the groove separating the pons and medulla. By the way, the seventh and eighth nerves exit more laterally in this same groove. The sixth cranial nerve continues anterolaterally through the pontine cistern dorsal to the cavernous sinus (this is occasionally referred to as Dorello's canal). It traverses the cavernous sinus lateral to the internal carotid artery, but moving to an inferolateral position as it goes forward. It then passes through the superior orbital fissure and finally innervates the lateral rectus muscle. Cranial nerve VI, with its relatively long free segment in the pontine segment, which is tethered at Dorello's canal, is especially vulnerable during transtentorial herniation or head trauma. Hence, lateral rectus palsy is a frequent physical finding in herniation or head trauma.

The facial nerve, CN VII, has three nuclei. The motor nucleus is relatively deep in the ventrolateral pontine tegmentum. The salivary nucleus is located slightly caudal and lateral to the motor nucleus, its function is autonomic. The solitary or sensory nucleus arises from the craniad aspect of the tractus solitarius in the medulla oblongata. Although much more complex, the seventh nucleus essentially lies anterolateral to the sixth nucleus. Its fibers swing medially around the sixth nucleus and then dorsally to the facial colliculus, a bulge in the floor of the fourth ventricle. From there the fibers head anterolaterally to exit along with the eighth nerve in the pontomedullary sulcus at the cerebellopontine angle. Cranial nerve VII crosses the cistern and enters the internal auditory canal, traveling in the anterior superior quadrant. It runs slightly forward to the geniculate ganglion, makes a sharp turn, and drops down the facial canal to exit at the stylomastoid foramen. It bifurcates in the parotid gland and then splits into multiple facial branches. There are other important branches of the facial nerve. The chorda tympani branches about 6 mm proximal to the stylomastoid foramen; it ascends to the tympanic cavity, running forward over the sphenoid and then deep to the lateral pterygoid to join the lingual nerve; it conveys taste from the anterior two-thirds of the tongue. The greater petrosal nerve arises from the geniculate ganglion and passes just beneath the trigeminal ganglion. At the foramen lacerum it joins with the deep petrosal (sympathetic) nerve to form the nerve of the pterygoid canal and ends in the pterygoid ganglion. It conveys taste from the palate and innervates the lacrimal gland.

The vestibulocochlear nerve, CN VIII, has two components; vestibular and cochlear. The cochlear nerve arises in the inferior cerebellar peduncle from dorsal and ventral cochlear nuclei. This sensory nerve travels around the lateral aspect of the peduncle and appears in the pontomedullary sulcus just lateral to the vestibular component. There are four vestibular nuclei—medial, inferior, lateral, and superior. They are found medial to the inferior cerebellar peduncle (restiform body). The nerve travels anteriorly between the restiform body and the trigeminal spinal tract and nucleus to exit just medial to the cochlear nerve in the pontomedullary sulcus adjacent to CN VII. From here the eighth nerve traverses the internal auditory canal, with the cochlear portion in the anterior inferior quadrant and the vestibular nerve occupying the posterior two quadrants. The cochlear nerve communicates with the spiral ganglion at the modiolus of the cochlea. The vestibular nerve extends to the vestibular ganglion in the lateral superior aspect of the internal auditory meatus.

The glossopharyngeal nerve, CN IX, has three nuclei. The rostral portion of the nucleus ambiguus contributes motor function. Sensory functions relate to the solitary tract nucleus in the deep reticular formation of the medulla oblongata. Finally, the inferior salivary nucleus, which has a parasympathetic function, lies just caudal to the solitary nucleus. Its fibers emerge in the groove between the olive and the inferior cerebellar peduncle; it then crosses the basal cistern to pass near the opening of the cochlear aqueduct and rest on the jugular tubercle. From here it bends inferiorly, invested in its own dura, and passes through the anterior medial part (pars nervosa) of the jugular foramen. The partially bony septum between the pars nervosa and pars vascularis of the jugular foramen can be detected on CT. After exiting the skull base, it runs in the carotid space to supply the posterior tongue and pharynx, but it has two important branches. Jacobsen's nerve provides sensation to the middle ear and the sinus nerve supplies the carotid body.

The vagus nerve, CN X, arises from four nuclei in the medulla oblongata. The dorsal nucleus of the vagus has mixed functions and lies in the lower gray matter of the medulla oblongata. The nucleus ambiguus is also a player and again controls motor function. The lower part of the solitary tract nucleus mediates sensation. The spinal nucleus of the trigeminal nerve has some involvement with somatic afferent fibers. The vagus emerges in the groove between the inferior cerebellar peduncle and the olive as eight to ten rootlets, which appear just below the glossopharyngeal root. It follows the same path as the ninth nerve to the jugular foramen, where it descends with the eleventh nerve in the same dural sleeve through the pars vascularis. From here there is a long course in the carotid sheaths. The area distal to these segments differ on each side and is beyond the scope of this topic. Functionally, CN X supplies motor innervation to the soft palate, middle pharynx, inferior pharynx, and vocal cords as well as sensation above the true cord level.

The spinal accessory nerve, CN XI, is composed of spinal roots that come from the inferior aspect of the nucleus ambiguus and probably the dorsal vagal nucleus and emerges just below the vagus, then ascending along the vagal path to the jugular foramen. The spinal root is more substantial and emanates from the spinal nucleus located in the lateral anterior gray column of the cervical roots and then ascending to the jugular foramen along a similar path. It may extend as low as the fifth cervical vertebra. These fibers emerge between the ventral and dorsal cervical roots and then ascend to the jugular foramen along a similar path. Cranial nerve XI traverses the pars vascularis of the jugular foramen just posterior to the vagus nerve. From here it travels in the carotid space and then along the sternomastoid muscle. It innervates the sternomastoid and trapezius muscles and also communicates with the recurrent laryngeal nerve.

The hypoglossal nerve, CN XII (its nucleus of the same name), extends from the hypoglossal triangle of the floor of the fourth ventricle and extends caudal to the ventral gray matter of the closed portion of the medulla oblongata. This is a motor nucleus, which innervates the tongue. It emerges as a series of 10 to 15 rootlets in the anterolateral sulcus between the olive and the pyramid. From here they form two adjacent bundles, which pass dorsal to the vertebral artery and then pierce the dura to enter the hypoglossal (or anterior condylar) canal. Once it has exited the hypoglossal canal, the nerve descends in the carotid space to the hyoid bone and then turns up and forward to the sublingual space.

☐ PATHOLOGY

CONGENITAL

Cephaloceles Cephaloceles, representing approximately 10 to 20 percent of all craniospinal malformations, are protrusions of intracranial contents through a congenital defect in the calvarium and dura.

- Meningoceles involve the leptomeninges and subdural space.
- Meningoencephaloceles involve the meninges, subarachnoid space and a portion of the brain parenchyma.
- These lesions may either be of congenital or acquired. Acquired forms are most commonly due to either skull trauma or neurosurgical procedures.
- The most common presentation of these lesions is as a soft tissue mass protruding either under the scalp tissues or into the oral or nasal pharynx. The bony defect may be small, with a smooth, corticated aperture; it usually arises in the midline. Parasagittal defects may more commonly be seen in association with amniotic band syndrome.

Etiology Most often, these lesions are associated with failure of neural tube closure, but they may also arise within a persistent craniopharyngeal canal, or defects in major ossification centers, especially within the sphenoid region.

- Encephaloceles can occur anywhere within the calvarium most commonly along the midline either over the vertex or basilar regions.
- Encephaloceles occur in approximately one of every 4000 live births.
- Encephaloceles represent 10 to 20 percent of all craniospinal malformations and most commonly arise as follows:
  1. A defect in the fusion of the anterior neuropore at approximately the 25th gestational day.
  2. An expanding dural diverticulum extending through the craniopharyngeal canal or foramen cecum.
  3. From the failure of development of complex ossification centers, most commonly in the sphenoid area.
- The dura is usually continuous with the outer periosteal layer overlying the bony defect.
- Overlying soft tissue covering depends on location but most commonly is:
  1. Skin
  2. Nasal sinus mucosa
  3. Pharyngeal mucosa
- Acquired encephaloceles can arise at fracture sites or sites of dural laceration. They are most common in the basifrontal region as well as at craniotomy defects.

Incidence Cephaloceles occur in approximately 2 to 3 per 10,000 live births. Geographic and racial differences exist. Occipital cephaloceles occur most commonly in whites of European or North American extraction. Frontoethmoidal involvement is seen more commonly in the Southeast Asian population.

Types

- Occipital cephaloceles (70 to 80 percent) occur between the foramen magnum and lambdoid suture. This may be seen in association with:
  1. Chiari type II and type III malformations
  2. Klippel-Feil Syndrome
  3. Dandy-Walker malformation
  4. Cerebellar dysplasia
  5. Meckel's syndrome
- Parietal cephaloceles (5 to 10 percent) occur between the lambdoid and bregma sutures and are most commonly seen in association with:
  1. Dandy-Walker malformation
  2. Agenesis of the corpus callosum
  3. Chiari type II malformation
  4. Lobar holoprosencephaly
- Frontoethmoidal cephaloceles (5 to 10 percent) arise in the nasal ethmoid bones. These are developmentally not related to neural tube closure defects but instead to a failure of regression of a dural diverticulum during nasal development. Several variations may result, including:
  1. Dermoid
  2. Dermal sinus
  3. Heterotopic nasal glial tissue—"nasal glioma" (Fig. 2–1)
- Basal cephaloceles (1 to 2 percent) are commonly associated with a sellar/pituitary disorder; the lesion may present as a protruding mass into the pharynx or with a cerebrospinal fluid (CSF) leak. May be seen in association with agenesis of the corpus callosum.
- Subtypes of basal cephaloceles:
  1. Sphenopharyngeal
  2. Sphenoorbital
  3. Sphenoethmoidal
  4. Transethmoidal
  5. Sphenomaxillary

Arachnoid Cysts. Arachnoid or leptomeningeal cysts. These are benign congenital lesions that are believed to arise from a split or cleft within the pia-arachnoid tissue, with subsequent cyst formation. Size ranges from small to very large. The cyst typically contains CSF-like fluid that may be clear, xanthochromic, or frankly hemorrhagic. The cyst contents may communicate directly with the subarachnoid space or be entirely loculated. The cyst walls have no epithelial or glial components and hence, are not secretory.

- They represent 1 percent of intracranial space occupying lesions.
- There is a 3:1 male-female occurrence.
- Most are supratentorial, 90 percent
  Middle cranial fossa, 60 percent
  Quadrigeminal, 10 percent
  Suprasellar, 10 percent
  Convexity, 10 percent
  Intraventricular, less than 1 percent
- Posterior fossa, 10 percent. These occur most commonly at the cerebellopontine angle and at the cisterna magna.

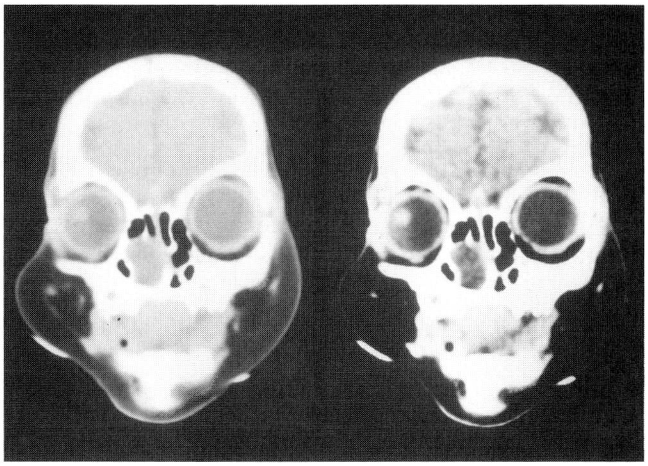

Figure 2–1 Nasal glial rest. Coronal CT in a child shows soft tissue mass in the nasal cavity.

Clinical

- Some 70 to 80 percent of the cysts eventually will become symptomatic, producing
  1. Seizures
  2. Headache
  3. Focal neurologic signs
- Most cysts remain unchanged in size, with a small subset that does increase in size with age. The mechanism is uncertain but is probably not secretory and may represent a ball/valve-type effect of fluid accumulation within the cyst.
- Arachnoid cysts may have either spontaneous or posttraumatic hemorrhage (Fig. 2–2).
- The cysts are occasionally seen in association with subdural hematomas.

Imaging COMPUTED TOMOGRAPHY

- The cyst invariably appears as a smooth, margined extraaxial mass of fluid density without associated calcification or contrast enhancement.
- Adjacent calvarial remodeling is common. Hypoplasia of the adjacent brain parenchyma is commonly seen, especially in the middle cranial fossa.

MAGNETIC RESONANCE IMAGING

- Typically, the cyst presents as an extraaxial mass with signal intensity paralleling that of CSF on all sequences.

Differential Diagnosis SUPRATENTORIAL

1. Dermoids/epidermoids. These tend to encase adjacent structures (arteries, nerves) whereas arachnoid cysts tend to displace them. Dermoid contains fatty tissue and is variably calcified. Epidermoid has a characteristic "dirty" CSF appearance.
2. Porencephalic cyst.

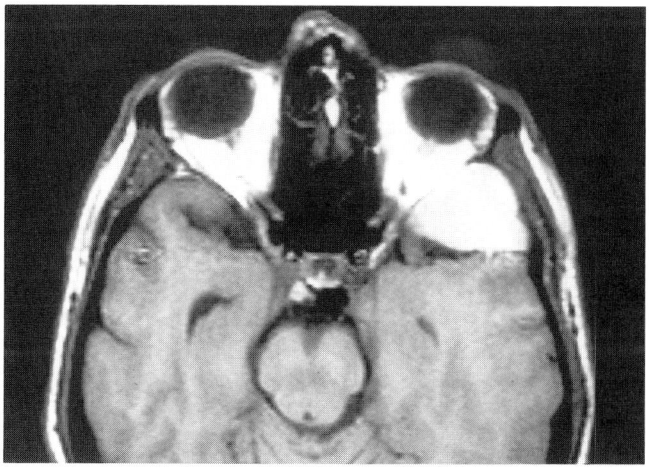

Figure 2–2 Hemorrhagic arachnoid cyst. Axial T1-weighted image demonstrates a high-signal-intensity extraaxial lesion in the anterior aspect of the left temporal fossa.

3. Cystic tumors. These always show a component with contrast enhancement, whereas the arachnoid cyst does not enhance.
4. Loculated hygroma.

INFRATENTORIAL

1. Mega cisterna magna
2. Dandy-Walker malformation
3. Dermoid/epidermoid

Dermoid Cysts Dermoid is a cystic mass of ectodermal origin. This benign lesion is typically a thick-walled cyst, often with partially calcified walls. The lesion will demonstrate varying contrast enhancement. Its contents typically are a viscous oily fluid derived from decomposed epithelial cells; it may also contain hair follicles, dental elements (including teeth), and portions of the mandible, sebaceous, and sweat glands.

Incidence The tumor is typically found at sites of closure along the neural tube or at sites of closure of cranial sutures.

Frequency of Occurrence

1. Midline, 40 percent
2. Frontal temporal, 45 percent
3. Parietal, 15 percent

- A midline dermoid is frequently associated with a dermal sinus. This is most frequently seen in the nasal and frontal regions but can also involve the parasellar and posterior fossa regions.
- Dermoids tend to slowly increase in size with time and have a tendency to encase rather than displace adjacent structures.
- Dermoids may spontaneously rupture, often causing an intense chemical meningitis.

Imaging COMPUTED TOMOGRAPHY

- Dermoids typically present as a well-circumscribed, low attenuating mass [−20 to −40 Hounsfield units (HU)].
- Calcification is frequently seen.

MAGNETIC RESONANCE IMAGING

- T1-weighted images are quite variable, ranging from isointense to skeletal muscle to hyperintense. T2-weighted images typically are hypo- to isointense, depending on the cyst contents.

Differential Diagnosis SUPRATENTORIAL

- Arachnoid cyst. It is important to recognize that arachnoid cysts tend to displace adjacent structures by mass effect as opposed to dermoids, which tend to encase adjacent structures without anatomic displacement.
- Porencephalic cyst
- Cystic tumors
- Loculated hygromas

INFRATENTORIAL

- Mega cisterna magna
- Dandy-Walker malformation

INFECTION

Mucocele ***Incidence*** Mucoceles are rather uncommon, whereas the mucous retention cyst, which is quite similar, is found in about 10 percent of the population.

Age and Gender Mucoceles are about equally distributed between the sexes, and they are broadly distributed across the age span from adolescent to elderly. Clinically, mucoceles present with mass effect, such as frontal bossing, proptosis, nasal obstruction, chronic headache, and (rarely) cranial nerve signs.

Location Primarily the frontal sinuses (60 percent), followed by the ethmoid sinuses (20 to 25 percent), about 10 percent in the antra, and 1 or 2 percent in the sphenoid sinuses. Very rarely, a mucocele will arise from the petrous apex and be confused with a cholesterol granuloma.

Pathology Mucoceles have a lining of cuboid epithelium and contain mucous secretions. Thus they are quite similar to a mucous retention cyst. The distinction lies in the fact that the mucocele represents an obstructed sinus or septated segment of a sinus that has become distended. The contents of the mucocele range from watery to so-called dried secretions. The latter become relatively high in protein content and occasionally even contain some hemorrhagic debris. As mucoceles continue to expand, they cause bone remodeling, which expansile process is the distinguishing characteristic of this lesion. Retention cyst is due to obstruction of small seromucinous gland, usually in the maxillary sinus.

Imaging **X-RAY** In the frontal sinus, a mucocele tends to appear as dense to slightly less dense than sinusitis. This is due to the erosion of bone, causing lucency, which balances the increasing density of the secretions in the mucocele. Erosion through the posterior wall of the frontal sinus is the primary concern for the surgeon. The ethmoid mucoceles tend to form in the smaller anterior ethmoid air cells. As they expand, they tend to erode through the cribriform plate into the frontal fossa or through the lamina papyracea, thus displacing the eye laterally. Sphenoid mucoceles tend to expand anterolaterally into the posterior ethmoids and orbital apex, where they impinge on the optic nerves. Little of this is identifiable on plain film. While antral mucoceles are rather dramatic on plain film, it is unlikely that they will involve skull-base structures.

COMPUTED TOMOGRAPHY

- The usual CT appearance of a mucocele is an expanded sinus cavity which has increased density due to mucus ranging from 10 to 20 HU but occasionally as dense as 40 HU.
- Mucoceles do not enhance; however, the infrequently occurring mucopyocele will demonstrate a fairly thick enhancing rim adjacent to the bony margins.
- Primarily, CT is useful to evaluate expansion through the skull base at the cribriform plate, the dorsum of the frontal sinuses, into the orbital recesses, and (rarely) into the cavernous sinus.

MAGNETIC RESONANCE IMAGING

- The appearance of mucoceles on MRI is essentially determined by the water content of the secretions. Recent lesions have more water, which diminishes as time passes, resulting in shortened T1-weighted images. T2-weighted images tend to remain high in signal until the secretions become desiccated and/or hemorrhagic, at which point they may appear as black as air.
- Fortunately, CT can resolve this problem. In most cases the lesion is quite uniform in density pattern internally.
- Enhancement of mucoceles is limited to a very thin margin adjacent to bone. A thick margin suggests infection and irregular enhancement suggests that you are entertaining the wrong diagnosis.

Fungal Sinusitis ***Incidence*** A large number of diverse fungi have been reported in cases of fungal sinusitis. Fortunately, two entities account for the vast majority of fungal sinus infections which traverse the skull base. These are aspergillosis and mucormycosis, which are invasive in diabetics, lymphomas, or patients who are immunosuppressed.

Location For an unknown reason, these fungal entities rarely involve the frontal sinuses. From the other sinuses, they invade through the skull base along vascular channels and emissary veins or into the orbit and then along the ophthalmic vessels into the cavernous sinus.

Pathology Aspergillosis is caused by the aspergillosis fungus, with *Aspergillus fumigatus* representing 90 percent of these infections. The spores are commonly found in the soil, plants, and decaying food. They are generally inhaled. These infections are often rather indolent and may form a fungus ball in the sinus. As they grow, usually in the maxillary antra, they may actually invade bone. In its most fulminant mode, *Aspergillus* invades the vascular walls, precipitating thrombosis, ischemia, and even hemorrhagic infarction.

Mucormycosis is caused by several fungi of the class Zygomycetes (Phycomycetes), which are inhaled. In diabetics and other immunocompromised patients, this is a highly aggressive, invasive fungus. In others, it behaves in a much more benign manner. Like *Aspergillus,* it attacks the vessels and spreads rapidly through the vessel walls, precipitating thrombosis and all its sequelae. Orbital invasion with dorsal extension along the ophthalmic vessels leads to cavernous sinus thrombosis. The entire process can be fatal within a few days. Clinically, crusted black tissue (eschar) is seen on the nasal mucosa and ischemic foci are common in immunocompromised patients. Those that survive the acute insult are often left blind, hemiparetic, or with cranial nerve palsies.

Imaging X-RAYS Plain-film findings are not very helpful, since they may demonstrate only some soft tissue density in a sinus or the nasal cavity. The sole exception may be concretions in the sinuses caused by very dense mycetomas; this is rare.

COMPUTED TOMOGRAPHY Computed tomography will demonstrate a soft tissue mass in the sinus or nasal cavity. Often there will be evidence of bone invasion in the less fulminant forms of the disease. There may be contrast enhancement along the margins of the lesion and within the cavernous sinus when it is invaded and thrombosed.

MAGNETIC RESONANCE IMAGING Imaging of mycetomas by MRI shows a low signal on all sequences since there is a paucity of mobile protons. Since a peripheral inflammatory response is usually elicited, you may see increased signal in these areas on T2-weighted images, and these same areas will enhance. Magnetic resonance imaging becomes very helpful when the absence of flow voids is apparent, especially in the cavernous sinus or ophthalmic vessels. Similarly, magnetic resonance angiography (MRA) will demonstrate thromboses in these areas. Obviously, in fulminant cases, evidence of infarcts and meningitis will often be demonstrated.

OSTEOMYELITIS

Osteomyelitis of the skull base is fortunately a rare event. Unfortunately, it can be devastating. Most of these cases arise from the area of the petrous bone, and are generally the sequelae of a malignant otitis externa caused by *Pseudomonas aeruginosa* which has been inadequately treated. Fungal invasion, as by *Aspergillus,* is covered above. Rarely, a child with pyogenic tonsillitis may undergo extension upward into the skull base. Occasionally, a sinus infection may extend into the skull base.

Clinical manifestations of the process include severe headache, hoarseness, aspiration, and difficulty swallowing secondary to cranial nerve involvement in the jugular fossa. Involvement of the petrous apex will be reflected by involvement of the fifth nerve at Meckel's cave and may involve the sixth nerve.

Imaging PLAIN FILM Plain film may demonstrate clouding of mastoid air cells, but frank, destructive bone changes are rarely seen.

COMPUTED TOMOGRAPHY This modality has become the most useful tool for evaluating osseous infection of the skull base, since it will demonstrate the destruction quite well. The lesion may extend through the petrous apex to the cavernous sinus, across to the opposite temporal bone, or into the jugular fossa.

MAGNETIC RESONANCE IMAGING This is probably the most useful technique for demonstrating one of the most devastating complications—venous sinus thrombosis. As one would expect, an absence of flow void would indicate a sinus thrombosis. The thrombus may present as increased signal in a venous sinus. Fluid in mastoid cells and/or cavities may be detected. Slow flow in the carotid canal will indicate invasion into the canal. Meningitis and brain abscess can also occur as further sequelae of skull-base osteomyelitis.

TRAUMA

This subject is covered in detail elsewhere in this text; however, a brief review of major aspects of trauma to the skull base is included here. Skull-base fractures are usually an extension of fractures in the cranial vault. They become significant when they involve one of the skull-base foramina and traumatize one of the nerves or vessels traversing the foramen in question. For instance, if the foramen ovale is fractured, one would anticipate involvement of the mandibular nerve (V_3). Similarly, trauma to the optic nerve would affect visual acuity. The three most common sites of skull-base fracture are the orbital roof, basiocciput, and petrous pyramid. Clinically, such fractures may present with periorbital hematomas, CSF otorrhea or rhinorrhea, hemotympanum, mastoid region ecchymosis, and cranial nerve lesions. Cerebrospinal fluid fistulas are generally diagnosed with thin-section CT augmented with intrathecal contrast, focusing on the sinuses or temporal bone, depending on the suspected clinical location of the leak. Carotid-cavernous fistula is an uncommon sequela of skull-base trauma. It usually presents with proptosis and chemosis. Computed tomography is useful to show the proptosis and may show enlarged superior ophthalmic veins with contrast enhancement. Magnetic resonance imaging will also demonstrate the increased blood flow as flow voids, and MRA will also demonstrate the findings. The definitive diagnosis still requires contrast angiography, and the treatment is usually accomplished with interventional techniques to ablate the fistula. Occasionally, an intimal vascular tear can result in thrombosis or embolization of small clots, which can lead to infarction.

☐ NEOPLASMS

JUGULAR FORAMEN

Glomus Jugulare Some 90 percent of all jugular foramen neoplasms are paragangliomas. The remaining 10 percent include schwannomas, meningiomas, carcinomas, chondrosarcomas, and nasopharyngeal tumors that extend cephalad. Glomus neoplasms represent slow-growing vascular tissue arising from neural crest derivatives. Glomus jugulare neoplasms or paragangliomas represent the second most common type of tumor to arise in the temporal bone,

Sites of Origin

- Tumor arises from paraganglial tissue in the jugular bulb adventitia.
- Tumor arises from paraganglial tissue of the tympanic branch of the glossopharyngeal nerve.
- Tumor arises from paraganglial tissue of the mastoid branch of the vagus nerve.

Incidence

- Male to female ratio of 3:1.
- Most common presentation is between the third and fourth decades.
- Some 10 percent of all patients may have multiple paragangliomas in the head and the neck region.

Differential Diagnosis

- Normal but prominent jugular bulb.
- Neural sheath tumor.
- Meningioma.
- Metastasis.

Imaging COMPUTED TOMOGRAPHY Typically, an enlarged or eroded jugular foramen is seen, and the margins may show evidence of direct invasion or pressure erosion, particularly of jugular spine.

MAGNETIC RESONANCE IMAGING

- A jugular foramen mass most commonly presents as a large, irregular, soft tissue lesion filling the foramen.
- The tumor may extend along normal tissue planes and potential spaces. T1-weighted signal intensity is isointense and shows dense contrast enhancement. T2-weighted signal intensity is generally heterogeneously hyperintense (salt-and-pepper appearance) (Fig. 2–3).
- In large lesions, foci of signal loss representing tumor vessels may be identified on T2-weighted images.

Angiography

- Usually supplied by ascending pharyngeal artery.
- Well-defined, dense vascular stain that persists into the late arterial phase.
- Arteriovenous shunting is seen with early filling of jugular vein.

Clinical Observations

- Enlarging paragangliomas may extend laterally, resulting in conductive hearing loss or pulsatile tinnitus.
- Medial extension can also involve cranial nerves IX, X, and XI.
- Enlarging tumor mass may also lead to the loss of pharyngeal or facial nerves.

Schwannomas These are benign, well-circumscribed solid masses arising from cranial nerves IX, X, or XI.

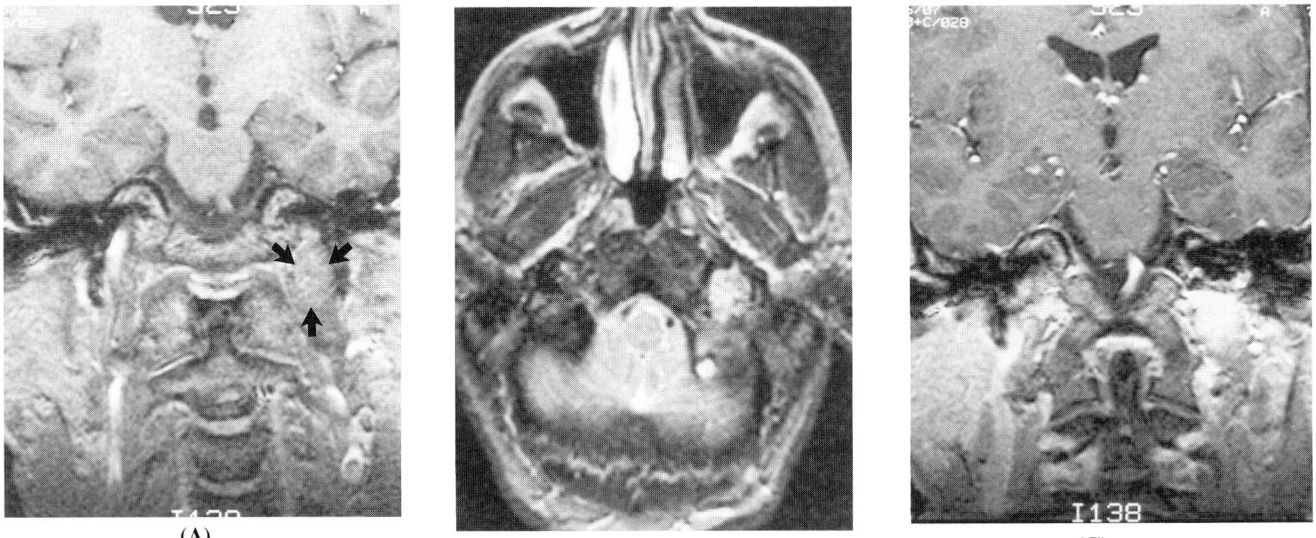

(A) (B) (C)

Figure 2–3 Glomus jugulare tumor. *A.* A coronal T1-weighted image shows a mass lesion in the left jugular fossa, which is isointense to adjacent muscle (*arrows*). *B.* An axial T2-weighted image reveals a mixed high-signal-intensity mass at the left jugular fossa (salt-and-pepper appearance), reflecting a vascular tumor with various internal flow velocities. *C.* A coronal gadolinium-enhanced T1-weighted image shows intense contrast enhancement.

They tend to expand centripetally within the jugular foramen by pressure erosion and without frank bony destruction. The margins generally appear to be more uniform and corticated than those seen with expanding paragangliomas within the same region. This is probably due to the slower growing nature of the tumor.

- These tumors may also involve the hypoglossal as well as facial nerves with a similar radiographic picture.
- Some 90 percent of all jugular foramen masses are paragangliomas.

Three types are identified:
Type A: Predominantly intracranial.
Type B: Predominantly occurring at the jugular foramen.
Type C: Predominantly occurring extra cranial with varying solid and cystic components.

Imaging MAGNETIC RESONANCE IMAGING The best choice for imaging these lesions is MRI. T1-weighted signal intensity is typically isointense with skeletal muscle. Postcontrast images generally show dense, uniform contrast enhancement. T2-weighted images show uniformly increased signal intensity.

Meningiomas Meningiomas of the jugular foramen are unusual and arise directly from arachnoid cells within the cranial nerve sheaths. The tumor tends to grow along the sheath, eroding the neural foramen due to pressure effect. The tumor mass may extend intracranially as well and become locally invasive. Caudad extension along the course of the jugular vein may also occur. Meningiomas can also arise within the acoustic meatus, in Meckel's cave, and along the greater or lesser petrosal nerve sulcus. Meningiomas can also rarely occur within the paranasal sinuses, most commonly the maxillary sinus.

Imaging COMPUTED TOMOGRAPHY

- Typically shows a uniformly enhancing soft tissue mass with localized erosive effects against the adjacent bone.
- Bony hyperostosis may be seen.

MAGNETIC RESONANCE IMAGING

- T1-weighted signal intensity tends to be hypo- or isointense. T2-weighting is highly variable but generally isointense. Contrast images generally show intense enhancement.

CLIVUS

Chordomas Chordomas represent slowly growing, rarely malignant (less than 10 percent) neoplasms arising from embryonic notochord ectopic rests. The majority of these tumors occur at three sites:

- The sacrococcygeal region (50 percent).
- The skull base (40 percent), where the neoplasm most commonly involves the clivus. Origination can also be seen from the petrous apex region.
- Cervical spine (10 percent).

Incidence

- 3:2 male to female ratio.
- There is a bimodal peak.
  1. The first peak occurs in the second to fourth decades and tends to be clival in location.
  2. The second peak tends to occur in the fourth to sixth decades and the sacrococcygeal region predominates.

Imaging COMPUTED TOMOGRAPHY

- Typically, a poorly enhancing destructive soft tissue mass with dystrophic calcifications is identified (Fig. 2–4). The mass is extraaxial and, in the skull base, commonly extends into the nasopharynx but may also be seen in the petrous apexes and sphenoid region. Typically there is destruction of the clivus.

MAGNETIC RESONANCE IMAGING

- This modality is more advantageous than CT examination in staging. T1-weighted signal intensity typically shows a mixed hypo- and isointense mass with mild to moderate enhancement. T2-weighted images typically show increased signal intensity.

Chondrosarcoma Chondrosarcoma is a slow-growing malignant cartilaginous neoplasm and represents approximately 10 to 20 percent of malignant bone tumors and 6 percent of skull-base tumors. Some 75 percent of all cranial chondrosarcomas occur within the skull base.

Tissue of Origin

- Cartilage
- Endochondral bone
- Mesenchymal rests within soft tissues, meninges, or brain
- May arise from preexisting fibrous dysplasia, Paget's disease, or osteochondroma

Sites of origin The most common location for chondrosarcoma of the skull base is the clivus, with lesser involvement at the cerebellopontine angle as well as the sphenoethmoidal, maxillary, and nasal sinuses.

Imaging COMPUTED TOMOGRAPHY

- Typically, the mass demonstrates a pathognomonic calcified matrix (50 percent).

MAGNETIC RESONANCE IMAGING

- T1-weighted images tend to be hypointense relative to skeletal muscle and show heterogeneous contrast enhancement. T2-weighted images tend to be hyperintense in signal intensity.

Figure 2–4
bony destruct
T1-weighted i

METASTAS

Skull-base i
skull-base 1
from an ext
Distal meta

- Lung—th
- Breast—1
- Prostate—
 sue mass

Skull-bas
most typica

Differe
- Osteomy
- Eosinopl
- Sarcoma
- Paget's d
- Radiatio

Imagin
- This mo
 destructi

MA
- Typically
 signal in
 contrast
 ically are

Plasmac

plasma cel
solitary for
temic mult

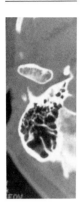

Primary nasopharyngeal lymphoma is predominantly non-Hodgkin's and of the histiocytic type. Disease limited to the nasopharynx is unusual. Findings on both CT and MRI are nonspecific and tend to mimic other common nasopharyngeal lesions, including squamous cell carcinoma. Lymphomatous masses, however, tend to be large, lobular, homogeneous soft tissue masses and most commonly involve concomitant disease within Waldeyer's ring.

Nasopharyngeal Rhabdomyosarcoma Please see the discussion under "Nasoethmoidal Rhabdomyosarcoma."

Pathology The tumor arises from rhabdomyoblasts in the nasopharynx.

- Nasopharyngeal involvement represents 15 percent of all head and neck rhabdomyosarcomas.
- Anterior skull-base infiltration or cavernous sinus involvement extension is seen in 35 percent of cases.
- Meningeal and neurovascular extension is common.
- Distal metastases and regional lymph node involvement are common.

Imaging COMPUTED TOMOGRAPHY

- Examination by CT typically shows a homogeneous, infiltrating soft tissue mass arising within the nasopharynx and commonly invading both the skull base and posterior maxillary sinus walls. Intracranial extra dural extension with cavernous sinus involvement may be seen.

MAGNETIC RESONANCE IMAGING

- Gadolinium-enhanced MRI with fat-suppression technique is useful in evaluating skull-base and intracranial extension as well as sinus involvement.

NASOETHMOIDAL

Esthesioneuroblastoma This tumor is also referred to as an olfactory neuroblastoma. It is an uncommon malignant tumor arising in the olfactory sensory receptors and is derived from cells of neural crest origin.

Incidence Tumors occur throughout the age range of 10 to 60 years, with slightly increased rates of occurrence seen at 10 to 20 years and from 50 to 60 years.

Pathology The tumor is histologically similar to adrenal neuroblastoma and arises from the sympathetic ganglion neuroblast. There are three histological types:

- Neuroblastoma with pseudorosettes (20 percent)
- Neuroepithelioma with true rosettes (40 percent)
- Neurocytoma without rosettes (40 percent)

Staging

- Stage A: Disease is confined to the nasal cavity (30 percent).
- Stage B: Disease involves the nasal cavity but also extends to the paranasal sinuses (40 percent).
- Stage C: Disease is found remote to the nasal cavity and paranasal sinuses (30 percent).

Some 20 to 30 percent of esthesioneuroblastomas demonstrate regional metastases.

Imaging Esthesioneuroblastomas most commonly originate as a polypoid soft tissue mass arising in the upper nasal cavity; this mass may extend into the paranasal sinuses, the orbit, or through the cribriform plate. Bone destruction is common although the tumor may extend microscopically through the cribriform plate without obvious destruction and manifest itself as a soft tissue mass intracranially.

COMPUTED TOMOGRAPHY

- Tumor presents as a homogeneous, enhancing soft tissue mass.
- Calcifications may be contained within the mass.
- Bone involvement is variable, ranging from changes secondary to pressure effects to gross destruction.

MAGNETIC RESONANCE IMAGING

- Tumor tends to be of intermediate signal intensity on T1-weighted images, with moderate inhomogeneous contrast enhancement.
- T2-weighted images generally show intermediate signal intensity.
- Magnetic resonance imaging with gadolinium enhancement is most useful for evaluation of intracranial extension.

Lymphoma This mesodermal sarcoma represents approximately 10 to 15 percent of all head and neck tumors. Non-Hodgkin's lymphoma is the second most common sinonasal malignancy after squamous cell carcinoma.

Incidence Approximately 5 percent of all lymphomas occur in the sinonasal area as a primary disease process.

- There is equal sex distribution.
- There is a low association with preexisting sinus disease (10 to 15 percent).
- Histiocytic lymphoma is the most common cell type.

Imaging Skull-base lymphoma is most commonly seen in the nasal cavity and maxillary sinuses. Occasionally it also arises in the ethmoidal sinuses and only rarely in the sphenoid and frontal sinuses. Isolated extranodal involvement generally cannot be separated in appearance from squamous cell carcinoma.

COMPUTED TOMOGRAPHY

- Examination by CT generally shows a large soft tissue mass demonstrating moderate enhancement.
- The degree of bone involvement is variable and extensive destructive involvement mimicking squamous cell carcinoma is occasionally seen.

MAGNETIC RESONANCE IMAGING

- Intermediate signal intensity on both T1- and T2-weighted sequences with moderate homogeneous contrast enhancement.
- Magnetic resonance imaging is good at delineating marrow replacement within the skull base as well as extension along nerve sheaths. Fat-suppressed post-contrast images are particularly useful in determining tumor margins, especially in the paranasal sinuses.
- Sinonasal masses will enhance uniformly, as opposed to rimlike enhancement associated with chronic sinus disease.

Nasoethmoidal Carcinomas Nasoethmoidal carcinomas originate from the paranasal sinuses or nasal cavity and represent approximately 3 percent of all head and neck tumors. They often extend into the anterior skull base and commonly present initially as advanced disease with a poor clinical prognosis. Tumor may be masked by symptoms associated with chronic sinusitis.

Incidence This tumor is predominantly seen to occur in males in the fifth and sixth decades, 20 percent of whom have a history of chronic sinusitis.

Pathology The most common tumor cell type is that of squamous cell carcinoma, although undifferentiated carcinoma, mixed salivary gland tumors, lymphoma, and esthesioneuroblastomas are also encountered.

Sites of origin:

- Nasal cavity (30 percent)
- Maxillary sinus (60 percent)
- Ethmoidal sinuses (10 percent)
- Frontal and sphenoid sinuses (less than 1 percent)
- Tumors tend to be highly aggressive, often clinically advanced when initially diagnosed; they have extensive skull-base involvement, including both anterior and middle cranial fossae as well as orbital and pterygopalatine fossa involvement.
- Metachronous head and neck lesions may occur in as many as 40 percent of cases.
- Metastatic spread is commonly seen to the retropharyngeal nodes (15 percent) as well as to the jugular digastric and submandibular node groups.

Imaging Plain films of the sinuses show a bulky soft tissue nasal mass with up to 80 percent incidence of associated bony destruction.

COMPUTED TOMOGRAPHY

- Bone-window settings are most useful for evaluating sinus wall involvement.
- Typically the soft tissue mass is small, showing mild enhancement with extensive adjacent bone destruction.

MAGNETIC RESONANCE IMAGING

- Intermediate signal intensity on both T1- and T2-weighted images is common.
- Sites of necrosis may occur as bright focal areas on T2-weighted imaging, but these may also reflect trapped mucus within the tumor mass.
- Sinus disease secondary to obstruction caused by the neoplasm usually exhibits high signal intensity on T2-weighted images, whereas the neoplasm is of intermediate signal intensity.

Inverted Papilloma This tumor is a benign, slow-growing neoplasm, typically arising at the juncture of the ethmoidal and maxillary sinuses along the lateral wall of the nasal cavity.

Incidence Inverted papillomas represent approximately 3 to 4 percent of all sinonasal tumors. Some 90 percent arise along the lateral nasal wall. Approximately 10 percent are found to arise from the nasal septum. There is 3 percent bilateral involvement. Male:female ratio is 3:1 and the tumor most commonly presents in the fourth to sixth decades.

Pathology

- The tumor is believed to arise from surface epithelium that extends endophytically into the submucosal stroma.
- Three distinct cell types of nasal papilloma are identified:

1. Inverted papilloma (47 percent)
2. Fungiform papilloma (50 percent)—most commonly seen to arise within the nasal septum.
3. Cylindrical papilloma (3 percent)—similar to the inverted type, with both endo- and exophytic forms of epithelial growth.

- There is a reported 10 to 20 percent incidence of concomitant squamous cell carcinoma.
- Inverted papillomas are not associated with chronic infection or a history of smoking.

Imaging Inverted papillomas most commonly present as a polypoid, homogeneous mass arising from the lateral nasal wall, often expanding the nasal cavity, secondary to extension into the adjacent sinuses with pressure erosion of the lateral nasal cavity walls. Sinus involvement, when it does occur, is primarily into the maxillary and ethmoidal cavities, although the tumor may extend superiorly through the cribriform plate.

- Approximately 30 to 40 percent of inverting papillomas will cause frank bony destruction secondary to pressure erosion and not direct invasion

COMPUTED TOMOGRAPHY

- Most useful for evaluation of paranasal sinus extension and bony involvement including extension through the cribriform plate.

MAGNETIC RESONANCE IMAGING

- Most useful in separating sinus tumor from inflammatory reaction and mucous secretions by demonstrating solid tumor enhancement with contrast.

The appearance on MRI, however, is not specific, and differentiation from other types of neoplasm cannot be made.

- Magnetic resonance imaging is also useful in evaluating extension through the cribriform plate into the cranial vault. T1-weighted images are isointense to skeletal muscle. Mild to moderate inhomogeneous contrast enhancement is noted within the tumor. Intermediate signal intensity is noted on T2-weighted images.
- Differential diagnosis includes squamous-cell carcinoma, esthesioneuroblastoma, melanoma, and lymphoma.

Nasoethmoidal Rhabdomyosarcoma Rhabdomyosarcoma represents a malignant mesenchymal tumor of striated muscle; in approximately 40 percent of cases, it originates in the head and neck region.

Incidence
- Represents 10 percent of all solid tumors seen up to age 15 years.
- Most common sarcoma seen in childhood.
- 70 percent present by age 10 years.
- Peak occurrence is from 2 to 6 years (45 percent).
- Approximately 10 percent of these tumors will occur in the second decade and beyond, with an annual recurrence of approximately 4 percent each decade thereafter.
- Most common pediatric extraaxial malignancy to involve the skull base.
- Intracranial extradural involvement in approximately 30 percent of cases, including cavernous sinus invasion.

Pathology Three cell types are known:
- Embryonal—Most commonly occurs in the first decade. Some 25 percent will occur over age 20 years, however, and 40 to 50 percent will occur in the head and neck area. This tumor is often metastatic to regional lymph nodes.
- Alveolar—This tumor most commonly occurs in the second and third decades, and 20 percent will occur in the head and neck area. The tumor is highly metastatic to both regional and distal lymph nodes.
- Pleomorphic—This tumor occurs most commonly in the fourth to sixth decades and is uncommonly seen in the pediatric population. About 10 percent of these tumors will occur in the head and neck region.
- Head and neck rhabdomyosarcomas are subdivided by site of origin into three diagnostic groups:
  1. Orbital
  2. Perimeningeal—This group has the worst overall prognosis due to its anatomic location, which includes the nasal cavity, paranasal sinuses, posterior nasal pharynx, and middle ear cavity.
  3. Other head and neck sites.
- Head and neck tumor distribution:
  1. Orbit, 45 percent
  2. Nasal pharynx, 25 percent
  3. Mastoid and middle ear cavities, 15 percent
  4. Sinonasal cavity, 15 percent

Imaging COMPUTED TOMOGRAPHY
- Tumor typically is a large, enhancing homogeneous soft tissue mass with extensive bone destruction.

MAGNETIC RESONANCE IMAGING
- T1-weighted images tend to be isointense to skeletal muscle. T2-weighted images are normally inhomogeneous and of increased signal intensity. There is moderate contrast enhancement.
- Magnetic resonance imaging is useful in accessing meningeal and cavernous sinus extension as well as occasionally demonstrating the mass to arise from muscle tissue.
- Differential diagnosis includes lymphoma and squamous cell carcinoma.

SUGGESTED READINGS

Skull base anatomy
1. Braun IF, Nadel L: The central skull base, in Som PM, Bergeron RT (eds): *Head and Neck Imaging.* St Louis, Mosby-Year Book 1991, pp 875–924.
2. Grant JCB et al: *Grant's Atlas of Anatomy.* Baltimore, Williams & Wilkins, 1962.
3. Grossman RC, Yousem DM: Sella and central skull base. in *Neuroimaging: The Requisites.* St Louis, Mosby-Year Book 1994, pp 305–334.
4. Grossman RC, Yousem DM: Temporal bone. in *Neuroimaging: The Requisites.* St Louis, Mosby-Year Book 1994, pp 335–358.
5. Harnsberger HR. Base of skull and cranial nerves: Normal anatomy. in Osborn A (ed): *Handbook of Neuroimaging.* St Louis, Mosby-Year Book 1991, pp 127–138.
6. Kucharczyk W et al: *Central Nervous System.* St Louis, Mosby Wolfe, 1994, pp 2.4–2.52.
7. Lustrin ES et al: Normal anatomy of the skull base, in Weber AL: Neuroimaging of the skull base. *Neuroimaging Clin North Am* 4:465–478, 1994.

Miscellaneous
1. Bradley WG: MR of the brain stem: A practical approach. *Imaging* 179:319–332, 1991.

2. Braun IF, Nadel L: in *Som and Bergeron's Head and Neck Imaging.* Mosby-Year Book 1991, pp 875–923.
3. Grossman RI, Yousem DM: Central skull base, in *Neuroimaging: the Requisites.* St. Louis, Mosby-Year Book 1994, pp 305–334.
4. Harnsberger HR: Base of skull and cranial nerves: Normal anatomy, in Handbook of Neuroimaging. St Louis, Mosby-Year Book 1991, pp 127–138.
5. Lanzieri CF: MR imaging of the cranial nerves. *AJR* 154:1263–1267, 1990.
6. Rubenstein S et al: Trigeminal nerve and ganglion in the Meckel cave: Appearance at CT and MR imaging. *Imaging* 193:155–159, 1994.
7. Warwick R, Williams PL: Neurology, in *Gray's Anatomy,* 35th ed. Longman Group, 1975, pp 996–1030.

☐ QUESTIONS (True or False)

1. Several important foramina consistently seen situitated at the medial aspect of sphenoid include the
- **a.** Foramen rotundum
- **b.** Foramen ovale
- **c.** Foramen of Vesalius
- **d.** Foramen spinosum
- **e.** Innominate canal

2. Regarding sphenoid bone,
- **a.** It consists of greater wing, lesser wing, and body.
- **b.** Fusion of sphenooccipital synchondrosis occurs near 16 years of age.
- **c.** The foramen lacerum is a fibrous structure through which nothing passes.
- **d.** The pterygoid canal is better seen on axial CT scans.
- **e.** The optic canal is seen medial to the anterior clinoid process.

3. Regarding occipital bone,
- **a.** The hypoglossal canal is seen between the occipital condyle and jugular tubercle.
- **b.** The posterior condylar canal contains a muscular branch of the vetebral artery.
- **c.** The occipital bone consists of the basiocciput, exocciput, and supraocciput.
- **d.** The groove for the transverse sinuses is seen immediately adjacent to lambdoid suture.
- **e.** Important structures passing through the foramen magnum include the medulla oblongata, spinal accessory nerve, vertebral arteries, etc.

4. Regarding temporal bone,
- **a.** The styloid process is located posteriorly and laterally to the stylomastoid foramen.
- **b.** The arcuate eminence covers the superior semicircular canal.
- **c.** The jugular foramen is situated anterior to the carotid canal.
- **d.** The pars nervosa of the jugular foramen contains cranial nerve IX and its sensory branch to the middle ear (Jacobson's nerve) and the inferior petrosal sinus.
- **e.** The vagus nerve is located medially in the pars vascularis of the jugular foramen.

5. Regarding cranial nerve III,
- **a.** It exits the midbrain on the medial aspect of the cerebral peduncles.
- **b.** It travels between the superior cerebellar artery and the posterior cerebral artery.
- **c.** It passes beneath the posterior communicating artery.
- **d.** The third nerve is found in the superior medial cavernous sinus.
- **e.** The third nerve supplies all the extraocular muscles except the lateral rectus and superior oblique muscles.

6. Regarding cranial nerve V,
- **a.** It is the motor nerve for the muscles of mastication and the sensory nerve for the face and much of the scalp.
- **b.** The gasserian ganglion is seen at Meckel's cave and three major branches exit the ganglion.
- **c.** V_1 travels through the cavernous sinus into the superior orbital fissure.
- **d.** V_2 also travels through the cavernous sinus into the foramen ovale.
- **e.** V_3 innervates the muscles of mastication and receives sensation from the lower face and jaw.

7. Regarding the facial nerve,
- **a.** It has three nuclei (the motor nucleus, salivary nucleus, and solitary or sensory nucleus).
- **b.** The seventh nerve nucleus lies anterolateral to the sixth nerve nucleus.
- **c.** The seventh nerve travels in the posterior superior quadrant of the internal auditory canal.
- **d.** The chorda tympani conveys taste from the anterior two-thirds of the tongue.
- **e.** The greater petrosal nerve arises from the geniculate ganglion.

8. Regarding vagus nerve,
- **a.** The vagus nerve arises from two nuclei in the medulla oblongata.
- **b.** The vagus nerve travels through the pars nervosa of the jugular foramen.
- **c.** The vagus nerve supplies motor innervation to soft palate, middle pharynx, inferior pharynx, and vocal cords.

d. The vagus nerve emerges in the groove between inferior cerebellar pedicle and the olive.
e. The vagus nerve follows the same path as the ninth nerve to the jugular foramen.

9. Regarding the glomus jugulare paraganglioma,
   a. Tumor arises from paraganglia tissue in the jugular bulb adventitia.
   b. The majority of jugular foramen neoplasms are paragangliomas.
   c. Some 60 percent of all patients may have multiple paragangliomas.
   d. This type of lesion is usually supplied by the ascending pharyngeal artery on angiography.
   e. Arteriovenous shunting is seen with early filling of the jugular vein.

10. Regarding esthesioneuroblastoma,
   a. It is also referred to as an olfactory neuroblastoma.
   b. Bone destruction is not seen.
   c. Gadolinium-enhanced MRI is most useful for the evaluation of intracranial extension.
   d. Histologically, the tumor is similar to an adrenal neuroblastoma and arises from the sympathetic ganglion neuroblast.
   e. It occurs in patients ranging from 3 to 10 years old.

☐ ANSWERS

1. a. T
   b. T
   c. F
   d. T
   e. T

2. a. T
   b. T
   c. T
   d. F
   e. T

3. a. T
   b. F
   c. T
   d. F
   e. T

4. a. T
   b. T
   c. F
   d. T
   e. T

5. a. T
   b. T
   c. T
   d. F
   e. T

6. a. T
   b. T
   c. T
   d. F
   e. T

7. a. T
   b. T
   c. F
   d. T
   e. T

8. a. F
   b. F
   c. T
   d. T
   e. T

9. a. T
   b. T
   c. F
   d. T
   e. T

10. a. T
   b. F
   c. T
   d. T
   e. F

CHAPTER

3 Orbit

Leonard Petrus
Chi S. Zee

☐ NORMAL ANATOMY OF THE ORBIT

BONY ORBIT

Orbital roof

- The orbital roof is triangular in shape and formed by the orbital plate of the frontal bone, which separates the orbit from the anterior cranial fossa.
- A fossa for the lacrimal gland is seen at the anterolateral aspect of the orbital roof.

Orbital Floor

- The orbital floor is triangular in shape and formed by the orbital plate of the maxilla, portions of the palatine bone, and the zygoma.
- Inferior blowout fractures usually occur in the region of the orbital plate of the maxilla.
- The infraorbital groove and infraorbital canal are seen in the floor of the orbit and contains the infraorbital nerve and vessels.

Medial Orbital Wall

- The medial orbital wall is rectangular in shape; it is the thinnest component of the bony orbit.
- The medial orbital wall is composed of the frontal process of the maxilla, the lacrimal bone, the lamina papyracea of the ethmoid, and the bony sphenoid.
- The lacrimal fossa is formed by the maxilla and lacrimal bone.

Lateral Orbital Wall

- The lateral orbital wall is formed by the zygoma anteriorly and greater wing of the sphenoid posteriorly.

Superior Orbital Fissure

- The superior orbital fissure is a space between the greater and lesser wings of the sphenoid; it connects the cavernous sinus with orbit.
- The superior ophthalmic vein and several cranial nerves—the oculomotor (CN III), trochlear (CN IV), abducens (CN VI), and the ophthalmic division of the trigeminal (CN V_1) nerve—pass through the superior orbital fissure.

Inferior Orbital Fissure

- The inferior orbital fissure connects the orbit with the pterygopalatine fossa and nasopharyngeal masticator space.
- It is formed by the maxilla, the palatine bone, and the greater wing of the sphenoid.
- The zygomatic nerve and the communication between the inferior ophthalmic vein and pterygoid plexus pass through the inferior orbital fissure.

Optic Canal

- The optic canal lies within the lesser wing of sphenoid and separated from the inferior medial aspect of the superior orbital fissure by the optic strut.
- The optic nerve and ophthalmic artery, surrounded by a dural sheath, pass through the optic canal.

SOFT TISSUE STRUCTURES OF THE ORBIT

Globe

- The wall of the globe consists of three layers: (1) retina; (2) choroid, ciliary body, and iris; (3) cornea anteriorly and sclera posteriorly.
- The lens lies between the iris and the vitreous humor.

- Between the cornea and the lens is a space containing the aqueous humor, which is divided by the iris into anterior and posterior chambers.

Optic Nerve and Sheath

- The optic nerve (CN II) extends from the papilla on the posterior surface of the globe to the optic chiasm.
- The optic nerve is approximately 45 mm in length and 3 to 4 mm in diameter.
- The optic nerve has three components: (1) orbital, (2) canalicular, and (3) intracranial.

Intraconal–conal Area

- Six extraocular muscles (the medial and lateral recti, the superior and inferior recti, and the superior and inferior oblique muscles) insert on the sclera.
- The levator palpebrae muscle lie under the roof of the orbit, above the superior rectus muscle.
- The four rectus muscles and the fibrous septa make up the muscle cone, which contains the optic nerve, ophthalmic artery, superior ophthalmic vein, and cranial nerves III, IV, VI, and V_1, surrounded by fat.
- Zinn's ligamentous ring is formed by the four recti, superior oblique, and levator palpebrae muscles.
- The optic nerve is surrounded by a meningeal sheath containing cerebrospinal fluid.

Extraconal Area

- The extraconal area is the space between the muscle cone and bony orbit, which contains fat.
- The lacrimal gland is located at the anterior aspect of the orbit, superolateral to the globe.

☐ LESIONS OF THE GLOBE

A bewildering array of pathologies affect the bony orbit and its contents. However, the evaluation of orbital disease is significantly aided by subdividing the orbit and its contents into anatomic compartments, placing a lesion into one of these compartments, and deriving a differential diagnosis based on image characteristics and relevant clinical information.

Both computed tomography (CT) and magnetic resonance imaging (MRI) play significant roles in orbital imaging. Computed tomograpy will detect 95 percent or more of surgically proven masses in the orbit. Magnetic resonance imaging does, however, provide significant improvement in the detection and characterization of subtle ocular lesions.

CONGENITAL ABNORMALITY

Persistent Hyperplastic Primary Vitreous During the first month of gestation, the space between the lens and the retina contains the primary vitreous. Made up of fibrillar ectodermal tissue and mesodermally derived tissue, it includes the hyaloid vessel and its branches. By the 14th gestation week, the secondary vitreous begins to fill the vitreous cavity, completely replacing it—except for a small central space—by the fifth or sixth month of development. This space is Cloquet's canal, which runs in an S-shaped course between the optic nerve and the posterior surface of the lens.

When the fibrovascular elements of the primary vitreous fails to regress, persistent hyperplastic primary vitreous (PHPV) occurs.

- Unilateral leukocoria in a microphthalmic eye
- May develop glaucoma and phthisis bulbi

Imaging COMPUTED TOMOGRAPHY

- Microphthalmia
- Deformity in globe configuration
- Increased attenuation of vitreous from previous hemorrhage
- Enhancement of abnormal intravitreal tissue
- Enhancement of a triangular density extending from the lens to the back of the orbit, which represents persistence of fetal tissue along Cloquet's canal
- No calcification

MAGNETIC RESONANCE IMAGING

- Hyperintense vitreous on T1- and T2-weighted images from hemorrhage in the subhyaloid or subretinal space.
- Hypointense to isointense tubular structure extending from the posterior lens to the optic disk region on T1-weighted images.
- Tubular structure enhances markedly following gadolinium.

Note: If changes in PHPV are present bilaterally, consider Norrie's disease (congenital progressive oculoacoustic cerebral degeneration) or Warburg's syndrome.

Retinopathy of Prematurity (Retrolental Fibroplasia)
This condition usually develops as a response to prolonged exposure to high concentration of oxygen in premature babies.

Pathology

- Patchy proliferation of capillaries within nerve fiber layer of the retina.

Imaging COMPUTED TOMOGRAPHY

- Bilateral microphthalmia
- Increased density in vitreous bilaterally from neovascular ingrowth
- Calcification rare

MAGNETIC RESONANCE IMAGING

- Abnormal retrolental soft tissue
- Hyperintense vitreous on both T1- and T2-weighted images; indistinguishable from PHPV

Coats' Disease This is a primarily vascular anomaly of the retina, characterized by idiopathic retinal telangiectasia and exudative retinal detachment.

- Invariably unilateral.
- Boys—6 to 8 years of age—are affected twice as often as girls.

Imaging COMPUTED TOMOGRAPHY

- Generalized increased density of involved globe caused by retinal detachment and proteinaceous subretinal exudate
- Normal globe size
- No calcification
- Compared to retinoblastoma, PHPV and toxocaral endophthalmitis, no distinct tumor mass present

MAGNETIC RESONANCE IMAGING

- Various signal intensities of involved globe on all pulse sequences due to the mixture of protein and lipid in the subretinal fluid that forms secondary to retinal detachment

Coloboma This is a congenital lesion due to a defect in the fusion of the fetal optic fissure in which tissue or portion of a tissue is lacking.

- Presents as localized defect in sclera, uvea, or retina.
- Imaging by CT or MRI usually demonstrates a posterior globe defect with optic disk excavation, usually at site of attachment of optic nerve to globe.
- Retroocular cyst may be associated.

Abnormalities of Globe Size The globe and optic pathways develop primarily from ectodermal tissues. Developmental abnormalities of the globe result in a spectrum of findings including cyclopia, synophthalmia, clinical anophthalmia, and microphthalmia.

Computed tomography demonstrates a small globe associated with a small, poorly developed orbit in developmental microphthalmia. An acquired form of microphthalmia is seen in adults as a shrunken, calcified globe, which may be secondary to trauma, surgery, or inflammation.

Macrophthalmia involves an enlargement of the globe and is most commonly a result of juvenile glaucoma or myopia. In its most severe form, it is called buphthalmos.

NEOPLASMS

Retinoblastoma

- Most common intraocular tumor of childhood. The tumor is congenital in origin but is usually not recognized at birth.
- Over 90 percent of all diagnoses are made in children under 5 years of age.
- Unilateral in about 70 percent of cases and bilateral in 30 percent.
- If bilateral, 90 percent of cases are inherited.
- Presents with leukocoria in 60 percent. (Table 3-1).

Pathology Retinoblastomas are derived from primitive embryonal retinal cells. The tumor is either undifferentiated or well differentiated and is composed of small round or ovoid cells with scant cytoplasm and relatively large nuclei. Some tumors display significant necrosis and prominent foci of calcification.

- Trilateral retinoblastoma = bilateral retinoblastoma + primitive neuroectodermal tumor in pineal region

Imaging COMPUTED TOMOGRAPHY

- Hyperattenuating intraocular mass.
- Tumor may be endophytic, exophytic, or (very rarely) diffuse.
- Calcification present in over 90 percent of cases (Fig. 3–1).
- Look for optic nerve invasion. This worsens prognosis significantly.

MAGNETIC RESONANCE IMAGING

- T1-weighted and proton-weighted scans demonstrate an isointense to slightly hyperintense mass relative to the vitreous.
- On T2-weighted images, tumor tissue is distinctly hypointense compared with the adjacent vitreous.

Medulloepithelioma This is a rare tumor of the ciliary body seen in young children. The tumor arises from the primitive unpigmented epithelial lining of the ciliary

Table 3–1
MOST COMMON CAUSES OF LEUKOKORIA

Pathologic Conditions	Frequency of Causing Leukokoria	Calcification	Subretinal Fluid
Retinoblastoma	58%	+ +	+
Persistent hyperplastic primary vitreous	28%	−	+
Toxocaral endophthalmitis	16%	−	+
Coats' disease	16%	−	+
Retinopathy of prematurity	5%	±	+
Retinal astrocytoma	3%	±	Uncommon

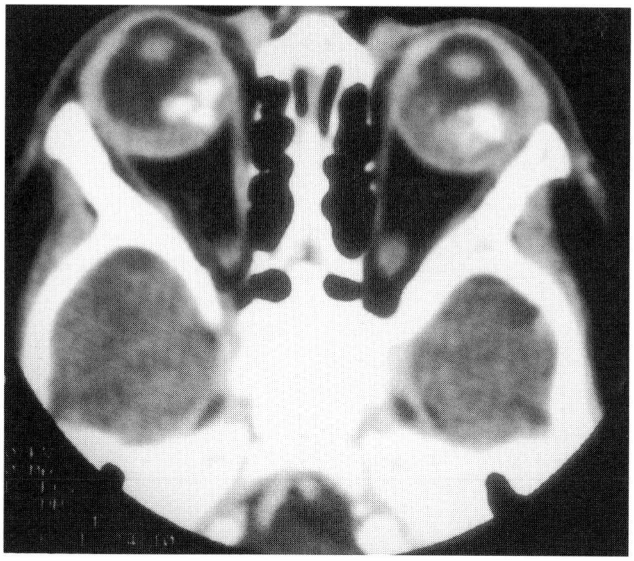

Figure 3–1 Retinoblastoma. An axial postcontrast CT scan shows calcification in both globes with an irregular enhancing mass.

body. On CT, a hyperdense mass is seen in the region of the ciliary body, and the tumor may spread along the iris or backward along the surface of the retina.

Choroidal hemangioma

- Usually seen in patients 10 to 20 years of age.
- Benign vascular lesion that may be isolated or seen in association with Sturge-Weber disease (encephalotrigeminal syndrome).
- Computed tomography demonstrates an ill-defined mass in the globe that undergoes marked enhancement on contrast infusion.
- Magnetic resonance imaging visualizes choroidal hemangioma as a hyperintense mass to vitreous on T1-weighted images, becoming isointense to vitreous on T2-weighted images.

Retinal Astrocytoma Retinal astrocytomas are low-grade neoplasms or hamartomas that arise from the nerve fiber layer of the retina or optic nerve. About 15 percent of patients have tuberous sclerosis, and 14 percent of retinal astrocytomas occur in patients with neurofibromatosis (NF) type I.

Imaging COMPUTED TOMOGRAPHY

- Single or multiple masses along the retina. Calcification may be present but, unlike retinoblastoma, there is no growth into the vitreous.
- Look for evidence of tuberous sclerosis in the brain and NF type I findings in the orbit.

Uveal Melanoma

- Most common primary intraocular malignancy in adults. These tumors typically affect Caucasians aged 50 to 70 years.
- Some 85 percent of these lesions arise from the choroid, where there may be accompanying retinal detachment. About 9 percent occur in the ciliary body and 6 percent arise from the iris.
- Tumor may be composed of either spindle or epithelioid cells or both. Some tumors are amelanotic.
- Diagnosis is usually made with combined ophthalmoscopic and ultrasound examinations.
- On CT and MRI, features vary with the presence or absence of accompanying retinal detachment.
- Melanotic melanomas have short T1 and T2 values; they appear moderately high-signal on T1-weighted images and as moderately low-signal-intensity masses on T2-weighted images.
- Magnetic resonance imaging is more sensitive than CT in distinguishing ocular tumors from fluid collections.
- If retinal detachment is present, high-signal subretinal fluid is seen in all pulse sequences in addition to the mass.

Ocular Metastasis Lung and breast carcinomas are the most common primary lesions to metastasize to the globe. Metastatic tumor to the globe tends to involve the uveal tract (vascular layer between the retina and sclera).

Imaging COMPUTED TOMOGRAPHY

- Multiple areas of increased density in the posterior portion of the uveal tract with associated subretinal fluid

MAGNETIC RESONANCE IMAGING

- Multiple lesions in the posterior portion of the uveal tract that are hyperintense to vitreous on T1-weighted images and hypo- to isointense to vitreous on T2-weighted images.
- Associated subretinal fluid can be separated from tumors on MRI.

INFLAMMATORY LESIONS OF THE GLOBE

Toxocaral Endophthalmitis *Toxocara canis* is the main ascarid causing disease in humans. It is spread by swallowing infective eggs from food contaminated by dog feces.

When a clinically recognizable disease occurs, the condition is called visceral larva migrans. When the larva infects the eye, a retinal granuloma may result, or it may cause retinal detachment associated with an organized vitreous.

- Usually affects children between 2 and 8 years of age.

Imaging COMPUTED TOMOGRAPHY

- Dense vitreous or an irregularly enhancing intravitreal mass with thickening of the uveoscleral coat is usually seen.
- No calcification.

- Normal-sized globe.

MAGNETIC RESONANCE IMAGING
- The granuloma is usually visible as a central mass with variable signal intensity.
- Subretinal exudate (high on T1- and T2-weighted images) may be present.

Note: The appearance of chronic retinal detachment on both CT and MRI often resembles *Toxocara* granuloma, Coats' disease, retinopathy of prematurity (ROP), PHPV, and retinoblastoma.

TRAUMA

Ocular trauma may take the form of (1) contusion or concussion, with or without rupture of the outer coats, and (2) direct injury, simple or penetrating, with possible foreign bodies.

Computed tomography is ideally suited to image the bony orbit and its contents in the traumatized victim. It accurately localizes the site of a foreign body, intra- or extraocular, and can also detect lens dislocation and disruption of the wall of the globe.

Magnetic resonance imaging is excellent in evaluating the eye when retinal or choroidal detachment is suspected following trauma. It utilized its tremendous contrast-resolution capabilities in detecting hemorrhage or transudate in the subretinal or suprachoroidal potential spaces in retinal and choroidal detachments respectively.

DEGENERATIVE

Disk Drusen ***Pathology***
- Cellular accretion of hyalinelike material on the surface of the optic disk.

Imaging COMPUTED TOMOGRAPHY
- Shows a globe with discrete, flat calcifications of the optic nerve disk.
- Some 75 percent are bilateral.

Phthysis Bulbi
- Involves atrophy of the globe with thickening of the walls, sometimes accompanied by scleral and lenticular calcification.
- Computed tomography will demonstrate a dense, shrunken globe.

☐ LESIONS OF THE OPTIC NERVE/SHEATH

ENLARGED OPTIC NERVE/SHEATH COMPLEX (TABLE 3-2)

Optic Nerve Glioma
- About 75 percent of tumors detected by age 10 and 90 percent by age 20.
- Peak age of presentation is between 2 and 6 years.
- Some 33 percent of patients show evidence of NF type I
- About 15 percent of patients with NF type I have optic or chiasmal glioma

Pathology
- Tumor is usually derived from astrocytes and tends to be limited by the dural covering of the optic nerve.
- Childhood optic glioma is most commonly pilocytic astrocytoma; it has a good prognosis for life and poor prognosis for vision.

Table 3–2
OPTIC NERVE/SHEATH ENLARGEMENT

Conditions	Findings
Optic nerve glioma	Association with neurofibromatosis, type I Chiasm (and optic pathway) involvement Big optic canal Occasional enhancement
Optic nerve meningioma	Association with neurofibromatosis, type II Calcification Chiasm usually uninvolved Normal-sized canal with sclerosis Tram-track sign on postcontrast images
Sarcoidosis	Disk edema in 5% of cases Optic nerve involvement unusual
Optic neuritis	Idiopathic or occurrence with demyelinating disease such as multiple sclerosis Enhancement of the optic nerve that may or may not be enlarged.
Increased intracranial pressure	Bilateral

- Adult optic gliomas tend to be glioblastomas with aggressive behavior (rare).

Imaging COMPUTED TOMOGRAPHY

- Well-defined, fusiform enlargement of the optic nerves
- Lucent areas secondary to mucinous or cystic change
- Intense contrast enhancement following infusion of contrast media

MAGNETIC RESONANCE IMAGING

- Enlargement of the nerve with characteristic kinking and buckling.
- The mass demonstrates T1 and T2 prolongation; post-gadolinium fat-suppressed images exquisitely demonstrate the intensely enhancing tumor (Fig. 3–2).
- Gadolinium-enhanced MRI is superior to CT in the evaluation of intracranial extension of the optic glioma.

Optic Nerve Sheath Meningioma Meningiomas usually arise in middle-aged (35- to 60-year-old) women. They also occur in children with NF type II.

Pathology

- The meningothelial variety is the most common type of meningioma within the orbit.
- Pediatric meningiomas tend to be more aggressive than those in adults. Intratumoral psammomatous calcifications may be present, particularly within highly cellular areas of the tumor.

Imaging COMPUTED TOMOGRAPHY

- Most common feature is a well-defined tubular thickening of the optic nerve.
- Fusiform enlargement of the optic nerve is also occasionally seen.
- Stippled calcification is common within the tumor, helping to differentiate it from optic nerve glioma.
- May also show sclerotic changes at the apex of the orbit, which is an indication of intracranial extension of meningioma.
- Post-contrast, there is moderate to marked enhancement of the tumor, producing the so-called tram-track sign of perioptic meningioma.
- Tram-track sign also present in cases of optic neuritis and pseudotumor.

MAGNETIC RESONANCE IMAGING

- Demonstrates uniform thickening of the intraorbital segment of the optic nerve.
- The tumor shows hypointensity relative to normal brain tissue on T1-weighted images and iso- to slightly hyperintensity on T2-weighted images.
- Postgadolinium fat-suppressed images demonstrate marked enhancement of the tumor, often depicting the tram-track sign (Fig. 3–3).
- Intracranial extension usually stops at the prechiasmatic optic nerve sheath.

Other Tumors

- Hemangiopericytoma and hemangioblastoma can originate from the optic nerve/sheath.
- Lymphoma/leukemia rarely infiltrates the optic nerve/sheath complex exclusively.
- Metastases to the optic nerve may also occur.

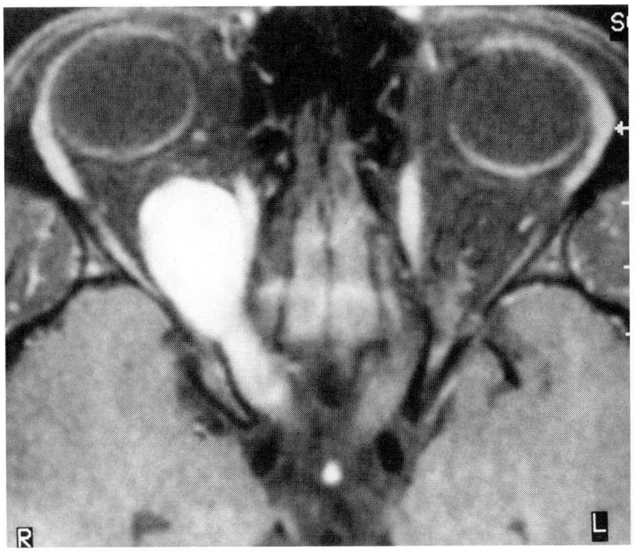

Figure 3–2 Optic nerve glioma. A gadolinium-enhanced, fat-suppressed T1-weighted image demonstrates an enhancing mass of the right optic nerve.

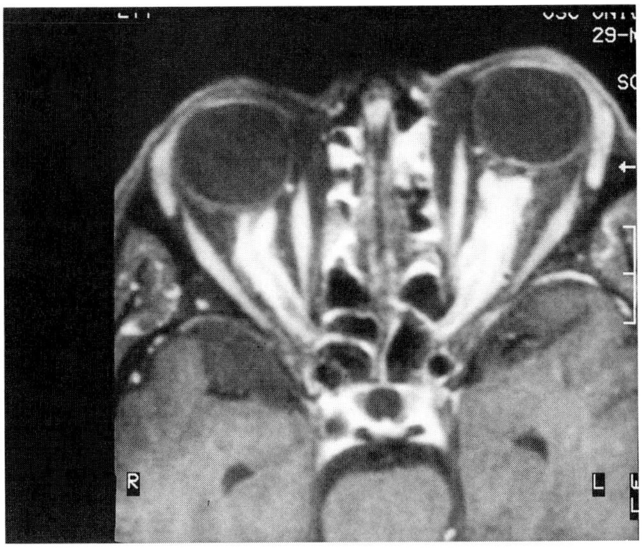

Figure 3–3 Bilateral optic nerve meningioma. A gadolinium-enhanced, fat-suppressed T1-weighted image demonstrates enhancement of optic nerves. The tram-track sign, typical of optic meningioma, is seen on the right side.

Systemic Diseases
- Systemic diseases with secondary or primary involvement of the optic nerve include sarcoidosis, toxoplasmosis, tuberculosis, and syphilis.
- The CT and MRI findings of the above mimic an optic nerve meningioma.

Optic Neuritis
- Usually an acute, idiopathic inflammatory process.
- There is diffuse and smooth expansion of the optic nerve.
- Optic neuritis is sometimes an early manifestation of multiple sclerosis (MS).
- Approximately 50 percent of patients with optic neuritis develop MS.
- Contrast-enhanced CT may show the tram-track sign described for optic nerve meningioma.
- On MRI, the optic nerves may appear hyperintense on T2-weighted images.
- Gadolinium-enhanced images with fat-suppression technique show enhancement of the optic nerve, which may or may not be enlarged.

Trauma Trauma in or around the optic nerve may result in edema or hematoma formation and consequent optic nerve enlargement.

HYPOPLASIA OF THE OPTIC NERVE

- Diagnosed when the nerve measures less than 2 mm.
- May be an isolated congenital anomaly or may be associated with other ocular, cranial, facial, or systemic abnormalities.
- If associated with absence of the septum pellucidum, dysplasia of the third ventricle, hypothalamic hypopituitarism, and growth hormone deficiency, the condition is referred to as septooptic dysplasia of de Morsier.

☐ CONAL AND INTRACONAL LESIONS

VASCULAR LESIONS

Venous Varix
- May be congenital or acquired.
- Acquired lesions may be seen in association with either intraorbital or intracranial arteriovenous malformations.
- The congenital variety represents congenital venous malformation characterized by a proliferation of venous elements and massive dilation of one or more orbital veins, presumably associated with a congenital weakness in the venous wall.
- On non-contrast CT scans, phleboliths may be seen.
- Contrast-enhanced CT reveal densely enhancing round or tubular structures located within the muscle cone.
- These structures enlarge with the Valsalva maneuver.
- Magnetic resonance imaging documents all levels of flow characteristics of blood, from signal-void lesions in fast-flowing varices to flow-related enhancement in slow-flowing varices.

Superior Ophthalmic Vein (SOV) Thrombosis
- Often occurs in conjunction with septic or aseptic cavernous sinus thrombosis.
- Computed tomography reveals an enlarged SOV with an enhancing rim and a low-density central thrombus. The ipsilateral cavernous sinus is usually enlarged.
- Magnetic resonance imaging demonstrates the enlarged SOV without the central flow void. Thrombus will manifest varied appearances depending on its age.

Carotid Cavernous (CC) Fistula
- May result from trauma or surgery or may occur spontaneously.
- Presents clinically with proptosis, chemosis, venous engorgement, pulsating exophthalmos, and an auscultable bruit.
- Both CT and MRI reveal enlargement of the superior ophthalmic vein and the extraocular muscles of the involved orbit.
- Angiographic demonstration of exact location of the CC fistula is essential and aids in planning definitive therapy.

INFLAMMATORY LESIONS

Idiopathic Orbital Inflammatory Syndrome (Orbital Pseudotumor)
- Nonspecific, idiopathic inflammatory condition for which no local identifiable cause or systemic disease can be found.
- The patient can be of any age with pain and signs of inflammation usually evident, especially in the acute phase.
- Most common cause of intraorbital mass in adults (Table 3-3).
- Orbital pseudotumor may be associated with Wegener's granuloma, fibrosing mediastinitis, thyroiditis, and cholangitis.

Pathology
- In the acute form, there is a relatively hypocellular but polymorphic infiltrate.
- Lymphocytes predominate.
- The acute phase is very responsive to steroids.
- The chronic or subacute form also exhibits a hypocellular polymorphic infiltrate, but in addition, there is a prominent fibrotic stroma.
- Lymphoid follicles are often present.

Imaging Findings on CT depend upon which tissue is involved by the orbital pseudotumor.

Table 3–3
INFILTRATIVE LESIONS

Conditions	Findings
Endocrine ophthalmopathy	Uniform, even thickening of extraocular muscle (EOM) Increased fat Spares tendinous insertion on globes No mass
Pseudotumor	Amorphous mass EOM involvement extends to tendinous insertion Scleral thickening Good responses to steroids
Orbital Tumors	
Hemangioma	Most frequent benign tumor Bulky high-attenuation mass Contrast enhancement variable (marked in cavernous type) Possible phleboliths
Lymphoma	Older age groups Irregular amorphous mass May encase/infiltrate globe Bone erosion frequent
Metastatic	Bone destruction Extraconal mass

Two types, myositic and tumefactive.

1. *Myositic form*

- The inflammatory process involves one or more of the extraocular muscles.
- Scan by CT or MRI demonstrates enlargement of the involved muscles, which may extend anteriorly to involve the inserting tendon (unlike Graves' disease).

2. *Tumefactive form (diffuse orbital pseudotumor)*

- Manifests as streaky density obliterating the fat and becoming homogeneous in later phases.
- The lesion can completely replace the retrobulbar fat.
- Marked enhancement (unlike lymphoma).
- No preseptal inflammation.
- No bone erosion.
- Rarely has sharp borders.
- Process may involve the orbital apex or present with typical orbital apical syndrome of pain, minimal proptosis, and restricted extraocular muscle movements.
- Pseudotumor may also involve the lacrimal gland, causing diffuse enlargement of the gland on CT.
- When the sclera is involved, CT demonstrates thickening of the posterior wall of the globe, extending to involve the most anterior portion of the optic nerve.
- When the optic nerve sheath is involved, CT demonstrates thickening of the margin of the nerve, with streaky densities extending into the adjacent orbital fat.
- The MRI is quite specific: low signal intensity on T2-weighted images probably due to hypercellularity and little free water.
- Enhancement of the involved tissue is seen on both contrast-enhanced CT and MRI.

Retrobulbar Cellulitis and Abscess Formation Retrobulbar cellulitis and abscess formation within the muscle cone is usually seen in the context of a diffuse infection of the orbit. The image findings will be discussed in the section dealing with pathologies of the extraconal space.

ENDOCRINE LESIONS

Thyroid Ophthalmopathy

- Most common cause of proptosis in adults.
- Orbit problems may precede the actual thyroid abnormality or occur when the thyroid disease has been brought under control.
- In 70 percent of patients, there is clinical and biochemical evidence of hyperthyroidism.

Imaging **COMPUTED TOMOGRAPHY AND MAGNETIC RESONANCE IMAGING**

- Usually bilateral disease (80 percent) with multiple muscles affected.
- The inferior and medial rectus muscles are most commonly involved, followed by the superior muscle complex and the lateral rectus.
- The enlargement tends to involve the muscle bellies, with sparing of the tendons.

- In 10 percent, one isolated muscle belly is involved.
- There may be an overall increase in the volume of the retroocular fat.

TUMORS

Capillary Hemangioma

- Some 95 percent occur in infants less than 6 months of age.
- The tumor often increases in size for 6 to 10 months and then gradually involutes.
- Female predominance.

Pathology The tumor is composed of endothelial and capillary vessel proliferation with benign endothelial cells surrounding small, capillary-sized vascular spaces.

Imaging COMPUTED TOMOGRAPHY

- Enhanced CT reveals a fairly well marginated mass spanning the conal-intraconal space and also involving the extraconal space.
- The mass may extend intracranially through the superior orbital fissure, optic canal, and orbital roof.

MAGNETIC RESONANCE IMAGING

- Slightly hyperintense to muscles with areas of signal void (vessels) on T1-weighted images.
- Heterogeneously hyperintense to fat on T2-weighted images.
- Contrast enhancement is seen.

Cavernous Hemangioma

- Most common benign orbital tumor.
- Occurs from second to fourth decades.
- Unlike the capillary hemangiomas, these tumors show slow, progressive enlargement.
- Female predominance.

Pathology The tumors are composed of large, dilated vascular channels lined by thin, attenuated endothelial cells. They tend to possess a distinct fibrous pseudocapsule, giving rise to a well-defined mass.

Imaging COMPUTED TOMOGRAPHY

- Appear as sharply circumscribed, homogeneous, round to oval masses that enhance uniformly.
- Some 83 percent of these masses are found in the intraconal space, but they may occur anywhere in the orbit.
- The orbit may be expanded.
- Calcification in phlebolith may be seen in the lesion.
- The lesions usually do not deform the globe.

MAGNETIC RESONANCE IMAGING

- Features are nonspecific and demonstrate a well-defined intraconal mass exhibiting isointensity to muscle on T1-weighted images and hyperintensity on T2-weighted images.
- Contrast enhancement is usually uniform but may be heterogeneous.

Lymphangioma

- About 1 to 2 percent of orbital childhood masses.
- Occurs in the first decade.
- Associated with lesions on lid, conjunctiva, cheek.

Pathology The lesion is made up of dilated lymphatics, dysplastic venous vessels, smooth muscle, and areas of hemorrhage.

Imaging COMPUTED TOMOGRAPHY

- Mild to moderate enlargement of the orbit.
- Poorly defined multilobulated inhomogeneous lesion with intra- and extraconal components.
- Single/multiple cystlike areas with rim enhancement.
- Rarely contains phleboliths (differential diagnosis: hemangioma, orbital varix).

MAGNETIC RESONANCE IMAGING

- Multiloculated, poorly marginated lesions.
- Heterogeneous in signal intensity.
- Magnetic resonance imaging is more sensitive than CT in identifying subacute, old hemorrhage and defining the various components of hemorrhage within the lesion.
- Partial, heterogeneous enhancement may be seen.

Lymphoma

- Mean age is in the fifties in immunologically normal patients and in the thirties in AIDS patients.
- Secondary malignant lymphoma as part of a systemic disease occurs in a younger age group.
- Some 75 percent have or will have systemic lymphoma.

Pathology

- Most common cytologic forms are histiocytic and lymphocytic in various degrees of differentiation.
- Orbital lymphoma may involve any component of the orbit.
- The lacrimal gland (extraconal space) is the most common site, followed by the conal-intraconal space and the optic nerve sheath complex.

Imaging COMPUTED TOMOGRAPHY

- The lesions tend to mold themselves to preexisting structures without eroding bone or enlarging the orbit.
- Retrobulbar lymphomas have a varied radiographic appearance.
- Some have sharply circumscribed borders or may appear infiltrative and obliterate normal tissue planes.
- There is variable enhancement with intravenous contrast.
- The differential diagnosis includes tumefactive pseudotumor and retrobulbar metastatic focus.
- Lacrimal gland lymphoma displaces the globe medially forward and appears as a moderately enhancing mass in the lacrimal gland. Further discussion of lacrimal gland tumors will follow.

MAGNETIC RESONANCE IMAGING

- Lymphomas have an intermediate or hypointense signal on T1-weighted and proton-density-weighted images and appear hyperintense on T2-weighted images. Intense contrast enhancement is seen.

Rhabdomyosarcomas

- Some 90 percent occur in patients under 16 years of age.
- The tumors arise from extraocular muscles or from pluripotential mesenchymal elements.
- The most common site is the superonasal quadrant of the orbit but many tumors are also found in a central location behind the globe.

Pathology Rhabdomyosarcomas are classified into one of three histologic types: embryonal, differentiated, or alveolar. Either type may occur in the orbit, with embryonal rhabdomyosarcoma being the most common and differentiated rhabdomyosarcoma the least frequent. Histologically, the tumor may be difficult to differentiate from neuroblastoma and retinoblastoma.

Imaging COMPUTED TOMOGRAPHY

- Radiologic features are varied.
- Early rhabdomyosarcomas are often extraconal and may involve the preseptal compartment
- Advanced rhabdomyosarcomas usually extend into the intraconal space.
- Bone destruction may be associated with rhabdomyosarcoma, and the tumor may extend into the paranasal sinuses.
- Look for intracranial extension.
- Histiocytosis X—look for other lytic calvarial lesions.

MAGNETIC RESONANCE IMAGING

- Isointense to muscle on T1-weighted images and hyperintense on T2-weighted images.
- Rhabdomyosarcoma can be differentiated from capillary hemangioma on MRI by identifying the signal void areas (vessels) within the capillary hemangioma and bone destruction associated with rhabdomyosarcoma.

Metastases

- Metastatic disease to the eye and orbit is found in 12 percent of patients with metastatic carcinoma.
- In children, the primary tumors, in descending order of frequency, are neuroblastoma, Ewing's sarcoma, and Wilms' tumor.
- In adults, the primary tumor is usually breast or lung, with less cases from genitourinary or gastrointestinal primary sites.
- The globe is most commonly involved by metastatic disease. Detachment of the retina often accompanies these lesions.
- Extraocular muscle metastasis present as a segmental or more rarely diffuse widening of the involved muscle. Isolated lateral rectus muscle enlargement is invariably due to metastasis.
- Intraconal metastatic tumor generally presents on CT as an infiltrating contrast-enhancing mass, which often involves the globe margin or extraocular muscles.
- Extraconal metastasis may involve the extraconal tissue or the contiguous bony orbit or periorbital area. The lacrima gland may be enlarged by metastatic involvement.

□ EXTRACONAL LESIONS

A number of conditions mentioned in the preceding discussion, although primarily occurring within the muscle cone, may transgress the extraocular muscles to involve the extraconal space. These include most of the neoplastic lesions mentioned earlier and also pseudotumor.

There are, however, a number of disease entities that appear to arise primarily within the extraconal space. These include the following.

INFLAMMATORY CONDITIONS

Subperiosteal Cellulitis/Abscess

- Orbital infection accounts for about 60 percent of primary orbital disease.
- The majority are sinus in origin.
- In the early stage, the infection is confined to the paranasal sinus, but it causes congestion of the venous outflow of the eyelid and conjunctiva, resulting in preseptal cellulitis.
- Computed tomography reveals a diffuse increase in density and thickening of the lid and conjuctiva.
- As the reaction of the orbital periosteum begins and gradually advances, the edema of the eyelids and conjunctivae becomes more generalized and the eye begins to protrude. Inflammatory tissue and edema collect beneath the periosteum to form a subperiosteal abscess.
- If unchecked, the inflammatory process extends to involve the periorbital and retroorbital fat, resulting in true orbital cellulitis. Intraconal or extraconal loculation and abscess formation may then occur.

TUMORS

Epidermoid and Dermoid Tumors

- These are the most frequent developmental cysts involving the orbit and periorbital structures.
- Most appear during childhood.

- The tumors usually arise anteriorly between the globe and the orbital periosteum in the superolateral quadrant of the extraconal orbit.

Pathology

- Both cysts result from inclusion during closure of the neural tubes.
- Epidermoid tumors contain only squamous debris and cholesterol, while dermoid tumors may contain, in addition, fat, sebaceous glands, teeth, and hair.

Imaging COMPUTED TOMOGRAPHY

- The lesions are seen as low-density, extraconal, well defined masses with smooth margins.
- Fat may be seen in dermoid cysts.

MAGNETIC RESONANCE IMAGING

- Similar signal intensity features to dermoid, or epidermoid elsewhere.
- Enhancement of the cyst wall may be seen.

Lacrimal Gland Tumors

- A number of inflammatory and neoplastic conditions result in enlargement of the lacrimal gland.
- Tumors of the lacrimal gland may be epithelial, lymphoid, or metastatic.
- Benign mixed tumor and adenoid cystic carcinoma accounts for 50 percent of lacrimal gland tumors.
- Non-Hodgkin's lymphoma and metastases may affect the lacrimal gland.
- Findings on CT and MRI are nonspecific. Both modalities display diffuse glandular enlargement with oblong contouring.
- Epithelial neoplasms tend to be associated with bone remodeling and destruction.
- Inflammatory lymphoid lesions tend to mold themselves to preexisting orbital structures without eroding bone or enlarging the orbit.

LESION OF THE BONY ORBIT

- Primary or metastatic lesions to the bony orbit may extend into the extraconal space.
- Squamous-cell carcinoma of the maxillary or ethmoid sinuses may also spread into the orbit.
- The tumor gains access to the orbit through the weaker inferior and lateral walls.
- Involvement of the posterior maxillary sinus wall may give rise to the orbital apex syndrome.

TRAUMA

- Any type of orbital trauma, blunt or penetrating, may cause hemorrhage and edema in the extraconal space.
- Computed tomography will exquisitely demonstrate the fractures, which may be complex or isolated.

CONGENITAL

Cephalocele

- Consists of a protrusion of intracranial contents through a congenital defect in the calvarium and dura.
- Some 15 percent of all encephaloceles arise around the nose and orbit.
- Computed tomography is excellent at demonstrating the bony margins of the defect.
- Magnetic resonance imaging is the best modality for identifying the presence of brain tissue in a cephalocele.

SUGGESTED READINGS

Lesions of the Globe

1. Harnsberger HR: State of the art orbital imaging. *Semin Ultrasound CT MR* 9:379–483, 1988.
2. Hopper KD et al: Abnormalities of the orbit and its contents in children: CT and MRI imaging. *AJR* 156:1219–1224, 1991.
3. Hopper KD et al: CT and MR imaging of the pediatric orbit. *Radiographics* 12:485–503, 1992.
4. Smirniotopoulous JR et al: Differential diagnosis of leukokoria: Radiologic-pathology correlation. *Radiographics* 14:1059–1079, 1994.

Optic Nerve/Sheath Lesions

1. Azar-Kia B et al: CT and MRI of the optic nerve and sheath. *Semin Ultrasound CT MR* 9:443–454, 1988.
2. Rothfus WE et al: Optic nerve/sheath enlargement: A differential approach based on high resolution CT morphology. *Radiology* 150:409–415, 1984.

Conal and Intraconal Lesions

1. Armington WG, Bilaniuk NT: The radiologic evaluation of the orbit: Conal and intraconal lesions. *Semin Ultrasound CT MR* 9:455–473, 1988.
2. Flanders AE et al: CT characteristics of orbital pseudotumors and other orbital inflammatory processes. *J Comput Assist Tomogr* 13:40–47, 1989.

Extraconal Lesions

1. Hesselink JR et al: CT of masses of the lacrimal gland region. *Radiology* 131:143–147, 1979.

☐ QUESTIONS (True or False)

1. Intraorbital calcification occurs in:
   a. Trichinosis
   b. Pseudotumor
   c. Retinoblastoma
   d. Lymphoma
   e. Carcinoma of the lacrimal gland

2. Bony destruction of the orbit is frequently seen in:
   a. Orbital lymphoma
   b. Hemangiomas
   c. Dermoid cysts
   d. Neurofibroma
   e. Pseudotumor

3. Subretinal fluid is seen with:
   a. PHPV
   b. Coats' disease
   c. Optic nerve drusen
   d. Coloboma
   e. Retinal astrocytoma

4. Regarding Graves' disease:
   a. Patients are usually hyperthyroid
   b. There is good correlation with lab values
   c. Usually unilateral
   d. Involves the tendinous insertion on the globes
   e. Isolated muscle belly involvement occurs

5. Regarding pseudotumor:
   a. Never occurs in children
   b. Associated with fibrosing mediastinitis
   c. Usually bilateral
   d. The globe is spared
   e. The mass is well defined

☐ ANSWERS

1. a. T
   b. F
   c. T
   d. F
   e. T

2. a. F
   b. F
   c. F
   d. F
   e. F

3. a. T
   b. T
   c. F
   d. F
   e. T

4. a. T
   b. F
   c. F
   d. F
   e. T

5. a. F
   b. T
   c. F
   d. F
   e. F

C|H|A|P|T|E|R

4 Paranasal Sinuses and Nose

Steven Epner
Chi S. Zee

☐ NORMAL ANATOMY AND DEVELOPMENT

The paranasal sinuses all arise as evaginations from the nasal fossa and lined by a similar pseudostratified columnar ciliated epithelium. There is much anatomic variation to the conchae or turbinates, the respective meatus of each, and the sinus ostia.

The inferior meatus has only one major ostium, that of the nasolacrimal duct.

The middle meatus has an anteriorly located frontal recess into which the nasofrontal duct drains the frontal sinus 50 percent of the time. In the other 50 percent, the nasofrontal duct drains into the anterior ethmoid air cells, which then drain into the frontal recess. The maxillary sinus drains into the ethmoid infundibulum lateral to the uncinate process of the inferior turbinate and inferior to the ethmoid bulla arising from the lateral wall of the middle meatus. The ethmoid infundibulum communicates with the nasal fossa by coursing superiorly and around the uncinate process via the hiatus semilunaris. Accessory antral ostia are often present, which drain into the infundibulum. Anterior ethmoid air cells drain into the anterior aspect of the hiatus semilunaris. The majority of the middle ethmoid air cells empty through the ethmoid bulla into the middle meatus through the midportion of the hiatus semilunaris. The term *ostiomeatal complex* refers to the uncinate process, ethmoid infundibulum, maxillary sinus ostium, middle turbinate, frontal recess, and ethmoid bulla. (See Diagram 4–1.)

The superior meatus drains the posterior ethmoid air cells via the posterior ethmoid ostia. A supreme meatus and concha is present in 60 percent of patients and often drains a posterior ethmoid air cell. The sphenoid sinus lies superior and posterior to the superior concha and drains into the sphenoethmoidal recess.

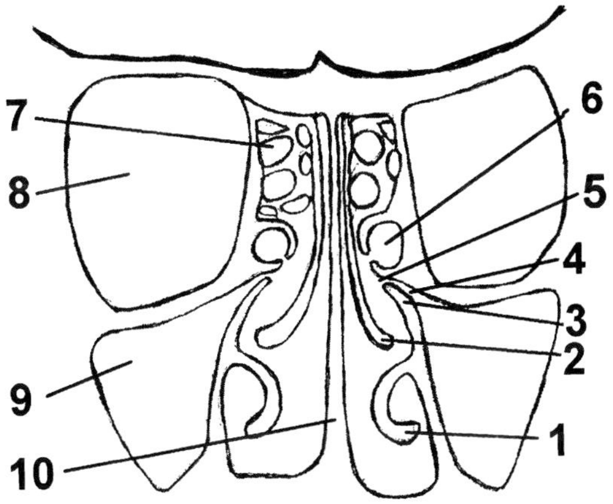

Diagram 4–1

1. Inferior turbinate
2. Middle turbinate
3. Uncinate process
4. Maxillary ostium
5. Hiatus semilunaris
6. Ethmoid bulla
7. Ethmoid air cells
8. Orbit
9. Maxillary sinus
10. Nasal septum

The frontal sinuses are the only ones to be absent at birth. They develop after the first year and often remain pea-sized until 7 years of age. The sphenoidal sinuses are tiny nonpneumatized mucosal evaginations at birth and remain small before the age of 3, developing fully by 15 years of age. The ethmoid sinuses are aerated at birth but rapidly develop after 7 years of age, reaching maturity between 12 and 14 years of age. The maxillary sinuses are relatively well developed at birth, rapidly expanding to adult proportions and configuration after 7 years of age. Before the age of 1 year, sinus opacification cannot be given any clinical significance; it should be interpreted with caution before 3 years of age.

INFLAMMATORY DISEASES

ACUTE SINUSITIS

- Often begins as a viral infection: Rhinoviruses, parainfluenza viruses, influenza viruses, adenovirus, and respiratory syncytial virus are the most common agents.
- Mucosal thickening may obstruct ostia, changing the oxygen tension and the normal flora. Bacterial sinusitis may then superinfect. Common organisms include *Streptococcus pneumoniae, Haemophilus influenzae, beta-hemolytic streptococcus,* and rarely *Staphylococcus aureus* and *Pseudomonas.*
- Any physiologic or anatomic deviation may predispose one to develop obstructed drainage of the paranasal sinuses. This may include enlargement of the ethmoid bulla, an air cell within the uncinate process, or simply edematous changes of the mucous membranes.
- Acute sinusitis is usually associated with single or unilateral sinus disease, however, pansinusitis may occur.
- Allergic sinusitis, found in 10 percent of the population, tends, in comparison, to be a symmetrical, bilateral process, reflecting its systemic nature. In addition, multiple polyps are associated with allergic sinusitis, while solitary polyps are more often inflammatory in etiology.

Imaging

- Acute sinusitis cannot be diagnosed on the basis of a single exam. Only in the appropriate clinical setting with findings of air-fluid levels should the diagnosis be confidently made.
- Normal mucosa on plain film, computed tomography (CT), or magnetic resonance imaging (MRI) is so thin that it is not visualized.
- Mucosal thickening may be seen with infection, fibrosis, allergies, chemically induced inflammation, tumor, or any combination of the above.
- Plain film and CT may demonstrate washout of the mucoperiosteal white line about the sinuses secondary to hyperemia.
- Computed tomography with contrast shows enhancement of thickened mucosa with underlying low attenuation of submucosal edema. Low-density mucoid secretions may be entrapped within the central portion of the sinus.
- Magnetic resonance imaging shows thick, inflamed mucosa to follow the characteristics of water: low signal on T1-weighted imaging, intermediate signal on proton-density, and high signal on T2-weighted imaging, while fibrosis gives low to intermediate signal on all sequences.

FUNGAL SINUSITIS

- Most commonly involves the maxillary and ethmoid sinuses.
- The most common causes are aspergillosis, mucormycosis, and candidiasis. Patients are usually immunocompromised, diabetic, or on antibiotic therapy.

Imaging Radiologic findings can vary from nonspecific to characteristic of fungal disease.

PLAIN FILM AND COMPUTED TOMOGRAPHY

- Air-fluid levels are rare.
- Bone may become thickened and sclerotic with erosive changes (remodeled) and may be confused with an aggressive malignant lesion.
- Intrasinus concretions may develop and have high density on CT and plain films.

MAGNETIC RESONANCE IMAGING

- Mycetomas have few free protons and typically are hypointense on T1-weighted images and markedly hypointense on T2-weighted images. Iron or manganese content may also contribute the marked hypointensity. Extreme cases may cause confusion with normal aeration (Fig. 4–1).

CHRONIC SINUSITIS

- Most common cause of sinus opacification; however, this is hardly specific.
- Results from persistent acute inflammation or repeated episodes.
- Anaerobes predominate as the pathologic agents with chronic sinusitis as opposed to acute sinusitis. Common organisms include *streptococci, Bacteroides,* and *Fusobacterium.*
- The mucosa can become atrophic, sclerosing, or hypertrophic

Imaging PLAIN FILM AND COMPUTED TOMOGRAPHY

- Thickened mucosa, sclerotic osseous reaction, and sinus wall thickening.

COMPLICATIONS OF SINUSITIS

Inflammatory Polyps and Retention Cysts

- Polyps result from mucous membrane hyperplasia due to chronic inflammation, mostly affecting the maxillary antra and nasal fossae.
- Mucous retention cysts are the result of obstruction of a mucin-secreting gland and are thus lined by epithelium.
- Intrasinus polyps and retention cysts cannot be distinguished on radiographic examination.
- As previously mentioned, inflammatory polyps tend to involve fewer of the sinuses and to be less symmetrical than allergic polyps.

Imaging PLAIN FILM AND COMPUTED TOMOGRAPHY

- May opacify the sinus if large.
- Usually small, from 3 to 10 mm.

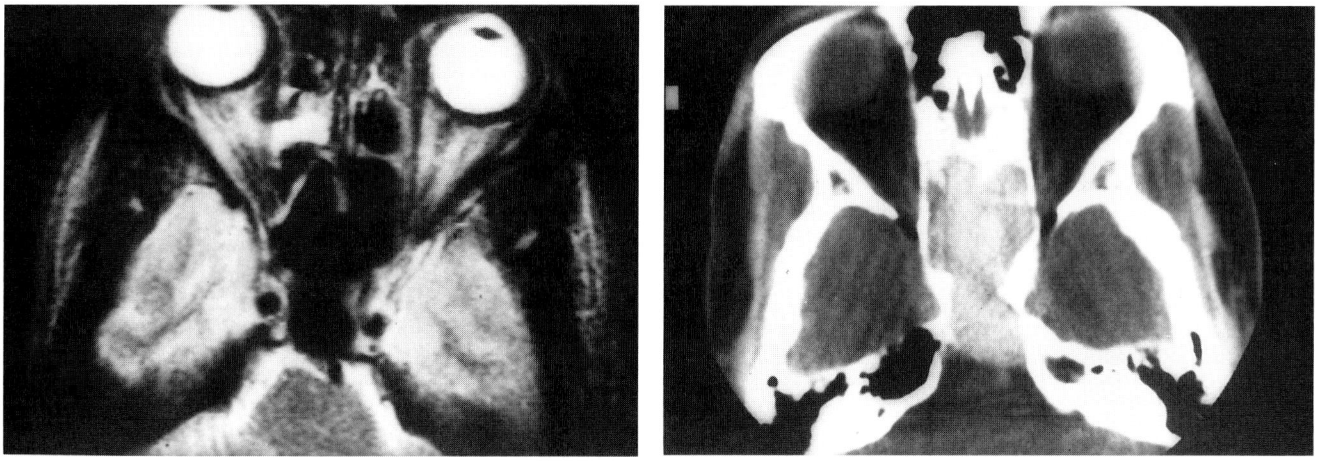
(A) (B)

Figure 4–1 Mucormycosis of sphenoid sinus. *A.* An axial T2-weighted image shows marked hypointensity within the sphenoid sinus. This very low signal intensity is due to mucormycosis but cannot be distinguished from a normal aerated sinus. Slight high-signal mucosal disease is seen in the right ethmoid sinus. *B.* An axial CT scan with contrast demonstrates the presence of an enhancing mass in the sphenoid sinus with bony destruction of the clivus.

- Often have a convex border, distinguishing them from air-fluid levels.
- When large, they may expand the sinus.

MAGNETIC RESONANCE IMAGING

- Usually low to intermediate signal intensity on T1-weighted images and high intensity on T2-weighted images, reflecting high water content.
- May have high signal on T1-weighted images, secondary to high protein content.

Mucoceles

- Develop as a result of obstruction of a sinus ostium, most commonly from mucosal disease. Obstruction from tumor, trauma, or septated sinus may also lead to mucocele formation.
- Most common cause of expansile lesions of any paranasal sinus.
- Approximately two-thirds of cases involve the frontal sinus, followed by ethmoid > maxillary > sphenoid.
- Present with frontal bossing, proptosis, or change in voice.
- Pain suggests infection-pyomucocele.

Imaging PLAIN FILM

- Opacification of the sinus with loss of the mucoperiosteal white line.
- Contour of the sinus may be expanded, displacing the orbital roof or frontal sinus septum.

COMPUTED TOMOGRAPHY

- Low-density expansile lesion that may become hyperdense if secretions become inspissated.

MAGNETIC RESONANCE IMAGING

- Usually reflect high water content: low signal on T1-weighted images, high signal on T2-weighted images.
- May develop higher proteinaceous content: high signal on T1- and T2-weighted images.
- With time, inspissation and even higher protein content develops and there will be low signal on both T1- and T2-weighted images. Signal loss may be so profound as to simulate a normally aerated sinus.

Osteomyelitis

- Often develops in patients with partially treated sinusitis.
- Maxillary sinus osteomyelitis often secondary to dental disease.
- Frontal sinus osteomyelitis in adults often secondary to trauma or direct spread of frontal sinusitis; in children, it is usually secondary to hematogenous spread.
- Pott's puffy tumor is a subgaleal abscess over the frontal sinus, which may be associated with osteomyelitis.

Imaging PLAIN FILM AND COMPUTED TOMOGRAPHY

- Initially localized osteopenia, with loss of the mucoperiosteal white line.
- Sinus wall thickening, focal destructive changes, sequestrum formation.

Orbital Complications Usually from ethmoid or sphenoid disease.

- Orbital cellulitis.
- Orbital abscess.
- Optic neuritis.
- Superior orbital fissure syndrome, usually from sphenoid sinusitis. May develop orbital pain, ophthalmoplegia, exophthalmos. Cranial nerve (CN) VI usually involved first, followed by CN III, CN IV, and CN V_1.

Intracranial Complications Usually from frontal sinusitis:

- Meningitis

- Epidural and subdural abscess
- Cerebritis
- Cerebral abscess
- Cavernous sinus thrombosis
- Superior sagittal sinus thrombosis
- Rarely, intracranial extension of polyposis

Spread may be secondary to:

- Trauma
- Congenital osseous defects
- Direct invasion through the sinus wall
- Tracking along the olfactory nerves
- Diploic veins with retrograde thrombophlebitis
- Valveless angular and ethmoidal veins to the cavernous sinus

GRANULOMATOUS DISEASE

- A diverse group of entities lead to the formation of granulomatous disease:
  1. Infections—i.e., tuberculosis, syphilis, leprosy, yaws, and so on
  2. Collagen vascular—Wegener's
  3. Lymphoma-related—midline granuloma
  4. Idiopathic—sarcoid
  5. Irritants—cocaine, beryllium
- The nasal fossa tends to be involved first and the diagnosis should be questioned if no nasal septum involvement exists.
- Sinus involvement usually occurs only after septal disease.
- The nasal septum may be thickened or a frank bulky soft tissue mass may be present.
- Focal septal cartilage or bone erosion may occur.
- Osseous structures may become thickened and sclerotic.
- Mild enhancement may be present on evaluation.
- Magnetic resonance imaging may show variable signal characteristics on T2-weighted imaging of mixed areas of fibrosis (low signal) and granulation tissue (high signal).

Wegener's Granulomatosis

- Autoimmune/hypersensitivity reaction.
- Necrotizing vasculitis with granulomatous inflammation.
- Involves paranasal sinuses, lungs, skin, and kidneys.
- Begins as a chronic inflammatory process of the nose and sinuses, usually involving the septum first—saddle nose.
- Males outnumber females 2:1; disease appears in fourth or fifth decade.
- Renal involvement in 90 percent of cases.
- Secondary bacterial infection may develop.
- Some 90 percent respond to cyclophosphamide and steroids during active phases.

Idiopathic Midline Granuloma

- Possibly a lymphoma-related process, a lymphoreticular disorder.
- Chronic necrotizing inflammation of the nose, sinuses, facial tissues, and upper airway—often mutilating in form, with massive osseous destruction.
- Granulomas may or may not be present.
- Primary vasculitis not present (not in lungs or kidneys), in contrast with Wegener's.
- Females outnumber males; disease appears in fifth or sixth decade.
- Radiation therapy is the treatment of choice, with some reported cases of long-term remission.
- Surgery is of questionable value and may actually hasten the process.

Cocaine Nose

- Cocaine-induced granuloma of the nasal septum.
- Similar imaging features to idiopathic midline granuloma.

☐ NEOPLASMS AND MASS LESIONS

- Sinonasal carcinomas are rare and represent less than 1 percent of all malignancies.
- Physician must be aware of potential pathway of tumor extension to help direct therapy.
- Tumor may spread from sinus to sinus, the anterior or middle cranial fossa, orbits, pterygopalatine fossa, or palate.
- Nodal disease is a poor prognostic sign. Retropharyngeal, upper internal jugular, and submandibular nodes are most frequently involved.
- Postcontrast CT and especially MRI T2-weighted scans are indispensable to help differentiate soft tissue neoplasms from accompanying inflammatory disease and obstructed sinus secretions.
- The overwhelming majority of sinonasal tumors are densely cellular and of intermediate signal, while the higher water content of mucosal disease and secretions is high in signal on T2-weighted images.
- Aggressive bony destruction is most indicative of squamous-cell carcinoma as well as metastatic disease, only a few of the aggressive sarcomas, and rarely aggressive fungal disease.
- Mucoceles—along with most sarcomas, polyps, inverting papillomas, lymphoma, and minor salivary gland tumors—tend to remodel bone.

COMMON BENIGN MASS LESIONS

Papillomas Three distinct histologic papillomas unique to the nasal vault exist: inverted, fungiform, and cylindric-cell papillomas.

Inverted Papillomas–47 percent

- Usually appear in adult males.
- Characteristically involve the lateral nasal wall in approximately 90 percent of cases.
- Inverted papillomas may invade into the ethmoid or maxillary sinus and rarely into the sphenoid or frontal sinus.
- Endophytic growth of epithelium into stroma.
- High recurrence rate—approximately 30 percent. Extensive resection must be done.
- Approximately 10 percent associated with malignancy, usually squamous-cell carcinoma.

Fungiform papillomas—50 percent

- Usually appear in adult males.
- Nasal septum—characteristically involved in approximately 95 percent of cases.
- Exophytic growth with verrucous appearance.
- Not premalignant.

Cylindric-Cell Papillomas—3 percent

- Similar characteristics as inverted papilloma.
- Have endophytic and/or exophytic growth.

Imaging Radiographically, all three types of papillomas tend to expand and remodel the nasal fossa.

- Extension into sinuses is common and causes destructive sinusitis.
- The nasal septum is usually intact but bowed to opposite side of mass.
- Small calcifications may be seen within the polypoid mass.

Angiofibroma (Juvenile Nasopharyngeal Angiofibroma)

- Rare, histologically benign, but highly aggressive, highly vascular polypoid mass.
- May present with epistaxis, nasal obstruction, or nasopharyngeal mass.
- Occurs almost exclusively in males.
- Typically appears between 10 and 18 years of age.
- Originates from a fibrovascular stroma on the posterolateral nasal wall near the sphenopalatine foramen.
- Close to 90 percent extend into the pterygopalatine fossa and expand it. Then, it may extend laterally through the pterygomaxillary fissure into the nasopharyngeal masticular space.
- Sphenoid > maxillary > ethmoid extension commonly seen.
- Intracranial extension present in 5 to 20 percent of cases, usually through the inferior and superior orbital fissures, vidian canal, and foramen rotundum into the middle cranial fossa.
- Due to vascularity, biopsy is hazardous and should be done only in an operating room setting and only if diagnosis cannot be established radiographically.

Imaging PLAIN FILM

- Soft tissue nasopharyngeal mass.
- Widening of the pterygopalatine fossa.
- Anterior bowing of the posterior wall of the maxillary sinus.

COMPUTED TOMOGRAPHY

- Dynamic scanning demonstrates marked enhancement.

MAGNETIC RESONANCE IMAGING

- Low to intermediate heterogeneous signal intensity on T1-weighted images and intermediate to high heterogenous signal intensity on T2-weighted images, with flow voids seen corresponding to tumor vascularity (Fig. 4–2*A* and *B*).
- Intense enhancement is seen after contrast injection.

ANGIOGRAPHY

- Internal maxillary and ascending pharyngeal artery are the major feeding vessels.
- May also be supplied from contralateral external carotid branches as well as feeding vessels from the internal carotid artery. Rarely, the vertebral artery may be a source if the tumor is large enough.
- A lobulated, highly vascular mass is seen during the arterial phase and persists into the late venous phase (Fig. 4–2*C*).

Differential Diagnosis

- Antrochoanal polyps
- Embryonal rhabdomyosarcoma

Treatment

- Embolization greatly reduces blood loss during resection.
- Radiation therapy used for intracranial extension.
- Estrogen has variable response in decreasing tumor size and vascularity.

Antrochoanal Polyps

- Most are unilateral, solitary lesions, usually not associated with chronic sinusitis or allergy.
- Comprise only 6 percent of all nasal polyps.
- Arise from mucosa of maxillary sinus and extend through the ostium into the nasal fossa and nasopharynx.
- Occur most commonly in teenagers and young adults.
- May widen the infundibular region and destroy the medial antral wall.

Imaging PLAIN FILM

- Soft tissue opacification of the sinus and nasal fossa, which may extend to the nasopharynx.

COMPUTED TOMOGRAPHY

- Mucoid density of approximately 10 to 18 HU filling the maxillary sinus and ipsilateral nasal fossa with ostial widening.

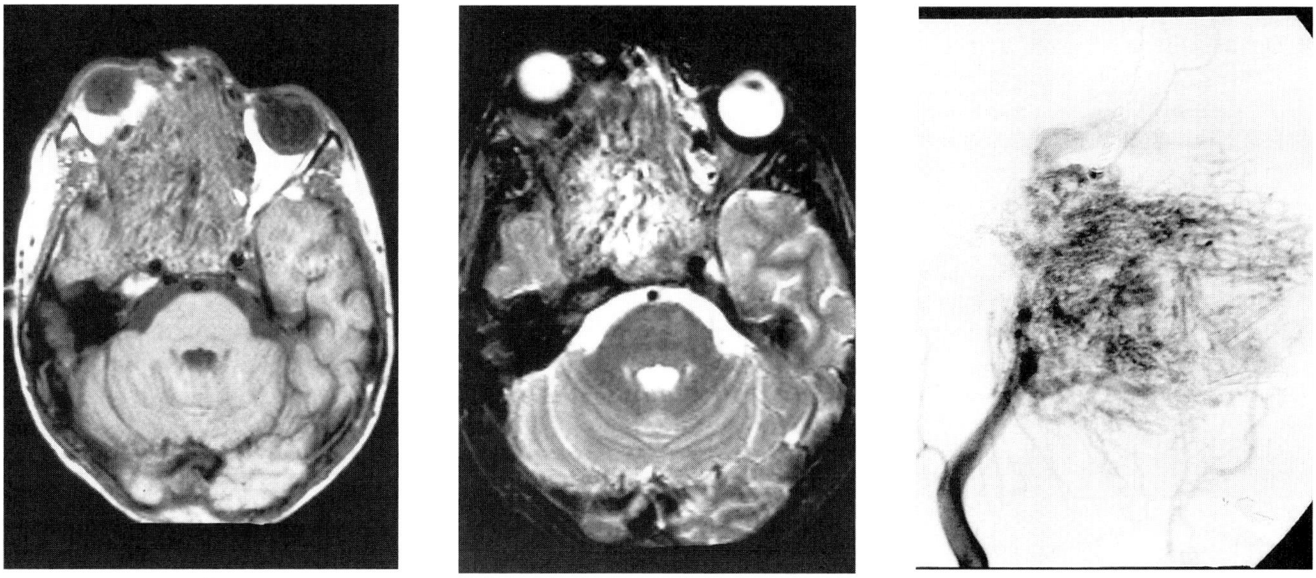

(A) (B) (C)

Figure 4–2 Juvenile angiofibroma. *A.* An axial T1-weighted image demonstrates a heterogeneous low-signal-intensity mass involving the nasal cavity and sphenoid sinus; extension into both orbits and the right cavernous sinus as well as the right temporal fossa seen. Curvilinear areas of signal void and high signal represent tumor vascularity with varying flow velocity. *B.* An axial T2-weighted image reveals a mixed, predominantly high-signal-intensity mass with curvilinear areas of signal void representing tumor vascularity. *C.* An internal maxillary angiogram (*lateral view*) demonstrates extensive tumor vascularity with an early draining vein superiorly.

MAGNETIC RESONANCE IMAGING

- Typically low to intermediate signal on T1-weighted images and high on T2-weighted images, demonstrating their high water content and helping to differentiate them from more worrisome masses such as squamous-cell carcinoma.

Nasal Polyps

- Most common expansile lesions of the nasal cavity.
- Pathogenesis is uncertain but most often associated with allergies. Other associations include infection, vasomotor rhinitis, cystic fibrosis, aspirin intolerance, nickel exposure, and diabetes mellitus.
- Usually multiple and bilateral but may be unilateral and solitary.
- Nasal polyps are generally uncommon in children except with cystic fibrosis.

Imaging PLAIN FILMS

- Unique soft tissue density of the nasal vault, which may be expanded.

COMPUTED TOMOGRAPHY

- Mass of mucoid density (10 to 18 HU).
- An overall mass effect may cause confusion with malignant lesions. Two appearances are, however, suggestive of its benignity: a polypoid mucocele may expand the intercellular septa of the ethmoid complex without osseous destruction. The other finding suggestive of polyposis is a soft tissue density surrounded by mucoid secretions in a curvilinear or looping configuration, which may enhance minimally. This latter finding has also been described with aspergillosis.

MAGNETIC RESONANCE IMAGING

- Typically reflects high water content and low signal on T1-weighted images and high signal on T2-weighted images.
- Signal may become variable from chronicity, leading to desiccation and increasing protein concentration.
- Intracranial extension can rarely occur and often extends with a polypoid contour.

Osteoma

- Dense, compact bone or lamellar bone with intertrabecular fibrous tissue.
- Majority (80 percent) are found in the floor of frontal sinus.
- Osteoma may block the nasofrontal duct, causing mucocele formation.
- Osteoma may erode the posterior wall of the frontal sinus, causing pneumocephalus.

UNCOMMON BENIGN MASS LESIONS

Meningioma

- Less than 1 percent of meningiomas arise as primary lesions outside the central nervous system (CNS).
- Most extra-CNS meningiomas occur in the head and neck, such as bony skull, bony orbit, nose or paranasal sinuses, oral cavity, middle ear, skin of the scalp.
- A mass lesion that remodels bone and has similar imaging features as meningiomas elsewhere.

Schwannoma

- A benign encapsulated nerve sheath tumor.
- Occurs in patients 30 to 60 years of age.
- Female-to-male ratio = 2–4 to 1.
- Sinonasal schwannomas are rare. Most of the cases occur in the nasal fossa, maxillary sinuses, and ethmoid sinuses.
- Bone remodeling with destruction.
- Pathology and imaging features are similar to those of schwannomas elsewhere.
- Malignant schwannoma (rare) is associated with neurofibromatosis in 25 to 50 percent of cases and is the malignant counterpart of neurofibroma.

COMMON MALIGNANT NEOPLASMS

Squamous-Cell Carcinoma *Incidence*

- The most common malignancy of sinonasal origin, accounting for approximately 80 percent of cases.
- Association with nickel, chromium, radium, and mustard gas exposure, radiotherapy, chemotherapy, and rhinoscleroma.
- Some 10 percent of patient with inverted papilloma will have association.

Age and Gender

- Primarily occur in males in sixth and seventh decades.

Location

- Maxillary sinus involved in 80 percent of cases either directly or by invasion.
- Nasal cavity origin in approximately 30 percent of cases.
- Ethmoid origin in approximately 10 percent of cases.
- Approximately 15 percent of cases have nodal metastases.

Imaging PLAIN FILM AND COMPUTED TOMOGRAPHY

- Aggressive osseous destruction by unilateral soft tissue mass with little if any enhancement.

MAGNETIC RESONANCE IMAGING

- Low to intermediate signal typically on T1-weighted images and predominantly intermediate to high signal intensity on T2-weighted images.
- In contrast to the high signal intensity of associated mucosal disease, the neoplasm is of relatively lower signal intensity on T2-weighted images.
- Mild, patchy enhancement is seen.

Differential Diagnosis

- Lymphoma
- Glandular malignancy
- Other malignancy

Treatment

- Radiation therapy and surgery.
- Poor survival rate: around 30 percent with local recurrence common.
- Synchronous or metachronous lesions of head and neck origin as well as a variety of other malignancies are seen in approximately 15 percent of patients.

Glandular Tumors

- Approximately 10 percent of all sinonasal neoplasms.
- Includes minor salivary gland tumors as well as adenocarcinoma.
- Occurs in decreasing frequency—adenoid cystic carcinoma, adenocarcinomas, mucoepidermoid carcinoma, undifferentiated carcinoma.
- Adenoid cystic carcinoma can spread by perineural invasion despite apparent total resection, leading to high local recurrence and poor prognosis.
- Adenocarcinoma associated with hardwood and shoe industry workers. A similarly poor prognosis exists.
- Radiographic appearance similar to squamous-cell carcinoma.

Lymphoma

- Approximately 8 percent of sinonasal malignancies and 80 percent of the sinonasal sarcomas.
- Usually non-Hodgkin's lymphoma of the histiocytic type.
- Nasal fossa and maxillary sinus involved most frequently.
- Tend to be bulky soft tissue masses that expand the nasosinal cavity and only occasionally erode bone.
- Radiosensitive and chemosensitive.

Imaging COMPUTED TOMOGRAPHY

- Moderate enhancement on CT.
- An associated mass in Waldeyer's lymphatic ring or lymphoadenopathy in the neck can suggest the diagnosis.

MAGNETIC RESONANCE IMAGING

- Low to intermediate signal on all MRI sequences.

Esthesioneuroblastoma

- Neural crest origin arising from olfactory epithelium.
- Bimodal peak of second and fifth decades, with reported age range from 3 to 88 years.
- Usually has unilateral involvement of the nasal fossa but often extends into the paranasal sinuses and intracranially via the cribriform plate.
- Cure rates may be high if resection is aggressive, including dura and olfactory bulb, as microscopic tumor invasion is present even in the radiographic absence of invasion or bone remodeling.

Imaging COMPUTED TOMOGRAPHY

- Enhancing, often homogenous mass, which may remodel or erode the bone, including the cribriform plate and sometimes the paranasal sinuses (Fig. 4–3*A*).
- Calcification may occasionally be seen.
- Adjacent bony hyperostosis may be seen.

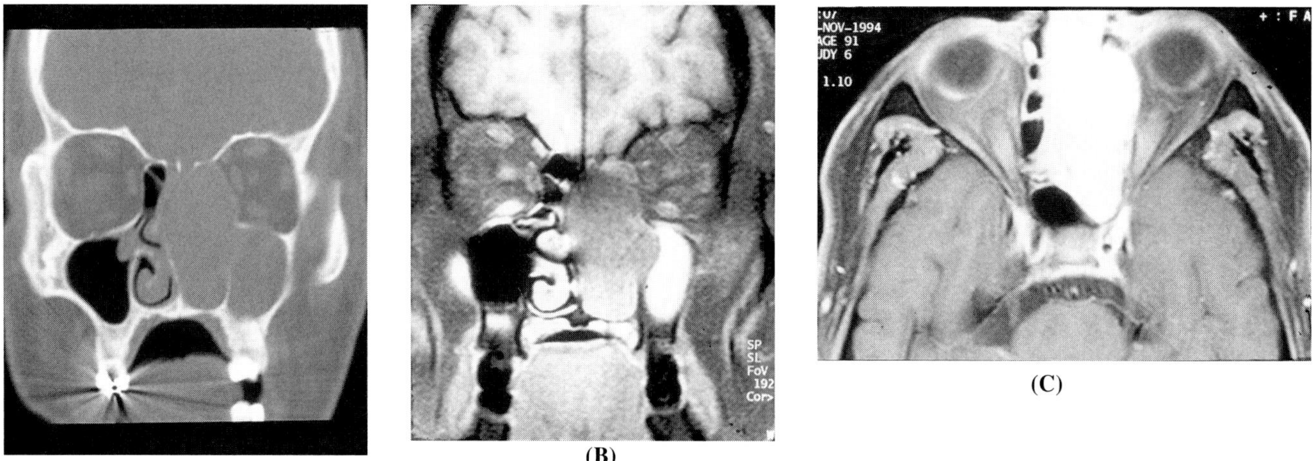

(A) (B) (C)

Figure 4–3 Esthesioneuroblastoma. *A* Coronal CT scan show an expansile mass in the left side of the nasal cavity, with bony erosion. Deviation and remodeling of the nasal septum to the right of the medial left orbital wall and of the medial left maxillary sinus wall to the left is seen with bony erosion. Extension of the soft tissue mass into the left maxillary and left ethmoid sinuses is seen. *B.* A coronal, fat-suppressed, T1-weighted image reveals an intermediate-signal-intensity mass in the left nasal cavity with extension into the left ethmoid and maxillary sinuses. The mucus in the left maxillary sinus shows high signal intensity. *C* Enhanced, fat-suppressed axial T1-weighted images show an intensely enhancing mass. Note the enhancement of normal rectus muscles.

MAGNETIC RESONANCE IMAGING

- Variable MRI appearance, which can be homogenous or heterogenous in nature.
- Generally hypointense on T1-weighted images and isointense to mildly hyperintense on T2-weighted images as compared with gray matter (Fig. 4–3 *B*).
- Tumoral cysts at the margin of the intracranial extent of disease is a rare but suggestive finding for esthesioneuroblastoma.
- Intense enhancement is seen (Fig. 4–3 *C*).
- Differential diagnosis includes lymphoma, squamous-cell carcinoma, adenocarcinoma, melanoma, plasmacytoma, rhabdomyosarcoma, metastasis, Wegener's granulomatosis, cocaine granuloma, and bacterial or fungal sinusitis.

UNCOMMON MALIGNANT NEOPLASMS

Osteosarcoma

- Most frequently seen in maxillary sinus, mandible, and calvarium.
- Osteosarcoma arises from undifferentiated connective tissue of bone, producing osteoid matrix.
- Most maxillary osteosarcomas arise from the alveolar ridge.
- Soft tissue mass with osteoid or chondroid tumor matrix calcification and aggressive bone destruction is seen on CT.

Chondrosarcoma

- Sinonasal chondrosarcoma is rare.
- Chondrosarcomas arise from the wall of the maxillary sinus, at the junction of the nasal septum vomer with the sphenoid and ethmoid sinuses.
- Large, sharply demarcated mass with matrix calcification, bony erosion, and destruction is seen on CT.

Malignant Melanoma.

- Sinonasal melanomas arise from melanocytes that have migrated from the neural crest to the mucosa of the sinuses and nose during embryologic development.
- Most frequently arise from nasal septum.
- Peak age: 60 to 70 years.
- Bone remodeling and erosion may be seen.
- In some cases, melanotic melanomas may have high signal intensity on T1-weighted images.
- Enhancement is seen on both CT and MRI.

Granulocytic Sarcoma (Chloroma)

- A rare malignant tumor composed of immature myeloid elements.
- Granulocytic sarcoma occurs in 3 percent of patients with acute or chronic myeloid leukemia.
- Tumors may be intraosseous or extramedullary in location.
- Computed tomography shows homogenously enhancing mass.
- MRI shows low to intermediate signal intensity on T1-weighted images and high signal intensity on T2-weighted images.

Plasma Cell Dyscrasia

- In the head and neck, soft tissue masses occur in the nose, paranasal sinuses, nasopharynx, and tonsils.
- Lytic lesions involving the bony structure in the head and neck are found in 85 percent of patients.

Extramedullary Plasmacytoma

- A rare soft tissue malignant tumor of plasma cells.
- Some 80 percent of these tumors occur in the head and neck.
- About 3 to 4 percent of all sinonasal tumors.
- The majority of these tumors occur in patients over the age of 40.
- Some 20 percent associated with multiple myeloma.
- Male:female = 4:1.
- On CT, enhancing mass that remodels bone.
- MRI shows low to intermediate signal on T1-weighted image and variable, but predominantly indeterminate signal on T2-weighted images.

Rhabdomyosarcoma

- Represents about 35 to 45 percent of soft tissue tumors in the head and neck.
- Some 78 percent occur in pediatric patients under 12 years of age.
- There are three types of rhabdomyosarcoma:
  1. Embryonal (occur under 10 years of age; 79 percent arise from head and neck or genitourinary tract).
  2. Alveolar (occur between 15 to 25 years of age; 18 percent in head and neck).
  3. Pleomorphic (occur between 40 to 60 years of age; 7 percent in the head and neck).
- The common sites for head and neck rhabdomyosarcomas are:
  Orbit (36 percent)
  Nasopharynx (15.4 percent)
  Middle ear and mastoid (13.8 percent)
  Sinonasal (8.1 percent)
  Face (4.5 percent)
  Neck (4.1 percent)
  Larynx (4.1 percent)

Fibrosarcoma

- About 15 percent of fibrosarcomas occur in the head and neck region.
- Sinonasal cavities are the most common site of head and neck disease, followed by larynx, neck and face.
- Patients' age ranges from 20 to 60 years.
- Pathologically, these tumors may vary from well-differentiated to poorly differentiated (grades I through IV).

Fibrous Histiocytoma

- Most fibrous histiocytomas of soft tissue or osseous origin are malignant.
- Only about 3 percent occur in the head and neck, with the majority in the skin, orbit, and sinonasal cavity.
- Slight male predominance of 3:2.
- Occurs in adult patients.
- On CT, an enhancing mass with bone destruction.
- On MRI, low to intermediate signal intensity on both T1- and T2-weighted images.

Hemangiopericytoma

- Some 15 percent occur in the head and neck.
- In the head and neck region, 55 percent arise from the nose.
- Middle-aged patients.
- Computed tomography shows an expansile mass with bone remodeling and homogenous contrast enhancement.
- Magnetic resonance imaging shows low signal intensity on T1-weighted images and intermediate to high signal intensity on T2-weighted images. Contrast enhancement is seen.

CONGENITAL ABNORMALITIES

Nasal Dermoids

- Abnormal embryonic development with various theories of residual fibrous connection of dura herniating from the foramen cecum to cutaneous elements drawing in dermal tissue—hair, sweat, and sebaceous glands or possibly from failure of degeneration of ectodermally derived elements within the nasal septum. Histologically, may be a dermoid, epidermoid, or simply have a thin epithelial lined dermal sinus with or without a cyst.
- Usually presents at birth or infancy, with male predominance.
- May present as an extra- or intranasal mass, rarely with intracranial extension, usually with a sinus tract that may exit from the glabella to the nasal tip.
- Tuft of hair and discharge from the sinus tract is clinically diagnostic.
- Complete removal is required, as progressive growth or infection can occur.

Imaging

- Both CT and MRI help to determine extent of the mass and sinus tract.
- Fusiform mass of fat density or signal intensity in the nasal septum.
- Broadened nasal septum may be seen with a dermal sinus tract.
- Computed tomography may demonstrate bony canals through the nasal bones, septum, and possibly skull base.
- Enlarged foramen cecum and distorted crista galli are suggestive of intracranial extension; however, this is not specific. Surgical studies propose extracranial excision and craniotomy, performed only if the cephalic portion of dissection contains dermal elements.

Nasal Gliomas

- Rare lesions of neurogenic origin.
- Glioma is a misnomer, as *glial heterotopia in extradural sites* better describes these lesions.
- Various theories exist as to the pathogenesis of nasal gliomas. Faulty closure of the anterior neuropore with

abnormal separation of epithelial tissue precludes proper migration of mesoderm to form bone. Osseous defect may occur, causing an encephalocele lined by leptomeninges and surrounded by cerebrospinal fluid (CSF). These meningocephaloceles may become "pinched off" by constricting dura and bone, becoming benign nonneoplastic heterotopias—nasal gliomas.

- Usually present at birth or infancy with male predominance.
- Some 60 percent are extranasal, 30 percent intranasal, and 10 percent intra-/extranasal location.
- About 15 percent have a fibrous stalk attaching to the dural plate, most commonly with intranasal gliomas (35 percent), suggesting common etiology with encephalocele development.
- No reported cases of aggressive growth or metastasis.

Nasal Encephaloceles

- Extracranial herniation of meninges and brain through a cranial defect, which is always present.
- As with nasal gliomas, several theories exist as to the embryogenesis of nasal encephaloceles, including defects in the closure of the anterior neuropore, as described above, or possibly defects in neural crest/mesodermal migration.
- Anterior encephaloceles are of two varieties: sincipital and the less common basal encephaloceles.
- Sincipital encephaloceles are associated with a visible external mass and are subdivided as to the cranial extent of the defect: nasofrontal, nasoethmoidal, and nasoorbital.
- Basal encephaloceles appear as internal masses forming between the anterior border of the cribriform plate and either the superior orbital fissure or the posterior clinoid fissure. The encephaloceles may extend into the nasal cavity, nasopharynx, or orbit and are subdivided as transethmoidal, sphenoethmoidal, transsphenoidal, and sphenoorbital.
- Suspicion for encephalocele should exist for any child with suspected nasal polyp, nasopharyngeal mass, recurrent meningitis, and possible CSF rhinorrhea.

Imaging

- Axial CT and coronal imaging defines the osseous defect (Fig. 4–4*A*.)
- Better definition of the soft tissue components and dural defect by MRI (Fig. 4–4*B*).

Choanal Atresia or Stenosis

- Secondary to failure of the nasobuccal membrane to perforate normally during early gestation.
- Prominence in females 2:1.
- Unilateral to bilateral 2:1.
- Atresia plates are bony in 90 percent and membranous in 10 percent.
- Associated congenital anomalies in approximately 50 percent, more frequently with bilateral choanal atresia.
- Newborns are obligate nose breathers, mouth breathing being a learned response that takes days to weeks to learn. Unilateral atresia usually causes no acute respiratory distress but does cause unilateral nasal discharge. Bilateral atresia causes nasal obstruction with respiratory distress in the newborn.
- Immediate management is placement of an oral airway.

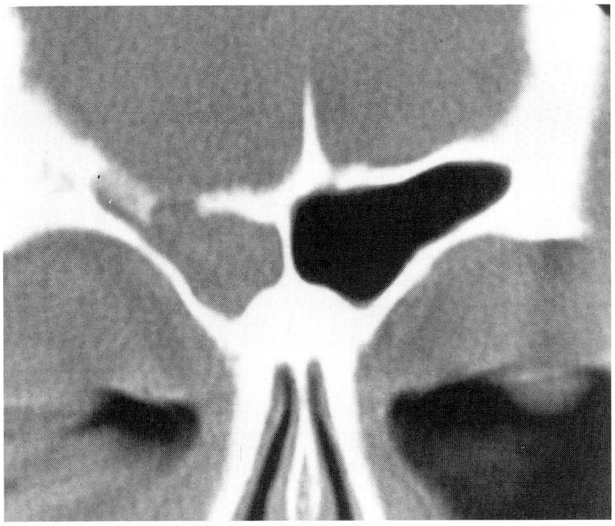

(A)

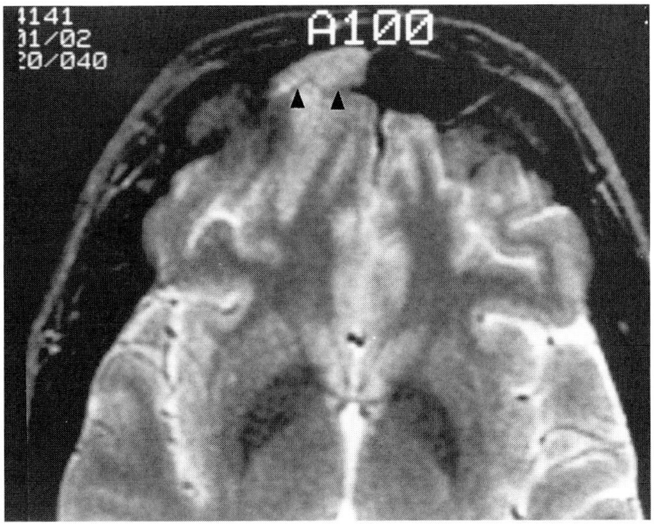

(B)

Figure 4–4 Encephalocele into the frontal sinus. *A.* A coronal CT demonstrates a defect at the superior margin of the frontal sinus and soft tissue density within the frontal sinus on the right side. *B.* An axial T2-weighted image reveals an insointense mass in the right side of the frontal sinus (*arrowheads*).

- Surgical correction is usually through a transpalatal approach, which is preferred over the more precarious transnasal approach. Surgery is usually delayed until the patient is at least 12 months old.

Imaging

- CT scanning (paralleling the posterior hard palate) is the preferred method for diagnosis and surgical planning.
- May see thickening and medial bowing of the lateral wall of the nasal cavity and an enlarged vomer. Bony fusion of these elements may be present versus a soft tissue mass or membrane, with often minimal narrowing of the choana.

SUGGESTED READINGS

1. Ballenger JJ: The nose and accessory sinuses, in Ballenger JJ (ed): *Diseases of the Nose, Throat, Ear, Head and Neck,* 13th ed. Philadelphia, Lea & Febiger, 1985.
2. Batsakis, JG: *Tumors of the Head and Neck, Clinical and Pathological Considerations.* Baltimore, Williams & Wilkins, 1979. pp 177–187.
3. Diament MJ et al: Prevalence of incidental paranasal sinus opacification in pediatric patients: A CT study. *J Comput Assist Tomogr* 11:426–431, 1987.
4. Feldman BA, Feldman DE: The nose and sinuses, in Lee KJ (ed): *Essential Otolaryngology Head and Neck Surgery,* 5th ed. New York, Elsevier, 1991.
5. Harner S: The anatomy of congenital atresia. *Otolaryngol Head Neck Surg* 89:7–9, 1981.
6. Hengerer AS, Newburg JA: Congenital malformations of the nose and paranasal sinuses, in Bluestone CD et al (eds): *Pediatric Otolaryngology,* 2nd ed. Philadelphia, Saunders, 1990.
7. Hyams VJ: Papillomas of the nasal cavity and paranasal sinuses: A clinicopathologic study of 315 cases. *Ann Otol Rhinol Laryngol* 80:192, 1971.
8. Lloyd GA et al: Magnetic resonance imaging in evaluation of nose and paranasal sinus disease. *Br J Radiol* 60:957–968, 1987.
9. Lund VJ, Lloyd GAS: Radiological changes associated with inverted papilloma of the nose and paranasal sinuses. *Br J Radiol* 57:455–461, 1984.
10. Pashley NRT: Congenital anomalies of the nose, in Cummings CW et al (eds): *Otolaryngology Head and Neck Surgery.* St Louis, Mosby, 1986.
11. Schatz CJ, Becker TS: Normal CT anatomy of the paranasal sinuses. *Radiol Clin North Am* 22:107–118, 1984.
12. Schuster JJ et al: MR of esthesioneuroblastoma and appearance after craniofacial resection. *AJNR* 15:1169–1177, 1994.
13. Silver AJ et al: The opacified maxillary sinus: CT findings in chronic sinusitis and malignant tumor. *Radiology* 163:205–210, 1987.
14. Slovis TL et al: Choanal atresia: Precise CT evaluation. *Radiology* 155:345–348, 1985.
15. Som PM: Sinonasal cavity, in Som PM, Bergeron RT (eds): *Head and Neck Imaging,* 2d ed. St Louis, Mosby-Year Book, 1991.
16. Som PM et al. Chronically obstructed sinonasal secretions: Observations on T1 and T2 shortening. *Radiology* 172:515–520, 1989.
17. Som PM et al: Benign and malignant sinonasal lesions with intracranial extension: Differentiation with MR imaging. *Radiology* 172:763–766, 1989.
18. Som PM et al: CT appearance distinguishing benign nasal polyps from malignancies. *J Comput Assist Tomogr* 11:129–133, 1987.
19. Som PM et al: Sinonasal tumors and inflammatory tissues: Differentiation with MR imaging. *Radiology* 167:803–808, 1988.
20. Som PM, et al: Sinonasal esthesioneuroblastoma with intracranial extension: Marginal tumor cysts as a diagnostic MR finding. *AJNR* 15:1259–1262, 1994.
21. Tassel PV et al: Mucoceles of the paranasal sinuses: MR imaging with CT correlation. *AJNR* 10:607–612, 1989.
22. Towbin R, Dunbar JS: The paranasal sinuses in childhood. *Radiographics* 2:253–279, 1982.
23. Zinreich SJ et al: Fungal sinusitis: Diagnosis with CT and MR imaging. *Radiology* 169:439–444, 1988.
24. Harnsberger HR: Handbook of Head and Neck Imaging, 2nd ed. St. Louis, Mosby, 1995.

☐ QUESTIONS (True or False)

1. Regarding normal anatomy of the nose,
  - **a.** The inferior meatus drains the nasolacrimal duct.
  - **b.** The anterior ethmoid air cells drain into the anterior aspect of the hiatus semilunaris.
  - **c.** The majority of middle ethmoid air cells empty through the ethmoid bulla into the middle meatus.
  - **d.** The superior meatus drains the sphenoid sinus.
  - **e.** The frontal sinuses are absent at birth.

2. Regarding fungal sinusitis,
  - **a.** It most commonly involves the maxillary and ethmoid sinuses.
  - **b.** It commonly occurs in nonimmunocompromised patients.
  - **c.** Air-fluid level is common.
  - **d.** May be confused with aggressive malignant lesions.
  - **e.** Mycetomas show marked hypointensity on T2-weighted images.

3. Mucoceles
   a. Develop as a result of obstruction of a sinus ostium.
   b. Are the most common cause of expansile lesions of any paranasal sinuses.
   c. Most commonly found in the frontal sinus.
   d. Signal intensity on MRI is variable.
   e. Calcification is commonly seen.

4. Wegener's granulomatosis
   a. Involves paranasal sinuses only.
   b. In saddle nose is due to involvement of the nasal septum.
   c. Is more commonly seen in males.
   d. Is best treated surgically.
   e. Causes necrotizing vasculitis with granulomatous inflammation.

5. Juvenile nasopharyngeal angiofibroma
   a. Occurs almost exclusively in males.
   b. Originates from a fibrovascular stroma on the posterolateral nasal wall near sphenopalatine foramen.
   c. Does not involve the pterygopalatine fossa.
   d. Seen with intracranial extension, usually involves extreme bony destruction.
   e. Is a highly vascular mass with stain persisting into venous phase.

6. Squamous cell carcinoma
   a. Is the most common malignancy of sinonasal origin.
   b. Is associated with inverted papilloma.
   c. Occurs in males in the sixth and seventh decades.
   d. Commonly involves the maxillary sinus.
   e. Shows high signal intensity lesion on T2-weighted MRI, similar to mucosal disease.

7. Esthesioneuroblastoma
   a. Is seen exclusively in adults.
   b. Usually has unilateral involvement of the nasal fossa.
   c. Occasionally contains calcification.
   d. Is never seen with adjacent bony hyperostosis.
   e. Differential diagnosis include lymphoma, squamous cell carcinoma, adenocarcinoma, melanoma, and plasmacytoma.

8. Nasal dermoids
   a. Usually present at birth or in infancy.
   b. Show male predominance.
   c. Commonly develop intracranial extension.
   d. Cause discharge from sinus tract.
   e. Are a fusiform mass with fat in the nasal septum.

☐ ANSWERS

1. a. T
   b. T
   c. T
   d. F
   e. T

2. a. T
   b. F
   c. F
   d. T
   e. T

3. a. T
   b. T
   c. T
   d. T
   e. F

4. a. F
   b. T
   c. T
   d. F
   e. T

5. a. T
   b. T
   c. F
   d. F
   e. T

6. a. T
   b. T
   c. T
   d. T
   e. F

7. a. F
   b. T
   c. T
   d. F
   e. T

8. a. T
   b. T
   c. F
   d. T
   e. T

CHAPTER

5

Nasopharynx, Oropharynx, Oral Cavity, Larynx, and Hypopharynx

Dale Sue

Imaging of the pharynx, oral cavity, larynx and hypopharynx may seem both complex and intimidating even to an experienced neuroradiologist. The following chapter provides a review and study guide in the anatomy and pathology of the nasopharynx, oropharynx, oral cavity, and larynx. Although the chapter is not totally comprehensive, this information should make imaging and differential diagnosis of these areas less intimidating for the radiologist/neuroradiologist.

☐ NORMAL ANATOMY

TRADITIONAL CLASSIFICATION

Nasopharynx The nasopharynx is lined by squamous epithelium mucosa and occupies the most superior extent of the aerodigestive tract. It is bounded superiorly by the sphenoid sinus and upper clivus, posteriorly by the lower clivus and upper cervical spine, anteriorly by the posterior nasal margin, and laterally by the medial pterygoid plates, muscle, and deep tissues surrounding the airway. The inferior boundary of the nasopharynx is the soft palate, which acts as a division between the nasopharynx and the oropharynx. Although the nasopharynx is a relatively small area of the extracranial head and neck, vital neurovascular structures at the skull base are in close proximity to the nasopharynx, including the jugular fossa, foramen ovale, carotid canal, sella turcica, and cavernous sinus. Other important nonneurovascular structures in close proximity include the torus tubarius and opening of the eustachian tube.

Oropharynx The oropharynx predominantly contains muscle, lymphoid tissue, and fat. As mentioned above, the oropharynx is demarcated from the nasopharynx above by the soft palate. It is delineated from the oral cavity by the circumvallate papillae of the tongue and includes the posterior one-third of the tongue or tongue base, the palatine tonsils, the soft palate, and the oropharyngeal mucosa and constrictor muscles. The oropharynx extends inferiorly from the level of the soft palate to the top of the epiglottis.

Oral Cavity As in the oropharynx, the oral cavity predominantly contains muscle, lymphoid tissue, and fat. The oral cavity consists of the anterior two-thirds of the tongue, floor of the mouth, buccal mucosa, mandible, and maxilla. It is demarcated from the oropharynx posteriorly by the circumvallate papillae of the tongue.

Larynx Detailed anatomy of the larynx is beyond the scope of this review chapter. A comprehensive account of laryngeal anatomy can be found in a chapter written by Hugh D. Curtin in *Head and Neck Imaging* (see "Suggested Readings").

The skeleton of the larynx is composed of cartilage and fibrous bands. The main cartilaginous structures of the larynx include the cricoid, thyroid, arytenoid, and epiglottic cartilage. The cricoid cartilage is the foundation of the larynx and has a "signet" shape with the larger signet portion posteriorly called the quadrate laminae. Perched upon the upper margin of the quadrate laminae are the two paired arytenoid cartilages. The pyramid-shaped arytenoid cartilages are important surgical and radiologic landmarks. The arytenoid has a muscular process projecting laterally and a vocal process projecting anteriorly, which serves as a point of attachment for the posterior vocal cord. Both the cricoid and thyroid cartilages act as a protective shield for the inner larynx.

The epiglottic cartilage is held in place by the hyoepiglottic and thyroepiglottic ligaments. Most of the epiglottis resides behind the anterior aspect of the thyroid cartilage, with only a small portion extending above the hyoid bone. The larynx is suspended from the hyoid bone via the posterior thyrohyoid ligament and thyrohyoid membrane.

The mucosal surface of the larynx has important landmarks, especially to the otolaryngologist, including the epiglottis, false and true cords, aryepiglottic folds, and pyriform sinuses. The paraglottic and preepiglottic spaces, which lie between the mucosal surface and the cartilaginous skeleton, contain loose areolar tissue, muscular structures, and lymphatics.

Branches of the vagus nerve innervate the larynx. The intrinsic muscles of the larynx are innervated by the recurrent laryngeal nerve. The course of the recurrent laryngeal nerves should be noted, since the right and left sides follow different paths and any pathology along the course of these nerves can cause a paralysis of the intrinsic muscles. The left recurrent laryngeal nerve loops around the aorta on the left side from the anterior to the posterior direction and then ascends in the tracheoesophageal groove at the lateral margin of the esophagus. The right recurrent laryngeal nerve loops around the subclavian artery from the anterior to the posterior direction and then ascends in the tracheoesophageal groove also at the lateral margin of the esophagus. The cricothyroid muscle, which is the sole extrinsic laryngeal muscle, is innervated by the external branch of the superior laryngeal nerve. The internal branch of the superior laryngeal nerve supplies sensation to the inner laryngeal mucosa.

Blood supply roughly follows the course of the nerves. The superior and inferior laryngeal arteries supply the larynx. The inferior laryngeal artery, which is a branch of the thyrocervical trunk, courses with the recurrent laryngeal nerve into the larynx. The superior laryngeal artery, which is a branch of the superior thyroid artery of the external carotid system, follows the internal branch of the superior laryngeal nerve.

The lymphatic drainage for the larynx is different for the upper and lower mucosal surfaces. The supraglottic larynx drains into upper jugular nodes. The preepiglottic and paraepiglottic spaces are rich in lymphatics. Lymphatic drainage from the true cord is sparse. The subglottic larynx drains into the pretracheal and paratracheal lymph nodes and eventually into the lower jugular nodes. The Delphian node is located immediately anterior to the cricothyroid membrane and receives lymphatic drainage from the region of the anterior commissure and subglottic larynx. The deep larynx, which excludes the mucosal surfaces, drains only superiorly into the upper jugular nodes.

Anatomic regions are important in discussing pathology of the larynx, since most surgery is described in reference to these terms. The supraglottic region on the larynx extends from the level of the laryngeal ventricle superiorly to the free edge of the epiglottis and aryepiglottic folds. The subglottic region extends from the lower margin of the glottic region down to the lower margin of the cricoid cartilage. The glottic region is defined as an area that begins from an imaginary horizontal plane, which divides the laryngeal ventricle into upper and lower halves down to 1 cm below the apex of the ventricle.

Hypopharynx The hypopharynx is below the oropharynx and above the larynx. The hypopharynx is a caudal continuation of the pharyngeal mucosal space extending from nasopharynx and oropharynx. It consists of pyriform sinus, postcricoid area, and posterior hypopharyngeal wall.

The anteromedial margin of the pyriform sinus is the posterolateral wall of the aryepiglottic fold. The lateral wall of the pyriform sinus is adjacent to the posterior thyroid cartilage ala. The posterior wall of the pyriform sinus is the lateral aspect of the posterior hypopharyngeal wall. The postcricoid area is the anterior wall of the lower pharynx, which extends from the level of arytenoid cartilages to the inferior border of cricoid cartilage. The posterior pharyngeal wall extends from the level of valleculae to the level of the cricoarytenoid joint.

SPACE-ORIENTED CLASSIFICATION

The fascial layers of the neck consist of the superficial and deep cervical fascia. The superficial cervical fascia contain blood vessels, lymphatics, hair follicles, and cutaneous nerves. With cross-sectional imaging, structures that are routinely identified include the platysmas and the anterior and external jugular veins. The deep cervical fascia consists of three layers (superficial or investing, middle, and deep or prevertebral layers); these are both important and convenient because they cleave the neck into functional spaces, which can help the radiologist in localizing and forming a differential diagnosis of a lesion based on its space of origin. The neck can be further subdivided into suprahyoid and infrahyoid areas. The suprahyoid area includes the deep spaces between the skull base and hyoid bone and the infrahyoid area extends inferiorly from the hyoid bone to the clavicles.

Strictly Suprahyoid Spaces A lesion in the suprahyoid region can be assigned to a space of origin by determining the central point of the lesion and evaluating its effect on or displacement of the parapharyngeal space fat, since this space is surrounded by the pharyngeal mucosal, masticator, parotid, and carotid spaces.

Parapharyngeal Space This is a centrally located space of the deep face which is filled predominantly with fat and extends from the skull base to the hyoid bone. This space also contains branches of cranial nerve (CN) V, and the pterygoid venous plexus. As mentioned above, most lesions will be localized in relation to their effect upon the parapharyngeal space. A lesion localized within the parapharyngeal space fat must be surrounded totally by fat.

Pharyngeal Mucosal Space This space is located medial to the parapharyngeal space and thus displaces the parapharyngeal space laterally. The pharyngeal mucosal space contains mucosa, lymphoid tissues of Waldeyer's ring, the eustachian tube, the superior and middle constrictor muscles, the levator palatine muscles, the pharyngobasilar fascia, and minor salivary glands.

Masticator Space The masticator space lies anterior to the parapharyngeal space; thus a lesion would displace the parapharyngeal space fat posteriorly. The masticator space has a suprazygomatic component. The masticator space extends from the suprazygomatic component inferiorly to the inferior margin of the mandible. Structures within this space include the muscles of mastication, masticator and inferior alveolar nerves, inferior alveolar artery and vein, and the ramus and posterior body of the mandible. A malignancy within this space can spread perineurally along the third division of CN V intracranially into the middle cranial fossa.

Parotid Space The parotid space is lateral to the parapharyngeal space; thus the lesion within the parotid space displaces the parapharyngeal space medially. This space contains the parotid gland, intraparotid facial nerve, retromandibular vein, external carotid artery, and lymph nodes. A large mass in this space usually widens the stylomandibular notch. Analogous to the masticator space, a malignancy may spread perineurally via CN VII into the temporal bone. A more detailed discussion of the parotid space can be found in Chapter 6.

Submandibular Space The submandibular space is inferolateral to the mylohyoid muscle and superior to the hyoid bone. This space contains the anterior belly of the digastric muscle, superficial portion of the submandibular gland, submandibular and submental lymph nodes, facial artery and vein, inferior loop of CN XII, and fat. There is no fascial boundary between the submandibular space and the parapharyngeal space above; thus a large parapharyngeal space lesion may present as a submandibular space mass.

Sublingual Space The sublingual space is superomedial to the mylohyoid muscle. No fascia separates the posterior sublingual space from the submandibular space; thus lesions may spread posteriorly into the submandibular space. The contents of the sublingual space include the anterior aspect of the hypoglossal muscle, lingual nerve, CN IX and XII, lingual artery and vein, sublingual glands and ducts, deep portion of the submandibular gland, and submandibular gland duct (Warton's duct).

Strictly Infrahyoid Spaces ***Visceral Space*** The major structures within the visceral space include the hypopharynx, larynx, thyroid and parathyroid glands, trachea, esophagus, periesophageal lymph nodes, and recurrent laryngeal nerves within the tracheoesophageal grooves. Thyroid gland disease predominates within this space.

Spaces Common to Both Suprahyoid and Infrahyoid Neck ***Carotid Space*** The carotid space is posterior to the parapharyngeal space; thus a lesion in this space would displace the parapharyngeal space fat anteriorly. All three layers of the deep cervical fascia contribute to the carotid sheath, which defines this space. The carotid space extends from the base of the skull to the aortic arch. The structures within the suprahyoid compartment include the internal carotid artery, jugular vein, CN IX through XII, and deep cervical lymph nodes. Structures within the infrahyoid carotid space include the common or internal carotid arteries, internal jugular vein, and vagus nerve. The sympathetic plexus is embedded within the medial wall of the carotid sheath. Common diseases within the carotid space involve the neural vascular structures (carotid body paragangliomas, neurogenic tumors, thrombophlebitis) mentioned above; nodal disease is also common.

Retropharyngeal and Danger Spaces Pathologic processes within these spaces cannot be differentiated from each other with imaging. The retropharyngeal space extends from the skull base to approximately the T3 level. The danger space extends from the skull base down to the level of the diaphragm and thus represents a pathway by which retropharyngeal disease may spread into the posterior mediastinum. Danger space is situated between the retropharyngeal space and prevertebral space between two leaves of the deep layer of deep cervical fascia. A retropharyngeal space abnormality can be differentiated from a prevertebral space abnormality by noting its relationship to the prevertebral muscles. A retropharyngeal space lesion would displace the prevertebral muscle posteriorly, while a prevertebral space lesion would displace the muscles anteriorly. Common diseases involving the retropharyngeal and danger spaces include infection, hematomas, lipomas, extranodal metastasis, edema from the jugular vein, and lymphatic obstruction.

Prevertebral Space The prevertebral space contains prevertebral, paraspinal, and scalene muscles along with the vertebral body, spinal cord, and vertebral artery and vein. A lesion within the prevertebral space would displace the prevertebral muscles anteriorly.

Anterior Cervical Space The anterior cervical space contains primarily fat. It is deep to the sternocleidomastoid muscle and superficial to the visceral and carotid spaces. Isolated disease of this space includes lipomas and second branchial cleft cysts.

Posterior Cervical Space The posterior cervical space also contains primarily fat. In addition, it contains the spinal accessory lymph node chain and thus is commonly involved by both inflammatory and malignant nodal disease. Other abnormalities within this space include cystic hygromas/lymphangiomas, lipomas, liposarcomas, and third branchial cleft cysts.

☐ IMAGING

MAGNETIC RESONANCE IMAGING VERSUS COMPUTED TOMOGRAPHY

Nasopharynx and Oropharynx Most authorities agree that magnetic resonance imaging (MRI) is the imaging study of choice for evaluating the nasopharynx and oropharynx because of its superior soft tissue resolution and multiplanar capabilities. A cooperative patient is required, since any motion—including swallowing, talking, and snoring—will degrade images. Imaging of the naso- and oropharynx are performed with routine head coils. Imaging of the neck requires an anterior and/or posterior neck coil. Computed tomography scanning is complementary to MRI in evaluating the bony structures of the skull base and face.

Imaging of the oral cavity tends to be more sensitive to patient-induced motion artifact. Therefore, CT is the preferred modality for the examination of the oral cavity.

Larynx CT is used more commonly than MRI in the imaging evaluation of the larynx. More so than in the oral cavity, MRI is limited secondary to patient-induced motion artifact. Motion artifact tends to be less of a problem with low- or midfield-strength units. However, MRI still has some potential advantages over CT because of its multiplanar capabilities and high-resolution imaging. Once again, a highly cooperative patient is required, along with a surface or anterior neck coil. The appearance of the laryngeal skeleton is variable with both CT and MRI, depending upon the amount of ossification/mineralization.

☐ PATHOLOGY OF THE NASOPHARYNX

BENIGN MUCOSAL LESIONS

Thornwaldt's Cyst This entity is related to the normal transient descent of the notochord into the nasopharynx. When the notochord ascends back into the skull, a small portion of the developing nasopharyngeal mucosa may follow and create a midline track or pit. This is usually located between the longus capitis muscles and may close over and result in a midline cyst, which can become infected.

- It is usually hyperintense in signal on both the T1- and T2-weighted images.
- On CT, it is isodense relative to surrounding muscle and adenoidal tissue.
- An infected cyst can potentially lead to a retropharyngeal abscess.

Adenoidal Hypertrophy Usually seen in children and young adults. It is not invasive, occupying the mucosal side of the nasopharynx, and is usually homogenous and isodense to the surrounding musculature.

Teratoma
- These congenital three-germ-layer tumors usually occur in the midline or lateral wall of the nasopharynx.
- There is a female predominance.
- A midline mass containing both fat and calcifications is diagnostic.
- Appearance on CT is variable, depending on the contents of the teratoma.

INFLAMMATORY LESIONS

Masticator Space Infections
- Usually caused by uncontrolled dental infection leading to osteomyelitis of the mandible.
- Thus common causes include actinomycosis of the mandible, hemotogenous osteomyelitis of the mandible, and inferior extension of the malignant otitis externa.
- Differentiated from tumors within the masticator space by the presence of adjacent soft tissue cellulitis and clinical history.

Mucosal Infections Usually a result or extension of infections from surrounding areas (i.e., adenoidal or tonsillar infection in children).

Malignant Otitis Externa
- Usually occurs in elderly diabetic patients with opportunistic infection (usually *pseudomonas aeruginosa*) of the external auditory canals.
- Can rapidly lead to osteomyelitis of the temporal bone and skull base.
- Ominous clinical findings include a jugular foramen syndrome and facial palsy.
- On MRI, contrast enhancement of the surrounding musculature and periosteum.

Retropharyngeal Abscess Secondary to tonsillar infection in children and perforation of the posterior pharyngeal wall or retropharyngeal adenitis in adults. An area of hypodensity on CT and hyperintense signal intensity on T2-weighted images with MRI anterior to the prevertebral muscles. On MRI, contrast may differentiate between frank abscess and cellulitis, with different enhancing patterns.

Parapharyngeal Space Abscess Usually a result of tonsillar infection or perforation of the pharynx and may extend into the submandibular space. With cross-sectional imaging, the adjacent airway is displaced medially and the medial pterygoid muscle laterally. If undrained, a mycotic aneurysm can develop rapidly, within days.

NEOPLASTIC LESIONS

Mucosal Space Masses ***Squamous-Cell Carcinoma***

- Male:female = 2:1.
- Represent 80 percent of all superficial epithelial carcinomas of the nasopharynx.
- More prevalent in Asian countries, especially in southern provinces of China.
- Tobacco and alcohol abuse is not strongly associated.
- Genetic factors as well as the Epstein-Barr virus are associated with nasopharyngeal carcinoma.
- The lateral pharyngeal recess is the most common site of origin.
- Unilateral middle ear fluid accumulation should raise suspicion for nasopharyngeal carcinoma.
- On MRI, a mass lesion that is hypointense on T1-weighted images and hyperintense on T2-weighted images. Intense, inhomogenous contrast enhancement is seen.
- The presence of lower cervical adenopathy decreases survival dramatically.
- In posttherapy imaging, MRI may be useful, since this modality can potentially distinguish between the post-radiation changes of mucosal fibrosis (hypointense on both T1- and T2-weighted images) and recurrent or residual tumor.
- Treatment usually consists of radiation therapy unless adenopathy is present, for which neck dissection is performed.

Lymphoma

- Usually non-Hodgkin's type.
- Indistinguishable from squamous cell carcinoma but tends to be more bulky.
- Treatment consists of radiation therapy and chemotherapy.

Rhabdomyosarcoma

- Seen primarily in young children below 6 years of age.
- The most frequent sites in the head and neck include the orbit and nasopharynx, followed by the paranasal sinuses and middle ear.
- Skull base invasion along with cavernous sinus syndrome are common.
- May also appear similar to squamous cell carcinoma, but may not involve the mucosal space, since it arises from muscle.

Minor Salivary Gland Carcinoma Rare. Appearance similar to squamous cell carcinoma. Perineural spread is common, especially with adenoid cystic carcinoma.

Carotid Space Masses ***Paraganglioma***

- Benign tumors that arise from the APUD cells (amine precursor uptake and decarboxylation cells), which produce bioactive amines such as norepinephrine, epinephrine, and serotonin.
- Female:male = 3:1.
- The majority of the patients are in their fourth and fifth decades.
- Commonly seen in the carotid bifurcation, jugular bulb, middle ear, and nodose ganglion of vagus nerve (Table 5-1).
- Multiple in 3 to 5 percent of patients and familial in 20 to 30 percent.
- The patient may present with pulsatile tinnitus, neck mass with bruit, jugular fossa syndrome, or hearing loss.
- Enhances intensely on CT and may cause bony erosion, which is irregular and permeative.
- On MRI, larger paragangliomas may demonstrate intermediate signal on T1-weighted images and heterogenous high signal on T2-weighted images ("salt and pepper"), reflecting slow flow (or hemorrhage) and flow voids.
- There is also intense contrast enhancement with MRI.

Table 5-1
FOUR TYPES OF PARAGANGLIOMAS

Name	Location	Origin	Clinical Symptoms
Glomus tympanum	Cochlear promontory (middle ear)	Jacobsen's nerve	Hearing loss, pulsatile tinnitus
Glomus jugulare	Jugular foramen	Jugular ganglion	Various neuropathy of cranial nerves IX through XII. Pulsatile tinnitus, hearing loss
Glomus vagale	Carotid space below skull base and above bifurcation	Nodose ganglion of the vagus nerve	Neck mass with bruits, cranial neuropathy
Carotid body tumor	Carotid bifurcation	Carotid body	Neck mass with bruits

Modified from Table 5-2, "Types of Paraganglioma," in HR Harnsberger: *Handbook of Head and Neck Imaging,* 2d ed. Mosby, 1995.

- The differential diagnosis of a pulsatile intratympanic mass includes tympanic tumor, glomus jugulare tumor, aberrant carotid artery, and exposed jugular bulb.

Schwannoma
- Benign encapsulated tumor that has both a cellular and mixed component (Antoni A or B cells), which differentiate schwannomas from neurofibromas.
- Occur in the third through sixth decades of life and may present as either a painless neck mass or with pain and cranial neuropathy related to the nerves within the jugular foramen.
- Nerve sheath tumor masses can be seen within the parapharyngeal space, masticator space, or carotid space.
- As opposed to the more invasive jugular paraganglioma, its slow growth may cause smooth, bony expansion and erosion.
- Contrast enhancement is seen on both CT and MRI images.
- A well-defined homogenous signal mass is seen, which becomes progressively hyperintense with more T2 weighting.
- Occasionally, a vascular schwannoma may not be differentiated from paraganglioma on imaging studies.
- Treatment is surgical excision.

Neurofibroma
- Benign, nonencapsulated, but well-circumscribed tumors of the peripheral nerves.
- Solitary neurofibromas are found in patients between 20 and 30 years of age.
- Nine percent of patients have von Recklinghausen's disease.
- Usually presents as a solitary subcutaneous mass but may expand a larger nerve in a fusiform fashion.
- Neurofibromas may enhance on CT or MRI.
- Characteristically, a central, hypointense-signal, fibrous core surrounded by hyperintense areas may be seen on T2-weighted MRI.
- Neurofibromas rarely show cystic or necrotic changes, which could be seen in schwannomas.

Meningioma
- Usually originates from the jugular fossa and may extend caudally to involve the carotid space.
- Enhances intensely on both CT and MRI; may be frankly calcified and slightly hyperdense on unenhanced CT.
- On MRI, the typical signal characteristics of a meningioma are similar to those intracranially, with a meningioma paralleling the signal of gray matter.
- Because of the absence of hyperintense signal on T2-weighted images, a meningioma can be differentiated from a schwannoma, with the latter demonstrating hyperintense signal with more T2 weighting.

Parapharyngeal Space Masses ***Lipomas*** Usually asymptomatic and incidental; display imaging characteristics of fat on CT and MRI. Lipomas may extend out of the carotid or retropharyngeal space.

Minor Salivary Gland Tumors Minor salivary gland tumors arise from ectopic cell rests. Although 50 percent are benign mixed-cell tumors, neither CT nor MRI can differentiate between benign and malignant types of salivary gland tumors or other malignancies.

Masticator Space Masses As mentioned previously, the parapharyngeal space is displaced posteromedially. Both primary and metastatic tumors may involve the masticator space. The most common metastatic neoplasms within this space include lung, kidney, and breast carcinomas. Extension of dental lesions from the mandible, such as dentigerous cysts or ameloblastoma, may also involve the masticator space. Involvement of the skull base and cavernous sinus can be seen from masticator space neoplasms via perineural spread along the mandibular nerve of the third division of the fifth cranial nerve. Differential from infectious diseases can be made by clinical history and absence of intense cellulitis and gas formation.

☐ PATHOLOGY OF THE OROPHARYNX AND ORAL CAVITY

INFLAMMATORY LESIONS

Infections of the Teeth, Mandible, Salivary Glands, and Tonsils These are responsible for most inflammatory disease of the oral cavity. Dental infections may potentially lead to deep soft tissue infections and subsequent involvement of the maxillary sinus, mandible, and masticator space. Submandibular gland infection and abscess are usually caused by a calculus obstructing the submandibular duct.

Ludwig's Angina
- An eponym assigned to an infectious process where there is extensive involvement of the floor of the mouth.
- Usually originates from a dental or salivary gland infection and can lead to mediastinal involvement if untreated.
- Streptococcal or staphylococcal bacteria are the common offenders.
- Associated with a clinical syndrome, which includes submandibular and intraoral cellulitis, trismus, and airway obstruction.

Tonsillar Abscess
- *Beta-hemolytic streptococcus, Staphylococcus, Pneumococcus*, and *Hemophilus* are the common offenders.
- Occurs usually in adolescents or young adults and is usually self-limited. However, it can potentially lead to peritonsillar or tonsillar abscesses.

- Appearance on cross-sectional imaging may simulate tumor.

Ranula

- A ranula is a postinflammatory retention cyst of the sublingual glands or minor salivary glands of the sublingual space.
- There is usually pain and swelling of the sublingual space.
- If the ranula is confined to the sublingual space, it is a simple ranula.
- If the ranula ruptures and extends poteriorly into the submandibular space, it is called a diving ranula. The diving ranula is actually a pseudocyst and has no epithelial lining. With imaging, there is a characteristic "tail sign" within the sublingual space, with the bulk of the pseudocyst seen within the submandibular space.
- The differential diagnosis includes cystic hygroma and epidermoid.

BENIGN LESIONS

Thyroglossal Duct Anomalies ***Thyroglossal Duct Cyst***

- Midline neck mass anterior to and at the level of hyoid bone.
- Bimodal presentation: first peak, before the age of 10 years; second peak, between 20 and 30 years.
- During embryogenesis the anlage of the thyroid and parathyroid glands descends from the foramen at the cecum base of the tongue to the anterior visceral space of the infrahyoid neck. A tract of epithelial tissue (thyroglossal duct) is left along the pathway, and this may give rise to a thyroglossal duct cyst.
- Pathologically, the thyroglossal duct cyst is made up of squamous-cell mucosa.
- On CT or MRI, a characteristic midline or paramedian cystic mass is seen at the level of hyoid bone (Fig. 5-1).

Lingual Thyroid Embryologic failure of thyroidal tissue to descend from the foramen cecum of the tongue. The most common site is the dorsal posterior third of the tongue. Usually an asymptomatic reddish mass and more prevalent in women. Usually enhances with iodinated contrast on CT, as does normal thyroid tissue in the neck.

Hemangioma

- Usually presents as a reddish mass at the base of the tongue but may also involve the face.
- It is the most common cervical mass in children.
- The cavernous type is the most common and pathologically consists mostly of stagnate nonclotted blood.
- With CT imaging, a muscle density soft tissue mass is seen and phleboliths, if present, are diagnostic.
- On MRI, an infiltrative lesion with inhomogenous signal with both isointense and hyperintense areas of signal intensity. On T2-weighted images, areas of hyperintense signal are seen, reflecting areas of increased blood pooling.

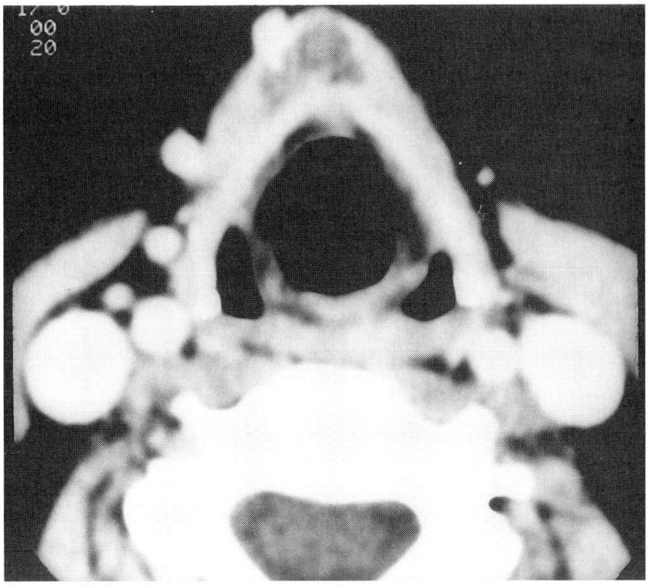

Figure 5-1 Thyroglossal duct cyst. An axial CT image shows a midline cystic lesion anteriorly at the level of hyoid bone.

Skeletal Muscle Mass Lesions ***Rhabdomyoma*** A rare benign skeletal tumor. Rhabdomyomas of the head and neck do not have an association with tuberous sclerosis. They are well-circumscribed lesions that have the density or signal intensity of normal muscle on cross-sectional imaging.

Benign Masseteric Hypertrophy Idiopathic enlargement of the masseteric muscle, more common in males and approximately 50 percent bilateral. Masseteric enlargement may be either congenital or acquired, with the latter commonly resulting from dental malocclusion or chronic, excessive teeth grinding. On cross-sectional imaging, focal enlargement of the masseter muscle is seen, with preservation of surrounding fatty and fascial planes.

Neurogenic Lesions ***Schwannoma*** The most frequent sites orally are the tongue, palate, and floor of the mouth. Imaging characteristics were previously described.

Neurofibroma Although most commonly peripheral within the neck and associated with von Recklinghausen's syndrome, a neurofibroma involving the oral cavity can occur (rarely), with the most frequent site being the tongue. A characteristic finding is unilateral macroglossia.

Granular Cell Tumors

- Histologically benign lesions that contain neurogenic, skeletal, and histiocytic elements.
- Although histologically benign, these lesions are infiltrative and recurrences are common if surgical resection is not complete.
- These tumors are called granular-cell myoblastomas in adults; the lesion usually presents as a mass within the dorsum and tip of the tongue.

- On CT, it is indistinguishable from carcinoma of the tongue.
- Magnetic resonance imaging may be more specific, with hypointense signal on both T1- and T2-weighted images reflecting the fibrous and/or skeletal components.

Minor Salivary Gland Tumors

- Malignancy is greater with minor salivary gland tumors as opposed to the major salivary glands.
- Adenoid cystic carcinoma is the most common malignancy of the minor salivary gland tumors within the oropharynx.
- Early invasion of the cranial nerves is common with adenoid cystic carcinoma.
- On the other hand, benign mixed-cell tumors present as well-marginated masses that displace rather than infiltrate the surrounding soft tissues.

MALIGNANT LESIONS

Squamous-Cell Carcinoma

- Over 90 percent of malignant lesions within the oral cavity and oropharynx are squamous-cell carcinomas.
- These carcinomas are associated with cigarette smoking, alcohol, and chewing tobacco abuse. In addition, exposure to betel nut and the HTLV-III virus, which is seen with acquired immunodeficiency syndrome (AIDS).
- Early in the disease, the patient is relatively asymptomatic. Unfortunately, the carcinoma is advanced at the time of diagnosis.
- Signs and symptoms include otalgia (referred pain to the external auditory canal), ill-fitting dentures, dysphagia with nasal speech, or a palpable cervical lymph node.
- Squamous-cell carcinomas of the oropharynx tend to spread submucosally along the deep musculofascial planes. Only 5 percent become exophytic.
- Invasion of the skull base can eventually occur, along with retrograde perineural spread with more aggressive lesions and recurrent squamous-cell carcinomas.
- The mandible may be involved by direct invasion or retrograde perineural spread along the inferior alveolar nerve (Fig. 5-2).
- The most common cranial nerves involved include the twelfth and branches of the fifth.
- In general, the incidence of cervical node metastasis depends on the size of the primary lesion, larger lesions being associated with more extensive nodal metastasis.
- Tonsillar carcinoma is the most common malignancy of the oropharynx and oral cavity.
- Carcinoma of the tongue has a higher incidence of bilateral nodal disease because of the rich lymphatics of the tongue.
- Regarding carcinoma of the tongue, an important observation must be made as to whether the disease has spread across the midline to determine whether a hemiglossectomy as opposed to a total glossectomy can be performed, since the latter is poorly tolerated and results in chronic aspiration. Assessment of crossing the midline is best with T2-weighted MRI.
- Of special note are the MRI characteristics of carcinoma of the soft palate. The soft palate normally demonstrates hyperintense signal on T1-weighted images because of the presence of fat and mucous glands, which contain proteinaceous material. Therefore, this normal hyperintense signal on the T1-weighted images is replaced by lower-signal tissue.

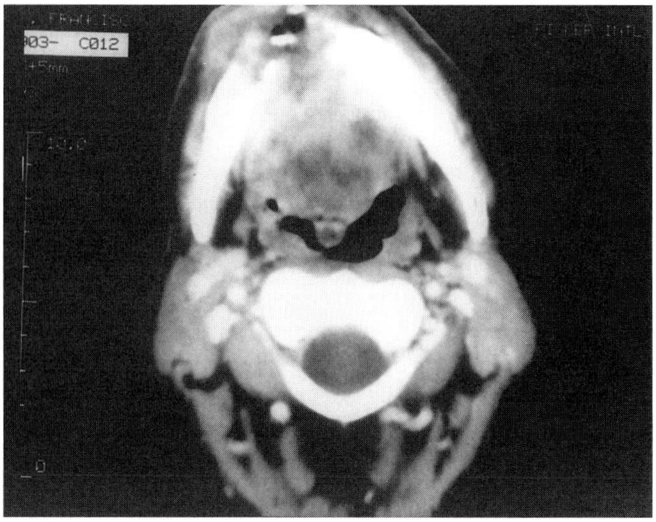

Figure 5-2 Carcinoma of the tongue and floor of the mouth. Axial postcontrast CT shows a slightly hyperdense mass at the anterior aspect of floor of the mouth and the tongue, crossing the middle and invading the adjacent mandible with bony destruction seen. Tumor mass is also seen anterior to the destroyed mandible.

Non-Hodgkin's Lymphoma Represents 5 percent of malignancies in this region and is the second most common malignancy of the oropharynx. Usually develops in the palatine and lingual lymphoid tissues. It is indistinguishable from squamous-cell carcinoma on cross-sectional imaging.

Carcinomas Other than Squamous Cell Originate from minor salivary glands. The majority of minor salivary glands are located posterior to the second molars; thus carcinomas of the minor salivary glands have their highest frequency in the posterior soft palate. Minor salivary gland tumors include malignant mixed-cell, adenoid cystic, mucoepidermoid, and adenocarcinomas. Characteristic of adenoid cystic carcinoma is the tendency for early invasion and infiltration along nerves and recurrence of disease within 10 to 15 years regardless of treatment. Adenocarcinoma has the worse prognosis of any of the minor salivary gland malignancies.

Melanoma and Sarcoma Rare. Melanomas may be multicentric, grow rapidly, and can be distinguished from undifferentiated carcinoma only by using special melanin-specific stains on histology.

☐ DIFFERENTIAL DIAGNOSIS BASED UPON SPACE OF ORIGIN

Please see Table 5-2.

☐ PATHOLOGY OF THE LARYNX

INFLAMMATORY DISEASE

Croup Inflammation of the subglottic larynx is referred to as croup. The causative organism is usually type I parainfluenza virus. It usually occurs in younger children of approximately 6 months to 3 years of age. The child usually presents with a characteristic barking cough and stridor. It appears to occur in children as opposed to adults because the mucosal tissue is looser and thus the swollen wall can more easily impinge on the airway. Radiographs demonstrate a "steeple-shaped" airway with loss of the subglottic angle. There may be associated distention or ballooning of the pharynx and pyriform sinuses if the film is taken at inspiration.

Epiglottitis Occurs in older children, and the causative pathogen is *Haemophilus influenzae*. Patients present with sore throat; inability to swallow, including saliva; and airway compromise. A lateral radiograph is characteristic, but should be obtained only in an area where there is constant observation as well as personnel and equipment necessary for doing an emergency tracheostomy. These radiographs should therefore be performed in either the emergency department or operating room. On the lateral radiograph, the epiglottis is thickened and indistinct in outline, blending into the aryepiglottic folds, which are also enlarged.

Table 5-2
DIFFERENTIAL DIAGNOSIS ACCORDING TO SPACE OF ORIGIN

Space of Origin	Differential Diagnosis
Strictly suprahyoid spaces	
Parapharyngeal	Nerve sheath tumors, lipoma, minor salivary gland tumors
Pharyngeal mucosal	Tonsillitis/abscess, minor salivary gland tumors, Thornwaldt cysts, squamous cell carcinoma, non-Hodgkin's lymphoma
Masticator	Benign masseteric hypertrophy, hemangioma/lymphangioma, dental lesions including abscesses, nerve sheath tumors, sarcomas, non-Hodgkin's lymphoma, and metastatic disease
Parotid	First branchial cleft cyst, hemangiomas/lymphangioma, abscess, benign lymphoepithelial cysts (AIDS), salivary gland tumors, Warthin tumor, metastatic disease
Submandibular	Second branchial cleft cysts, cystic hygroma/lymphangioma, hemangioma, Ludwig's angina, cellulitis/abscess, diving ranula, submandibular gland inflammation, lipoma, epidermoid/dermoid, benign mixed tumor of the submandibular gland, tail of the parotid gland tumor, lymphoma, submandibular gland malignancy, direct invasion or nodal metastasis of squamous cell carcinoma
Sublingual	Epidermoid/dermoid, hemangioma, cystic hygroma/lymphangioma, lingual thyroid tissue, Ludwig's angina, abscess, simple or diving ranula, benign mixed salivary gland tumor, sublingual gland malignancy, direct extension from squamous cell carcinoma
Strictly infrahyoid spaces	
Visceral	Thyroglossal cyst, thyroid disease; less commonly, parathyroid and esophageal disease
Spaces common to both suprahyoid and infrahyoid neck	
Carotid	Ectatic or asymmetrical vessels, aneurysms of the carotid vessels, abscess, nerve sheath tumors, paraganglioma, non-Hodgkin's lymphoma, nodal metastasis
Retropharyngeal/danger space	Infection/abscess, edema from jugular vein or lymphatic obstruction, lipoma, hemangioma, nodal metastasis
Prevertebral space	Vertebral artery aneurysm or ectasia, anterior vertebral osteophytes, vertebral body abscess/osteomyelitis, chordoma, neurogenic tumors, non-Hodgkin's lymphoma, vertebral body tumors including metastatic disease
Anterior cervical space	Lipomas, second branchial cleft cysts
Posterior cervical space	Lipoma, liposarcoma, cystic hygroma, lymphangiomas, third branchial cleft cyst, nodal disease

Modified from Table 1, "Differential Diagnosis of Deep Facial Lesions Based on Their Space of Origin," in HR Harnsberger and AG Osborn: Differential diagnosis of head and neck lesions based on their space of origin. 1. The suprahyoid part of the neck. *AJR* 157:147–154, 1991.

Granulomatous Disease ***Tuberculosis*** Rare. Lateral radiographs may show a nodular, thickened epiglottis. Ulceration and necrosis of the epiglottis may occur, along with perichondritis and fixation of the cricoarytenoid joint.

Sarcoid Radiographic findings are nonspecific. Sarcoid may cause diffuse thickening or nodular lesions. Other systemic manifestations of this disease would be present.

Wegener's Granulomatosis, Syphilis, and Leprosy Rare.

Rheumatoid and Collagen Vascular Disease Since the cricoarytenoid and cricothyroid joints are synovial joints, they can be involved by rheumatoid disease. There is usually hoarseness and potential fixation of the cricoarytenoid joints. On CT, there may be irregular erosions and sclerosis of these joints along with adjacent soft tissue swelling.

Perichondritis Seen with radiation therapy and tuberculosis.

TRAUMA

The most common cause of trauma to the larynx is a motor vehicle accident. The larynx is usually crushed against the cervical spine. Adults are more vulnerable to laryngeal fractures because of the larynx's lower position. In children, the mandible protects the larynx. Fractures of the larynx are best evaluated with CT scanning after the patient's airway has been managed. Evaluation for fragments of cartilage that may impinge upon the airway or perforate the mucosa should be performed, along with identifying any hematomas that may compromise the airway. With perforation, extraluminal air can be seen dissecting within the soft tissues. Hyoid fractures should also be identified. Arytenoid dislocation can also be seen and is usually associated with fracture of one of the larger laryngeal cartilages. Dislocations of the cricothyroid joint can also be seen as a rotational malalignment of the thyroid and cricoid cartilages. Unless the patient has already been tracheotomized in the field, laryngotracheal separation is usually not seen in the radiology department because it is usually fatal.

CONGENITAL LESIONS

A combination of plain radiographs and CT is useful in evaluating the size and length of the residual or malformed airway.

Laryngomalacia An abnormality where the structures are present but are too soft to keep the laryngeal airway open. Tracheostomy may be needed, but the child eventually outgrows this abnormality as the cartilages mature.

Subglottic Stenosis Another abnormality that is usually outgrown. There is narrowing of the subglottic larynx from the true cord down to the lower cricoid, secondary to soft tissue thickening in the subglottic area between the cricoid cartilage and airway lumen. The cricoid cartilage may be elliptical rather than round. The diagnosis is made by endoscopy as opposed to radiography because the cartilage is not calcified at this age.

Webs and Atresia Webs are usually at the level of the true cords and are associated with cricoid anomalies. Atresia of the larynx results from incomplete recanalization at this level; thus there is no airway within the larynx. Tracheostomy is required for the newborn. Radiographs are obtained to exclude other causes or airway abnormality.

Clefts Clefts are a result of incomplete fusion of the tracheoesophageal septum as the trachea separates from the esophagus during development. The patient usually presents with aspiration symptoms and multiple pneumonias.

Hemangiomas Subglottic hemangiomas cause nonspecific narrowing of the airway on lateral radiographs. Hemangiomas are discussed in further detail under "Benign Lesions," below.

BENIGN LESIONS

Vocal Cord Nodules These nonneoplastic lesions are seen with vocal abuse. They occur on the free margin of the true vocal cord.

Papillomas
- Occur most often in children.
- Although they are benign and noninvasive, recurrence after treatment is common.
- The trachea and bronchial tree are also involved; in severe cases, there may be airway compromise and obstructive pneumonia.
- Cavitation of the nodules can occur.

Hemangiomas
- Occur in both children and adults.
- In children, airway compromise is more common and there is a predilection for the subglottic area.
- Partial airway obstruction usually occurs within the first year of life, and the airway compromise is exacerbated by any inflammation (such as croup) and by crying, which causes venous engorgement.
- Diagnosis may be suggested by lateral radiographs but is usually made by endoscopy.

Lipoma Characteristic appearance on both CT and MRI because of the high signal fat content on T1-weighted images.

Neurogenic Tumors Paragangliomas, neurofibromas, and granular cell tumors have been reported but are uncommon. Paragangliomas demonstrate significant enhancement on CT because of their high vascularity.

Laryngocele

- Laryngoceles are benign but often result from a malignant process such as carcinoma of the true vocal cord or ventricle.
- The laryngeal saccule is normally a collapsed potential air space passing superiorly from the ventricle of the larynx. However, an obstructing lesion to the ventricular opening may cause dilatation of this small diverticulum, forming a laryngocele or saccular cyst, the former being filled with air and the latter with fluid.
- An internal laryngocele is within the confines of the thyroid cartilage and thyrohyoid membrane.
- An external laryngocele protrudes through the thyrohyoid membrane. Internal or mixed types are the most common.
- On CT and MRI, appearance depends on whether the laryngocele or saccular cyst is filled with air or fluid. Once again, a tumor should be excluded if a laryngocele is present.

MALIGNANCY

Squamous-Cell Carcinoma

- Approximately 95 percent of malignancies of the larynx are squamous-cell carcinomas.
- The less common malignancies of the larynx include adenocarcinoma, verrucous carcinoma, anaplastic carcinoma, spindle cell carcinoma, and sarcoma. These malignancies usually cannot be differentiated from each other or squamous cell carcinoma with imaging.
- Pathologic diagnosis is usually made by endoscopy and biopsy.
- However, imaging has an important role in accurately determining the extension of the malignancy so that the most appropriate therapy and surgical procedure can be implemented (Fig. 5-3).
- Voice conservation is the goal whenever possible.
- The multiplanar imaging capabilities of MRI along with its higher sensitivity and soft tissue resolution can be very helpful provided that the patient is cooperative. Sole axial imaging may underestimate the full extent of the patient's disease.
- Imaging is used to determine whether the malignancy is supraglottic, glottic, subglottic, or transglottic.
- Depending upon the involvement of certain important structures and anatomic regions, a determination can be made as to whether the patient undergoes a supraglottic laryngectomy, vertical frontolateral hemilaryngectomy, or total laryngectomy.

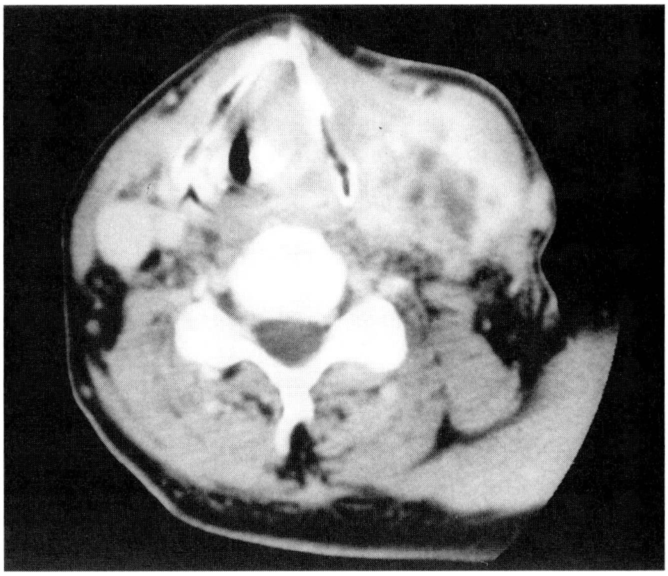

Figure 5-3 Laryngeal squamous-cell carcinoma. Axial postcontrast CT demonstrates a left vocal cord mass with involvement of the anterior commissure, posterior commissure, cricoid cartilage, and arytenoid cartilage. Extensive nodal disease is seen on the left side of the neck with enhancing, matted, necrotic lymph nodes.

- Radiation therapy is also a form of voice conservation therapy but can be used only with superficial lesions. Radiation perichondritis and necrosis are potential complications.
- The treatment of nodal disease is controversial at this time; thus the importance of detecting metastatic nodes with CT or MRI is not definitely known. Most believe that it is still worth performing.
- A patient with squamous-cell carcinoma of the larynx (especially supraglottic) has a relatively good chance of developing a second primary lesion. Therefore the workup of a patient with head and neck squamous cell carcinoma should also include an evaluation of the lungs, esophagus, and stomach.

Supraglottic Squamous-Cell Carcinoma

- The supraglottic larynx is defined as the upper larynx extending down to the ventricle and including the false cords, aryepiglottic folds, and epiglottis. The voice conservation surgery for a supraglottic malignancy would be a supraglottic laryngectomy.
- Supraglottic squamous-cell carcinoma constitutes approximately 30 percent of all laryngeal carcinomas.
- Early nodal metastasis to the deep cervical nodal chain is common because of the lush lymphatic network within the supraglottic larynx.
- Three major clinical blind spots for evaluating supraglottic laryngeal carcinoma include the preepiglottic space, paraglottic space, and thyroid cartilage (Fig. 5-4).

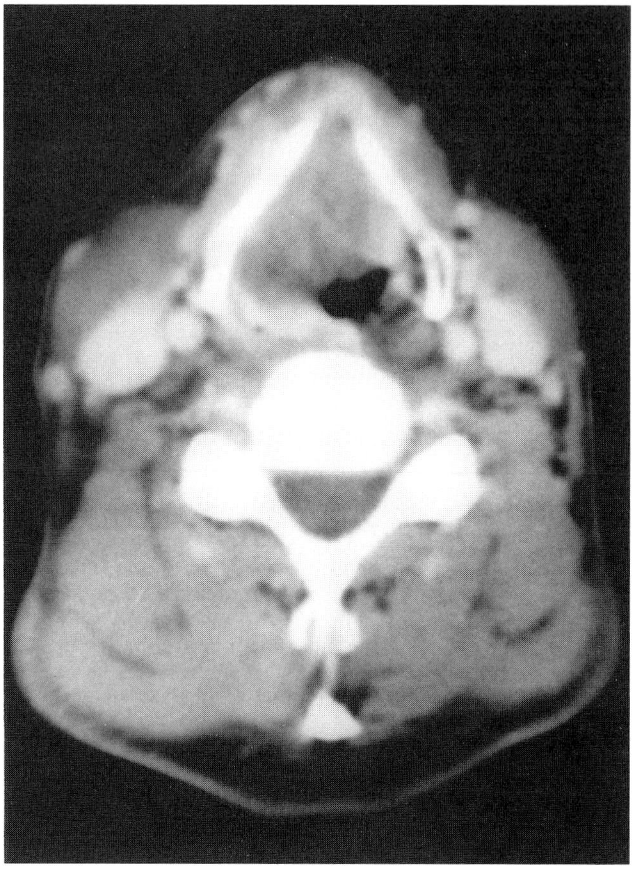

Figure 5-4 Supraglottic laryngeal squamous cell carcinoma. Axial postcontrast CT image demonstrates a right supraglottic tumor. Involvement of the preepiglottic space, and paraglottic space is seen.

Glottic Squamous-Cell Carcinoma

- Glottic squamous cell carcinoma constitutes approximately 60 percent of laryngeal carcinomas.
- Glottic carcinomas are detected early due to clinical symptom of hoarseness.
- Isolated glottic tumors rarely present with nodal metastasis because the true vocal cord is relatively alymphatic.
- Glottic tumors can spread anteriorly to involve the anterior commissure; posteriorly to involve the arytenoid cartilage, cricoid cartilage, and posterior commissure; inferiorly to involve the subglottic region; and superiorly to involve the paraglottic space.

Subglottic Squamous-Cell Carcinoma

- Subglottic squamous-cell carcinoma constitutes only 5 percent of all laryngeal carcinomas.
- The infraglottic region is defined as an arbitrary line 1 cm below the lateral extent of the apex of the ventricle. The speech conservation surgery in this region is the vertical frontolateral hemilaryngectomy. This involves removal of one false cord, one true cord, the ventricle, and the ipsilateral thyroid ala.

Vocal Cord Paralysis ***Recurrent Laryngeal Nerve*** The muscles of the larynx except for the cricothyroid muscle are innervated by the recurrent laryngeal nerve. With CT imaging, atrophy of the thyroid arytenoid muscle, vocal cord thinning, and dilatation of the pyriform sinus and valleculae ipsilaterally are seen. There is also lack of movement of the cord with special maneuvers. With recurrent laryngeal nerve paralysis, the path of the vagus nerve and recurrent laryngeal nerve must be evaluated for pathology.

Superior Laryngeal Nerve The cricothyroid thyroid muscle is innervated by the superior laryngeal nerve. With paralysis, the posterior larynx is deviated toward the side of the nerve lesion. With a superior laryngeal nerve paralysis, the course of the upper vagus should be thoroughly examined, which includes the pars nervosa of the jugular foramen, and the carotid space.

SUGGESTED READINGS

1. Becker M et al: Neoplastic invasion of the laryngeal cartilage of MR imaging and CT with histopathologic correlation. *Radiology* 194:661–669, 1995.
2. Harnsberger HR: *Handbook of Head and Neck Imaging*, 2nd ed. St Louis, Mosby-Year Book, 1995.
3. Harnsberger HR, Osborn AG: Differential diagnosis of head and neck lesions based on their space of origin: 1. The Suprahyoid part of the neck. *AJR* 157:147–154, 1991.
4. Lawson W et al: Cancer of the larynx, in Suen JY, Myers E (eds): *Cancer of the Head and Neck*. New York, Churchill Livingstone, 1989.
5. Mancuso AA et al: *Workbook for MRI and CT of the Head and Neck*. Baltimore, Williams & Wilkins, 1989.
6. Lufkin RB et al: *MRI of the Head and Neck: The Raven MRI Teaching File*. New York, Raven Press, 1991.
7. Smoker WRK, Harnsberger HR: Differential diagnosis of head and neck lesions based on their space of origin: 2. The infrahyoid portion of the neck. *AJR* 157:155–159, 1991.
8. Som PM et al: *Head and Neck Imaging*. St Louis, Mosby-Year Book, 1991.

☐ QUESTIONS (True or False)

1. Regarding the nasopharynx,
- **a.** It is bounded superiorly by the sphenoid sinus and upper clivus.
- **b.** The posterior boundary is the lower clivus and upper cervical spine.
- **c.** The inferior boundary is the base of the tongue.
- **d.** The eustachian tube opens into the nasopharynx.
- **e.** It is lined by squamous epithelium.

2. Regarding the larynx,
- **a.** The main cartilaginous structures of the larynx include the cricoid, thyroid, arytenoid, and epiglottic cartilages.
- **b.** The arytenoid has a muscular process projecting anteriorly and a vocal process projecting posteriorly.
- **c.** The intrinsic muscles of the larynx are innervated by the recurrent laryngeal nerve.
- **d.** The inferior laryngeal artery is a branch of the thyrocervical trunk; the superior laryngeal artery arises from the superior thyroid artery.
- **e.** There is an anterior commissure and a posterior commissure.

3. Regarding squamous cell carcinoma of the nasopharynx,
- **a.** The lateral pharyngeal recess is the least common site of origin.
- **b.** It is the most common superficial epithelial carcinoma of the nasopharynx.
- **c.** Unilateral middle ear fluid accumulation should suggest the possibility of nasopharyngeal carcinoma.
- **d.** The presence of lower cervical adenopathy decreases survival dramatically.
- **e.** Radiation therapy is the treatment of choice unless adenopathy, which is treated with dissection, is present.

4. Regarding thyroglossal duct cysts,
- **a.** They are lateral neck masses at the level of hyoid bone.
- **b.** They frequently contain aberrant thyroid tissue.
- **c.** Pathologically, they are made up of squamous cell mucosa.
- **d.** Some 50 percent of cases seen before the age of 10 years.
- **e.** The thyroglossal duct involutes by the eighth fetal week.

5. Regarding ranula,
- **a.** A ranula is a postinflammatory retention cyst of the sublingual glands or minor salivary glands of the sublingual space.
- **b.** If the ranula is confined to the sublingual space, it is a simple ranula.
- **c.** If the ranula extends posteriorly into the submandibular space, it is called a diving ranula.
- **d.** The diving ranula is lined by squamous epithelium.
- **e.** The diving ranula can present as a pseudocyst within the submandibular space, with a "tail sign" within the sublingual space.

6. Regarding laryngocele,
- **a.** Laryngoceles are benign lesions and are not associated with malignancies.
- **b.** An internal laryngocele is seen within the confines of the thyroid cartilage and thyroid membrane.
- **c.** An external laryngocele protrudes through the thyrohyoid membrane.
- **d.** A laryngocele is filled with air.
- **e.** A saccular cyst is filled with fluid.

7. Regarding malignancy of larynx,
- **a.** Approximately 95 percent of malignancies of the larynx are squamous-cell carcinomas.
- **b.** Axial imaging may underestimate the full extent of the patient's disease.
- **c.** Nodal metastasis to the deep cervical chain is common in isolated glottic tumor.
- **d.** Glottic squamous-cell carcinoma constitutes approximatly 60 percent of laryngeal carcinomas.
- **e.** A patient with squamous-cell carcinoma of the larynx has a relatively good chance of developing a second primary lesion.

8. Lesions in the carotid space include
- **a.** Aneurysms of the carotid vessels.
- **b.** Nerve sheath tumors
- **c.** Paraganglioma
- **d.** Nodal metastasis
- **e.** Branchial cleft cyst

☐ ANSWERS

1. **a.** T
b. T
c. F
d. T
e. T

2. **a.** T
b. F
c. T
d. T
e. T

3. **a.** F
b. T
c. T
d. T
e. T

4. **a.** F
b. F
c. T
d. T
e. T

5. **a.** T
b. T
c. T
d. F
e. T

6. **a.** F
b. T
c. T
d. T
e. T

7. **a.** T
b. T
c. F
d. T
e. T

8. **a.** T
b. T
c. T
d. T
e. F

CHAPTER

6 Salivary Glands

Terry S. Becker

DIAGNOSTIC IMAGING TECHNIQUES

Manifestations of salivary gland disease are usually noted clinically (swelling, single or multiple masses, pain or tenderness). Because the clinical presentation and physical examination cannot differentiate between benign and malignant processes, biopsy is frequently required.

Multiple imaging techniques are utilized. The purposes of imaging are as follows: (1) confirmation of salivary gland origin—i.e., differentiation of intrinsic lesions from lesions of the parapharyngeal space, masticator space, subcutaneous and deep soft tissues, submandibular space, submental space, and mandible; (2) differentiation of neoplasms from masses of other origin; (3) differentiation of benign neoplasms from malignant neoplasms (although fine needle aspiration biopsy or incisional or excisional biopsy is often required); (4) definition of anatomic extent, and, (5) aiding in the performance of aspiration biopsy guided by computed tomography (CT) or magnetic resonance imaging (MRI) when the lesion is difficult to localize clinically.

PLAIN-FILM RADIOGRAPHY

Plain-film radiography is of limited value. It is useful in the evaluation of sialolithiasis, calcific and bony lesions that may mimic salivary gland disease, and calcification in tumor masses, but it is less sensitive than CT. The gland being studied should be imaged by multiple views to isolate calcification and calculi from the bony mandible.

SIALOGRAPHY

Since the advent of CT and MRI, sialography has played a limited but still valuable role in the evaluation of chronic inflammatory processes involving the ductal system of the parotid and submandibular glands. It can rarely be utilized for the sublingual glands as the ducts are numerous and small.

Sialography has been replaced by CT and MRI in the evaluation of salivary gland and adjacent tumor masses. Indications for sialography are suspicion of (1) chronic, recurrent, and nonspecific sialadenitis; (2) Sjögren's syndrome, Mikulicz syndrome, and other forms of autoimmune disease; (3) submandibular or parotid gland sialolithiasis; and (4) posttraumatic or postoperative fistula, stricture, or cyst. Sialography is contraindicated in the presence of acute salivary gland infection.

Sialography is of limited value for the evaluation of salivary gland neoplasms. Extrinsic masses displace the gland. Lesions are more likely to be intrinsic when parotid parenchyma surrounds the greater portion of the mass. Other features of intrinsic origin are irregular destruction of the gland, punctate sialectasis, and gross enlargement of the gland. Irregular contrast pooling and ductal obstruction or destruction are considered features of malignancy but are nonspecific.

COMPUTED TOMOGRAPHY

Computed tomography of the salivary glands is obtained by using thin-section (5-mm) axial (or occasionally coronal) images, usually following intravenous injection of contrast solution.

Parameters evaluated include tumor borders, homogeneity, density, and enhancement. A well-defined homogenous mass suggests a benign process.

COMPARISON OF MAGNETIC RESONANCE IMAGING AND COMPUTED TOMOGRAPHY

Magnetic resonance imaging has several advantages over computed tomography in the evaluation of parotid masses. It can better distinguish parotid and extraparotid pathology, such as parapharyngeal masses and may differentiate a single multilobulated mass from multiple adjacent masses. T2-weighted images appear superior to T1-weighted images in differentiating tumor from normal parotid tissue, since most tumors have high signal on T2-weighted images. However, MRI is less valuable in demonstrating tumor calcification, which is easily seen on CT. The signal characteristics of MRI with the exception of tumor hemorrhage are relatively nonspecific. Complexity of signal does not differentiate benign from malignant neoplasms. Although not recommended for routine parotid imaging, gadolinium is valuable in selected cases. Gadolinium cannot differentiate benign from malignant lesions but may help to define infiltration of the borders of a lesion. Gadolinium may also identify the facial nerve by its relation to the retromandibular vein.

Magnetic resonance imaging and CT are morphologically comparable in the evaluation of parotid and submandibular gland masses. Magnetic resonance imaging may be better in the differentiation of intrinsic lesions of parotid gland from lesions of the parapharyngeal and masticator space. Computed tomography may be of greater value in inflammatory lesions of the parotid and submandibular glands, particularly in the presence of calcification or calculi. The CT and MRI imaging appearance of parotid and submandibular gland tumors is generally nonspecific. There is a variably enhancing mass with the central low to moderate density on CT. A malignant or more aggressive process may be suspected in the presence of marked irregularity of the margin of the mass and/or infiltration of the mass into the parapharyngeal space, masseter muscle, or subcutaneous soft tissues. Ulceration or bone erosion is occasionally present. The MRI appearance of tumors is also nonspecific, appearing mildly hypointense to intermediate signal intensity on T1-weighted images with increased signal intensity on T2-weighted sequences. Cystic areas in Warthin's tumor or cysts are represented as high-signal areas on T2-weighted images.

ULTRASONOGRAPHY

High resolution (7.5- to 10-MHz transducer) real time ultrasonographic images of the parotid or submandibular salivary gland are frequently useful for the identification of a mass and to determine whether a mass is solid or cystic. Small focal fluid cysts or abscess may be identified. Ultrasound-guided aspiration is a simple and inexpensive procedure.

Ultrasonography is limited in the evaluation of neoplasms, although ultrasound is excellent in defining the relationship of the carotid artery and internal jugular vein to a parotid mass. Aneurysm, which rarely mimics a parotid gland or parapharyngeal space neoplasm, is readily identified with ultrasound. Paraganglioma (carotid body and glomus vagale tumors) have an echogenic appearance. Carotid body tumors will separate the internal and external carotid artery.

Ultrasound is less specific than CT or MRI in the evaluation of neoplasms. Although the superficial portion of the parotid gland is easily visualized with ultrasound, the deep lobe tends to be obscured because of the ramus of the mandible.

Pleomorphic adenomas are hypoechoic and fairly well defined with posterior acoustic enhancement. Warthin's tumors are more echogenic. Lymph nodes tend to hypoechoic. Calculi are echogenic with acoustic shadowing. Occasionally dilated ducts may be identified by ultrasound.

RADIONUCLIDE IMAGING (SCINTIGRAPHY)

Radionuclide scanning is occasionally used in the evaluation of the salivary glands, although it is less sensitive and specific than CT or MRI. Sodium 99m pertechnetate is concentrated and excreted by the salivary glands (as well as the thyroid gland). A tumor appears as a filling defect. Salivary gland oncocytes in Warthin's tumor and oncocytoma readily take up the pertechnetate, demonstrating a "hot spot." In patients with ductal obstruction, diffuse increased uptake in the gland will be present. Accumulation of gallium 67 citrate is noted in inflammatory or neoplastic processes as well as sarcoidosis, melanoma, and lymphoma. Gallium may be limited, however, because of normal uptake in oral and pharygeal mucosa by minor salivary glands and secretory glands.

Pertechnetate-labeled red blood cells are useful in the diagnosis of hemangioma. Bone scanning agents such as technetium 99m methylene diphosphorate (MDP) are useful in studying involvement of the mandibular and facial skeleton and in the early detection of skeletal metastasis. Indium-111-labelled white blood cells accumulate in the parotid and lacrimal glands in Sjögren's syndrome.

ANGIOGRAPHY

Therapeutic angiography is frequently used in the preoperative embolization of highly vascular neoplasms such as paraganglioma or arteriovenous malformation. Diagnostic angiography is less important since the advent of CT and MRI.

IMAGING AND FINE NEEDLE ASPIRATION

Diagnostic imaging and fine needle aspiration cytology are complementary procedures in the evaluation of salivary gland masses. Fine needle biopsy is easy to perform, inexpensive, and highly accurate. Biopsy guided by CT, MRI, or ultrasound is utilized when the mass is either not readily evident on physical examination or where "blind" aspiration cytology or biopsy would be difficult or dangerous because of overlying vascular or neural structures.

☐ NORMAL ANATOMY ON COMPUTED TOMOGRAPHY AND MAGNETIC RESONANCE IMAGING

The axial CT images obtained are visualized with soft tissue windows (approximate width/level of 350/50 HU).

PAROTID GLAND

The parotid gland, the largest of the major salivary glands, is arbitrarily divided into the deep and superficial lobes by the facial nerve. The superficial lobe is that portion lateral to the medial margin of the ramus and abuts the posterior aspect of the masseter muscle, extending for a variable degree anterior and lateral to the masseter muscle. Posteriorly, the superficial lobe abuts the sternocleidomastoid muscle at the posterior belly of the digastric muscle, noted anteromedially. The tail of the parotid extends inferiorly from the superficial lobe for a variable distance. The deep lobe extends behind the ramus of the mandible. The deep lobe is bordered medially by the parapharyngeal space, internal carotid artery, and internal jugular vein. The deep lobe extends to the parapharyngeal space via the stylomandibular tunnel (between the ramus of the mandible and the styloid process).

The facial nerve leaves the skull at the stylomastoid foramen, traveling through a fat pad and entering the posterior aspect of the parotid gland between the posterior belly of the digastric and sternocleidomastoid muscles. The fat pad may be identified on CT or MRI. The intrinsic portion of the facial nerve lies just posterior and lateral to the retromandibular vein and external carotid artery and divides into major branches overlying the ramus of the mandible. The facial nerve runs between the deep and superficial portions of the parotid gland. The facial nerve is not identified on CT but has been described on thin-section MRI.

The parotid ductal system empties into Stenson's duct, which is approximately 7 cm long. It extends anteriorly from the gland, crossing the masseter muscle, where it extends medially, piercing the buccinator muscle and entering the mouth opposite the second upper molar. Accessory lobes of the parotid gland may be present overlying the masseter or adjacent to the main portion of the gland. An accessory duct has been described in as many as 90 percent of patients.

PARAPHARYNGEAL SPACE

The parapharyngeal space is divided into the prestyloid and poststyloid components by a line from the medial apsect of the medial pterygoid plate to the styloid process. Prestyloid lesions tend to be of salivary gland origin, either from the deep lobe of the parotid gland or a minor salivary gland. Poststyloid masses usually represent paraganglioma, neuroma, or lymphadenopathy. The masticator space containing the masseter muscle, temporalis muscle, medial and lateral pterygoid muscles, ramus, and mandibular nerve is separated from the prestyloid parapharyngeal space by a fascial layer extending to the skull base. Salivary gland tumors do not occur in the masticator space.

SUBMANDIBULAR GLAND

The submandibular glands are noted in the submandibular space (or triangle) against the submandibular depression on the inner surface of the body of the mandible posterior and inferior to the mylohyoid muscle, separated from the parotid gland by the stylomandibular fascia. A portion of the gland extends superiorly over the posterior margin of the mylohyoid muscle. The submandibular gland ductal system drains via Wharton's duct, which runs between the mylohyoid and hyoglossus muscles, opening into the mouth adjacent to a small papilla lateral to the frenulum.

Multiple minor salivary glands are noted in the oral cavity, nasal cavity, paranasal sinuses, pharynx, and larynx.

The CT and MRI appearance of the parotid gland is related to its variable but generally high fat content, with intermediate density between fat and muscle. Mild enhancement of the parotid gland occurs after intravenous contrast infusion. The MRI signal intensity is intermediate between fat and muscle on T1-weighted images, becoming closer to fat on T2-weighted images. The submandibular glands generally have less fat than the parotid glands and are closer to muscle density or intensity on CT MRI (on both T1- and T2-weighted images).

Resolution on MRI may be superior to that on CT, differentiating primary parotid neoplasm from a mass arising in the parapharyngeal space. The presence of a fat plane between a mass and the parotid gland is indicative of its origin outside the parotid gland—i.e., in the parapharyngeal space. Fat plane obliteration suggests that the lesion is intraparotid. A pedunculated mass arising within the deep lobe may suggest that the fat plane is intact on all but one or two images. In differentiating prestyloid from poststyloid parapharyngeal space masses, displacement of the parapharyngeal fat plane is important. A prestyloid lesion (i.e., deep lobe minor salivary gland tumor) will displace the fat plane posteromedially. A poststyloid parapharyngeal space neoplasm—such as paraganglioma, neuroma, or lymphadenopathy—will displace the fat plane anterolaterally.

After administration of gadolinium, the normal parotid gland shows marked glandular enhancement. The retromandibular vein the facial nerve may be identified as a structure of low signal intensity. Both benign and malignant neoplasm show variable enhancement. Extraglandular tumor infiltration may be better defined with gadolinium. Gadolinium offers no advantage over conventional unenhanced T2-weighted images in inflammatory disease. Gadolinium offers no advantage in Sjögren's syndrome, which shows high signal intensity on T2-weighted images and nonhomogenous signal on both T1- and T2-weighted images.

Lymphepithelial cysts do not enhance with gadolinium but are better defined because of the enhancement of the surrounding parenchyma.

In malignant lesions such as adenocarcinoma, adenoid cystic carcincoma, squamous-cell carcinoma and lymphoma, variable contrast enhancement is present. Gadolinium may define the extent of soft tissue infiltration, and it may be of value in differentiating recurrent neoplasm from fibrosis, since fibrosis enhances only slightly.

☐ INFLAMMATORY DISEASES OF THE SALIVARY GLANDS

SJÖGREN'S SYNDROME

Sjögren's syndrome is an autoimmune inflammatory process involving the salivary glands (usually the parotid glands) and the lacrimal glands, generally associated with rhematoid arthritis. The characteristic triad is that of dry eyes (keratoconjunctivitis sicca) and dry mouth (xerostomia)—together referred to as *sicca syndrome*—and autoimmune disease (most commonly rheumatoid arthritis). Sjögren's syndrome is 10 times more frequent in females, most commonly middle-aged or older.

While parotid glandular architecture may be preserved in Sjögren's syndrome, periductal mononuclear and dense lymphocytic cell infiltration is present. Complications include abscess formation, sialadenitis, salivary gland calcification, regional lymphadenopathy, non-Hodgkin's lymphoma, and pseudolymphoma.

Parotid sialography remains the most effective imaging procedure in the diagnosis of Sjögren's syndrome. Involvement is usually bilateral. The parotid gland is mild to markedly enlarged. Early in the disease, multiple punctate contrast collections are present throughout the gland. As the disease progresses, the punctate contrast collections become larger and more globular. Ultimately the parotid may become completely replaced by the circular contrast collections, becoming a cavitary mass with complete destruction of the salivary gland. Areas of tubular sialectasia or strictures may occur. Delayed films will demonstrate variable retention of contrast material, often remaining for long periods of time, particularly if oil-based contrast agents are used.

Since the imaging characteristics of Sjögren's syndrome are not distinguishable from recurrent parotitis of childhood, differentiation must be made clinically.

The CT appearance of Sjögren's syndrome is that of bilateral parotid gland (and less frequently submandibular gland) enlargement with multiple areas of low attenuation. Multilocular cysts and calcifications have also been noted. If Sjögren's syndrome is complicated by non-Hodgkin's lymphoma, an intraglandular mass will be evident.

Multiple small cysts up to 4 mm and/or multisepated cystic masses up to 3 cm in diameter have been described on ultrasound. It is not certain whether this represents the underlying pathologic change of dilated hypertrophic ducts or extravasation of salivary fluid secondary to destruction of the duct wall.

INFECTION OF THE SALIVARY GLANDS

Inflammation of the major salivary glands (sialadenitis) may be caused by retrograde extention of pathogens of the mouth or may be blood-borne. When acute, the diagnosis is readily made clinically and diagnostic imaging procedures are generally not necessary. Sialography is contraindicated in acute sialadenitis because of the possible accentuation of inflammatory disease. In acute sialadenitis, CT or MRI will demonstrate the fluctuant, enlarged gland as well as the extent of intraparotid and extraparotid inflammation involving the masseter muscles, subcutaneous soft tissues, masticator or parapharyngeal space (Fig. 6-1).

Abscess formation may complicate suppurative sialadenitis within the parotid gland or in the masticator or

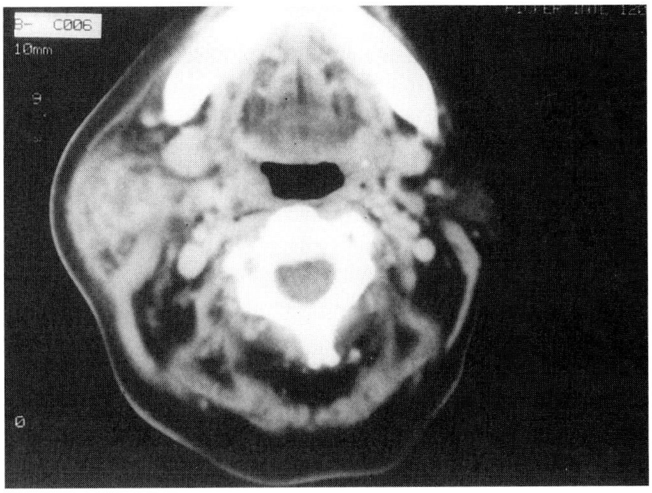

Figure 6-1 Parotitis. As seen on CT, the entire right parotid gland is enlarged and hyperintense. No abscess collection is present.

parapharyngeal space. The abscess is visualized by CT as a hypointense central region surrounded by a variably enhancing rim and by MRI as a central water-density collection (low or medium signal intensity on T1-weighted images with increase in signal intensity on T2-weighted images) in a bed of edema. Ultrasound will demonstrate a fluid collection and can be used for localization during aspiration drainage. The sialographic appearance of ductal displacement is nonspecific, noted in any mass involving the salivary gland.

Salivary gland fistulas complicating sialadenitis are best identified by sialography as extravasation of contrast into the oral cavity or through the skin. If the opening of the fistula is evident by physical examination, injection into this opening may demonstrate the salivary gland communication.

Lymphadenopathy secondary to salivary gland infection is best demonstrated by CT; it is seen as a low-density mass adjacent to or within the salivary gland.

SIALOLITHIASIS

The submandibular gland is involved in 80 percent of calculi and the parotid gland is involved in approximately 20 percent. Sublingular and minor salivary gland calculi account for less than 1 percent of symptomatic sialolithiasis.

Approximately 20 percent of calculi in the submandibular gland and 20 to 40 percent of calculi in the parotid gland are not visible on plain-film examination, even when multiple views are obtained.

Although sialography will identify intraductal calculi and sialectasia, small calculi are best demonstrated by CT as calcifications within the gland or along the course of Wharton's (submandibular gland) duct in the floor of the mouth or Stenson's (parotid gland) duct lateral to the masseter muscle.

RADIATION INJURY TO THE SALIVARY GLANDS

Radiation injury to the salivary glands results in decreased salivary gland function, decreased flow rate, and xerostomia.

Radiation injury causes increased CT density of the gland, the etiology of which is not certain. There is no evidence that chemotherapy results in change of appearance of the salivary glands.

☐ DIFFERENTIATING INTRINSIC PAROTID GLAND LESIONS FROM LESIONS OF THE MASSETERIC AND PARAPHARYNGEAL SPACE

The preoperative differentiation of intrinsic parotid lesions from tumors arising in the parapharyngeal space is important because primary parotid lesions are removed via a transparotid approach while extraparotid lesions are reached via a transcervical approach.

Both CT and MRI are frequently able to differentiate parapharyngeal masses from intrinsic parotid masses. The demonstration of a fat plane separating the normal parotid gland from the mass indicates parapharyngeal location. Lack of the fat plane implies a deep-lobe parotid tumor. This distinction can be difficult at times, however, particularly if the tumor is pedunculated, having only a small attachment to the gland.

Primary salivary gland tumors (most commonly deep-lobe pleomorphic adenomas) and minor salivary gland neoplasms displace the internal carotid artery posteriorly, while neuromas, schwannomas, and glomus tumors of the parapharyngeal space displace the internal carotid artery anteriorly. The MRI signal characteristics of these lesions are similar: a well-circumscribed lesion with intermediate signal on T1 weighting and increasing signal on T2 weighting. Focal areas of necrosis, hemorrhage, or calcification may alter this appearance. Paragangliomas are vascular and demonstrate signal flow voids, resulting in a salt-and-pepper appearance. Prestyloid lesions may pass through the stylomandibular tunnel and indicate salivary gland origin. Poststyloid compartment tumors include schwannoma, paraganglioma, retropharyngeal lymphadenopathy, or, less frequently, meningioma, hemangioma, chondrosarcoma, rhabdomyosarcoma, or perineural metastasis (as in adenoid cystic carcinoma). Lesions in the masticator space (lateral to the medial pterygoid fascia) may be meningioma, neurolemma, sarcoma, squamous-cell carcinoma, dentigerous cysts, or masseteric hypertrophy but not salivary gland lesions. Masticator space origin is indicated by (1) location anterior and lateral to the parapharyngeal fat; (2) limitation of tumor by boundaries of the masticator space—i.e., the sphenoid bone, posterior aspect of the mandible and zygomatic arch; (3) obliteration of the fat planes within the masticator space; and (4) tendency to spread through the foramen ovale.

☐ SALIVARY GLAND CYSTS

Cysts of the salivary gland are classified as congenital or acquired. Congenital cysts include branchial cleft cysts as well as dermoid and epidermoid cysts. Acquired cysts may be posttraumatic (sialocele), lymphepithelial cysts, or retention cysts (mucocele or ranula).

The imaging appearance of cysts, whether acquired or congenital, is similar. Sialography will demonstrate displacement of the ductal system around the nonspecific mass. Rarely, communication of contrast within the cyst occurs. Computed tomography demonstrates a well-circumscribed low-density (water content) mass. If infection has been present, the central density may be higher and an enhancing variable-thickness wall may be evident on postcontrast infusion scans. The MRI appearance is consistent with the water content of the cyst, with low signal on T1-weighted sequences, increasing on intermediately weighted scans and very bright signal on T2-weighted sequences. The signal characteristic may be altered if there has been previous infection or hemorrhage.

BRANCHIAL CLEFT CYSTS

First arch branchial cleft cysts, containing a lining of squamous or ciliated epithelium, may be present in the parotid gland. Characteristic fluid density is noted on CT (Fig. 6-2) and MRI (low signal on T1-weighted images and high signal on T2-weighted sequences) but may not be homogeneous if there has been prior infection or hemorrhage.

DERMOID AND EPIDERMOID

Dermoid and epidermoid cysts are slow-growing, variable in size, and usually identified in adulthood. They may be sublingual (between the geniohyoid and mylohyoid muscle), epihyoid (lying in the submental region between the skin and geniohyoid muscle), or lateral (under the mandible below the mylohyoid muscle).

LYMPHOEPITHELIAL CYSTS

Lymphoepithelial cysts present with painless swelling of the parotid glands and are most frequently seen in patients known to be HIV-positive, with or without the clinical signs of acquired immunodeficiency syndrome (AIDS). Although swelling may be unilateral, CT and MRI usually demonstrate that the process is bilateral, with multiple bilateral, well-circumscribed intraparotid masses. An enhancing rim may be evident on CT. The MRI appearance resembles that of cysts of other etiologies. Multiple small cervical lymph nodes up to 2 cm in diameter are noted in the posterior, submental, or submandibular triangles or internal jugular chain. Necrosis does not occur.

SIALOCELE

The sialocele (Fig. 6-3) is a posttraumatic cyst of the parotid or, less frequently, the submandibular gland, resulting from laceration or stricture with rupture of Stenson's or Wharton's duct. Extravasated mucinous or serous fluid accumulates within the gland or extends around the duct. The sialocele is also called a pseudocyst because no true epithelial lining is present. Sialocele may result from faulty dentures, buccal mucosal ulcerations, surgical sutures, or calculus removal. It is also seen following penetrating blunt trauma to the duct.

The differential diagnosis of sialocele includes other forms of congenital and acquired cysts. Abscess cannot be easily differentiated on imaging studies alone.

Fistula formation is usually a result of lacerating injury. Fistula communication with the oral cavity,

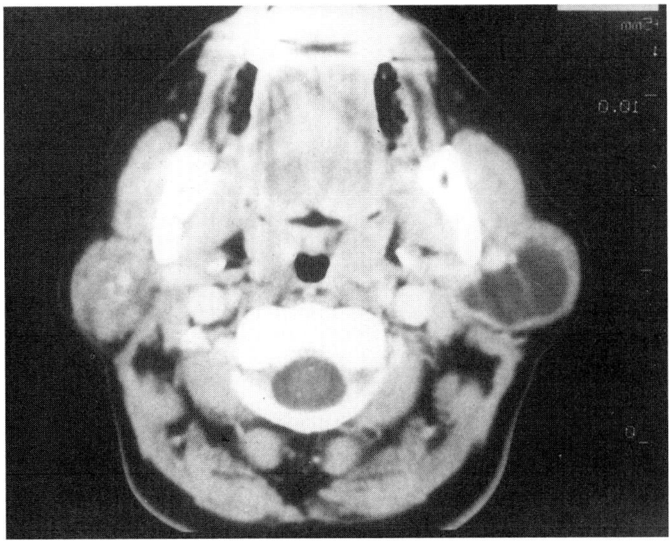

Figure 6-2 Branchial cleft cyst. As seen on CT, fluid density of well-marginated mass involves predominantly the superficial lobe of the left parotid gland.

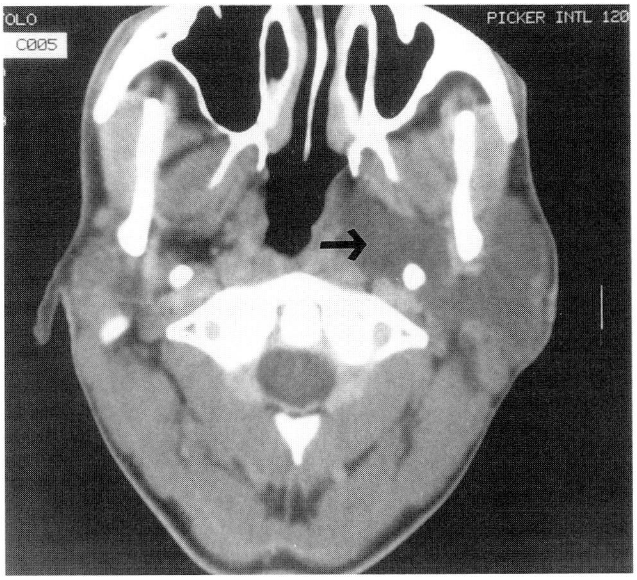

Figure 6-3 Sialocele. On CT, low-density mass involves most of the left parotid gland with marked extension into the parapharyngeal space (*arrows*).

oropharynx, hypopharynx, or skin may be demonstrated utilizing sialography.

Ranula (retention cyst or mucocele) results from obstruction of a sublingual or minor salivary gland duct in the floor of the mouth. It may be confined to the floor of mouth above the mylohyoid muscle or extend below the hyoid (plunging, deep, or diving ranula) into the submandibular or parapharyngeal space.

☐ SALIVARY GLAND NEOPLASMS

Although salivary gland neoplasms comprise less than 3 percent of all malignancies, the diagnosis is readily suspected clinically. Patients usually present with a progressive enlarging, painless mass in the region of the parotid or submandibular gland. Pain or facial weakness suggests malignancy.

Benign tumors appear well circumscribed on CT or MRI. Enhancement is variable but generally not marked. Low-grade malignant lesions such as mucoepidermoid carcinoma are difficult to differentiate from benign lesions. Malignant lesions cannot be differentiated from benign lesions based on the CT density, CT enhancment, MRI signal, or postgadolinum MRI enhancement. However, the presence of irregularity or infiltration into the soft tissues of the skin, masseter muscle, parapharyngeal space, or along the course of the parapharyngeal nerves or facial nerve (most frequently seen in the adenoid cystic carcinoma) suggests malignancy.

BENIGN NEOPLASMS

Pleomorphic Adenoma Pleomorphic adenoma (benign mixed tumor) accounts for approximately 60 to 70 percent of all benign tumors of the salivary glands. Pleomorphic adenoma occurs most commonly in the parotid

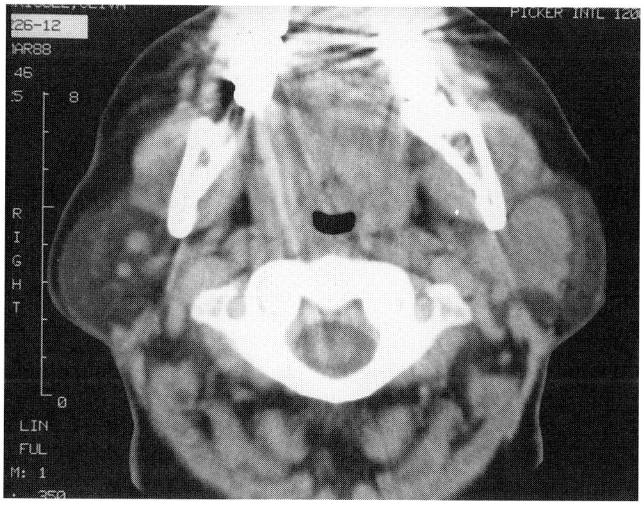

Figure 6-4 Pleomorphic adenoma. On CT, the well-circumscribed mass involves the superficial and, to a lesser extent, deep lobe of the left parotid gland.

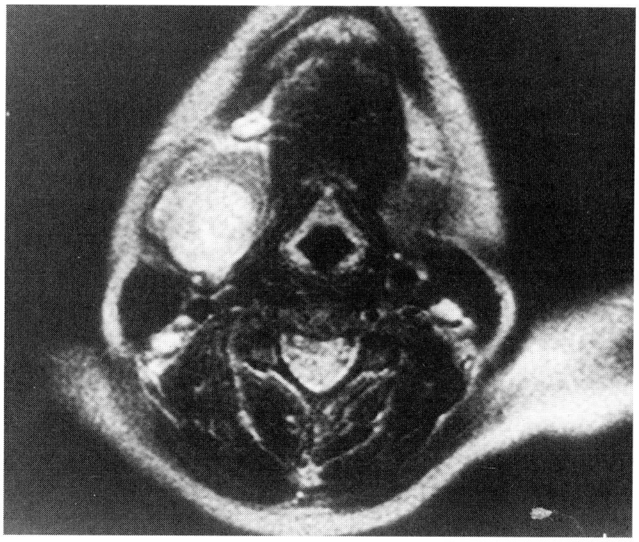

Figure 6-5 Pleomorphic adenoma. On MRI, T2-weighted sequence, the heterogenously bright, well-circumscribed mass is seen within the posterior aspect of the right submandibular gland.

glands and, to a lesser extent, in the submandibular and minor salivary glands. Sublingual pleomorphic adenoma is rare.

The sialographic appearance of pleomorphic adenoma is indistinguishable from other benign intraparotid neoplasms—i.e., smooth displacement of the salivary gland ducts and parenchyma. No abrupt truncation, focal irregularity, or extravasation of contrast material is present.

The CT appearance of pleomorphic adenoma (Fig. 6-4) is that of a well-circumscribed mass with homogenous to heterogenous density (related to fluid, fat, hemorrhage, or dystrophic calcification). Mild enhancement occurs but is nonspecific.

Magnetic resonance imaging will demonstrate a predominantly heterogenous, well-circumscribed mass of intermediate to low signal on T1-weighted images, with increasing signal on T2-weighted sequences (Fig. 6-5). If hemorrhage is present, there will be areas of high signal on both T1- and T2-weighted images. Calcification is generally not evident on MRI.

Warthin's Tumor and Oncocytoma Warthin's tumor (adenolymphoma or papillary cystadenoma lymphomatosum) accounts for less than 10 percent of parotid tumors. These tumors are invariably benign and occur only in the parotid gland. They contain oncocytic elements as well as cystic and lymphatic components and thus may represent heterotopic salivary gland epithelium trapped within intraparotid lymph nodes.

The sialographic appearance is identical with pleomorphic adenomas and other benign tumors of the parotid gland.

The CT appearance of Warthin's tumor is that of a homogenous, well-circumscribed mass in the parotid gland, frequently with hypodense or cystic areas. Calcification does not occur. The MRI appearance is that of a homogenous, well-circumscribed mass with intermediate low signal intensity on T1-weighted images and increase in signal on T2-weighted images. Approximately 10 percent of Warthin's tumors are bilateral.

Oncocytoma (Fig. 6-6*A* and *B*) is a benign tumor related to Warthin's tumor but composed entirely of oncocytes. Oncocytoma is a rare lesion occuring in less than 1 percent of all salivary gland tumors; it is most common in patients over the age of 55. Both oncocytoma and Warthin's tumor are unique in that they will accumulate technetium 99m pertechnetate.

Hemangioma and Lymphangioma Hemangiomata and lymphangiomata are benign nonepithelial tumors of the salivary glands, almost always involving the parotid gland. These tumors are composed of a network of epithelium-lined capillaries or lymphatic spaces, respectively. Dilated vascular channels may be identified. Hemangiomas are seen as well-circumscribed, benign-appearing lesions with displacement of the parotid ductal system on sialography. Plain films or CT may demonstrate multiple phleboliths. Tumor may extend to involve the surrounding musculature or parapharyngeal space, mimicking a malignant lesion.

Hemangioma has a heterogenous signal on both T1- and T2-weighted MRI sequences. Areas of signal void may occur secondary to tumor blood flow.

Lipoma and Liposarcoma Lipomas are rare lesions of the parotid gland and may be intraparotid or paraparotid. The characteristic CT and MRI appearance is related to the fat content: low attenuation on CT (−50 to −150 HU), high signal on T1-weighted MRI sequences, and intermediate signal on T2-weighted sequences. It is not possible to differentiate lipoma from liposarcoma on the basis of signal characteristics, since heterogenous signals occur in both lipoma (fibrosis) and liposarcoma (hemorrhage and/or necrosis).

Lipoma in the submandibular or paraparotid region may blend with normal fat.

MALIGNANT NEOPLASMS

Mucoepidermoid Carcinoma Mucoepidermoid carcinoma is the most common salivary gland malignancy, accounting for approximately 10 percent of salivary gland neoplasms. Low-grade mucoepidermoid carcinoma has CT and MRI characteristics resembling those of benign lesions, appearing well circumscribed and regularly marginated without infiltration into the adjacent soft tissues.

Homogenous to heterogenous density is present on CT (Fig. 6-7). There is low to intermediate signal on T1-weighted MRI images with increased signal on T2-weighted images.

Aggressive or cellular mucoepidermoid carcinoma will have irregular margination and infiltration into the soft tissues. Heterogenous CT density may occur but is not a reliable sign of aggressiveness. The MRI appearance of high-grade mucoepidermoid carcinoma reflects the greater cellularity and lower water content of the lesion: signal is intermediate on T1-weighted sequences and remains intermediate on T2-weighted images.

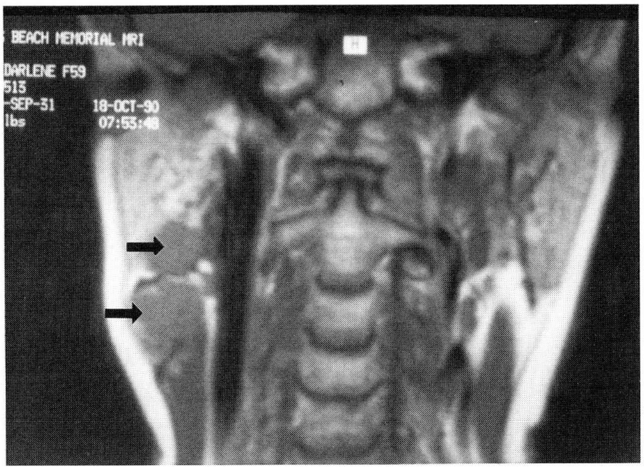

(A)

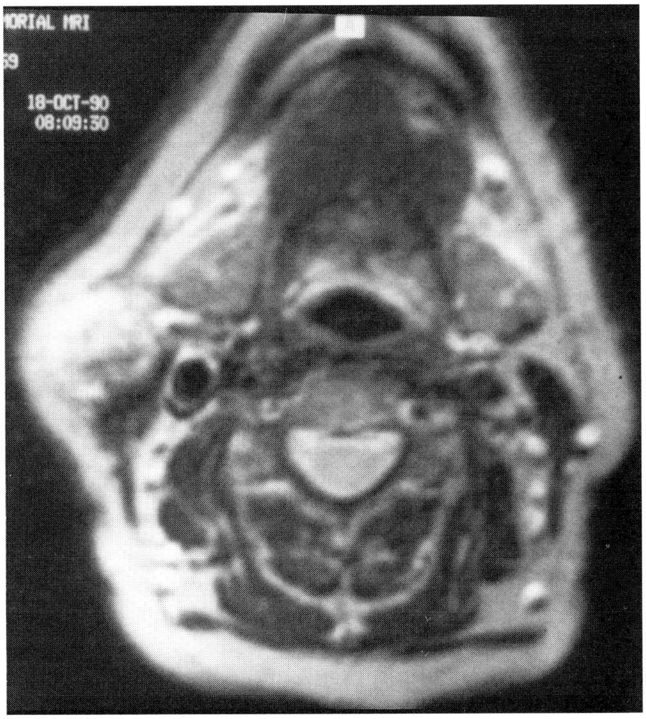

(B)

Figure 6-6 Oncocytoma of the parotid gland. *A*. Coronal T1-weighted MRI (TR/TE 555/20). Well-circumscribed bilobed mass (*arrows*) is intermediate in signal between muscle and normal parotid gland and extends from the tail of the gland. *B*. Axial T2-weighted MRI (TR/TE 2200/80). The mass is moderately and heterogenously increased in signal.

Adenoid Cystic Carcinoma Adenoid cystic carcinoma (Fig. 6-8) accounts for 30 percent of minor salivary gland tumors, 15 percent of submandibular gland tumors, and 2 to 6 percent of parotid gland neoplasms. Adenoid cystic carcinoma has a slow but prolonged course with frequent recurrences. Perineural extension, although seen in squamous-cell carcinoma and other malignancies, is most common in adenoid cystic carcinoma, allowing tumors to spread through the parapharyngeal space or intracranially. On CT, signs of perineural extension include obliteration of the normal fat plane beneath the stylomastoid foramen as well as tumor enhancement along the course of the facial nerve. When noninfiltrating adenoid cystic carcinoma is located within the parotid or submandibular glands, it is indistinguishable from other neoplasms. Tumors in the minor salivary glands will demonstrate diffuse vascular enhancement with variable infiltration into the adjacent soft tissues. Recurrent adenoid cystic carcinoma shows CT enhancement and increased T2-weighted MRI signal which may occur along the course of the facial or parapharyngeal nerves.

Squamous-Cell Carcinoma Squamous-cell carcinoma of the salivary gland occurs most commonly in the parotid gland and is usually the result of metastasis. Primary squamous-cell carcinoma may occur and be quite aggressive. The CT and MRI appearance is nonspecific. When of low grade, it resembles benign neoplasms. When aggressive, characteristic loss of margination, irregularity, and soft tissue infiltration may be identified.

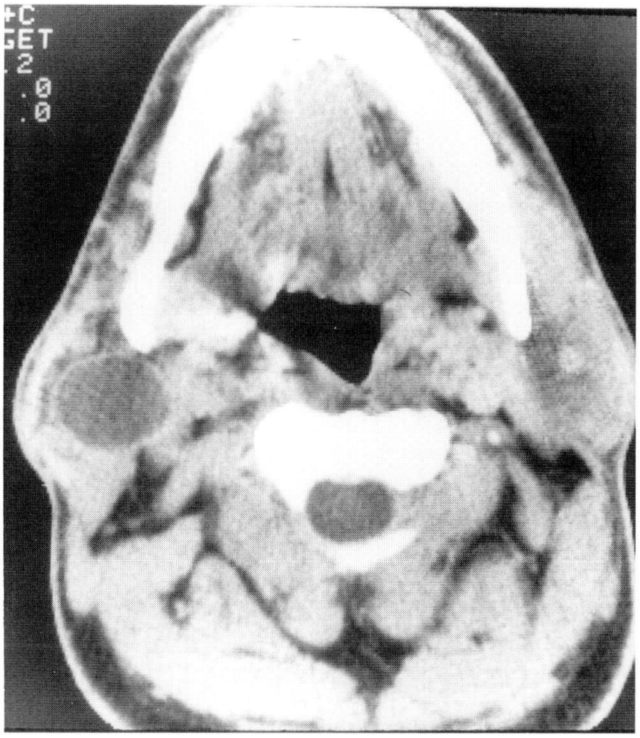

Figure 6-7 Mucoepidermoid carcinoma. On CT, the well-circumscribed low-density mass involves both the superficial and deep lobes of the right parotid gland. The tumor is not distinguishable from a benign lesion.

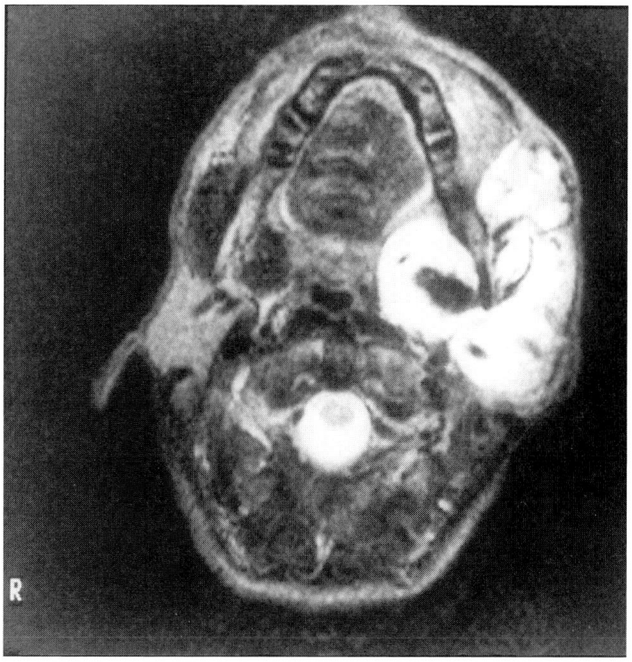

Figure 6-8 Adenoid cystic carcinoma. On MRI, T2-weighted sequence shows extensive heterogenous but very bright mass replacing the left parotid gland. Marked extension into the masseter muscle (*arrow*) and parapharnyngeal space (*arrowheads*).

Lymphoma Salivary gland lymphoma results from systemic lymphoma causing intraglandular and periglandular lymphadenopathy, although intrinsic submandibular gland lymphadenopathy is rare.

Computed tomography will show multiple well-circumscribed homogenous masses within the parotid gland and in the paraparotid region. Additional lymphadenopathy may be present in the submandibular, submental, and internal jugular spaces.

Lymphoma appears homogenous on MRI T1- and proton-density-weighted sequences. Variably increased signal is identified on T2-weighted images. The CT and MRI appearance will be altered in the presence of necrosis.

Inflammatory hyperplastic lymphadenopathy will resemble lymphomatous lymphadenopathy in its CT appearance. Diffuse infiltration of the subcutaneous soft tissue or periparotid region may give a clue as to the inflammatory nature. T2-weighted images on MRI may demonstrate brighter signal with inflammatory lymphadenopathy than in lymphoma.

Malignant Variations of Pleomorphic Adenoma These malignancies include carcinoma ex-pleomorphic adenoma, malignant mixed tumor, and benign metastasizing pleomorphic adenoma. Carcinoma ex-pleomorphic adenoma represents carcinoma, usually adenocarcinoma, of the parotid gland, occurring in 5 percent of benign pleomorphic adenoma, often years later. Metastasis to regional lymph nodes, lungs, bone, and brain may occur. Death usually occurs within 1 year. The malignant mixed tumor is rare. This tumor contains both epithelial and mesenchymal malignant elements and is therefore a true carcinosarcoma.

Both CT and MRI may be of value in demonstrating the progressive nature of carcinoma ex-pleomorphic adenoma and malignant mixed tumor when they are infiltrative. However, they are usually not distinguishable from other neoplasms of the parotid gland (Fig. 6-9).

Benign metastasizing pleomorphic adenoma is rare, manifested as a histologically benign tumor that is locally aggressive or undergoes hematogenous metastasis. It must be distinguished from recurrent pleomorphic adenoma or multicentric pleomorphic adenoma.

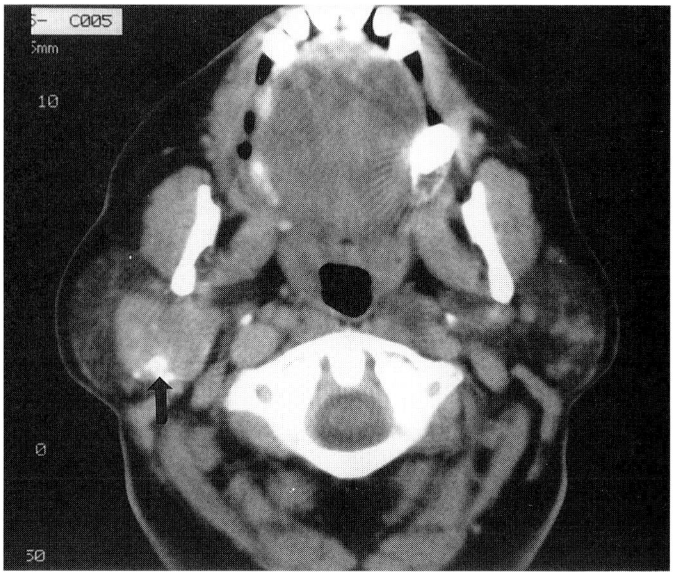

Figure 6-9 Carcinoma ex-pleomorphic adenoma. On CT, heterogenous, well-circumscribed mass involves both the superficial and deep lobe of the right parotid gland. Note the dense calcification (*arrow*) in the posterior aspect of the mass.

Metastasis Most metastases to the parotid or submandibular gland are from contiguous spread of squamous cell carcinoma of the pharynx and neck. Hematogenous metastases have been described in carcinoma of the breast, neck, lung, and kidney and in metastatic melenoma. Despite the vascularity of the parotid gland, blood-borne metastasis is rare.

SUGGESTED READINGS

1. March DE et al: Computed tomography of salivary glands in Sjögren's syndrome. *Arch Otolaryngol Head Neck Surg* 115:105, 1989.
2. Som PM et al: Tumors of the parapharyngeal space: Preoperative evaluation, diagnosis and surgical approaches. *Ann Otol Rhinol Laryngol* 90(suppl 80):3–15, 1981.
3. Som PM et al: Tumors of the parapharyngeal space and upper neck: MRI imaging characteristics. *Radiology* 164:823–829, 1987.
4. Tabor EK, Curtin HD: MR of the salivary glands. *Radiol Clin North Am* 27:379—392, 1989.
5. Teresi LM et al: Parotid masses: MR imaging. *Radiology* 163:405–409, 1987.

☐ QUESTIONS (True or False)

1. Regarding sialography,
- **a.** CT and MRI have replaced sialography in the evaluation of neoplasm of salivary gland.
- **b.** It is useful for evaluation of submandibular or parotid gland sialolithiasis.
- **c.** It is useful for evaluation of posttraumatic or postoperative fistula.
- **d.** It is useful for evaluation of acute salivary gland infection.
- **e.** It is useful for evaluation of chronic inflammatory processes.

2. Regarding parotid gland,
- **a.** A facial plane divides the parotid gland into superficial and deep lobes.
- **b.** The superficial lobe is lateral to the medial margin of the ramus and abuts the posterior aspect of the masseter muscle.
- **c.** Posteriorly the superficial lobe abuts the sternocleidomastoid muscle.
- **d.** The deep lobe extends behind the ramus of the mandible.
- **e.** The deep lobe is bordered medially by the parapharyngeal space, internal carotid artery, and internal jugular vein.

3. Regarding parapharyngeal space and masticator space,
   a. A parapharyngeal space mass arising from the parotid gland or minor salivary glands will displace the internal carotid artery posteriorly.
   b. Parapharyngeal space is divided into the prestyloid and poststyloid components.
   c. Poststyloid masses usually represent paraganglioma, neuroma, or lymphadenopathy.
   d. Salivary gland tumors commonly occur in masticator space.
   e. The masticator space contains the masseter muscle, temporalis muscle, medial and lateral pterygoid muscles.

4. Regarding pleomorphic adenoma,
   a. It is the most common neoplasm of the salivary glands.
   b. Pleomorphic adenoma occurs most commonly in the parotid glands.
   c. Pheomorphic adenoma is extremely rare in submandibular glands.
   d. The CT appearance of pleomorphic adenoma is that of a well-circumscribed mass with homogenous to heterogenous density.
   e. Hemorrhage, dystrophic calcification may be seen in pleomorphic adenoma.

5. Regarding Warthin's tumor,
   a. It accounts for less than 10 percent of parotid tumors.
   b. These tumors could be malignant.
   c. The CT appearance of Warthin's tumor is that of a homogenous well-circumscribed mass in the parotid gland.
   d. Approximately 10 percent of Warthin's tumors are bilateral.
   e. The MRI appearance is that of a homogeneous well-circumscribed mass with intermediate low signal intensity of T1-weighted images with increase in signal on T2-weighted images.

☐ ANSWERS

1. a. T
   b. T
   c. T
   d. F
   e. T

2. a. F
   b. T
   c. T
   d. T
   e. T

3. a. T
   b. T
   c. T
   d. F
   e. T

4. a. T
   b. T
   c. F
   d. T
   e. T

5. a. T
   b. F
   c. T
   d. T
   e. T

CHAPTER 7

Neck

John Go

NORMAL ANATOMY

In the past, for purposes of staging squamous-cell carcinoma, the suprahyoid neck has clinically been subdivided into three regions: the nasopharynx, oropharynx, and oral cavity. The nasopharynx and oropharynx are separated by an imaginary line drawn through the hard and soft palates. The borders of the nasopharynx are as follows:

- Anterior: posterior nasal cavity.
- Superior and posterior: sphenoid sinus and clivus.
- Laterally: The lateral nasopharyngeal wall. Found along the lateral wall is the torus tubarius, which separates the opening of the eustachian tubes and the mucosa lining the fossa of Rosenmuller (found along the posterolateral aspect of the neck).

The boundaries of the oropharynx include the following:

- Anterior: inferior to the ridge of circumvallate papillae on the tongue
- Posterior: constrictor muscles of the oropharynx
- Inferior: Separation from the hypopharynx by the pharyngoepiglottic folds and from the larynx by the epiglottis and glossoepiglottic folds

The oral cavity is the space within the mouth anterior to the circumvallate papillae of the tongue.

This subdivision of the suprahyoid neck is effective for the staging of squamous-cell cancers of the head and neck, but non-squamous cell cancer tends to spread along fascial enclosed spaces. These spaces, which, in the nineteenth century, were defined by anatomists who performed neck dissection on cadavers, were rediscovered by surgeons during drainage of neck abscesses. The abscesses were seen to be confined within these anatomically enclosed compartments within the neck. Harnsberger and coworkers have advocated this space-oriented subdivision of the neck, which separates the neck into spaces and correlates well with cross-sectional imaging.

The neck is basically enclosed by two fascial planes: the superficial and deep cervical fascia. The deep cervical fascia is composed of three layers:

1. Superficial layer
2. Middle or buccopharyngeal layer
3. Deep layer

These three layers subdivide the suprahyoid neck into seven spaces, as follows:

1. Pharyngeal mucosal space
2. Retropharyngeal space
3. Parapharyngeal space
4. Carotid space
5. Parotid space
6. Masticator space
7. Perivertebral space (for prevertebral space)

The superficial layer of deep cervical fascia invests the strap muscles of the neck, forms the posterior and lateral borders of the pharyngeal mucosal space, and contributes to parts of the posterior and the lateral borders of the carotid space.

The middle layer of deep cervical fascia surrounds the masticator and parotid spaces; it forms the posterolateral border of the carotid space and the lateral border of the parapharyngeal space as well as the anterior wall of the retropharyngeal space.

Table 7-1
DEEP SPACES OF THE SUPRAHYOID NECK

Fascia-Enclosed Space	Contents
Pharyngeal mucosal space[a]	Pharyngeal constrictor muscles Lymph nodes Minor salivary glands Levator veli palatini and eustachian tube Salpingopharyngeus muscle
Parapharyngeal space	Fat Branches of CN V_3 Ascending pharyngeal artery Internal maxillary artery Pharyngeal venous plexus
Masticator space	Muscles of mastication CN V_3 Ramus of mandible Inferior alveolar vein and artery
Carotid space	Lymph nodes Carotid artery and internal jugular vein Vagus nerve CN IX to XII (in area of nasopharynx) Sympathetic chain
Retropharyngeal space	Potential space between middle and deep layer of deep cervical fascia Fat
Parotid space	Lymph nodes Parotid gland Facial nerve External carotid Retromandibular vein
Perivertebral space	Prevertebral and paraspinal muscles Spinal column Vertebral arteries Phrenic nerve Brachial plexus

[a]The pharyngeal mucosal space is not totally enclosed by fascia, as its inner surface is the pharyngeal mucosa

Modified from Table 1-2, "Critical Contents of the Deep Spaces of the Suprahyoid Head and Neck," in HR Harnsberger: *Handbook of Head and Neck Imaging*, 2d ed. St. Louis, Mosby 1995.

The deep layer of deep cervical fascia (also called Cooper's fascia) surrounds the peripharyngeal and parapharyngeal space; it forms the medial aspect of the carotid space as well as the posterior boundary of the retropharyngeal space. Thus, the retropharyngeal space is a potential space between the middle and deep layers of deep cervical fascia. The portion of the deep layer that makes up the posterior border of the retropharyngeal space is composed of anterior and posterior slips. The potential space found between the two is called the danger space and extends from the skull base to the mediastinum, where the two slips merge. The importance of this space is that infection arising from the suprahyoid neck in the danger space may extend into the mediastinum. Both the retropharyngeal and danger spaces extend inferiorly to approximately the T3 vertebral body.

The infrahyoid neck may also be subdivided into fascial enclosed spaces by the three layers of deep cervical fascia. Like the suprahyoid neck, the three layers of deep cervical fascia are:

1. Superficial
2. Middle
3. Deep

The spaces formed are:

1. Visceral
2. Carotid
3. Posterior cervical
4. Retropharyngeal
5. Perivertebral

The superficial layer envelops the strap muscles and forms the anterior and lateral borders of the carotid space. The superior extension of this layer was discussed earlier, forming the masticator and parotid spaces.

The middle layer forms the visceral space and contributes to the medial, anterior, and lateral borders of the carotid space. The anterior border of the middle layer of

Table 7-2
DEEP SPACES OF THE INFRAHYOID NECK

Fascia-Enclosed Space	Contents
Carotid space, retropharyngeal space, and perivertebral space extend into the infrahyoid neck from the suprahyoid neck	Similar to suprahyoid neck CN X is the only cranial nerve extending into infrahyoid neck in carotid space
Visceral space (only space unique to infrahyoid neck)	Hypopharynx, larynx, trachea, esophagus Thyroid, parathyroid Lymph nodes Recurrent laryngeal nerves
Posterior cervical space (extends from a small superior tip at skull base to clavicle)	Fat CN XI Preaxillary branchial plexus Lymph nodes

Modified from Table 9-1, "Space and Contents of the Infrahyoid Neck," in HR Harnsberger: *Handbook of Head and Neck Imaging,* 2d ed. St. Louis, Mosby-Yearbook, 1995.

deep cervical fascia fuses with the superficial layer, which envelops the adjacent strap muscles. The anterior portion of the middle layer splits to invest the thyroid gland.

The deep layer of cervical fascia envelops and forms the perivertebral space and is the inferior extension of the same space as in the suprahyoid neck. This layer of deep cervical fascia also forms the posterior and posteromedial border of the carotid space and the posterior and lateral borders of the retropharyngeal space.

For a complete list of the various spaces of the suprahyoid neck, please refer to Chapter 5.

Of historical importance, another method of subdividing the neck is to subdivide the neck anatomically into "triangles" based on the neck muscles. The sternocleidomastoid muscle divides the neck into anterior and posterior triangles. The submental and submandibular triangles make up the suprahyoid component of the anterior triangle and are separated by the anterior and posterior bellies of the digastric muscles. The boundaries of these triangles are:

1. Submental triangle
   - Lateral—anterior belly of digastric
   - Superior—inferior border of mandible
   - Inferior—hyoid bone
2. Submandibular triangle
   - Medial—anterior belly of digastric
   - Lateral—posterior belly of digastric
   - Superior—lower border of the body of the mandible

The infrahyoidal components of the anterior triangle are as follows:

3. Muscular triangle
   - Medial—midline
   - Superior—hyoid bone
   - Inferior—sternocleidomastoid
   - Lateral border—superior belly of omohyoid and the sternocleidomastoid muscle
4. Carotid triangle
   - Superior—posterior belly of digastric muscle
   - Medial—superior belly of omohyoid muscle
   - Inferior and lateral—sternocleidomastoid muscle

The posterior triangle may be subdivided into two smaller triangles:

5. Occipital triangle
   - Lateral—trapezius muscle
   - Superior and medial—sternocleidomastoid muscle
   - Inferior—inferior belly of omohyoid muscle
6. Subclavian triangle
   - Inferior—clavicle
   - Superolateral—inferior belly of the omohyoid muscle
   - Medial—sternocleidomastoid muscle

□ CONGENITAL CYSTIC LESIONS OF THE NECK

THYROGLOSSAL DUCT CYST

Etiology The thyroid gland originates from the primitive pharynx as a focal area of thickening within the endoderm at approximately 24 days of gestation. This focal area of thickening is midline in position and caudal to the future tongue bud. Downward growth by this thyroid diverticulum occurs within the neck, ventral to the thyroid cartilage. During its descent, the thyroid diverticulum divides into two lobes connected by the isthmus. By 7 weeks, the developed gland has reached its final position in the inferior neck.

The thyroid diverticulum is connected via the thyroglossal duct to the tongue base. The foramen cecum is the cephalad opening of the thyroglossal duct. By the time the thyroid gland has reached its final position, the thyroglossal duct has disappeared (by 8 to 10 weeks). Occasionally, however, there may be persistence of the thyroglossal duct or, anywhere along the course of the embryonic thyroglossal duct, a cyst that presents as a neck mass.

Incidence Thyroglossal duct cysts (TDCs) are the most common midline neck masses, accounting for approximately 90 percent of congenital neck lesions. Ectopic thyroid tissue found along the course of the thyroglossal duct account for 0.6 to 36.5 percent of lesions.

Age and Gender About 50 percent of TDCs occur before the age of 10 years. A second peak is seen between 20 and 40 years. There is no sexual predominance.

Location About 75 percent of TDCs occur in the midline. By location, 20 percent are found in the suprahyoid region, 15 percent are associated with the hyoid bone, and 65 percent are located in the infrahyoid region deep to the strap muscles. The more inferior the cyst is in location, the more likely the cyst is midline. Because the path of the thyroglossal duct is initially anterior to the midportion of the hyoid bone and courses along the inferior and posterior surface before descending inferiorly, a TDC may involve the midportion of the hyoid bone, and this should be taken into consideration with regard to treatment.

Clinical Presentation Thyroglossal duct cysts present as palpable midline neck masses that may move superiorly, with tongue protrusion on physical exam. Complications include cyst rupture or infection. In some instances, sinus tract formation to the skin may form secondary to cyst perforation and infection forming a thyroglossal duct sinus.

There is a 1 percent incidence of carcinoma within a TDC which unsurprisingly, is of thyroid origin. About 85 percent of such cases are of the papillary type. Because of the risk of infection and carcinoma, TDCs are removed surgically.

The Sistrunk operation includes removal of the tract of the duct, resection of the base of the tongue, removal of the midportion of the hyoid bone, and pyramidal lobe of the thyroid gland.

Imaging *Computed Tomography*

- The cyst is of low density, with a thin wall that enhances with contrast.
- Attenuation of the cyst contents may be increased secondary to increased proteinaceous fluid.
- With infection, there may be wall thickening and loss of sharpness of the wall as well as infiltration of the surrounding fat.

Magnetic Resonance Imaging

- The cyst contents are of intermediate signal on T1-weighted images and hyperintense on T2-weighted images.
- With increasing proteinaceous fluid, the signal intensity on T1-weighted and T2-weighted images may increase.

As mentioned above, the incidence of ectopic thyroid tissue along the course of the thyroglossal duct varies from 0.6 to 26.5 percent. The most common location for ectopic thyroid tissue is in the lingual region. On CT, the ectopic thyroid behaves like normal thyroid; it is increased in attenuation precontrast secondary to its iodine content and enhances postcontrast.

BRANCHIAL APPARATUS ABNORMALITIES

Embryology Branchial apparatus abnormalities (BAAs) occur secondary to incomplete obliteration of the first or second branchial arch remnants, failure of the cervical sinus to obliterate during development, or failure of the second branchial apparatus to proliferate.

Incidence Some 95 percent of BAAs are derived from the second branchial arch. The most common abnormality is a cyst, though sinuses or fistulas may form. Abnormalities of the first branchial apparatus (BA) account for approximately 5 percent of all BAAs, with an equal number of cysts and sinuses occurring. Lesions of the third or fourth branchial apparatus are rare.

Age and Gender Branchial cleft cysts, the most common BAAs, usually present between the ages of 10 and 40 years; clinically, however, they may present at any age.

Location As mentioned above, abnormalities of the first BA present as cysts or sinuses with equal frequency.

- First branchial cleft cysts may be seen superficial to, within, or deep to the parotid gland.
- Abnormalities of the second BA are usually found at the angle of the mandible along the anterior margin of the sternocleidomastoid muscle. The most common form of this lesion is a cyst with a sinus or fistula tract.
- Abnormalities of the third BA are usually found in the posterior cervical space. Occasionally, cysts of the second BA may protrude posteriorly into the postcervical space; however, if the lesion is centered in the postcervical space, it is most likely an abnormality of the third BA.

Clinical Presentation

- Since most lesions are derived from the second branchial arch, the usual presentation is a painless fluctuant mass along the anterior border of the sternocleidomastoid muscle after an upper respiratory infection or trauma.
- First branchial cleft cyst often presents as "parotid abscesses" unresponsive to treatment. Otorrhea may be seen when the cyst connects to the bony-cartilaginous junction of the external canal.

Imaging *Computed Tomography*

- The cysts are thin-walled and unilocular with variable amounts of rim enhancement (Fig. 7-1).
- Septations are uncommon unless there is an associated infection.
- Cyst contents are usually between 10 and 25 HU, but this may be increased with infection.
- Large branchial cleft cysts may displace the carotid sheath structures posteromedially.

Magnetic Resonance Imaging

- The cyst contents are typically isointense or slightly hyperintense to cerebrospinal fluid (CSF) on T1- and T2-weighted images.
- Various degree of rim enhancement may be seen.

Differential Diagnosis Infected cysts may be confused with abscesses or necrotic lymph nodes, and clinical correlation is recommended to make the diagnosis.

CYSTIC HYGROMAS/LYMPHANGIOMAS

Embryology Lymphatic drainage of the neck originates from a number of lymphatic sacs that drain into the jugular venous system. Because of either agenesis or hypoplasia of the lymphatic sacs or obstruction of lymphatic drainage into the jugular venous system, cysts of varying sizes may form in the neck. Cystic hygromas/lymphangiomas (CH/L) represent a spectrum in this in utero form of lymphatic obstruction.

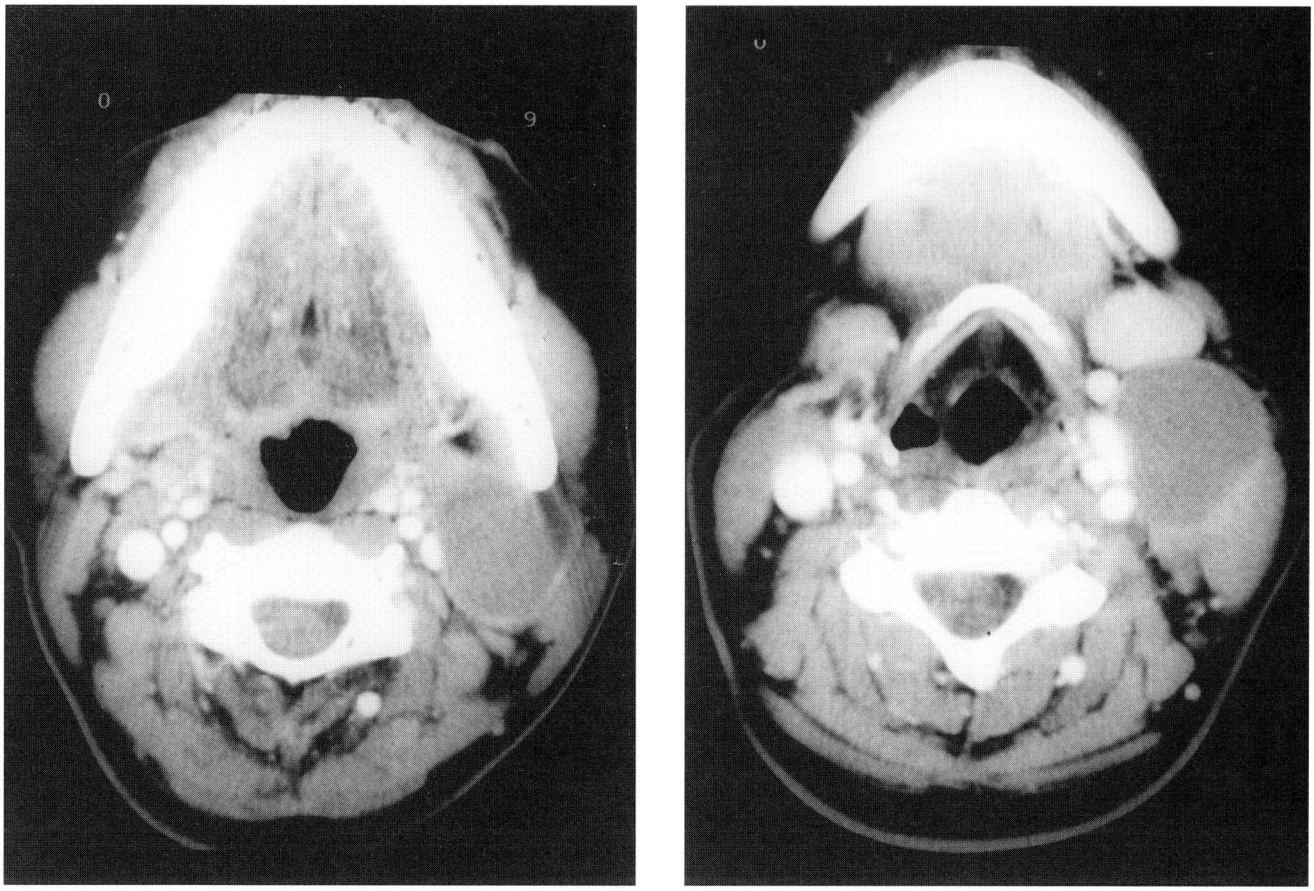

(A) (B)

Figure 7-1 Branchial cleft cyst. *A* and *B*. Axial postcontrast CT scan shows a cystic mass with faint rim enhancement, located at the angle of the mandible, posterior to the submandibular gland, anterior and medial to the sternocleidomastoid muscle, and lateral to the carotid artery and jugular vein.

Pathology Cystic hygromas/lymphangiomas are difficult to differentiate pathologically but may be subdivided into three types based on size:

1. Capillary lymphangiomas (small cystic areas)
2. Cavernous lymphangiomas (medium cystic areas)
3. Cystic hygromas (large cystic areas)

Incidence The incidence of cystic hygromas is 1:6500 pregnancies. Associated conditions with cystic hygromas include:

1. Turner's syndrome
2. Fetal alcohol syndrome
3. Noonan's syndrome
4. Familial pterygoid colli
5. Trisomy 13, 18, 21, 22
6. Distichiasis-lymphedema syndrome

Age and Gender Because CH represent a congenital functional/anatomic obstruction of lymphatic flow, 50 to 60 percent present at birth while 90 percent present by the age of 2.

Location Some 75 percent of CHs present in the neck, while 20 percent appear in the axillary region (3 to 10 percent present as mediastinal masses, extending from the neck). The remaining 5 percent are scattered in various areas such as the retroperitoneum, abdomen, scrotum, and bone.

The most common area within the neck is within the posterior cervical space, but CHs have been found within the submandibular, parotid, and sublingual spaces, with larger lesions extending by direct spread to other parts of the neck.

Clinical Presentation Cystic hygromas are painless, fluctuant, and easily compressible masses. The larger lesions may transilluminate with a light source on physical examination. With compression of the trachea, pharynx, or esophagus, larger lesions may present with symptoms of dyspnea or dysphagia.

Depending on the extent of lymphatic obstruction, prognosis may vary from 100 percent fatality secondary to fetal hydrops to spontaneous regression in 10 to 15 percent of cases.

Imaging *Ultrasound* In utero diagnosis may be made if multiloculated primarily cystic masses are seen. Echogenic masses may be present, representing small clusters of dilated cysts that are too small to resolve individually.

Computed Tomography

- Cystic hygromas are usually seen as fluid density masses with thin cyst walls with or without septations and typically without rim enhancement.
- Because these lesions are easily compressible, they do not exert mass effect (except larger lesions) and are frequently compressed by their surrounding structures. This fact may aid in differentiating these lesions from other cystic lesions such as branchial cleft cysts, necrotic lymph nodes, or abscesses.
- These lesions may rapidly increase in size because of secondary hemorrhage or infection, and there may be an increase in attenuation of the cyst contents.
- Secondary signs of infection may change the CT or MRI appearance of the lesion.

Magnetic Resonance Imaging

- Typically, cyst contents are hypointense on T1-weighted images and hyperintense on T2-weighted images (Fig. 7-2).
- Septations may be seen.
- After gadolinium injection, no rim enhancement is seen.

DERMOID CYSTS

Embryology Lesions derived from dermal elements (ecto-, meso-, or endoderm) may also present as cystic lesions, the most common being dermoid cysts. Classically, epidermoids were thought to originate from ectoderm, while dermoids were believed to arise from ecto- and mesodermal elements. Mesodermal products such as hair as well as sebaceous and sweat glands—which were thought to arise from mesoderm—actually arise from embryonic ectodermal elements within the mesoderm. Dermoids may therefore be referred to as ectodermal inclusion cysts.

Incidence Dermoid cysts are the least common type of congenital lesion. While 80 percent are found in the oral cavity or orbit, 7 percent are located in the head and neck regions.

Epidermoid cysts most commonly occur at birth. Dermoids may be found at birth but usually present at 1 to 2 year of age.

Locations Suprahyoid dermoid cysts are usually found in the midline and may occur in the floor of the mouth, the sublingual/submental regions, and the soft palate.

Clinical Presentation Unlike thyroglossal duct cysts, which are usually associated with the tongue or hyoid bone, dermoid cysts have no such predilection and do not move on tongue protrusion. Like other space-occupying lesions, dermoids may cause patients to present with dysphagia/dyspnea when the lesion compresses the trachea, pharynx, or esophagus, but these lesions are usually asymptomatic and are found incidentally.

Imaging *Computed Tomography/Magnetic Resonance Imaging* Without the presence of fat, epidermoids/dermoids cannot be distinguished. As they are normally low-density lesions, it may be hard to distinguish them from

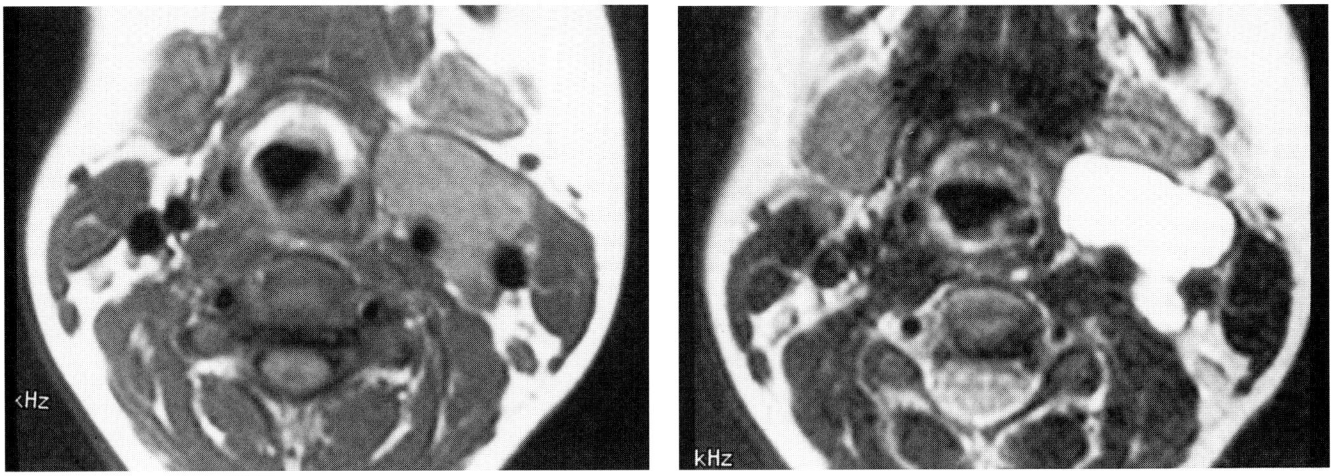

(A) (B)

Figure 7-2 Cystic hygroma. *A*. Axial T1-weighted image shows a hypointense cystic mass with internal septations in the submandibular space, with extension into the posterior cervical space. *B*. Axial T2-weighted image demonstrates a hyperintense cystic mass with internal septation.

ranulas, branchial cleft cysts, cystic hygromas, thyroglossal duct cysts, or abscesses.

On CT, epidermoids are similar to fluid in attenuation and exhibit fluid characteristics on MRI.

Dermoids may be of mixed signal on MRI secondary to their contents (increased protein content from the secretion from the glandular elements) and fat content.

INFLAMMATORY MASSES

On physical examination, it is difficult for the clinician to distinguish between cellulitis versus abscess in a clinically evident inflammatory process involving the neck. Computed tomography with contrast is currently the modality of choice to distinguish these two processes.

Cellulitis is an inflammatory process of the skin and underlying subcutaneous tissues without a definite focal fluid collection. On CT, there is skin thickening and increased streaky density in the subcutaneous tissue, which may represent a combination of dilated lymphatics, edema, and/or infiltration by inflammatory cells. There may also be loss of distinction of the fascial planes, with variable amounts of enhancement of the fascia surrounding adjacent muscles. Variable amounts of muscle thickening may also occur, depending on the extent of inflammation.

Abscesses, however, contain one or more areas of fluidlike density surrounded by rim enhancement as well as the changes seen with cellulitis. Loculations/septations may also be seen within the abscess. The wall surrounding the fluid collection is usually thick. Abscesses may occur as a progressive sequela of cellulitis, but they may also be secondary to other infectious sources, such as odontogenic infection, osteomyelitis, or trauma. The possibility of necrotic lymph nodes and infected congenital cysts should also be considered. Location of the lesion and clinical correlation is warranted.

The multiplanar capabilities of MRI may aid in determining the true extent and location of an abscess. They are typically of fluid signal intensity with thick walled rim enhancement plus or minus septation, with adjacent signal abnormalities within the adjacent subcutaneous tissue, skin, and muscle.

☐ MISCELLANEOUS CYSTIC LESIONS

RANULAS

Ranulas are mucous retention cysts that originate from an obstructed sublingual or minor solitary gland. They may be divided into the two types:

1. Simple—confined to the sublingual space and presenting as an intraoral mass
2. Plunging or diving—extension of the lesion around or through the mylohyoid muscle into the neck, usually in the submandibular region. This extension occurs secondary to cyst rupture and represents formation of a pseudocyst.

Imaging ***Computed Tomography/Magnetic Resonance Imaging*** The cyst contents are of fluid density (CT) and signal intensity (MRI). Differentiation between types I and II may be made depending upon the relationship of the lesion to the mylohyoid muscle. The cyst wall is typically thin and the lesion is usually multilocular in appearance.

LARYNGOCELE/PHARYNGOCELE

Laryngocele/pharyngocele is usually secondary to chronic increased pressure within the larynx or hypopharynx respectively. A laryngocele represents a dilated appendix of the laryngeal ventricle, while the less common pharyngocele represents herniation through the thyrohyoid membrane.

Edema or neoplasm within the laryngeal ventricle may obstruct the laryngeal appendix and by a ball-valve mechanism trap air in the appendix. Mucus secreted by the epithelium within the appendix may result in the formation of a fluid-filled laryngocele (a laryngeal mucocele).

Laryngoceles are usually confined to the perilaryngeal space.

Imaging ***Computed Tomography/Magnetic Resonance Imaging***

- A thin-walled, fluid-containing structure in a perilaryngeal location is usually seen in continuity with the laryngeal ventricle on cross-sectional imaging.
- With the less common pharyngocele, continuation with the pyriform sinus instead of the laryngeal ventricle is seen.

LYMPH NODES

Anatomy Of the 800 lymph nodes in the human body, approximately 300 are found in the cervical region. Based on the works of Rouviere, cervical lymph nodes were categorized into 10 anatomic locations based on which triangular space and adjacent neurovascular bundle they were near. This classification system has been simplified by the American Committee on Cancer (1994), subdividing lymph nodes by anatomic sites and then grouping by specific levels. The levels are as follows:

Level I.	Submandibular and submental nodes.
Level II.	Deep cervical chain: upper-jugular-chain-level (upper one-third); extends from the skull base to the level of the hyoid bone.
Level III.	Deep cervical chain: middle-jugular-chain level (mid one-third); extends from the level of hyoid bone to cricoid cartilage.

Level IV. Deep cervical chain: lower-jugular-chain level (lower one-third); extends from the level of cricoid cartilage to the clavicles.

Level V. Nodes in the posterior triangle, including lymph nodes along the course of the spinal accessary nerve and nodes that traverse the superior margin of the clavicles (transverse cervical chain).

Level VI. Precricoid, prelaryngeal, pretracheal, and paratracheal lymph nodes. (Note: lymph nodes are in the anterior compartment of the neck extending from the hyoid bone to the suprasternal notch.)

Level VII. Upper mediastinal lymph nodes.

Other groups of lymph nodes in the neck of less clinical significance are not included in the above classification system and are as follows:

1. Parotid.
2. Mastoids.
3. Occipital.
4. Submaxillary.
5. Facial—follows the facial artery and vein.
6. Sublingual—follows the lingual vessels.
7. Retropharyngeal.
   a. *Lateral group*—nodes follow the longus capitis muscle, medial to the carotid artery and CN IX through XII. (Also called nodes of Rouviere.)
   b. *Medial group*—nodes are near midline in position and in close proximity to the posterior wall, extending from the C1–2 articulation to the level of the hyoid bone.
8. Submental.
9. Nodes of the superior spinal accessory chain and superior aspect of the internal jugular chain.

The jugulodigastric node and Virchow's nodes are, respectively, the highest and lowest nodes along the internal jugular chain. Waldeyer's ring is an imaginary ring formed by the adenoids, palatine, and lingual tonsils, all of which contain lymphoid tissue. The clinical significance is that lymphoma of Waldeyer's ring cannot be differentiated from squamous cell carcinoma without biopsy. Infectious mononucleosis may have a similar appearance. The Delphian or prelaryngeal node, if enlarged in the setting of laryngeal carcinoma, signifies subglottic involvement.

Pathology and Radiology Lymph node pathology can be based on the following characteristics:

- Size—lymph nodes greater than 1 cm (measured on transverse scans along the short axis of the lymph node) are considered pathologic. The exception to this rule are the submental–submandibular and jugulodigastric nodes, which may be up to 1.5 cm in size. Adenopathy based on this criterion represents metastatic disease in 80 percent of cases, while 20 percent are due to reactive hyperplasia (Fig. 7-3).
- Contours—lymph nodes are fairly well circumscribed by the surrounding fat. Irregular or shaggy border suggests infiltration of the surrounding fat by tumor or inflammation.
- Density—nodes are of soft tissue density and fairly homogeneous. Central low density or low intensity on contrast-enhanced CT or T1-weighted MRI represents necrosis. Heterogeneous appearance of the nodes may signify infiltration or necrosis.
- Calcification—calcifications in lymph nodes are not common but may be seen in granulomatous disease, postradiation or chemotherapy of lymphoma, or metastatic disease, such as papillary carcinoma of the thyroid.

TUBERCULOUS ADENITIS (SCROFULA)

Organisms:

1. *Mycobacterium bovis* (classically)
2. *Mycobacterium tuberculosis*
3. Atypical mycobacteria:
   a. *Mycobacterium kansasii*
   b. *Mycobacterium avium-intracellulare*
   c. *Mycobacterium scrofulaceum*

Mycobacterium tuberculosis and atypical mycobacteria are the most common causes of tuberculous adenitis in the United States.

Incidence Tuberculosis lymphadenopathy represents about 5 percent of cases of cervical lymphadenopathy and is usually seen in patients from third-world countries, especially Southeast Asia.

Presentation ***Mycobacterium tuberculosis*** The lymphadenopathy seen is usually asymptomatic, firm, and nontender. If there is a concurrent infection, local inflammatory changes may be demonstrated. The age range is 20 to 30 years, and 50 percent of cases occur with concurrent systemic infection (previous exposure to tuberculosis). The nodal masses may occur from 2 weeks to 5 years after the initial infections.

Atypical mycobacteria Usually present with unilateral involvement and is more common in children. Areas of involvement are in the parotid, submandibular, upper cervical, and preauricular nodes.

Imaging ***Mycobacterium tuberculosis***—The distribution of nodes is primarily bilateral, in the posterior triangle. The more inferior the location of the nodes, the more likely that there is pulmonary involvement by *Mycobacterium tuberculosis*. Computed tomography demonstrates homogeneous soft tissue densities (plus or minus enhancement) with a thick rim of peripheral enhancement with or without central necrosis or calcification. With multiple nodes present and destruction of the walls of the masses, the lesions may coalesce, forming a cold abscess. There are usually inflammatory changes in the surrounding fat and skin.

CASTLEMAN'S DISEASE

A form of benign lymphoid hyperplasia of unknown etiology, Castleman's disease occurs in patients less than 30 years of age in 70 percent of cases. Also in 70 percent, the lesions occur in the mediastinum, but adenopathy may be present in the neck, axilla, shoulder, and abdomen. Computed tomography demonstrates the nodes to be homogeneous and of soft tissue density with a nonenhancing vascular rim.

Other causes for reactive lymphadenopathy include postinfectious (such as an adjacent abscess or postviral infection such as mononucleosis) and granulomatous disease.

LYMPHOMA

- Lymphomatous cervical adenopathy may be secondary to Hodgkin's or non-Hodgkin's lymphoma.
- Some 25 percent of cases of lymphomatous adenopathy are secondary to Hodgkin's disease.
- The following is a list of different features of Hodgkin's vs. non-Hodgkin's lymphoma.

	Hodgkin's	Non-Hodgkin's
Lymph node enlargement	Common	Common
Extranodal involvement	Rare	Common
Lymph node size	0.5–> 1 cm	0.5–> 1 cm
Necrosis	Less common	More common

- The non-Hodgkin's type (especially in AIDS patients) may demonstrate necrotic lymphadenopathy, seen as low-density nodes on CT scan.
- Lymph node enlargement is the common presentation for both non-Hodgkin's and Hodgkin's lymphoma.
- Based on imaging features, differentiation of nodal enlargement from non-Hodgkin's lymphoma, Hodgkin's lymphoma, or metastatic disease is not possible.

UNKNOWN PRIMARY TUMOR

Some 12 percent of patients with head and neck carcinoma and 5 percent of those with carcinoma may present with cervical lymphadenopathy, even though the site of origin of the neoplasm has not been discovered by the clinicians (Fig. 7-3). Based on the location of the lymphadenopathy, the following primary sites may be considered:

Level I.	(Submental nodes, submandibular nodes) Oral cavity, submandibular gland
Level II.	(Upper deep cervical chain nodes) Supraglottic larynx, nasopharynx, oropharynx, parotid gland
Level III.	(Middle deep cervical chain nodes) Oropharynx, hypopharynx, supraglottic larynx
Level IV.	(Lower deep cervical chain nodes) Subglottic larynx, hypopharynx, esophagus, thyroid
Level V.	(Spinal accessory nodes. Transverse cervical chain nodes) Nasopharynx, oropharynx
Level VI/VII.	(Pretracheal nodes, prelaryngeal nodes,

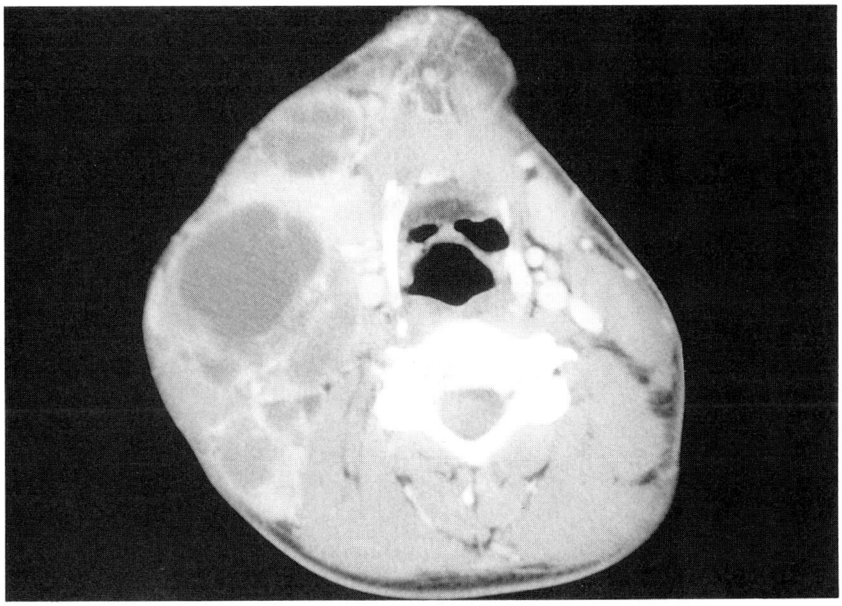

Figure 7-3 Metastatic lymph nodes with necrosis from unknown primary. Axial postcontrast CT scan shows multiple necrotic lymph nodes with poorly demarcated margin on the right side of the neck.

paratracheal nodes, and upper mediastinal nodes)
Thyroid, larynx, or lung

(Published with permission. RA Holliday. Neck Nodes and Masses. ASHNR 26th Annual Conference and Postgraduate Couse, Vancouver, BC, May 13–16, 1993, p95.)

In general, abnormal nodes found low in the neck have a worse prognosis than higher lymph nodes. Bilateral nodal metastases are usually secondary to nasopharyngeal, soft palate, tongue, or epiglottic primaries.

Necrotic lymphadenopathy in the left supraclavicular region may be secondary to metastases from the thyroid or from a primary neoplasm in the thorax or abdomen. Squamous cell nodal metastases spread by direct extension along the lymphatic chain. "Skip" lesions suggest that the primary is not from the neck.

INFECTION WITH HUMAN IMMUNODEFICIENCY VIRUS

Bilateral cervical lymphadenopathy with the presence of intraparotid lymphoepithelial cysts is highly indicative of human immunodeficiency virus (HIV) infection and may occur before the patient seroconverts. The lymph nodes seen are homogeneous and of soft tissue density. The parotid cysts are of fluid density on CT scan. The nodes may range in size from 0.5 to 2 cm.

SUGGESTED READINGS

1. Armington WG et al: Radiographic evaluation of brachial plexopathy. *AJNR* 8:361–367, 1987.
2. Babbel RW et al: The visceral space: The unique infrahyoid space. *Semin Ultrasound CT MR* 12:204–223, 1991.
3. Benson MT et al: Congenital anomalies of the branchial apparatus: Embryology and pathologic anatomy. *RadioGraphics* 12:943–960, 1992.
4. Curtin HD: Separation of the masticator space from the parapharyngeal space. *Radiology* 163:195–204, 1987.
5. Davis WL et al: Retropharyngeal space: Evaluation of the normal and disease with CT and MR imaging. *Radiology* 174:59–64, 1990.
6. Dillon WP et al: Magnetic resonance imaging of the nasopharynx. *Radiology* 152:731–738, 1984.
7. Hardin CW et al: CT in the evaluation of the normal and diseased oral cavity and oropharynx. *Semin Ultrasound CT MR* 6:131–153, 1986.
8. Hardin CW et al: Infection and tumor of the masticator space: CT evaluation. *Radiology* 157;413–417, 1985.
9. Harnsberger HR: CT and MRI of masses of the deep face. *Curr Probl Diagn Radiol* 16:141–173, 1987.
10. Harnsberger HR, Osborn AG: Differential diagnosis of head and neck lesions based on their space of origin: 1. The suprahyoid part of the neck. *Am J Roentgenol* 157:147–154, 1991.
11. Harnsberger HR: *Handbook of Head and Neck Imaging,* 2d ed. St. Louis, Mosby, 1995.
12. Holliday RA: Neck nodes and masses. ASHNR 26th Annual Conference and Posgraduate Course. Vancouver, BC, May 13–16, 1993.
13. Lindberg R: Distribution of cervical lymph node metastases from squamous cell carcinoma of the upper respiratory and digestive tracts. *Cancer* 29:1446–1449, 1972.
14. Mancuso AA et al: Computed tomography of cervical and retropharyngeal lymph nodes: Normal anatomy, variants of normal, and application in staging head and neck cancer: I. Normal anatomy. *Radiology* 148:709–714, 1983.
15. Mancuso AA et al: Computed tomography of cervical and retropharyngeal lymph nodes: Normal anatomy, variants of normal, and application in staging head and neck cancer: II. Pathology. *Radiology* 148:715–723, 1983.
16. Mancuso AA et al: CT of cervical lymph node cancer. *Am J Roentgenol* 136:381–385, 1981.
17. Reede DL et al: Computed tomography of cervical lymph nodes. *RadioGraphics* 3:339–351, 1983.
18. Som PM, Bergeron RT: *Head and Neck Imaging*, 2d ed. St Louis, Mosby-Year Book, 1991.
19. Som PM: Lymph nodes of the neck. *Radiology* 165:593–600, 1967.
20. Som PM: Detection of metastasis—Cervical lymph nodes: CT & MR criteria and differential diagnosis. *AJR* 158:961–969, 1992.

☐ QUESTIONS (True or False)

1. The following spaces are common to both the suprahyoid and infrahyoid neck:
   a. Carotid space
   b. Periventricular space
   c. Retropharyngeal space
   d. Parotid space
   e. Visceral space

2. Regarding thyroglossal duct cyst,
   a. Represents approximately 90 percent of congenital neck lesions.
   b. Is most commonly seen in the suprahyoid region.
   c. Carcinoma of thyroid origin can occur in a thyroglossal duct cyst.
   d. Cyst wall may enhance with contrast.
   e. Cyst fluid may contain various amounts of protein.

3. Regarding branchial cleft cyst,
- **a.** The majority of branchial cleft cysts derive from the first branchial arch.
- **b.** Branchial cleft cyst is the most common branchial arch anomaly (BAA).
- **c.** Second BAA are usually found along the anterior margin of the sternocleidomastoid muscle.
- **d.** Third BAA are usually found in the posterior cervical space.
- **e.** Differential diagnosis of branchial cleft cyst includes abscess, necrotic lymph nodes.

4. Cystic hygroma may be associated with
- **a.** Turner's syndrome
- **b.** Fetal alcohol syndrome
- **c.** Noonan's syndrome
- **d.** Trisomy 13
- **e.** Neurofibromatosis type I

5. Regarding cystic hygroma,
- **a.** Some 50 percent are present at birth.
- **b.** About 75 percent of cystic hygromas present in the neck.
- **c.** May present as a mediastinal mass.
- **d.** Most commonly seen in posterior triangle.
- **e.** Cystic hygromas are painful masses.

6. Regarding ranulas,
- **a.** They are congenital cysts.
- **b.** Simple ranula is confined to the sublingual space
- **c.** Plunging ranula extends from sublingual space to the submandibular space.
- **d.** The cyst contents are of fluid density or intensity.
- **e.** The cyst wall is very thick.

7. Regarding laryngocele,
- **a.** It is usually secondary to an acute increase in pressure within the larynx.
- **b.** A laryngocele represents a dilated appendix of the laryngeal ventricle.
- **c.** Laryngoceles are usually confined to the perilaryngeal space.
- **d.** Thin-walled, fluid-containing structure.
- **e.** Usually seen in continuity with the laryngeal ventricle.

8. Regarding lymph node pathology,
- **a.** Lymph nodes greater than 5 mm in diameter are considered pathological.
- **b.** Adenopathy may be due to metastatic disease or reactive hyperplasia.
- **c.** Lymph nodes are of soft tissue density and fairly homogeneous.
- **d.** Calcification in lymph nodes may be seen in certain metastatic diseases.
- **e.** Calcification in lymph nodes may be seen in granulomatous disease.

☐ ANSWERS

1. **a.** T **b.** T **c.** T **d.** F **e.** F

2. **a.** T **b.** F **c.** T **d.** T **e.** T

3. **a.** F **b.** F **c.** T **d.** T **e.** T

4. **a.** T **b.** T **c.** T **d.** T **e.** F

5. **a.** T **b.** T **c.** T **d.** T **e.** F

6. **a.** T **b.** T **c.** T **d.** T **e.** F

7. **a.** F **b.** T **c.** T **d.** T **e.** T

8. **a.** F **b.** T **c.** T **d.** T **e.** T

CHAPTER

8 Temporal Bone

William W.M. Lo
Leonard Petrus
Chi S. Zee

☐ NORMAL ANATOMY

TEMPORAL BONE

- Consists of five parts: squamous, mastoid, petrous, tympanic, and the styloid process.

Squamous Portion
- Forms part of the wall of the temporal fossa.
- Gives rise to the zygomatic process.

Mastoid Portion
- Develops after birth.
- Mastoid antrum is situated at the upper and anterior part of the mastoid portion.
- Continues inferiorly in adults as the mastoid process.
- Antrum communicates with the remainder of the mastoid cells and with the epitympanum via the auditus ad antrum.

Petrous Portion
- Resembles a toppled three-sided pyramid wedged between the sphenoid bone anteriorly and the occipital bone posteriorly.
- Has anterior, posterior, and inferior surfaces.

Anterior Surface
- Forms the posterior limit of the middle cranial fossa.
- Arcuate eminence, which marks the site of the underlying semicircular canal, is near its midposition.
- In front and lateral to eminence is the tegmen tympani that separates the tympanic and cranial cavities.

Posterior Surface
- Forms the anterior bony limit of the posterior fossa.
- Near the center is the opening of the internal auditory canal, the porus acousticus.
- Within the internal auditory canal (IAC), the lamina spiralis separates the fundus of the IAC from the vestibule.
- Fundus of the IAC divided into smaller upper and larger lower compartments by crista falciformis.
- Lateral portion of upper compartment separated into anterior and posterior portions by arachnoid tissue, which occasionally ossifies (Bill's bar).
- Vestibular aqueduct transmits the endolymphatic duct and opens above the sigmoid sulcus.

Inferior Surface
- Helps form the carotid canal and jugular foramen.
- Inferior tympanic canaliculus lies between the carotid canal and jugular fossa and transmits Jacobson's nerve.
- Mastoid canaliculus is located within the lateral part of the jugular fossa and transmits Arnold's nerve.
- Cochlear aqueduct transmits the perilymphatic duct and opens on this surface vertically beneath the porus acousticus.

Tympanic Portion
- Lies below the squamous part and in front of the mastoid process.
- Its posterior portion forms the anterior wall, floor, and posteroinferior aspect of the bony external auditory canal.

Styloid Portion

- Forms the styloid process.

NORMAL EXTERNAL AUDITORY CANAL

- Made up of fibrocartilage laterally and bone medially.
- The medial border of the external auditory canal (EAC) is formed by the tympanic membrane. The tympanic membrane (TM) attaches to the scutum superiorly and to the tympanic annulus inferiorly.

NORMAL MIDDLE EAR

- Consists of three parts: the epitympanum or attic, mesotympanum or tympanic cavity proper, and the hypotympanum.
- Has six important walls
- Roof (tegmental wall). The tegmen tympani separates the middle ear cavity from the middle cranial fossa.
- Floor (jugular wall). A thin plate of bone separates the cavity from the internal jugular vein. The bone may be deficient, with the jugular bulb present within the hypotympanum.
- Mastoid (posterior wall). The upper part of the posterior wall is absent and allows communication between the epitympanic recess and the mastoid antrum via the aditus ad antrum. The lower part of the mesotympanic portion of the posterior wall is made up of the pyramidal eminence (contains belly and tendon of stapedius), sinus tympani, and the facial nerve recess.
- Carotid (anterior wall). Contains the orifice of the semicanal for the tensor tympani muscle and the tympanic orifice of the eustachian tube, separated by the processus cochleariformis.
- Lateral (membranous wall).
- Medial (labyrinthine wall). The cochlear promontory and the oval and round windows are located on this wall.

Epitympanum

- Lies above the level of the tympanic membrane.
- Contains the head of the malleus and the body and short process of the incus.

Mesotympanum

- Tympanic cavity proper.
- Extends from inferior lip of the scutum above to a line drawn parallel to the inferior aspect of the bony EAC.
- Contains the manubrium of the malleus, long process of incus and stapes, and the two muscles of the middle ear—tensor tympani and stapedius.

Hypotympanum

- Lies in the floor of the middle ear.
- Contains no vital structures.

NORMAL INNER EAR

Bony Labyrinth

- Consists of vestibule, semicircular canals, cochlea, and vestibular and cochlear aqueducts.

Vestibule

- Largest part of membranous labyrinth.
- Leads anteriorly into the cochlea and posteriorly into the semicircular canals.
- Laterally, separated from the middle ear by the oval window niche.
- Medially, the lamina cubrosa separates it from the fundus of the IAC.

Semicircular Canals

- Project off the superior, posterior, and lateral aspects of the vestibule.
- Part of the superior semicircular canal forms a ridge (arcuate eminence) on the anterior surface of the petrous bone.
- Lateral semicircular canal projects as a ridge on the medial wall of the attic.

Cochlea

- Conical structure with its base lying on the IAC and its apex or cupola directed anteriorly, laterally, and slightly downward.
- Has approximately 2½ turns.
- Encircles a central bony axis, the modiolus.

Cochlear Aqueduct

- Extends from the basal turn of the cochlea to the cranial cavity anterosuperior to the pars nervosa of the jugular foramen.
- May regulate cerebrospinal fluid (CSF) and perilymphatic fluid pressures.

Vestibular Aqueduct

- Extends from the vestibule, coursing posteroinferiorly to the posterior wall of the petrous pyramid.
- Contains the endolymphatic duct and sac.

The membranious labyrinth consists of the vestibular sense organs (utricle and saccule), semicircular ducts, endolymphatic duct, cochlear duct, and multiple communicating channels.

ROUTE OF THE FACIAL NERVE

Cisternal Segment

- From brainstem to the porus acousticus.

Within IAC

- Occupies the anterosuperior portion of the canal.

Labyrinthine Segment

- Measures 3 to 4 mm in length.

Table 8-1
CAUSES OF PULSATILE TINNITUS

Congenital	Aberrant internal carotid artery Dehiscence of jugular bulb or high jugular bulb
Vascular	Arteriovenous (AV) malformation or AV fistula in the region of temporal bone Aneurysms in the region of temporal bone Dissections of petrous internal carotid artery
Tumor	Paraganglioma Glomus tympanicum Glomus jugulotympanicum Meningioma

- Passes forward and laterally over the top of the cochlea to terminate in the anterior genu (geniculate ganglion).

Tympanic Segment
- Around 12 mm in length.
- Extends from anterior to posterior genu.
- Travels just beneath the lateral semicircular canal in the medial wall of the middle ear cavity.

Mastoid Segment
- From posterior genu to the stylomastoid foramen.

There are three primary branches of the facial nerve: the greater superficial petrosal nerve (lacrimation), the nerve to stapedius, and the chorda tympani (taste in the anterior two-thirds of the tongue).

More than 50 percent of temporal bones exhibit bony dehiscence of part of the facial nerve canal.

□ CONGENITAL VASCULAR ANOMALIES

ABERRANT INTERNAL CAROTID ARTERY

- Some 90 percent occur in females.
- Clinically presents as pulsatile tinnitus (Table 8-1).
- Differential diagnosis of paraganglioma.

Imaging Computed Tomography
- Enhancing soft tissue mass in hypotympanum extending toward the oval window area, indenting promontory or displacing the TM laterally (Fig. 8-1*A*).
- May see an enlarged facial canal due to the presence of a stapedial artery that exits tympanic cavity with facial nerve.

Angiogram
- Lateral deviation of the ICA (Fig. 8-1*B*).

PARTIAL/COMPLETE ABSENCE OF INTERNAL CAROTID ARTERY

Imaging ***Computed Tomography***
- Absent vertical part of carotid canal with soft tissue mass in hypotympanum in partial absence and no carotid canal seen in complete absence.

HIGH JUGULAR BULB

Nondehiscent
- Jugular bulb ascends to or above the level of the floor of the EAC, with preservation of the bony plate that separates the bulb from the middle ear cavity.

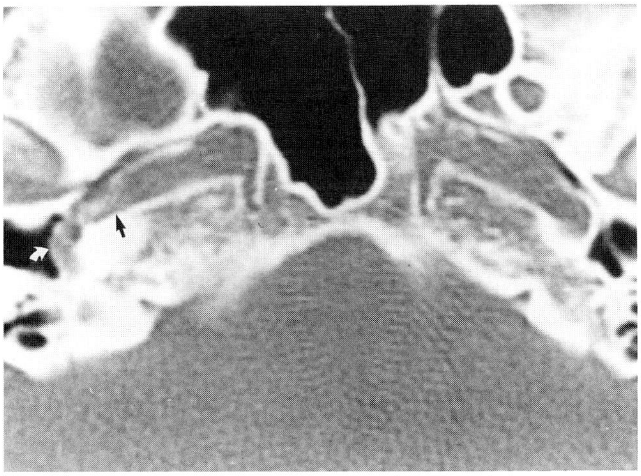

(A)

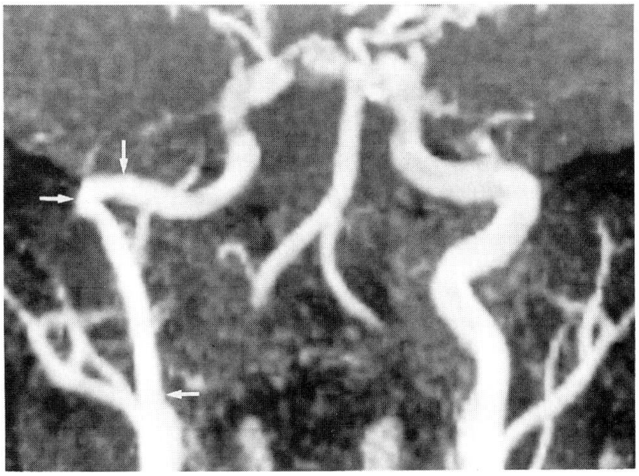

(B)

Figure 8-1 Aberrant carotid artery. A middle-aged woman was referred for evaluation of a pulsatile right retrotympanic mass found on physical examination. A paraganglioma was suspected. *A*. HRCT, A soft tissue mass (*curved arrow*) in right tympanic cavity extends anteriorly to enter the horizontal segment of the carotid canal through a dehiscence (*arrow*) in the carotid plate. The findings are diagnostic of an aberrant carotid artery. *B*. Magnetic resonance angiography, three-dimensional time of flight. The aberrant right carotid artery (*arrows*) is narrower than the normal left internal carotid artery and takes a slightly more lateral and posterior course to traverse the tympanic cavity before entering (*at vertical arrow*) the horizontal carotid canal.

- Most common vascular variant of the petrous bone.

Dehiscent

- Second most common vascular variant.
- Bluish mass behind TM on otologic exam (Table 8-2).
- Computed tomography shows an enhancing soft tissue mass in the middle ear as well as a bony defect above the jugular bulb in the floor of the hypotympanum.

JUGULAR DIVERTICULUM

- Situated more medially and posteriorly in the petrous bone compared to protruding jugular bulb.
- Does not invade middle ear.
- Computed tomography demonstrates the diverticulum extending superiorly into the petrous pyramid.

☐ CONGENITAL DEFORMITIES ASSOCIATED WITH DEAFNESS

DEFORMATION OF THE INTERNAL AUDITORY MEATUS

- The narrow (1- to 2-mm) canal of the internal auditory meatus (IAM) implies absence of the cochlear nerve and represents a contraindication to cochlear implantation.
- Widening of the canal is seen in neurofibromatosis type 1 (NF1) due to a general bone dysplasia and in NF2 from an acoustic neuroma.
- **X-linked progressive mixed hearing loss** is a rare congenital disorder associated with dilatation of the lateral aspect of the IAMs with an absent bony partition between the canal fundus and the basal turn of the cochlea. This seems to lead to a communication between the perilymph in the basal cochlear coil and the subarachnoid space in the IAM and the risk of developing a "stapes gusher" during stapes manipulation. This form of hearing loss should be recognized and stapes surgery avoided.

Table 8-2
INTRATYMPANIC VASCULAR MASSES

Congenital	Aberrant internal carotid High, dehiscent jugular bulb
Inflammatory	Cholesterol granuloma
Neoplasms	Paraganglioma Hemangioma Meningioma

MAJOR DEFORMITIES OF THE LABYRINTH

Michel's Aplasia

- Characterized by a complete lack of development of the inner ear (Fig. 8-2).
- Exceedingly rare.
- Probably due to an arrest of differentiation of the otic placode during the third gestational week.

Otocyst

- During the fourth week, the otic placode invaginates to form a simple cavity called the otocyst. A lack of normal differentiation beyond this stage results in a common cavity, with the cochlea and vestibule forming a cystic cavity with no internal architecture. This deformity probably precludes any eighth-nerve function.

Cochlea Dysplasia

- Arrest at the next stage of development, when there has been some differentiation into the cochlea and vestibular components of the labyrinth, is the most important deformity to recognize.
- Associated with a very real risk of translabyrinthine cerebrospinal fluid (CSF) fistula through a laterally tapered IAM which opens directly into a deformed cochleovestibular sac.
- Cerebrospinal fluid reaches the middle ear via a communication through a hole in the stapes footplate.
- Computed tomography reveals a wider than normal basal turn of cochlea, which communicates with a dilated vestibule.
- Children with this anomaly may present with recurrent attacks of predominantly pneumococcal meningitis.

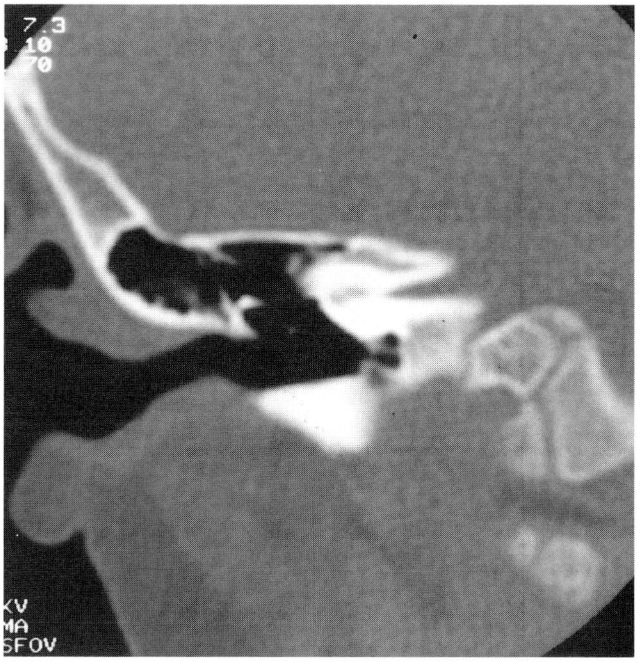

Figure 8-2 Michel's aplasia. Coronal CT of the right temporal bone shows a complete lack of development of the inner ear.

MINOR DEFORMITIES OF THE COCHLEA

Scheibe Malformation

- Most common hereditary congenital hearing loss.
- Involves the cochlea and saccule.
- No imaging abnormalities.

Alexander Malformation

- Aplasia of the cochlear duct, with a resultant effect on the adjacent organ of Corti and ganglion cells of the basal turn of the cochlea.
- No imaging abnormalities.

Mondini Malformation

- First described in 1791 by Carlo Mondini.
- Secondary to an arrest of development at the seventh week.
- Triad of incomplete partition of the middle and apical cochlear coils, dilation of the vestibule, and enlargement of the vestibular aqueduct (VA).
- In the United States, almost any congenital cochlear deformity is labeled a Mondini defect. *Please* avoid this, as a true Mondini deformity has *no* risk of CSF leak, but severe dysplasia of the cochlea is associated with such a risk.
- True Mondini dysplasias are eminently suitable for a cochlear implant.

DEFORMITIES OF THE VESTIBULES AND SEMICIRCULAR CANALS

- The semicircular canals develop between weeks 6 and 22. The short dysplastic lateral semicircular canal is a common deformity of the inner ear.
- Absent semicircular canals are a characteristic feature of the "CHARGE" association: a cluster of congenital abnormalities comprising coloboma, heart disease, atresia of the nasal choanae, retarded development, genital hypoplasia, and ear anomalies.

ABNORMALITIES OF THE COCHLEA AND VESTIBULAR AQUEDUCTS

Vestibular Aqueduct Syndrome

- "Large vestibular aqueduct syndrome" is the *most* common congenital inner ear anomaly demonstrated on imaging studies.
- The vestibular aqueduct (VA) is a bony canal that extends from the medial wall of the vestibule to an outer opening in the posterior surface of the petrous bone. An aqueduct is considered enlarged wherever its anteroposterior diameter is 1.5 mm or more measured at the midpoint of the postisthmic segment.
- This syndrome causes unilateral or bilateral high-frequency hearing loss, which is often progressive. Endolymphatic surgical procedures do *not* confer any benefit.

Abnormality of the Cochlear Aqueduct

- The entity of a wide cochlear aqueduct has been questioned by various authors and its link as a route for congenital CSF fistula should be viewed with skepticism.

ABNORMALITIES OF THE EXTERNAL AND MIDDLE EAR

- Unilateral or bilateral abnormalities of the external ear, including atresia of the external acoustic canal (EAC) and microtia, are regularly accompanied by developmental anomalies of the middle ear. In up to 10 percent of cases, there is an accompanying abnormality of the inner ear.
- High-resolution CT of the temporal bone will often determine a patient's candidacy for surgery. The radiologic evaluation of such a patient must take into account the following points:

1. The EAC may be narrow, short, and completely or partially atretic. It may lie in an abnormal direction. The atresia may be bony, membranous, or mixed.
2. Bony overgrowth about the deformed tympanic bone is referred to as the atresia plate. The completeness of this plate and its thickness should be evaluated.
3. The temporomandibular joint may be more posterior than usual and close to the mastoid process.
4. The size of the middle ear cavity is frequently reduced by encroachment of the atretic plate on the lateral side, a high jugular bulb inferiorly, and a descent of the middle cranial fossa and tegmen tympani, which form the roof of the middle ear cavity. This is a particular feature of first arch deformities like hemifacial microsomia and Treacher Collins syndrome.
5. Soft tissue opacification of the cavity is a frequent finding; this may be due to retained fluid, primitive mesenchymatous tissue, or cholesteatoma.
6. A normal ossicular chain is rarely found when there is atresia of the EAC, but complete absence of the ossicles is also unusual. Fusion of the malleus and incus is a frequent finding. The ossicles may be fixed to the walls of the middle ear cavity, the handle of the malleus may be attached to the atretic plate, or the ossicles may be situated more laterally than normal—a feature of hemifacial microsomia. The status of the stapes superstructure is important.
7. The oval window may be open or closed.
8. Surgeons need to know the relationship of the horizontal portion of the facial nerve to the oval window. The labyrinthine segment is usually unremarkable, but the tympanic and mastoid segments are often anomalous. The mastoid segment tends to have an abnormally anterior location.

☐ INFLAMMATORY DISEASES

EXTERNAL EAR

Malignant Otitis Externa Malignant otitis externa occurs in elderly insulin-dependent diabetic patients. Foul-smelling, purulent discharges from the patient's ear are seen. It is a very aggressive disease process and may mimic a malignant neoplasm. Invasion of the skull base may result in multiple cranial nerve palsies (VI, VII, IX, X, XI, and XII).

Pathophysiology Malignant otitis externa usually occurs at the bony cartilaginous junction of the external auditory canal. The main pathogen is *Pseudomonas aeroginosa*.

Imaging Computed tomography is the imaging modality of choice. Bone window images are useful in the evaluation of associated osteomyelitis, and soft tissue window images can demonstrate collections of pus in the carotid, masticator, and parapharyngeal spaces.

Keratosis Obturans

- Keratosis obturans occurs in middle-aged patients.
- It is usually a bilateral disease process.
- There is a known association with chronic sinusitis and bronchiectasis.
- Computed tomography shows a mass (keratin plug) in the EAC.

Cholesteatoma of the External Auditory Canal

- Usually occurs in patients over 40 years of age.
- Computed tomography shows a mass in the external auditory canal with evidence of bony erosion.

MIDDLE EAR

Otitis Media

- The most frequent causative agents are *Streptococcus*, *Haemophilus influenzae*, and *Pneumococcus*.
- Obstruction of the eustachian tube secondary to hypertrophy of lymphoid tissue in the nasopharynx is responsible for otitis media.
- Computed tomography shows fluid density filling the middle ear cavity.

Cholesteatoma of the Middle Ear A clinical history of recurrent otitis media, tympanic rupture, or tympanostomy tube placement is usually present.

Age Can occur at any age but is more frequently seen in younger patients.

Pathophysiology

- Acquired cholesteatoma in the middle ear cavity occurs as a result of ingrowth of squamous epithelium through the TM, which may have a perforation or retraction pocket.
- A mass composed of squamous and keratin debris erodes the bony middle ear cavity or ossicles.
- There are two types of acquired cholesteatomas:
  1. Pars flaccida cholesteatoma. The cholesteatoma begins as an inward growth of stratified squamous epithelium through a perforated eardrum at Prussak's space (between incus and the lateral wall of the epitympanum); it may extend into the posterolateral attic and into the mastoid antrum through the aditus ad antrum. The head of the malleus and the body of the incus are most susceptible to erosion by a pars flaccida cholesteatoma. The scutum is frequently eroded.
  2. Pars tensa cholesteatoma. The pars tensa cholesteatomas are much less common and they arise from the posterosuperior portion of the pars tensa of the tympanic membrane. The sinus tympani, pyramidal eminence, and facial nerve recesses are frequently involved. The long process of the incus and stapes may be eroded. The scutum is usually intact.

Imaging

- Computed tomography is the imaging modality of choice for cholesteatoma.
- A soft tissue mass associated with bony and/or ossicular erosion in appropriate location is most likely a cholesteatoma. Correlation with clinical findings—such as conductive hearing loss, retraction pockets, or perforated eardrum—are necessary.
- Computed tomography is useful not only to delineate the extent of the disease but also to detect associated bony changes, such as erosion of the lateral semicircular canal or facial nerve canal, tegmen tympani, or ossicular destruction (Table 8-3).
- Magnetic resonance imaging (MRI) is useful to detect intracranial complication of the cholesteatoma. On MRI, the cholesteatoma shows hypointensity on T1-weighted images and intermediate signal intensity on T2-weighted images.

Table 8-3
DIFFERENTIATION OF CHOLESTEATOMA VS. OTITIS MEDIA

CT Findings	Cholesteatoma	Otitis Media
Opacification of middle ear cavity	Yes	Yes
Erosion of scutum	Yes	No
Erosion and displacement of ossicles	Yes	No
Erosion of lateral semicircular canal, causing fistula	Yes	No
Perforation of tympanic membrane with retraction	Sometimes	Rare
Erosion of tegmen tympani	Sometimes	No

- It is not possible to differentiate globular inflammatory debris from early cholesteatoma.

INNER EAR

Labyrinthine Ossification

- The most common clinical presentation is deafness.
- Labyrinthine ossification may develop following chronic middle or inner ear infection, meningitis, trauma, or previous surgery.
- Bony replacement of the labyrinthine portion of the inner ear is seen on CT. (Fig. 8-3)

Petrous Apicitis

- Petrous apicitis is an inflammatory condition of the aerated petrous apex.
- Patients present with retroorbital pain, otorrhea, and sixth-nerve palsy.
- Computed tomography shows a destructive lesion at the petrous apex.
- Gradenigo's syndrome consists of irritation of the fifth cranial nerve, otorrhea, and sixth-nerve palsy.

Cholesterol Granuloma

- Cholesterol granulomas are probably caused by the rupture of a small vessel with hemorrhage in the petrous apex.
- A form of postinflammatory granulation tissue, which is a brownish fluid containing cholesterol crystals and blood.
- Cholesterol granulomas present as an expansile lytic lesion filled with soft tissue density at the petrous apex on CT (Fig. 8-4*A*).
- On MRI, a characteristic hyperintense mass on both T1- and T2-weighted images at the petrous apex is seen (Fig. 8-4*B*).
- The differential diagnosis includes a mucocele of the petrous apex, congenital epidermoid cyst, petrous apicitis, or a bony metastasis with hemorrhage.

□ TRAUMA

- Fractures of the temporal bone can be longitudinal, transverse, or mixed, depending on their orientation to the petrous ridge.
- Longitudinal fractures run along the axis of the temporal bone, extending from the EAC through the middle ear toward the sphenoid bone. Longitudinal fracture is more common and is seen in 80 percent of all temporal bone fractures. They are frequently associated with ossicular dislocation, especially in the incudostapedial joint. There is also a high incidence of hemotympanum (90 percent) and a moderate incidence of otorrhea (50 percent). Facial nerve injury is seen in 10 to 20 percent of the longitudinal fractures, usually at the geniculate ganglion.
- Transverse fractures are seen in 20 percent of the cases. Facial nerve injury is seen in up to 40 percent of the cases. Sensorineural hearing loss is not uncommon, and transection of the cochlear nerve can occur at the apex of the internal auditory canal. Hemotympanum is seen in 50 percent of transverse fractures.
- Most temporal bone fractures are actually of the mixed type.

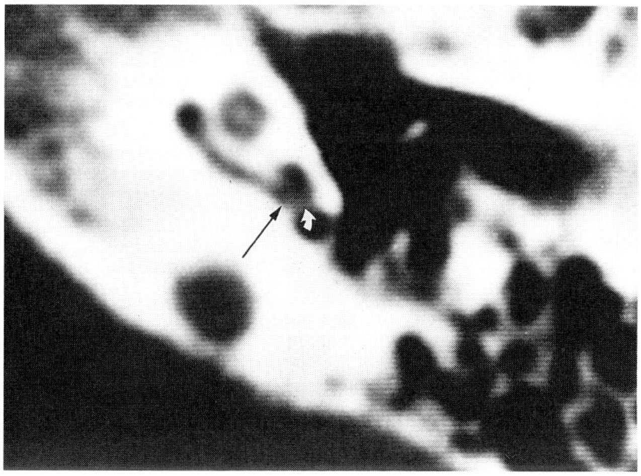

(A)

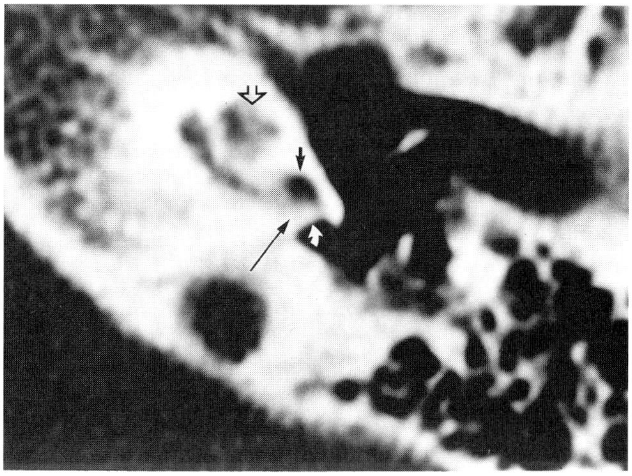

(B)

Figure 8-3 Labyrinthine ossification. A 23-year-old man developed bilateral profound sensorineural hearing loss following meningitis in 1987. *A*. High resolution computed tomography (HRCT) of right temporal bone performed in 1987 showed normal findings. Note complete absence of bone in scala tympani (*long arrow*) inside round window (*curved arrow*). *B*. HRCT of same temporal bone performed 2 years later showed ossification of proximal scala tympani (*long arrow*) at a typical location occluding previously patent round window (*curved arrow*) while preserving the scala vestibuli (*short arrow*). Note also thickening of the interscalar septum (*open arrow*) since the first study.

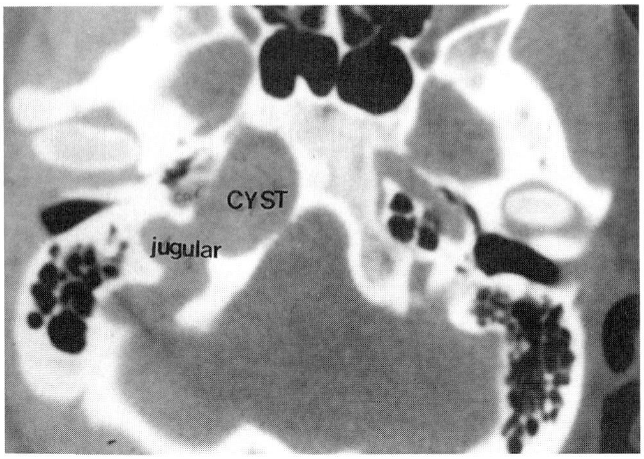

(A)

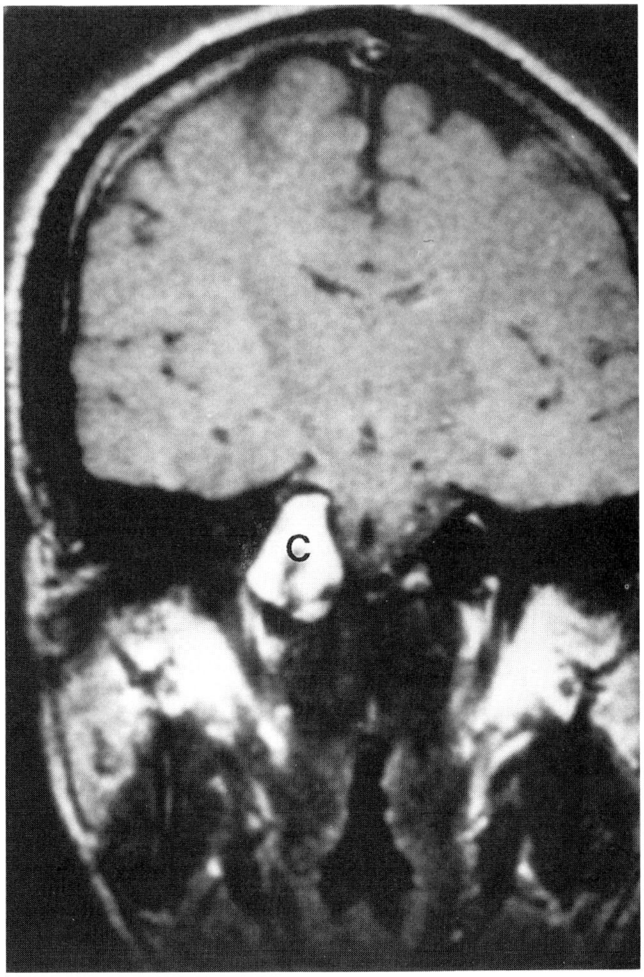

(B)

Figure 8-4 Cholesterol granuloma. A 40-year-old man with history of chronic otitis media. *A*. An axial CT shows bony erosion at the right petrous apex. (cyst-cholesterol granuloma; jugular-jugular foramen). *B*. A coronal T1-weighted image shows a predominantly high-signal-intensity mass (*C*) at the right petrous apex.

- Intracranial complications of temporal bone fractures include meningitis, venous sinus thrombosis, epidural hematoma, cerebrospinal fluid leakage, or traumatic meningocele.
- Computed tomography is the imaging modality of choice for evaluating temporal bone fracture. Both axial and coronal images should be obtained (Table 8-4).

☐ TUMORS OF THE TEMPORAL BONE

Neoplasms of the temporal bone can be subdivided into the following categories, according to their location. (See "Posterior Fossa Extraaxial Mass Lesions" in Chapter 12 for tumors in the cerebellopontine angle cistern.)

1. Internal auditory canal
2. Facial nerve canal
3. Petrous apex
4. Jugular foramen
5. Middle ear
6. Mastoid process
7. External auditory canal

In general, tumors medially located in the temporal bone present with cranial nerve symptoms and are best detected with MRI, but complete evaluation may require high-resolution computed tomography (HRCT) for bone detail. Laterally located tumors tend to cause conductive hearing loss and are best localized with HRCT; if the tumor extends beyond the external auditory canal or the middle ear, MRI may be required for complete evaluation. Tumors of the temporal bone are extremely diverse and numerous, but they tend to be specific to a particular anatomic region. Therefore, image analysis is better served by topographically rather than histologically based discussions.

INTERNAL AUDITORY CANAL

Vestibular schwannoma is by far the most common tumor within the internal auditory canal (IAC), as it is in the cerebellopontine angle. All other lesions are rare by comparison but should be carefully considered along with the history, as their management strategies may differ from that of vestibular schwannoma. Vestibular schwannomas cause sensorineural hearing loss, tinnitus,

Table 8-4
LONGITUDINAL AND TRANSVERSE FRACTURES

Findings	Longitudinal Fracture	Transverse Fracture
Frequency	80%	20%
Hearing loss	Conductive	Sensorineural
Ossicular disruption	Common	Rare
Facial nerve palsy	Uncommon (geniculate ganglion)	Common (horizontal portion)
Tympanic membrane perforation	Yes	No
Hemotympanum	Very common	Common

and disequilibrium but rarely facial twitching or weakness. In the IAC, the schwannoma is rounded or sausage-shaped, homogeneous, nearly isointense to gray matter on T1-weighted imaging and mildly hyperintense on T2-weighted imaging and markedly enhancing. Larger tumors protrude into the cerebellopontine cistern, widening the porus acousticus, and may contain cystic components.

Facial schwannomas in the IAC and the cerebellopontine angle (CPA) are, as a rule, indistinguishable from vestibular schwannomas both clinically and radiologically.

Hemangiomas may form intratumoral bone, or reticular bone in the adjacent wall of the IAC, better seen on CT than on MRI. On T2-weighted imaging, they tend to be more hyperintense than schwannomas. In the absence of such specific features, hemangiomas are radiologically indistinguishable from schwannomas. Clinically, however, they tend to cause a greater degree of nerve deficit for their size and are more often associated with facial palsy than are schwannomas.

Lipomas, characteristically hyperintense on T1-weighted images and hypointense on T2-weighted images, can be confirmed by fat-suppression techniques. Many authors urge conservative management for lipomas.

Osteomas vary in MRI intensities, depending on the presence or absence of marrow. Computed tomography is confirmatory.

Metastases, at times bilateral, can be distinguished from vestibular schwannomas and *neurofibromatosis type 2* by their rapid progression of symptoms and their frequent facial nerve involvement. They tend to enhance less than schwannomas on MRI.

Purely intracanalicular *meningioma*, *lymphoma*, *melanoma*, and *glioma* are extremely rare.

Rare but important nonneoplastic IAC mass lesions include *focal neuritis* of the acoustic nerve and *berry aneurysm* of the anterior inferior cerebellar artery.

Rarely, an *intralabyrinthine schwannoma* may also arise and appear as an enhancing lesion filling the cochlea or the vestibule.

FACIAL NERVE CANAL

Caveats in imaging evaluation of facial nerve tumors include the following:

- Moderate enhancement on MRI is seen along the facial nerve canal (FNC), especially the geniculate and tympanic segments in most of the *normal* subjects.
- Intense enhancement on MRI is seen along the FNC, especially proximally, in *inflammations*, such as idiopathic (Bell's) palsy and herpes zoster oticus (Ramsay Hunt syndrome), characteristically extending into the fundus of the IAC.
- Enlargement of the tympanic facial nerve canal on CT can be caused by a *persistent stapedial artery* rather than a tumor. The ipsilateral foramen spinosum is characteristically absent.

Facial Schwannoma

- Facial schwannomas can arise from any segment of the nerve.
- They vary greatly in configuration and differ in presenting symptoms, depending on the segment involved.
- On CT, the margins of bone erosion are smooth and well defined. (Fig. 8-5*A*).
- On MRI, facial schwannomas are similar to vestibular schwannomas in intensity—small tumors tend to be homogeneous and markedly enhancing (Fig. 8-5*B*), and large tumors often contain cystic components.
- In the CPA/IAC, facial schwannomas are in most cases indistinguishable radiologically and clinically from vestibular schwannomas.
- Facial schwannoma "dumbelling" from the posterior to the middle fossa across the mid–petrous bone through an enlarged labyrinthine FNC is distinctive in appearance and usually accompanied by acoustic and facial symptoms.
- Facial schwannomas arising from the geniculate ganglion balloon silently up into the middle fossa until they present with conductive hearing loss. They may simulate meningiomas in appearance.
- Facial schwannomas arising from the tympanic segment are small tumors causing conductive hearing loss and little facial weakness; they are differentiated from congenital cholesteatomas by enhancement on MRI.
- Facial schwannomas arising from the mastoid segment and those involving multiple segments cause facial palsy and tend to be sausage-shaped and often in multiple links, or they may appear as a string of beads, to be differentiated from perineural tumor spread.
- Facial schwannomas arising distal to the stylomastoid foramen appear as painless masses to be differentiated from parotid gland tumors.

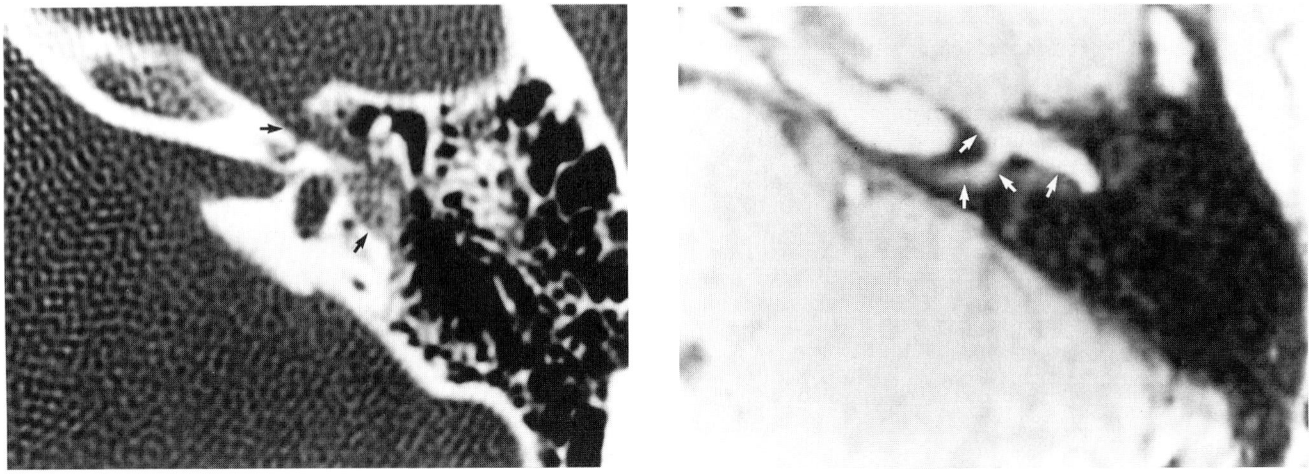

(A) (B)

Figure 8-5 Facial nerve schwannoma. A 40-year-old man developed progressive conductive and sensorineural hearing loss for 1 year followed by facial weakness. *A*. Transverse HRCT . The tumor has caused fusiform expansions with well-defined borders in the geniculate, and tympanic segments of the facial nerve canal (FNC) (*arrows*) but no apparent abnormality in the internal audity canal (IAC) or the labyrinthine FNC . *B*. Transverse gadolinium-enhanced T1-weighted MRI. A multisegment left facial nerve schwannoma appears as "links" of enhancing tumor (*arrows*) from fundus of IAC through tympanic portion of FNC. The tumor also involves the mastoid segment. Surgical exploration confirmed imaging findings.

Hemangioma/Vascular Malformation (Ossifying Hemangioma)

- Benign intratemporal vascular tumors along the course of the facial nerve are usually under 1 cm in diameter. They may form intratumoral bone spicules or reticular bone, better seen on CT than on MRI.
- The sites of predilection are IAC, geniculate ganglion, and posterior genu of the FNC (Table 8-5).
- Hemangiomas in the IAC have been discussed.
- Hemangiomas in the geniculate region may show heterogeneous intensities and enhancement that correlate with tumor-infiltrated reticular bone on CT.
- Hemangiomas in the posterior genu must be differentiated from small schwannomas.

Epidermoid Cyst (Congenital and Acquired Cholesteatoma)

- Supergeniculate congenital cholesteatomas cause facial palsy by erosion of the geniculate and labyrinthine FNC.
- Acquired middle ear cholesteatomas cause facial palsy by eroding the FNC as they extend medially from the anterior epitympanic space toward the petrous apex.
- On CT, their bone margins are sharply and smoothly defined; the lesions are hypodense and nonenhancing.
- On MRI, they are between gray matter and CSF in intensity on T1-weighted images (T1WI), isointense to CSF on T2-weighted images(T2WI), and nonenhancing.

Table 8-5
DIFFERENTIAL FEATURES OF COMMON GENICULATE GANGLION TUMORS ON COMPUTED TOMOGRAPHY

	Facial Schwannoma	Benign Vascular Tumor	Epidermoid
Size	Quite variable	Very small	Small
Shape	Round or sausage-shaped	Irregular	Unilocular or multilocular
Margins	Well defined	Ill defined	Extremely well defined
Location	Along IAC, FNC, or in MF	IAC, GG, or posterior genu	Supralabyrinthine
Density	Nearly isodense	Intratumoral bone	Hypodense to isodense
Enhancement	Yes	Yes	No

Abbreviations: IAC = internal auditory canal; FNC = facial nerve canal; MF = middle fossa; GG = geniculate ganglion.
Source: Adapted from Lo WWM: Tumors of the temporal bone and the cerebellopontine angle, in Som PM, Bergeron RT (eds): *Head and Neck Imaging*, 2d ed. St Louis: Mosby-Year Book, 1991, pp 1046–1108.

Paraganglioma (*glomus faciale*) may arise within the FNC from paraganglia along the distal portions of the nerves of Jacobson and Arnold and cause facial palsy or pulsatile tinnitus.

Choristoma, usually consisting of mature ectopic salivary tissue, can be found in the tympanic cavity attached to the facial nerve, often accompanied by incudostapedial deformity.

The descending facial nerve may be subject to invasion by papillary cystadenomatous tumors of the endolymphatic sac, jugular paragangliomas, squamous carcinoma of the external auditory canal, and perineural extension from carcinomas of the parotid gland, as well as by primary and metastatic carcinomas of the mastoid.

PETROUS APEX

Cystic masses include cholesterol cyst (cholesterol granuloma), congenital epidermoid cyst, and mucocele (Table 8-6).

- A *cholesterol cyst* is lined with fibrous tissue with chronic inflammatory reaction, foreign-body giant cells surrounding cholesterol crystals, red blood cells, and hemosiderin-laden macrophages; it contains a glistening greenish-brown liquid laden with cholesterol crystals.
- An *epidermoid cyst* (*cholesteatoma*) is lined with stratified squamous epithelium and contains cottage cheese–like grayish-white desquamated keratin.
- A *mucocele* is lined with columnar or cuboidal epithelium and contains mucus.
- Both cholesterol cyst and mucocele appear to be caused by obstruction of drainage in a pneumatized petrous apex, the former associated with repetitive cycles of hemorrhage and the latter unassociated with hemorrhage.
- Cholesterol cysts are far more common than the other cysts and are the most common primary mass lesion of the petrous apex.
- Cholesterol cysts and mucoceles can be treated by drainage; epidermoid cysts require resection.
- On CT, all three types of cysts appear as sharply and smoothly marginated, ovoid expansible nonenhancing masses posterior to the horizontal carotid canal. Cholesterol cysts are isodense with brain; the other two are isodense with CSF.
- On MRI, cholesterol cysts are uniquely hyperintense on both T1WI and T2WI, but they may contain hypointense debris and a hypointense rim on T2WI. Chemical shift artifact may be apparent.
- Epidermoid cysts are between CSF and gray matter in intensity on T1WI and hyperintense on T2WI. Lamination may be seen in the periphery on T1WI.
- Mucoceles are similar to epidermoid cysts in intensity but may vary according to the water and protein content of the mucus.

Solid tumors indigenous to the petrous apex include principally meningioma, chondrosarcoma/chordoma, and papillary cystadenomatous tumors of the endolymphatic sac. Tumors occasionally found here include, among others, myeloma, lymphoma, metastasis.

- *Meningiomas* (See Chapter 12) commonly arise from the posterior surface of the petrous bone in the form of a dura-based hemispheric mass. Less commonly, meningiomas spread along the dural surface in a plaque-like manner (en plaque). En plaque meningiomas are prone to infiltrate through the temporal bone from the posterior to the middle fossa and may be difficult to detect without paramagnetic contrast.
- *Chondrosarcoma* is the most common malignant neoplasm in the region of the petrous apex. Arising from cartilaginous rests and generally off midline, they may occasionally overlap with chordomas, which arise from notochord remnants and are generally midline. Both tumors are prone to be intermediate in intensity and relatively homogeneous on T1WI precontrast but inhomogeneous postcontrast and markedly inhomogeneous on T2WI, with many markedly hyperintense foci. Calcifications may be seen in both tumors on CT.
- *Endolymphatic sac tumor* causes irregular retrolabyrinthine bone destruction beginning from the region of

Table 8-6
DIFFERENTIAL FEATURES OF PETROUS APEX "CYSTIC" LESIONS

	Cholesterol Granuloma (Cholesterol Cyst)	Epidermoid (Congenital Cholesteatoma)	Mucocele
CT density	= brain	ω brain	< brain
T1WI intensity	> brain	ω brain	ω brain
T2WI intensity	> brain	> brain	> brain
Content arrangement	Homogeneous or with hypointense irregular debris	Lamination on T1WI	Homogeneous

Abbreviations: T1WI = T1-weighted images; T2WI = T2-weighted images.
Source: Adapted from Lo WWM: Tumors of the temporal bone and the cerebellopontine angle, in Som PM, Bergeron RT (eds): *Head and Neck Imaging*, 2d ed. St Louis: Mosby-Year Book, 1991, pp 1046–1108.

the cranial opening of the vestibular aqueduct. The tumor may then extend to the mastoid or the petrous or transdurally into the posterior fossa. Computed tomography shows spiculated or reticular intratumoral bone. On MRI, there is inhomogeneity with iso-, hypo- and hyperintense foci on precontrast T1WI and inhomogeneous enhancement in most cases.

- Most of the occasional tumors (*myeloma*, *lymphoma*, *metastasis*) show no specific features.
- *Trigeminal schwannoma*, congenital intradural *epidermoid cyst*, and *meningioma* in the region of the Meckle cave may erode the petrous apex.

Other lesions important in the differential diagnosis:

- *Giant petrous carotid aneurysm* may simulate a cystic mass. Laminated mural thrombi are usually present. Luminal enhancement is seen on CT and flow void on MRI.
- Marrow in *unilaterally unpneumatized petrous apex*, hyperintense on T1WI, may be mistaken as a lesion on MRI. Computed tomography provides the diagnosis.
- Similarly, *unilateral retained secretion* in petrous apical air cells, hyperintense on T2WI, may be misdiagnosed. Computed tomography shows no expansion.
- *Petrous apicitis* shows, in addition to presence of liquid, intra- and peripetrous enhancement.
- *Pseudomeningocele* through a dural defect may form in petrous apical air cells.

JUGULAR FORAMEN

Paraganglioma is the second most common tumor in the temporal bone after vestibular schwannoma; it is by far the most common tumor in the jugular foramen.

- Paragangliomas originate from paraganglia along the nerves of Jacobson and Arnold.
- Glomus tympanicum tumors are paragangliomas confined to the tympanic cavity and/or the mastoid; glomus jugulare tumors are those involving the jugular fossa and/or the skull base.
- Glomus vagale tumors originate from intravagal paraganglia at or below the skull base.
- Paragangliomas are three times more common in women than in men.
- The tumors may be multiple.
- Both tympanicum and jugulare tumors tend to cause pulsatile tinnitus and conductive hearing loss. Larger jugulare tumors cause deficits of CN VII, IX, X, and XI.
- The tumors tend to invade locally along vessels, air cell tracts, and foramina. Most jugulare tumors involve the jugular fossa, the hypotympanum, and the adjacent skull base.
- Computed tomography shows "moth-eaten" bone destruction.
- MRI shows "salt-and-pepper" inhomogeneity and arborizing flow voids in tumors larger than 2 cm.
- Angiography shows marked hypervascularity with enlarged feeding arteries and early draining veins.
- Scintigraphy with indium-111-octreotide may be used to detect multicentric, metastatic, or recurrent tumors.

PRINCIPAL DIFFERENTIAL DIAGNOSIS
(Table 8-7)

- *Schwannomas* of cranial nerve (CN) IX, X, and XI, when arising from the jugular foramen, cause sharp, smooth, rounded enlargement of the foramen on CT. They enhance homogeneously or contain cystic components on CT and MRI. They show only mild to moderate vascularity on angiography, with small scattered "puddles" of contrast in midarterial, capillary, and venous phases, and no early veins.
- *Meningiomas* of the jugular foramen, like glomus jugulare tumors, involve the foramen itself as well as the hypotympanum, the posterior cranial fossa, and the jugular vein. They cause a subtle loss of sharpness of the jugular cortex, ill-defined sclerosis, and sometimes focal hyperostosis on CT. On MRI, they are homogenous and moderately enhancing. On angiography, they show only minimal vascularity.

Table 8-7
DIFFERENTIAL DIAGNOSIS OF JUGULAR FORAMEN TUMORS

Tumor	CT Margin	Angiographic Vascularity	Typical MRI Appearance
Schwannoma	Well defined	Minimal to moderate	Homogeneous or cystic
Paraganglioma	Ill defined	Marked	"Salt and pepper"
Meningioma	Subtly ill defined	Minimal	Homogeneous
Malignant tumors (carcinomas, metastases)	Ill defined	Minimal to marked	Homogeneous
Chondrosarcoma	Ill defined	Minimal	Inhomogeneous T2
Nasopharyngeal carcinoma	Medial	Minimal	Infiltrative

Soure: Adapted from Lo WWM: Tumors of the temporal bone and the cerebellopontine angle, in Som PM, Bergeron RT (eds): *Head and Neck Imaging*, 2d ed. St Louis: Mosby-Year Book, 1991, pp 1046–1108.

- *Hemangiopericytoma* and *hypervascular metastases* from pheochromocytoma, hypernephroma, thyroid carcinoma, etc., may be indistinguishable from glomus jugulare tumors.
- *Other metastases* or *malignant tumors* may show bone changes similar to glomus jugulare tumors but are usually much less vascular and do not show the "salt-and-pepper" appearance or arborizing flow voids.
- *Chondrosarcoma* and extension from *nasopharyngeal carcinoma* may reach the medial aspect of the jugulare foramen.

MIDDLE EAR

Glomus tympanicum tumor is the most common neoplasm in the tympanic cavity. Like jugulare tumors, tympanicum tumors cause pulsatile tinnitus and conductive hearing loss. They originate from the cochlear promontory and, by definition, do not involve the skull base. They may extend into the external auditory canal or the mastoid but do not deform the ossicles.

- Glomus tympanicum tumor may be simulated clinically by an aberrant carotid artery or an exposed jugular bulb. Computed tomography is diagnostic of both.
- An *aberrant carotid artery*, after coursing through the tympanic cavity, enters the horizontal carotid canal through a dehiscence in the carotid plate. A *high jugular bulb* can be exposed by a dehiscence in the jugulare plate.
- *Other benign neoplasms* include *facial* and *chorda tympani schwannoma*, *hemangioma*, *adenoma* of the mixed pattern, and, very rarely, *meningioma*.
- *Nonneoplastic mass lesions* include *acquired cholesteatoma*, *cholesterol granuloma*, *congenital cholesteatoma*, *meningoencephalocele*, and *choristoma*.
- *Malignant neoplasms* include *squamous carcinoma*, *adenocarcinoma*, *rhabdomyosarcoma*, *lymphoma*, *metastasis*, etc. They usually also involve the external auditory canal or the mastoid and are seldom confined to the tympanic cavity at the time of presentation.

MASTOID

Aside from *fibrous dysplasia*, *osteoma*, and tumors arising from the descending facial nerve canal (*schwannoma* and *paraganglioma*), most tumors in the mastoid are malignant. These include squamous, adeno-, and undifferentiated *carcinomas*, *lymphoma*, *myeloma*, and *metastasis* in adults; *embryonal rhabdomyosarcoma* in young children; and *Langerhans cell histiocytosis* in children, adolescents, and young adults. They tend to cause irregular bone destruction. Computed tomography is helpful in estimating the growth rate of the lesion and differentiating malignancies from fibrous dysplasia and schwannoma. Histiocytosis may or may not show the classic "punched-out" borders. The MRI intensity patterns are generally nonspecific.

EXTERNAL AUDITORY CANAL

Benign Tumors

- *Exostoses* are sessile multinodular bone masses arising deep in the EAC; they are most often caused by frequent excessive contact with cold seawater for many years (surfer's ear).
- *Osteomas* are sporadic, solitary, unilateral, pedunculated growths of mature bone in the outer portion of the EAC.
- *Fibrous dysplasia*, usually involving a substantial portion of the temporal bone except the otic capsule, may markedly narrow the EAC. On CT, the lesion classically shows "ground-glass" density but may be sclerotic, lytic, or mixed; the bone is enlarged but the margins are always smooth and well defined. On MRI, the intensity is variable.

Malignant Tumors

- *Squamous carcinoma* is by far the most common. With a 5-year morality rate of about 50 percent, it is far more lethal than squamous carcinoma of the skin elsewhere. Early, the tumor may consist of a soft tissue mass with or without focal bone destruction in the EAC. It then invades the middle ear, the mastoid, the middle cranial fossa, and the various soft tissues inferior to the temporal bone.
- *Adenoid cystic carcinoma* is of more indolent growth but may be difficult to distinguish from squamous carcinoma on imaging.
- *Malignant external otitis* is important in the differential diagnosis.

SUGGESTED READINGS

Normal Anatomy and Congenital Malformation

1. Bergeron RT: The temporal bone, in Som PM, Bergeron RT (eds): *Head and Neck Imaging*, 2d ed. St Louis, Mosby-Year Book, 1991; pp 927–944.
2. Bergeron RT: The temporal bone, in Bergeron RT et al (eds): *Head and Neck Imaging, Excluding the Brain*. St Louis, Mosby-Year Book, 1991.
3. Lo WWM, Solti-Bohman LG: High resolution CT of the jugular foramen: Anatomy and vascular variants and anomalies. *Radiology* 150:743, 1984.
4. Phelps PD: Imaging for congenital deformities of the ear. *Clin Radiol* 49:663–669, 1994.
5. Swartz JD: Current imaging approach to temporal bone. *Radiology* 171:309–317, 1989.
6. Swartz JD, Harnsberger HR: *Imaging of the Temporal Bone*. New York, Thieme, 1992.

Inflammatory Diseases

1. Johnson DW et al: Cholesteatomas of the temporal bone: Role of computed tomography. *Radiology* 148:733–737, 1983.
2. Mendelson DS et al: Malignant external otitis: The role of CT and radionuclides in evaluation. *Radiology* 149:745–749, 1983.
3. Swartz JD et al: Labyrinthine ossification: Etiologies and CT findings. *Radiology* 157:395–398, 1985.

Trauma

1. Holland BA, Brant-Zawadzki M: High resolution CT of temporal bone trauma. *AJNR* 5:291–295, 1984.
2. Johnson DW et al: Temporal bone trauma: High resolution CT evaluation. *Radiology* 151:411–415, 1984.

Temporal Bone Tumors

1. Chandrasekhar SS et al: Imaging of the facial nerve, in Jackler DE (ed): *Neurotology*, St Louis, Mosby-Year Book, 1994, pp 341–359.
2. Hirsch WL Jr, Curtin HD: Imaging of the lateral skull base, in Jackler RK, Brackmann DE (eds): *Neurotology*, St Louis, Mosby-Year Book, 1994, pp 303–340.
3. Lo WWM: Imaging of the cerebellopontine angle, in Jackler RK, Brackmann DE (eds): *Neurotology*, St Louis, Mosby-Year Book, 1994, pp 361–398.
4. Lo WWM: Tumors of the temporal bone and the cerebellopontine angle, in Som PM, Bergeron RT (eds): *Head and Neck Imaging*, 2d ed. St Louis, Mosby-Year Book, 1991, pp 1046–1108.

Internal Auditory Canal Tumors

1. Cohen TI et al: MR appearance of intracanalicular eighth nerve lipoma. *AJNR* 13:118–190, 1992.
2. Dalley RD et al: Computed tomography of anterior inferior cerebellar artery aneurysm mimicking an acoustic neuroma. *J Comput Assist Tomogr* 10:881–884, 1986.
3. Dort JC, Fisch U: Facial nerve schwannomas. *Skull Base Surg* 1:51, 1991.
4. Han MH et al: Nonneoplastic enhancing lesions mimicking intracranial acoustic neuroma on gadolinium-enhanced MR images. *Radiology* 179:795, 1991.
5. Kasantikul V et al: Intracanalicular neurilemmomas: Linicopathologic study, *Ann Otol* 89:29, 1980.
6. Langman AW et al: Meningioma of the internal auditory canal, *Am J Otol* 11:201, 1990.
7. Lo WWM et al: Intratemporal vascular tumors: Detection with CT and MR imaging, *Radiology* 171:445–448, 1989.
8. Lo WWM et al: Intratemporal vascular tumors: Evaluation with CT. *Radiology* 159:181–185, 1986.
9. Mark AS: Vestibulocochlear system, in Kelly WM (ed): *Cranial Neuropathy. Neuroimaging Clin North Am* 3:153–170, 1993.
10. Neely JG, Alford BR: Facial nerve neuromas. *Arch Otolaryngol* 100:298–301, 1974.
11. Nelson DR, Dolan KD: Cerebellopontine angle metastatic lung carcinoma resembling an acoustic neuroma. *Ann Otol Rhinol Larynol* 100:685–686, 1991.
12. Saunders JE et al: Lipomas of the internal auditory canal. *Laryngoscope* 101:1031–1037, 1991.
13. Sundaresan N et al: Hemangiomas of the internal auditory canal. *Surg Neurol* 6:119–121, 1976.
14. Wong ML et al: Lipoma of the internal auditory canal. *Otolaryngol Head Neck Surg* 107:374, 1992.
15. Yuh WTC et al: Metastatic lesions involving the cerebellopontine angle. *AJNR* 14:99–106, 1993.

Facial Nerve Canal Tumors

1. Bottrill LS et al: Salivary gland choristoma of the middle ear. *J Laryngol Otol* 106:630–632, 1992.
2. Curtin HD et al: "Ossifying" hemangiomas of the temporal bone: Evaluation with CT, *Radiology* 164:831–835, 1987.
3. Dutcher PO Jr, Brackmann DE: Glomus tumor of the facial canal. *Arch Otolaryngol Head Neck Surg* 112:986–987, 1986.
4. Gebarski SS et al: Enhancement along the normal facial nerve in the facial canal: MR imaging and anatomic correlation. *Radiology* 183:391–394, 1992.
5. Guinto FC Jr et al: Radiology of the persistent stapedial artery, *Radiology* 105:365–369, 1972.
6. Inoue Y et al: Facial nerve neuromas: CT findings. *J Comput Assist Tomogr* 11:942–947, 1987.
7. Ishii K et al: Middle ear cholesteatoma extending into the petrous apex: Evaluation by CT and MR imaging. *Am J Neuroradiol* 12:719–724, 1991.
8. Kienzle GD et al: Facial nerve neurinoma presenting as middle cranial fossa mass: CT appearance. *J Comput Assist Tomogr* 10:391–394, 1986.
9. Lane JI: Facial nerve disorders, in Kelly WM (ed): Cranial neuropathy. *Neuroimag Clin North Am* 3:129–151, 1993.
10. Latack JT et al: Epidermoidomas of the cerebellopontine angle and temporal bone: CT and MR aspects. *Radiology* 157:361–366, 1985.
11. Latack JT et al: Facial nerve neuromas: Radiologic evaluation. *Radiology* 149:731–739, 1983.
12. Lo WWM et al: Intratemporal vascular tumors: Detection with CT and MR imaging. *Radiology* 171:445–448, 1989.
13. Lo WWM et al: Intratemporal vascular tumors: Evaluation with CT. *Radiology* 159:181–185, 1986.
14. May M: Tumors involving the facial nerve, in May M (ed): *The facial nerve*. New York, Thieme, 1986, pp 455–467.
15. Neely JG, Alford BR: Facial nerve neuromas. *Arch Otolaryngol* 100:298–301, 1974.
16. Parker GD, Harnsberger HR: Clinical-radiologic issues in perineural tumor spread of malignant diseases of the extracranial head and neck. *Radiolographics* 11:383–399, 1991.
17. Sartoretti-Schefer S et al: Idiopathic, herpetic and HIV-associated facial nerve palsies: Abnormal MR enhancement patterns. *AJNR* 15:479–485, 1985.

Petrous Apex Tumors

1. Batsakis JG, El-Nagger AK: Papillary neoplasms (Heffner's tumors) of the endolymphatic sac. *Ann Otol Rhinol Larynol* 102:648–651, 1993.
2. Bourgouin PM et al: Low-grade myxoid chondrosarcoma of the base of the skull: CT, MR and histopathology. *J Comput Assist Tomogr* 16:268–273, 1992.
3. Greenberg JL et al: Cholesterol granuloma of the petrous apex: MR and CT evaluation, *AJNR* 9:1205–1214, 1988.
4. Griffin C et al: MR and CT correlation of cholesterol cysts of the petrous bone. *AJNR* 8:825–829, 1987.
5. Grossman RI, Davis KR: Cranial computed tomographic apperance of chondrosarcoma of the base of the skull. *Radiology* 141:403–408, 1981.
6. Haynes RC, Amy JR: Asymmetric temporal bone pneumatization: An MR imaging pitfall. *AJNR* 9:803, 1988.
7. Ishii K et al: Middle ear cholesteatoma extending into the petrous apex: Evalution by CT and MR imaging. *Am J Neuroradiol* 12:719–724, 1991.
8. Larson TL, Wong ML: Primary mucocele of the petrous apex: MR appearance. *AJNR* 13:203–204, 1992.
9. Latack JT et al: Epidermoidomas of the cerebellopontine angle and temporal bone: CT and MR aspects. *Radiology* 157:361–366, 1985.
10. Latack JT et al: Giant cholesterol cysts of the petrous apex: Radiologic features. *AJNR* 6:409–413, 1985.
11. Lee YY et al: Intracranial dural chondrosarcoma. *Am J Neuroradiol* 9:1189–1193, 1988.
12. Lo WWM et al: Endolymphatic sac tumors: Radiologic diagnosis. *Radiology* 189:199–204, 1993.
13. Lo WWM et al: Cholesterol granuloma of the petrous apex: CT diagnosis. *Radiology* 153:705–711, 1984.
14. Lo WWM: Endolymphatic sac tumor: More than a curiosity. *AJNR* 14:1322–1323, 1993.
15. Meyer JR et al: Cerebellopontine angle invasive papillary cystadenoma of endolymphatic sac origin with temporal bone involvement. *AJNR* 14:1319–1321, 1993.
16. Meyers SP et al: Chondrosarcomas of the skull base: MR imaging features. *Radiology* 184:103–108, 1992.
17. Meyers SP et al: Cordomas of the skull base: MR features. *AJNR* 13:1627–1639, 1992.
18. Oot RF et al: The role of MR and CT in evaluating clival chordomas and chondrosarcomas. *AJNR* 9:715–723, 1988.
19. Reid CBA et al: Low-grade myxoid chondrosarcoma of the temporal bone: Differential diagnosis and report of two cases. *Am J Otol* 15:419–422, 1994.
20. Rosenberg AE et al: Chondroid chordoma—A variant of chordoma: A morphologic and immunohistochemical study. *Am J Clin Pathol* 101:36–41, 1994.
21. Sham JST et al: Nasopharyngeal carcinoma: CT evaluation of patterns of tumor spread. *AJNR* 12:265–270, 1991.
22. Tsuruda JS et al: MR evaluation of large intracranial aneurysms using cine low flip angle gradient-refocused imaging. *AJNR* 9:415–424, 1988.

Jugular Foramen Tumors

1. Abramowitz J et al: Angiographic diagnosis and management of head and neck schwannomas. *AJNR* 12:977–984, 1991.
2. Chakeres DW, LaMasters DL: Paragangliomas of the temporal bone: High-resolution CT studies. *Radiology* 150:749–753, 1984.
3. Harvey SA et al: Chondrosarcoma of the jugular foramen. *Am J Otol* 15:257–263, 1994.
4. Hesselink JR et al: Selective arteriography of glomus tympanicum and jugulare tumors: Techniques, normal and pathological arterial anatomy. *AJNR* 2:289–297, 1981.
5. Horn KL et al: Schwannomas of the jugular foramen. *Laryngoscope* 95:761–765, 1985.
6. Kaye AH et al: Jugular foramen schwannomas. *J Neurosurg* 60:1045–1053, 1984.
7. Kwekkeboom DJ et al: Octreotide scintigraphy for the detection of paragangliomas. *J Nucl Med* 34:873–878, 1993.
8. Lo WWM et al: High resolution CT in the evaluation of glomus tumors of the temporal bone. *Radiology* 150:737–742, 1984.
9. Miyachi S et al: Myeloma manifesting as a large jugular tumor: case report. *Neurosurgery* 52:133–136, 1990.
10. Molony TB et al: Meningiomas of the jugular foramen. *Otolaryngol Head Neck Surg* 106:128–136, 1992.
11. Mukherji SK et al: Irradiated paragangliomas of the head and neck: CT and MR appearance. *AJNR* 15:357–363, 1994.
12. Olsen WL et al: MR imaging of paragangliomas. *AJNR* 148:201–204, 1987.
13. Vogl TJ et al: Glomus tumors of the skull base: Combined use of MR angiography and spin echo imaging. *Radiology* 192:103–110, 1994.
14. Weber AL, McKenna MJ: Radiologic evaluation of the jugular foramen, vascular variants, anomalies, and tumors. *Neuroimaging Clin North Am* 4:579–598, 1994.

Middle Ear Tumors

1. Benecke JE Jr et al: Adenomatous tumors of the middle ear and mastoid. *Am J Otol* 11:20–26, 1990.
2. Bottrill LS et al: Salivary gland choristoma of the middle ear. *J Laryngol Otol* 106:630–632, 1992.
3. Larson TC III et al: Glomus tympanicum chemodectomas: Radiographic and clinical characteristics. *Radiology* 163:801–806, 1987.
4. Lo WWM, Solti-Bohman LG: High resolution CT of the jugular foramen: Anatomy and vascular variants and anomalies. *Radiology* 150:743–747, 1984.
5. Lo WWM et al: Aberrant carotid artery: Radiology diagnosis with emphasis on high resolution computed tomography. *Radiographics* 5:985–993, 1985.
6. Martin N et al: Cholesterol granulomas of the middle ear cavities: MR imaging. *Radiology* 172:521–525, 1989.

Mastoid Process Tumors

1. Bonafé A et al: Histiocytosis X of the petrous bone in the adult: MRI. *Neuroradiology* 36:330–333, 1994.
2. Cunningham MJ et al: Histiocytosis X of the temporal bone: CT findings. *J Comput Assist Tomogr* 12:70–74, 1988.
3. Friedman DP, Rao VM: MR and CT of squamous cell carcinoma of the middle ear and mastoid complex. *Am J Neuroradiol* 12:872–874, 1991.
4. Wiatrak BJ, Pensak ML: Rhabdomyosarcoma of the ear and temporal bone. *Laryngoscope* 99:1188–1192, 1989.
5. Yousem DM et al: Rhabdomyosarcoma in the head and neck: MR imaging evaluation. *Radiology* 177:683–686, 1990.

External Auditory Canal Tumors

1. Arriaga M et al: The role of preoperative CT scans in staging external auditory meatus carcinoma: Radiologic-pathologic correlation study. *Otolaryngol Head Neck Surg* 105:6–11, 1991.
2. Di Bartolomeo JR: Exostoses of the external auditory canal. *Ann Otol* 88 (suppl 61):2–20, 1979.
3. Sheehy JL: Diffuse exostoses and osteomata of the external auditory canal: A report of 100 operations. *Otolaryngol Head Neck Surg* 90:337–342, 1982.

☐ QUESTIONS (TRUE OR FALSE)

1. Regarding the facial nerve,
  a. It occupies the anterosuperior portion of the internal audity canal.
  b. The labyrinthine segment passes forward and laterally over the top of the cochlea to terminate in the anterior genu.
  c. The tympanic segment travels just above the lateral semicircular canal in the medial wall of the middle ear cavity.
  d. The greater superficial petrosal nerve is functionally related to lacrimation.
  e. The chorda tympani is functionally related to taste in the anterior two-thirds of the tongue.

2. Lesions causing pulsatile tinnitus include
  a. Dehiscence of the jugular bulb
  b. Aberrant internal carotid artery
  c. Glomus tympanicum tumor
  d. Cholesteatoma
  e. AVM or AV fistula in the region of temporal bone

3. Regarding the Mondini malformation,
  a. Any congenital cochlear deformity is a Mondini defect.
  b. Secondary to an arrest of development at the seventh week.
  c. Triad consists of incomplete partition of the middle and apical cochlear coils, dilation of vestibule, and enlargement of the vestibular aqueduct.
  d. True Mondini malformations are eminently suitable for a cochlear implant.
  e. First described in 1791 by Carlo Mondini.

4. Regarding cholesteatoma of the middle ear,
  a. Acquired cholesteatoma in the middle ear cavity occurs as a result of ingrowth of squamous epithelium through the tympanic membrane, which may have a perforation or retraction pocket.
  b. The mass may erode the bony middle ear cavity or ossicles.
  c. Two types of acquired cholesteatoma exist: pars flaccida and pars tensa cholesteatomas.
  d. Sometimes it is not possible to differentiate globular inflammatory debris from early cholesteatoma.
  e. In the evaluation of cholesteatoma, MRI is superior to CT.

5. Regarding trauma of the temporal bone,
  a. Longitudinal fractures run along the plane of the temporal bone.
  b. Longitudinal fractures are less common than transverse fractures.
  c. Longitudinal fractures are frequently associated with ossicular dislocation.
  d. Facial nerve injury is seen in up to 40 percent of the transverse fractures.
  e. Computed tomography is the imaging modality of choice for evaluating temporal bone fractures.

6. Regarding cystic masses at the petrous apex,
  a. A cholesterol cyst is lined with fibrous tissue and contains a glistening greenish-brown liquid laden with cholesterol crystals.
  b. An epidermoid cyst is lined with stratified squamous epithelium and contains cottage cheese–like grayish white desquamated keratin.
  c. A mucocele is lined with columnar or cuboidal epithelium and contains mucus.
  d. Cholesterol cysts are less common than other cysts.
  e. On MRI, cholesterol cysts are uniquely hyperintense on both T1- and T2-weighted images.

7. Jugular foramen masses include
  a. Paraganglioma
  b. Schwannoma
  c. Meningioma
  d. Hemangiopericytoma
  e. Cholesteatoma

8. Regarding mass in the tympanic cavity,
  a. Glomus tympanicum tumor is the most common neophasm.
  b. Aberrant carotid artery may simulate glomus tumor clinically.
  c. Facial and chorda tympani schwannoma may be seen.
  d. Meningioma is commonly seen.
  e. A high jugular bulb with bony dehiscence can simulate a glomus tumor clinically.

☐ ANSWERS

1. **a.** T
  b. T
  c. F
  d. T
  e. T

2. **a.** T
  b. T
  c. T
  d. F
  e. T

3. **a.** F
  b. T
  c. T
  d. T
  e. T

4. **a.** T
b. T
c. T
d. T
e. F

5. **a.** T
b. F
c. T
d. T
e. T

6. **a.** T
b. T
c. T
d. F
e. T

7. **a.** T
b. T
c. T
d. T
e. F

8. **a.** T
b. T
c. T
d. F
e. T

CHAPTER 9

Normal Neuroanatomy

Alyssa T. Watanabe
George P. Teitelbaum

☐ THE BRAIN AND ITS COVERINGS

The brain is made up of the cerebrum, brainstem, and cerebellum. The cerebrum may be further categorized into the cerebral hemispheres, the diencephalon, and deep gray nuclei. The brain contains a ventricular system, which is filled with cerebrospinal fluid (CSF). The calvarium and meninges encase the brain, which is bathed in CSF.

CEREBRAL HEMISPHERES

The cerebral hemispheres comprise an outer mantle of gray matter with underlying subcortical white matter tracts. There are four true anatomic lobes in each hemisphere: frontal, parietal, temporal, and occipital. The frontal and occipital lobes of the cerebral hemispheres are separated by the falx cerebri. The hemispheres are partially connected centrally by the corpus callosum. The convolutions of the brain are termed gyri and are separated by invaginations called sulci. The two most important sulci are the sylvian fissure (also called the lateral sulcus) and the central sulcus (Fig. 9-1). The central sulcus is the only long sulcus to pass over the lateral surface of the brain to the medial surface. The insula is the cortical involution of brain deep to the sylvian fissure beneath the frontal, parietal, and temporal lobe opercula.

Frontal Lobe The frontal lobe is the largest of the four lobes.

Anatomy The frontal lobe extends from the frontal pole to the central sulcus. It is separated inferiorly from the temporal lobe by the sylvian fissure. There are four main gyri: the precentral gyrus (which is situated transversely between the precentral sulcus and central sulcus) and the superior, middle, and inferior frontal gyri (which follow a parasagittal course). The gyrus rectus abuts the anterior cranial fossa in parallel with the olfactory bulb (Fig. 9-2). The cingulate gyrus curves superiorly around the corpus callosum.

The central sulcus is a very important surgical landmark because it separates the primary motor cortex (anteriorly) from the primary sensory cortex (posteriorly). The central sulcus can usually be identified on axial computed tomography (CT) and magnetic resonance imaging (MRI) as the largest of the three laterally directed sulci that are seen at the convexity. The axial method is the most reliable method unless three-dimensional reformatting is available. On axial images, the superior frontal sulcus will form a right angle with the precentral sulcus (Fig. 9-3). The next sulcus posteriorly is the central sulcus. The central sulcus is immediately anterior to the marginal ramus of the cingulate sulcus. At the convexity, the cingulate sulcus appears as a short transverse sulcus on the medial surface of the hemispheres. The V-shaped merging of the intraparietal sulcus with the postcentral sulcus is another useful landmark on axial images. On lateral sagittal images, there is a consistent Y-shaped involution (formed by the anterior horizontal and anterior ascending rami of the sylvian fissure) (Fig. 9-1). The descending sulci posterior to the "Y" represent the precentral sulcus and then the central sulcus. The central sulcus is the only major sulcus that can be traced all the way to the midline. On midline sagittal images, the cingulate sulcus ascends to the vertex immediately posterior to the central sulcus (Fig. 9-4).

Function The primary motor area or "motor strip" is located in the precentral gyrus. Damage to this area

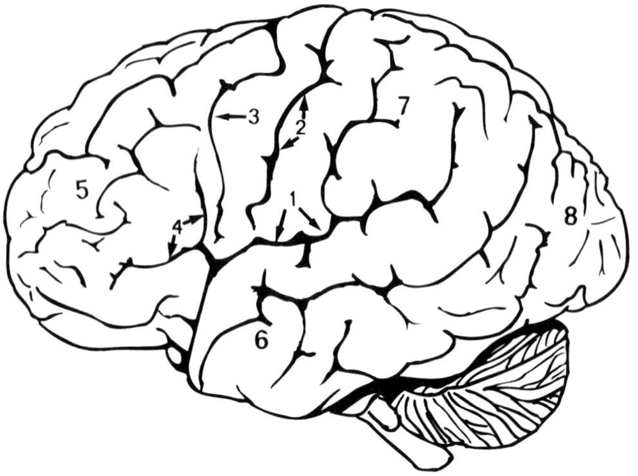

Figure 9-1 Lateral surface anatomy of the brain. Sylvian fissure (1). Central sulcus (2). Precentral sulcus (3). "Y"-shaped rami of the sylvian fissure (4). Frontal lobe (5). Temporal lobe (6). Parietal lobe (7). Occipital lobe (8). (*Adapted with permission from DeArmond et al.*[1])

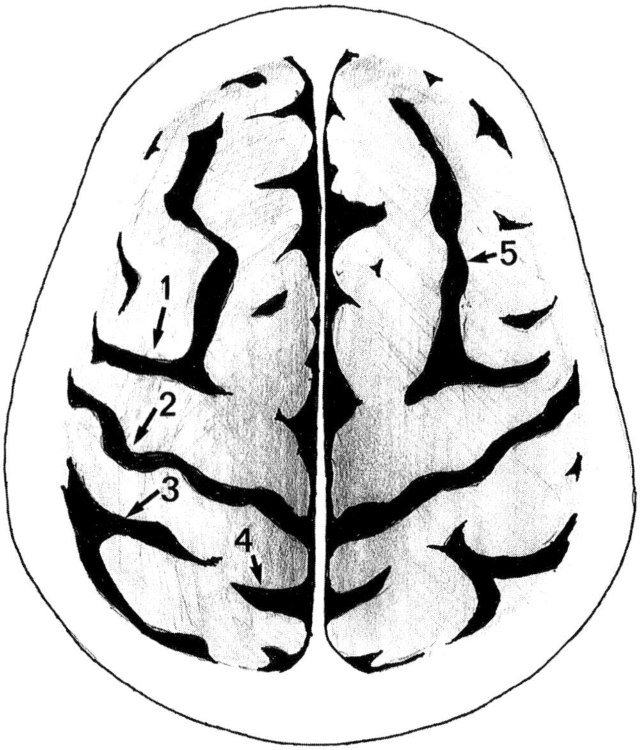

Figure 9-3 Axial anatomy of the convexity. Precentral sulcus (1). Central sulcus (2). Postcentral sulcus (3). Marginal ramus of the cingulate sulcus (4) is a short, paired sulcus on the medial surface posterior to the central sulcus. Superior frontal sulcus (5), which intersects with the precentral sulcus.

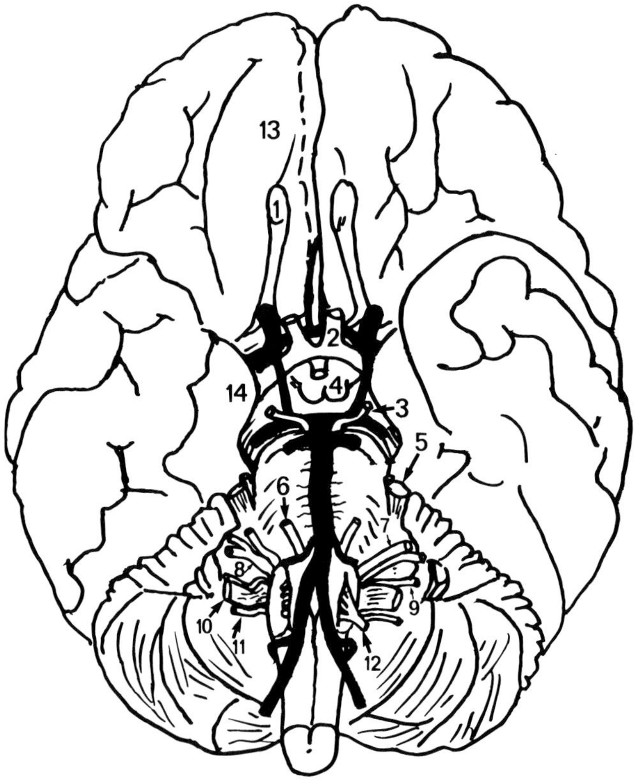

Figure 9-2 Axial surface anatomy of the base of the brain. Olfactory nerve (1). Optic nerve (2). Oculomotor nerve (3). Mamillary body (4). Trigeminal nerve (5). Abducens nerve (6). Facial nerve (7). Vestibulocochlear nerve (8). Glossopharyngeal nerve (9). Vagus nerve (10). Spinal accessory nerve (11). Hypoglossal nerve (12). Gyrus rectus (13). Uncus (14). (*Adapted with permission from DeArmond et al.*[1])

may result in contralateral hemiparesis. The supplementary motor area is situated more broadly in the rostral medial frontal lobe. The motor speech area (Broca's area) is located in the posterior inferior frontal gyrus of the dominant hemisphere (usually the left hemisphere in a right-handed person) (Fig. 9-21). The anterior frontal lobe contains the frontal eye fields, which control some voluntary eye movements. The olfactory bulbs and nerves arise from the inferior surface of the frontal lobe.

Parietal Lobe ***Anatomy*** At the convexity, the central sulcus separates the parietal lobe from the frontal lobe. The parieto-occipital sulcus marks the medial parietal lobe boundary. The other margins of the parietal lobe are not as clear cut. On axial CT and MRI, the level of the mid-atrium is a gross boundary for the occipital lobe caudally and the more cephalad parietal lobe.

Function The primary sensory area is situated within the postcentral sulcus of the parietal lobe. Selective speech and interpretative functions are located in the parietal lobe (Fig. 9-21). Lesions in the angular gyrus may result in difficulty with reading and writing. A lesion in the supramarginal gyrus may result in apraxia (inability to execute purposeful movements).

Temporal Lobe ***Anatomy*** This is the second-largest lobe. It is separated from the frontal lobe by the sylvian

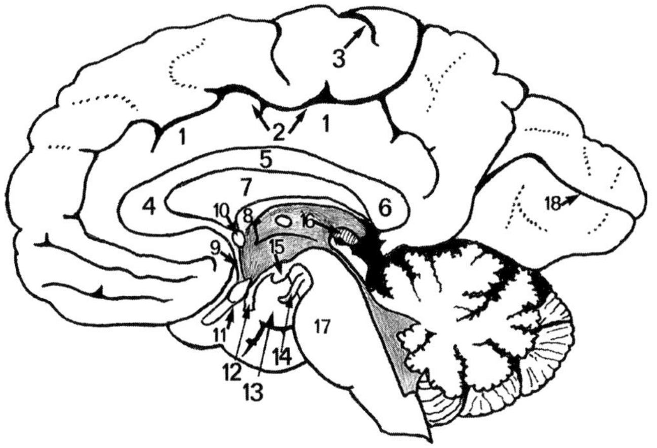

Figure 9-4 Sagittal midline anatomy of the brain. Cingulate gyrus (1). Cingulate sulcus (2). Central sulcus (3). Genu (4), body (5), and splenium (6) of the corpus callosum. Septum pellucidum (7). Fornix (8). Lamina terminalis (9). Anterior commissure (10). Optic chiasm (11). Infundibulum (12). Uncus (13). Third nerve (14). Mamillary body (15). Pineal gland (16). Pons (17). Calcarine sulcus (18). (*Adapted with permission from DeArmond et al.*[1])

fissure. The superior, middle, and inferior temporal gyri make up the lateral temporal lobe and course in the anterior-to-posterior direction. The inferior temporal lobe is formed by the parahippocampal gyrus, occipitotemporal gyrus, and inferior temporal gyrus. The uncus is the medial protrusion of the parahippocampal gyrus (Fig. 9-2).

The anatomy of the hippocampus is extremely complex but is becoming increasingly relevant in neuroimaging. The hippocampal formations include the hippocampus, dentate gyrus, subiculum, and associated gyral and white matter tracts (fimbria, alveus) (Fig. 9-5). The hippocampus is an invagination of cortex which is continuous with the subiculum of the parahippocampal gyrus (Fig. 9-5). The anterior hippocampus (also known as the pes) is medial to the temporal horn, caudal to the amygdala, and lateral to the choroidal fissure. The hippocampus is a unique part of brain in that gray and white matter are inverted (that is, the white matter overlies the gray). The gray matter of Ammon's horn is continuous with the cortex of the subiculum but is surrounded by the white matter of the dentate gyrus. The alveus continues as a white matter tract (the fimbria), which connects the hippocampus with the fornix.

Function The primary auditory cortex is contained within the insula in the superior temporal gyrus. The parahippocampal gyrus and hippocampal formations are an important part of the limbic system. The limbic system plays an important role in memory functions, particularly recent memory. Alzheimer's dementia may be related to hippocampal dysfunction. The Ammon's horn (also known as Sommer's sector) of the anterior hippocampus is a compaction of gray matter that is most sensitive to hypoxia (Fig. 9-5). It is frequently found to be abnormal

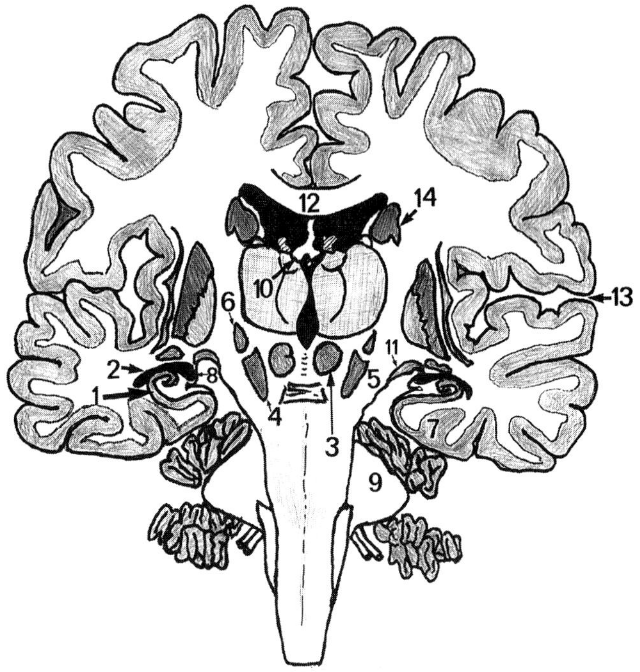

Figure 9-5 Midcoronal anatomy of the brain. Region of Ammon's horn of the hippocampus (1). Choroidal fissure (2). Red nucleus (3). Substantia nigra (4). Cerebral peduncle (5). Subthalamic nucleus (6). Parahippocampal gyrus (7). Temporal horn (8). Middle cerebellar peduncle (9). Fornix (10). Lateral geniculate (11). Corpus callosum (12). Sylvian fissure (13). Caudate nucleus (14). (*Adapted with permission from DeArmond et al.*[1])

in patients with temporal lobe epilepsy. The sensory speech area (Wernicke's area) is located in the posterior superior temporal gyrus, usually in the dominant hemisphere. The primary olfactory cortex is located in the uncus and other parts of the parahippocampal gyrus.

Occipital Lobe This is the smallest lobe.

Anatomy The lateral parieto-occipital transition is not anatomically defined. The parieto-occipital sulcus on the medial surface separates these two lobes. The occipital lobe rests on the tentorium cerebelli, which separates the cerebrum from cerebellum. The paired occipital lobes are separated medially by the interhemispheric fissure and falx cerebri. The calcarine sulcus separates the occipital lobe medially into the cuneus and the lingual gyrus.

Function The primary visual cortex lines the calcarine sulcus, involving both cuneus and lingual gyrus. The visual cortex receives input from the ipsilateral half of each retina (contralateral visual field). Injury to the visual cortex may result in contralateral homonymous visual field defects. The lateral occipital gyri contain visual association areas (Fig. 9-26).

Limbic System ***Anatomy*** The limbic system is considered by some anatomists to represent a lobe in a functional sense. The limbus includes the subcallosal, cingulate, and parahippocampal gyri; the hippocampal formations; nuclei of the amygdala and thalamus; the hypothalamus; the epithalamus; and parts of the basal ganglia. The cingulate gyrus wraps around the splenium and is actually contiguous with the parahippocampal gyrus. The indusium griseum is a thin gray matter band, closely apposed to the corpus callosum, which is contiguous with the parahippocampal gray matter. The parahippocampal gyrus, hippocampal formations, and amygdala are intimately related.

Function The limbic system serves many complex functions, including emotional behavior and memory formation.

WHITE MATTER

The Centrum Semiovale The main central masses of white matter, the centrum semiovale, contain commissural, projection, and association fibers. Motor and sensory fibers of the centrum converge toward the brainstem as the corona radiata. Short association fibers (subcortical U fibers) connect adjacent gyri. Abnormalities of the U fibers may sometimes be seen on MRI in association with multiple sclerosis. The long association fibers connect different lobes within the same hemisphere.

The Internal Capsule The anterior limb of the internal capsule separates the caudate head and the globus pallidus (Fig. 9-6). The pyramidal (descending motor) tracts pass through the corona radiata to the genu and anterior two-thirds of the posterior limb of the internal capsule. The genu contains the corticobulbar fibers that connect to the nuclei of cranial nerves (CN) III to XII in the brainstem tegmentum. The posterior limb contains the corticospinal tract fibers that control contralateral motor movement. The face and arms are topographically anterior to the legs. The pyramidal fibers continue caudally into the crus cerebri of the ventral cerebral peduncles and then to the medullary pyramids, where the fibers decussate. General sensory fibers, which synapse in the thalamus, are located in the posterior limb of the internal capsule lateral to the pyramidal fibers. The auditory and optic radiations traverse the most posterior part of the internal capsule (Fig 9-6).

Corpus Callosum and Other Commissural Fibers The cerebral hemispheres are connected by commissural (transverse) fibers. The corpus callosum is a large central white matter structure that partially connects the two hemispheres (Fig. 9-4). The corpus callosum forms the roof of the lateral ventricles. The corpus callosum is divided into the rostrum, genu, body, and splenium (from anterior to posterior). The fibers of the genu projecting into the frontal cortex form the forceps minor. The fibers of the splenium projecting into the occipital cortex form the forceps major.

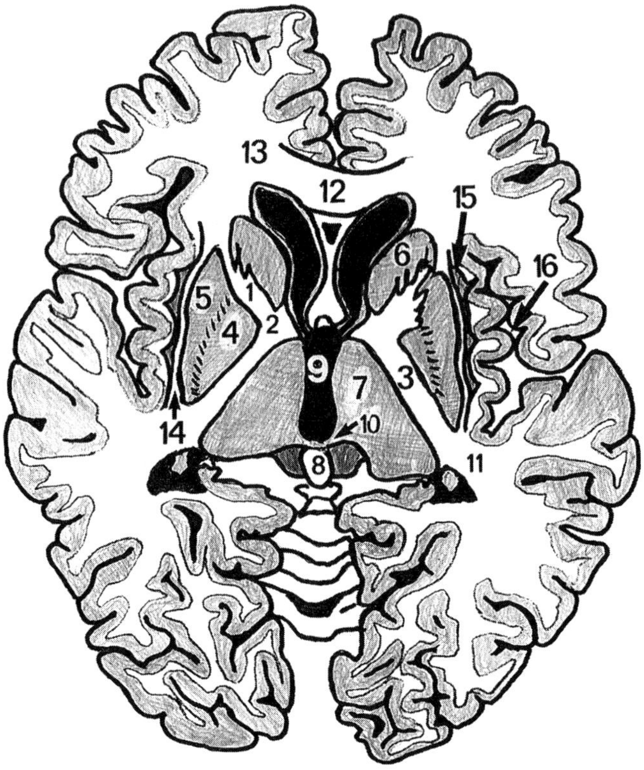

Figure 9-6 Axial anatomy through the basal ganglia and internal capsule. Anterior limb (1), genu (2), and posterior limb (3) of the internal capsule. Globus pallidus (4). Putamen (5). Caudate head (6). Thalamus (7). Pineal gland (8). Third ventricle (9). Posterior commissure (10). Optic and auditory radiations (11). Genu of corpus callosum (12). Forceps minor (13). External capsule (14). Claustrum (15). Insula (16). (*Adapted with permission from DeArmond et al.*[1])

The anterior commissure crosses the midline just rostral to the fornix and connects the olfactory bulbs and temporal lobes. The posterior commissure crosses the midline just anterior to the pineal gland and connects the superior colliculi. The hippocampal commissure connects the crura of the fornix. These transverse fibers run beneath the splenium and are of variable size. The fornix is a white matter tract that connects the mamillary bodies and the hippocampus. The fornix, therefore, plays a role in memory.

DEEP GRAY NUCLEI (BASAL GANGLIA)

The term *basal ganglia*, poorly defined, refers to the deep gray nuclei. The basal ganglia include the corpus striatum (caudate, putamen, and globus pallidus) as well as other gray areas (such as the claustrum and amygdala). *Lentiform nucleus* is an alternate term for the globus pallidus and putamen (Fig. 9-6).

Anatomy The internal capsule separates the caudate and lentiform nucleus. The head of the caudate protrudes into the anterolateral aspect of the frontal horn. The caudate curves inferiorly along the temporal horn and terminates at the amygdala. The amygdala is anterior to the temporal horn and cephalad to the pes hippocampus (Fig. 9-9).

With aging, the lentiform nucleus may partially calcify and progressively accumulate iron. The globus pallidus forms the medial part of the lentiform nucleus. It normally appears more hypointense than the putamen on T2-weighted MRI. This is due to slower iron accumulation within the putamen, which eventually approaches the iron level of the globus pallidus in the elderly.

The external (medial) and extreme (lateral) capsules are thin layers of white matter separated by a thin layer of gray matter known as the claustrum. These three layers are sandwiched between the putamen and the insula (Fig. 9-6).

Function Diseases of the basal ganglia may result in extrapyramidal disorders (unintentional motor movements) such as tremor, chorea, and athetosis. Caudate atrophy is associated with Huntington's disease. Pathology of the globus pallidus and putamen is associated with Parkinson's disease and Parkinson-like disorders. The amygdala is part of the limbic system.

DIENCEPHALON

The diencephalon is made up of multiple structures that contain the word *thalamus*: the thalamus, epithalamus (pineal gland and habenulae), hypothalamus, and subthalamus. The diencephalon plays some key roles, particularly in regulatory functions and the visual pathway. The majority of the optic nerve nuclei are in the thalamus.

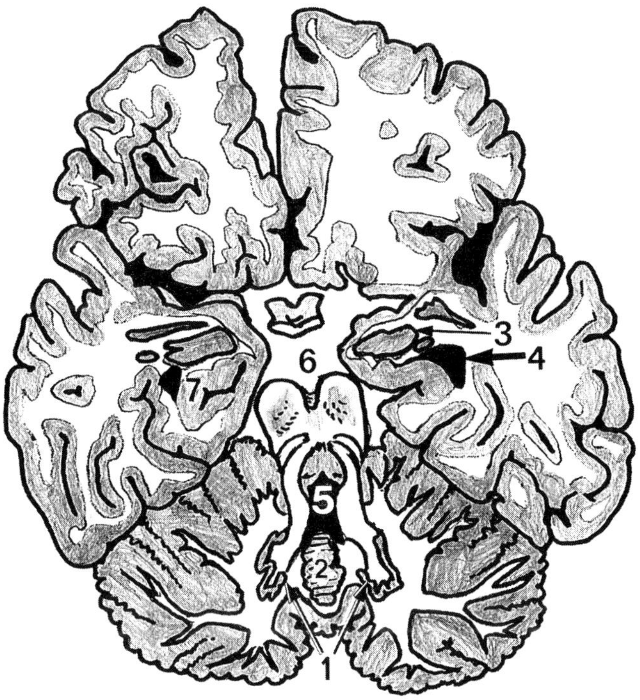

Figure 9-7 Axial anatomy of the inferior cerebrum and cerebellum. Dentate nuclei (1). Vermis (2). Amygdala (3). Temporal horn (4). Fourth ventricle (5). Interpeduncular cistern (6). Pes hippocampus (7). (*Adapted with permission from DeArmond et al.*[1])

Thalamus ***Anatomy*** The thalamus is situated between the internal capsules and forms the lateral walls of the third ventricle (Fig. 9-6). The massa intermedia describes the midline continuity of the thalamus, which exists in 80 percent of people.

Function The thalamus is a relay and integrative center that contains sensory, motor, and limbic nuclei. The medial and lateral geniculate bodies are thalamic sensory nuclei that are dorsolateral to the upper midbrain. These nuclei are part of the auditory and visual pathways respectively. The thalamus is felt to be crucial in certain types of sensation, particularly pain. A pure sensory stroke may occur because of a thalamic lacuna. The thalamic motor nuclei are part of the pathway from the cerebellum and globus pallidus to the primary motor cortex. The limbic nuclei interconnect with other parts of the limbic system, such as the amygdala, olfactory cortex, and hypothalamus.

Hypothalamus ***Anatomy*** The hypothalamus forms the floor and inferior walls of the third ventricle. It includes the optic chiasm, lamina terminalis, infundibulum (pituitary stalk), tuber cinereum, and mamillary bodies. There are numerous hypothalamic nuclei, which have complex connections to the limbic system. The lamina terminalis, optic chiasm, and median eminence of the hypothalamus are directly contiguous. The median eminence forms a portion of the floor of the third ventricle and continues in the suprasellar cistern as the infundibulum. The infundibulum extends to the posterior lobe of the pituitary gland through the diaphragma sella. The infundibulum normally enhances with contrast due to its lack of a blood-brain barrier. The tuber cinereum and mamillary bodies make up the posterior hypothalamus. The mamillary bodies project ventral and medial to the cerebral peduncles (Figs. 9-2 and 9-4).

Function The hypothalamus serves important regulatory functions. The neurohypophysis (median eminence and infundibulum) contains nerve fibers that control the secretion of the posterior pituitary hormones: vasopressin and oxytocin. The hormones of the anterior pituitary are controlled indirectly by hypothalamic releasing hormones, which are transported via the portal circulation. The mamillary bodies are connected to the limbic system and are associated with memory.

Pineal Gland and Habenulae ***Anatomy*** The epithalamus comprises the pineal gland and paired habenulae. The pineal gland is attached to the posterior wall of the third ventricle (Fig. 9-4). It is posterior and superior to the posterior commissure, to which it is attached. It is anterior and inferior to the splenium of the corpus callosum. It is superior to the superior colliculi of the midbrain tectum. Habenular and pineal calcifications are a frequent normal finding. The habenular calcifications are slightly ventral to the pineal. The pineal gland lacks a blood-brain barrier and therefore normally enhances with intravenous contrast.

Function These structures serve an unknown function in humans.

Subthalamus *Anatomy* The subthalamic nucleus makes up the main body of the subthalamus. This nucleus is situated medial to the internal capsule and ventral to the inferior thalamus.

Function Damage to this area may result in hemiballismus.

BRAINSTEM

The brainstem comprises the midbrain, pons, and medulla. The brainstem can also be divided longitudinally as the basis (ventral), tegmentum (dorsal brainstem), and tectum (dorsal midbrain). The descending (motor) tracts pass through the ventral brainstem. The brainstem tegmentum contains cranial nerve nuclei (III through XII), the reticular activating system (RAS), and ascending (sensory) spinal tracts. The RAS regulates state of consciousness, and cardiorespiratory functions. The cranial nerves are summarized in Table 9-1. Note is made that some of the cranial nerve nuclei traverse the tegmentum: CN VII and VIII nuclei traverse the pontomedullary junction. The CN V nuclei are widely positioned in the midbrain, pons, medulla, and cervical cord.

Midbrain The midbrain forms a transition between the brainstem and cerebrum. The ventral midbrain is made up of two cerebral peduncles (crus cerebri), which are separated by the interpeduncular cistern. The cerebral peduncles contain corticospinal, corticobulbar, and corticopontine fibers. The paired paramedian red nuclei are immediately dorsal to the substantia nigra. The red nucleus is important in motor coordination. It has fiber connections to the cerebellum, thalamus, and rubrospinal tract. The aqueduct of Sylvius runs through the dorsal tegmentum, surrounded by periaqueductal gray matter. The third, fourth, and portions of the fifth cranial nerve nuclei are located in the midbrain. The oculomotor nerve (CN III) nuclei are in the midbrain tegmentum situated just medial to the medial longitudinal fasciculi (MLF) and ventral to the periaqueductal gray matter. The fibers of CN III course through the red nucleus, substantia nigra, and cerebral peduncle (Fig. 9-8).

The midbrain tectum (roof) is dorsal to the tegmentum and aqueduct. The tectum contains four dorsal protuberances (quadrigeminal plate), the paired superior and inferior colliculi. The superior colliculi are a part of the visual pathway, involved in ocular reflexes. A few of the optic nerve nuclei are located here. The inferior colliculi are involved in auditory reflexes and integration. The superior and inferior colliculi project respectively to the lateral and medial geniculate nuclei of the thalamus. The geniculate nuclei are located dorsolateral to the midbrain.

Pons The descending motor tracts (corticospinal fibers) pass through the ventral pons. The ventral pons, which is protuberant, is also known as the "pontine belly." The main sensory nuclei of the trigeminal (CN V) nerve are in the upper pons. The inferior pontine tegmentum contains the abducens (CN VI) and facial (CN VII) nuclei. The CN VI nuclei are in the pontine tegmentum just ventral to the fourth ventricle. The CN VI nucleus may be seen as a small bulge into the fourth ventricle, the facial colliculus. The colliculus is so named since it is here that CN VII wraps around the CN VI nucleus. The cochlear nuclei are located in the inferior cerebellar peduncles (also known as restiform bodies) at the pontomedullary junction. The MLF are situated in the paramedian dorsal pons, adjacent to the fourth ventricle and medial to the CN VI nuclei. Internuclear ophthalmoplegia (INO) results from injury to the MLF and has a high clinical association with multiple sclerosis (Fig. 9-9).

Medulla The descending corticospinal (motor) tracts in the pyramids of the ventral medulla decussate at the craniocervical junction. The vestibular nuclei and cochlear nuclei of the eighth nerve are located in the tegmentum, the pontomedullary junction, partly in pons,

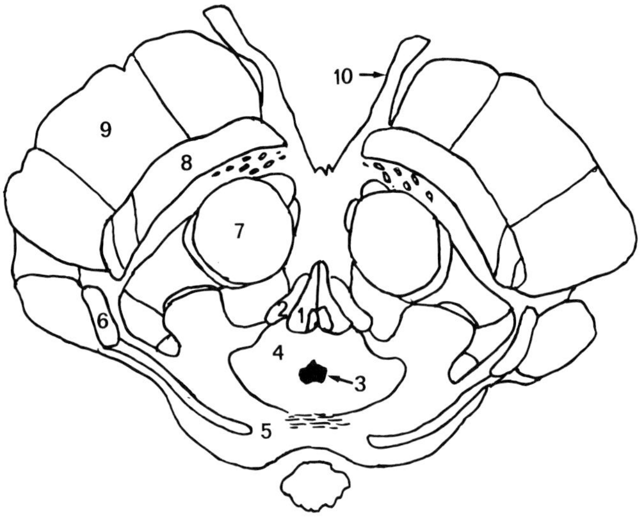

Figure 9-8 Axial anatomy of the midbrain. Oculomotor nucleus (1). Medial longitudinal fasciculus (2). Aqueduct of Sylvius (3). Periaqueductal gray matter (4). Superior colliculus (5). Medial geniculate (6). Red nucleus (7). Substantia nigra (8). Pyramidal tract of cerebral peduncle (9). Oculomotor nerve (10). (*Adapted with permission from DeArmond et al.*[1])

Table 9-1
THE CRANIAL NERVES

	Type	Nuclei	Function	Cranial Passage
CN I Olfactory	Sensory	Cerebrum	Olfaction	Cribriform plate
CN II Optic	Sensory	Diencephalon	Vision	Optic canal
CN III Oculomotor	Motor	Midbrain	EOM—pupillary constriction, visual accommodation	SOF
CN IV Trochlear	Motor	Midbrain	EOM	SOF
CN V Trigeminal	Mixed	Midbrain to cervical cord	Facial sensation, muscles of mastication, gustation	V_1: SOF V_2: foramen rotundum V_3: foramen ovale
CN VI Abducens	Motor	Pons	EOM	SOF
CN VII Facial	Mixed	Pons	Facial muscles, gustation, salivation, lacrimation, acoustic dampening	IAC Stylomastoid foramen
CN VIII Vestibulocochlear	Sensory	Pons	Hearing, balance	IAC
CN IX Glossopharyngeal	Mixed	Medulla	Gustation, salivation, swallowing, carotid receptors	Jugular foramen (pars nervosa)
CN X Vagus	Mixed	Medulla	Gustation, swallowing, palatal elevation, speech (vocal cords), visceral parasympathetic motor supply	Jugular foramen (pars vascularis)
CN XI Spinal accessory	Motor	Medulla	Neck muscles (trapezius, sternocleidomastoid)	Jugular foramen (pars vascularis)
CN XII Hypoglossal	Motor	Medulla	Tongue muscles	Hypoglossal canal

Abbreviations: EOM = extraocular muscles; SOF = superior orbital fissure; IAC = internal auditory canal.

and partly in medulla. The spinal nucleus of CN V (the trigeminal nerve) is in the medulla. The nuclei of CN IX, X, XI, and XII are all in the caudal medulla below the level of the fourth ventricle. The gracilis and cuneatus tubercles form the dorsal surface of the medulla. These longitudinal ridges can sometimes be seen on MRI. These tubercles are an extension of the corresponding spinal cord fasciculi, the posterior columns. The medially located gracilis tubercle contains sensory information from the lower body and the laterally situated cuneatus contains sensory information from the upper body (Fig. 9-10).

THE CRANIAL NERVES

Cranial Nerve I (Olfactory) ***Anatomy*** The olfactory nerve (CN I) fibers arise from the olfactory mucosa and traverse the perforations of the cribriform plate of the ethmoid bone. The olfactory nerve (CN I) nuclei are located in the olfactory bulb, which runs along the undersurface of the inferior frontal lobe. The olfactory tracts are white matter extensions of the brain which enter the uncus, anterior commissure, and amygdala (Fig. 9-2).

Function Cranial nerve I is a sensory nerve devoted to olfaction (smell).

Cranial Nerve II (Optic Nerve) ***Anatomy*** The optic nerve (CN II) arises from the retina and courses through the optic canal (which is superomedial to the superior orbital fissure). The nerve fibers then pass through the optic chiasm, which is part of the hypothalamus. The CN II fibers continue as the optic tracts to the lateral geniculate bodies (sensory nuclei) of the thalamus. A few of

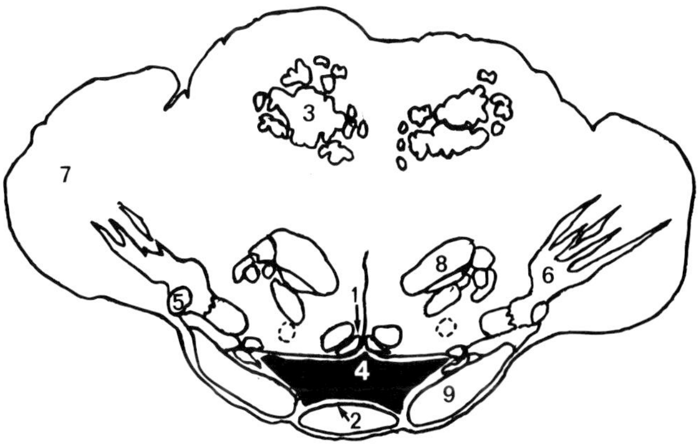

Figure 9-9 Axial anatomy through the pons. Medial longitudinal fasciculus (1). Superior medullary velum (2). Pyramidal tracts (3). Fourth ventricle (4). Sensory nucleus of CN V (5). Trigeminal nerve (6). Middle cerebellar peduncle (7). Medial lemniscus (8). Superior cerebellar peduncle (9). (*Adapted with permission from DeArmond et al.*[1])

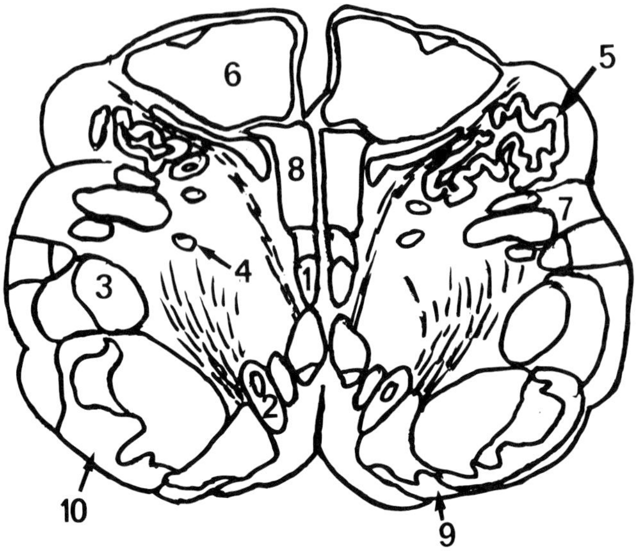

Figure 9-10 Axial anatomy through the medulla. Medial longitudinal fasciculus (1). Hypoglossal nucleus (2). Spinal nucleus of CN V (3). Nucleus ambiguus, CN X (4). Olivary nuclei (5). Pyramidal tracts (6). Spinothalamic tracts (7). Medial lemniscus (8). Fasciculus gracilis (9). Fasciculus cuneatus (10). (*Adapted with permission from DeArmond et al.*[1])

the CN II fibers continue to nuclei in the superior colliculus and pretectal area. The optic radiations are white matter tracts that continue posteriorly to the visual cortex in the occipital lobes. Each occipital lobe processes data from the contralateral visual field.

Function Cranial nerve II is a sensory nerve solely devoted to vision. Prechiasmatic lesions may result in monocular blindness, chiasmatic lesions are associated with bitemporal hemianopsia, and retrochiasmatic lesions may result in homonymous hemianopsia.

Cranial Nerve III (Oculomotor Nerve) ***Anatomy*** The oculomotor nerve (CN III) can be consistently seen on MRI as it exits into the interpeduncular cistern. The third nerve passes between the posterior cerebral and superior cerebellar arteries and runs parallel and inferior to the posterior communicating artery (Fig. 9-2). Mass effect from a posterior communicating aneurysm may produce a CN III palsy. The third cranial nerve traverses the superolateral cavernous sinus and enters the orbit through the SOF.

Function Cranial nerve III is a motor nerve. Its fibers innervate most of the extraocular muscles (EOM): medial rectus, superior rectus, inferior rectus, inferior oblique, and levator palpebrae. This nerve also controls intrinsic muscles of the eye which control pupillary constriction and accommodation.

Cranial Nerve IV (Trochlear Nerve) ***Anatomy*** The trochlear (CN IV) nerve is the only cranial nerve to decussate and it is the only cranial nerve to exit from the dorsal surface of the brainstem. Cranial nerve IV, like CN III, enters the cavernous sinus and exits through the SOF. It is not usually visible on standard imaging studies due to its small size.

Function Cranial nerve IV, a motor nerve, innervates the superior oblique muscle.

Cranial Nerve V (Trigeminal Nerve) ***Anatomy*** The trigeminal nerve (CN V) is the largest of the cranial nerves and has three divisions: V_1, V_2, and V_3. Cranial nerve V has a large sensory root and a smaller motor root. The motor fibers arise from the pontine tegmentum. The sensory nuclei are broadly situated throughout the brainstem tegmentum and upper cervical cord.

The fifth nerve exits from the lateral pons at the level of the middle cerebellar peduncles (Fig. 9-8). The trigeminal fibers join to form the trigeminal (also called gasserian) ganglion, which is contained in a dural fold (Meckel's cave) posterolateral to the cavernous sinus. The fibers of the trigeminal nerve traverse the skull through three different skull openings: the superior orbital fissure (V_1, the ophthalmic division), the foramen rotundum (V_2, the maxillary division), and the foramen ovale (V_3, the mandibular division). The cutaneous branches of V_2 (the infraorbital branch) enter the orbital floor through the infraorbital foramen and enter the skull through the inferior orbital fissure (IOF).

Function Cranial nerve V is a mixed nerve. Cranial nerve V_3 innervates most of the muscles of mastication and the tensor tympani muscle of the middle ear. All three divisions of CN V contribute to facial sensation.

Cranial Nerve VI (Abducens Nerve) ***Anatomy*** Cranial nerve VI exits the ventral pontomedullary junction and then courses to Dorello's canal in the clivus. It and Dorello's canal can occasionally be seen on MRI axial images. Cranial nerve VI enters the inferolateral cavernous sinus and exits into the orbit through the SOF.

Function Cranial nerve VI is a motor nerve which innervates the lateral rectus. The lateral rectus palsy is the most common EOM palsy due to the long course of CN VI.

Cranial Nerve VII (Facial Nerve) ***Anatomy*** The facial (CN VII) nerve exits the ventral midbrain and runs parallel with the vestibulocochlear nerve through the cerebellopontine angle cistern to the internal auditory canal. Cranial nerve VII takes a complex course through the temporal bone before it exits through the stylomastoid foramen. The cell bodies for the taste fibers are located in the geniculate ganglion in the temporal bone.

Function The facial nerve (CN VII) has motor and sensory functions. Functions include motor innervation to the muscles of facial expression, the platysma, and the stapedius muscle in the inner ear, which is important in acoustic dampening. Cranial nerve VII also innervates the lacrimal gland as well as the sublingual and submandibular glands. The sensory fibers of the facial nerve connect to the trigeminal sensory nuclei and supply sensation of the external ear and taste fibers of the anterior two-thirds of the tongue.

Cranial Nerve VIII (Vestibulocochlear Nerve) ***Anatomy*** The vestibulocochlear nerve (CN VIII) runs in parallel in the cerebellopontine angle cistern with CN VII from the internal auditory canal to the pontomedullary junction.

Function Cranial nerve VIII is a sensory nerve. The cochlear division transmits hearing. It is part of the acoustic pathway, which includes the inferior cerebral peduncle, pontine tegmentum and tectum, medial geniculate, and superior temporal gyrus. The auditory cortex in each hemisphere processes data from both ears. Thus, a solitary cortical lesion does not result in significant hearing loss. The superior and inferior vestibular divisions are related to equilibrium. Tumors of CN VIII may result in sensorineural hearing loss or vertigo.

Cranial Nerve IX (Glossopharyngeal Nerve) ***Anatomy*** The glossopharyngeal nerve (CN IX) exits the lateral medulla in the postolivary sulcus. Cranial nerve IX immediately joins CN X and CN XI to form the CN IX–XI nerve complex (Fig. 9-2). Cranial nerve IX exits through the pars nervosa (which is ventral to the pars vascularis) of the jugular foramen.

Function Cranial nerve IX is a mixed nerve. The pharyngeal branch of CN IX supplies sensation to the pharynx and soft palate; therefore it is responsible for the afferent gag reflex. Cranial nerve IX taste fibers from the posterior tongue connect with the trigeminal system, and CN IX receptors in the carotid body and sinus are involved in the cardiorespiratory regulatory reflex. Although CN VII passes through the parotid, it is CN IX that controls parotid secretions. Motor innervation is to the stylopharyngeus muscle. Injury to this muscle may result in dysphagia. The nerves of Arnold and Jacobson (which are CN X and CN IX branches, respectively) may give rise to the glomus jugulare tumor. Solitary CN IX palsies are rare.

Cranial Nerve X (Vagus Nerve) ***Anatomy*** The vagus (CN X) nerve exits in the retroolivary sulcus of the lateral medulla. Cranial nerve X exits with CN XI through the pars vascularis of the jugular foramen. The left vagus courses down to the level of the aorticopulmonic window in the chest. This is about the level of the fifth thoracic vertebra. The right CN X loops around the right subclavian artery. This is about the level of the clavicle. Both ascend to the larynx in the tracheoesophageal groove.

Function Cranial nerve X supplies the muscles of the soft palate and pharynx and therefore controls the efferent gag reflex. The vagus also supplies the intrinsic muscles of the larynx via the recurrent laryngeal nerve. Cranial nerve X also conveys parasympathetic motor supply to the viscera and stimulates peristalsis, gastric secretions, and pancreatic secretions. Hoarseness due to vocal cord paralysis is a sign of vagus nerve malfunction.

Cranial Nerve XI (Spinal Accessory Nerve) ***Anatomy*** The spinal accessory nerve (CN XI) is part cranial nerve and part spinal nerve. The spinal motor fibers ascend from the C1–5 anterior horn cells of the cervical cord and ascend through the foramen magnum to join the cranial component, which exits from the medulla. The spinal root then exits through the pars vascularis of the jugular foramen.

Function The spinal fibers supply the sternocleidomastoid and trapezius muscles.

Cranial Nerve XII (Hypoglossal Nerve) ***Anatomy*** The hypoglossal nerve (CN XII) exits from the medulla in the preolivary sulcus. The nerve exits through the hypoglossal canal. The motor fibers of CN XII loop as far caudal as the hyoid before ascending to innervate the tongue muscles.

Function Cranial nerve XII innervates the tongue and strap muscles. A sensory branch innervates the dura of the posterior fossa.

THE VENTRICULAR SYSTEM

The cerebral hemispheres contain central fluid-filled cavities, which are lined by ependyma. The fluid, surrounds the brain and spinal cord (Fig. 9-11).

Lateral Ventricles The paired lateral ventricles are made up of the frontal (anterior) horns, occipital (posterior) horns, and temporal (inferior) horns. The trigone (also known as the atrium) connects the occipital and temporal horns to the body of the ventricle. The frontal horns and ventricular bodies are separated by the septum pellucidum. During early life or as a normal variant, there may be CSF cavities within the septum (the cavum septum pellucidum and cavum vergae). These CSF cavities may persist as a normal variant.

The lateral ventricles are bordered by the corpus callosum above and the caudate nucleus laterally. The choroidal fissure is the medial wall of the inferior horn and body where the ependyma and pia abut. The floor of the ventricles is bordered by the thalamus and the fornix. The choroid plexus of the lateral ventricles is highly vascularized and produces the bulk of CSF.

Third Ventricle The third ventricle is the cavity of the diencephalon. The lateral walls of the midline third ventricle are formed by the thalamus (Fig. 9-6). The lower walls and floor are formed by the hypothalamus. The anterior commissure and lamina terminalis form the

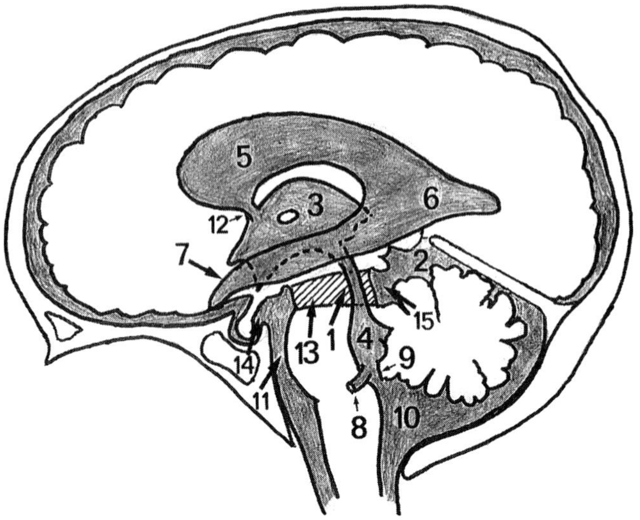

Figure 9-11 Lateral diagram of the ventricles and CSF spaces. Aqueduct (1). Superior cerebellar cistern (2). Third ventricle (3). Fourth ventricle (4). Frontal (5), occipital (6), and temporal (7) horns of the lateral ventricles. Foramina of Luschka (8) and Magendie (9). Cisterna magna (10). Prepontine cistern (11). Foramen of Monro (12). Ambient cistern (13). Suprasellar cistern (14). Quadrigeminal plate cistern (15).

anterior wall. The third ventricle has several recesses: the optic recess (between the optic chiasm and lamina terminalis), the infundibular recess (inferior to the optic recess), the pineal recess, and the suprapineal recess. These recesses are of variable size but may markedly expand in the presence of hydrocephalus.

Aqueduct of Sylvius The aqueduct is a narrow cavity which runs through the dorsal midbrain between the tegmentum and tegmen (Fig. 9-11). It does not contain any choroid.

Fourth Ventricle The fourth ventricle is the cavity of the pons and upper medulla (Figs. 9-9 and 9-11). The fourth ventricle is dorsal to the pontomedullary tegmen. The obex is the caudal midline termination of the fourth ventricle. The roof of the fourth ventricle is formed by the superior and inferior medullary vela of the cerebellum. The choroid plexus of the tela choroidea projects into the caudal fourth ventricle. The CSF of the fourth ventricle empties into cisterna magna via the foramina of Luschka and Magendie.

Foramina of Luschka and Magendie The foramina of Luschka (lateral apertures) are the openings for the lateral recesses of the fourth ventricle into the cerebellopontine angles (Fig. 9-11). The choroid plexus may be found in the foramina or lateral recesses.

The foramen of Magendie (medial aperture) is in the caudal roof of the fourth ventricle. The majority of CSF exits through the foramen of Magendie into the subarachnoid space.

THE CEREBELLUM

Anatomy The cerebellum is separated from the cerebrum by the tentorium cerebelli. The cerebellum is connected to the brainstem via three white matter peduncles: superior (brachium conjunctivum) which connects to midbrain; middle (brachium pontis), which connects to the pons; and inferior (restiform body), which connects to the medulla. The middle cerebellar peduncle is the largest of the three.

There are two paired lateral cerebellar hemispheres and a midline vermis. The hemispheres are divided into many lobes and lobules. The flocculus projects into the cerebellopontine angle and may mimic an extraaxial mass. The cerebellar tonsils (inferior aspect of the hemispheres) may project up to 2 mm caudal to the foramen magnum. There are four paired deep cerebellar nuclei. The paired dentate nuclei are readily identified on T2-weighted MRI due to iron deposition. The dentate nuclei are located in the white matter of the cerebellar hemispheres (Fig. 9-7).

Function The cerebellum is involved in motor coordination, equilibrium, and maintenance of muscular tone. Signs and symptoms of cerebellar disorder include ataxia, nystagmus, tremor, and incoordination.

THE COVERINGS OF THE CENTRAL NERVOUS SYSTEM

The brain and its coverings are protected by the bony skull. The brain is separated from the skull by three membranes: the dura, arachnoid, and pia. The arachnoid and pia are also known as the leptomeninges. These membranes surround the entire central nervous system (CNS): brain, spinal cord, and optic nerve. The CNS is bathed in cerebrospinal fluid, which is constantly circulating.

The Dura The dura consists of an outer periosteal layer and an inner meningeal layer. The periosteal layer of dura is strongly adherent to the inner surface of the skull. The meningeal dura has many infoldings and is less adherent. The meningeal dura continues through the foramen magnum into the spinal canal, forming the outer layer of the thecal sac. The epidural space is a potential space in the cranium. It represents the space between the two layers of dura. In the spine the epidural space separates the meningeal dura and the vertebrae.

A midline infolding of the meningeal layer of the dura is the falx cerebri. The falx is continuous with the folds of the tentorium cerebelli, which separates the cerebrum from the cerebellum. The free borders of the tentorium are called the tentorial incisura. The brainstem passes through the tentorium incisura. The diaphragma sella represents another dural infolding, which separates the pituitary fossa from the suprasellar cistern. The infundibulum of the hypothalamus traverses the diaphragma sella. The large venous sinuses (dural sinuses) are contained within these two dural layers. Dural calcifications are a frequent normal finding on CT.

The cranial dura is mainly innervated by branches of CN V. The infratentorial cranial dura and upper cervical dura is supplied by CN X and CN XI.

The Arachnoid The arachnoid, an avascular membrane, surrounds the brain and spinal cord. The arachnoid villi (granulations) protrude through the dura into the superior sagittal sinus. Arachnoid granulations progressively increase in size with age and may calcify. The arachnoid villi are a major source of CSF resorption.

The subarachnoid space, between the arachnoid and the pia, is filled with cerebrospinal fluid (CSF). The basal and lumbar cistern are widenings of the pia and arachnoid. In these regions, the arachnoid and dura are closely apposed. Vessels and nerves traverse the subarachnoid space. The ambient cistern contains the great vein of Galen as well as the posterior cerebral, anterior choroidal, and superior cerebellar arteries. The basilar artery runs in the prepontine cistern. The interpeduncular cistern and superior cerebellar cisterns are important anatomic landmarks.

The Pia The pia is intimately apposed to the brain and spinal cord. The filum terminale is the caudal continuation of the pia, which attaches to the distal thecal sac and extends to the coccyx as the coccygeal ligament. The dentate ligaments are bilateral projections of the pia which traverse the arachnoid at intervals to attach to the dura. The dentate ligaments and filum along with the spinal roots fixate and stabilize the spinal cord.

The Cerebrospinal Fluid Pathway The CSF is clear and colorless. It is mainly formed in the choroid plexus within the ventricles. The normal CSF volume is about 150 mL, with CSF formation rate of 500 to 750 mL per day. The CSF flows from the paired lateral ventricles through the foramina of Monro, into the midline third ventricle, through the aqueduct of Sylvius, and into the midline fourth ventricle. The CSF then passes outside of the brain through the foramen of Magendie or the foramina of Luschka. It then enters the subarachnoid space, including the basal cisterns of the brain and the lumbar cistern. Cerebrospinal fluid does not normally circulate in the central spinal canal in adults. The CSF eventually flows back up to the convexity, where it is resorbed in the arachnoid granulations in the superior sagittal sinus. The CSF pressure varies with cardiac and respiratory fluctuations.

☐ THE SPINAL CORD

The spinal cord is continuous with the medulla. It terminates as the conus at the level of the L1 vertebra in the adult. The spinal cord contains central gray matter surrounded by peripheral white matter. The ventral columns (also known as the anterior horns) of white matter contain descending (motor) tracts. The dorsal (posterior) columns contain the ascending (sensory) tracts. The lateral columns contain both ascending and descending tracts. The central canal of the spinal cord is a potential space that does not normally contain CSF.

THE SPINAL NERVES

There are 31 pairs of spinal nerves: 8 cervical, 12 thoracic, 5 lumbar, 5 sacral, and 1 coccygeal. The cervical nerve roots exit above the corresponding vertebral body. For example, C1 exits between the occiput and C1, and C8 exits between C7 and T1. The remaining spinal nerves exit below their corresponding vertebrae. That is, the L5 root exits beneath the L5 pedicle, just above the L5-S1 disk space. The nerve roots exit through the superior portions of the foramina.

The spinal cord ends at L1-2 in the adult. The cauda equina is the continuation of the spinal nerves of L2-S5, which continue caudally in the thecal sac. Thus, the sacral nerves originate at the termination (also known as the conus) of the spinal cord at the L1-2 vertebral level and traverse caudally through the subarachnoid space of the lumbar cistern to exit at the corresponding sacral vertebrae.

☐ NEUROVASCULAR ANATOMY

BRANCHES OF THE AORTIC ARCH

The usual branching order of the great vessels from the aortic arch is the innominate, left common carotid (CCA), and left subclavian arteries (Fig. 9-12). The most common anatomic variants and anomalies of the arch include common origin of the innominate and left CCAs (25 percent), origin of the left CCA from the proximal innominate artery (bovine left CCA) (5 to 10 percent), separate origin of left vertebral artery (VA) from the arch (5 percent), and aberrant right subclavian artery origin from the arch (0.5 percent).

THE EXTRACRANIAL CAROTID ARTERIES

Usually the right CCA arises from the bifurcation of the innominate artery. The left CCA typically arises separately from the aortic arch just distal to the origin of the innominate artery. However, the left CCA may have a common origin with the innominate artery. The common carotid bifurcation into the internal and external carotid arteries is usually located at the C4-5 level, although this is variable. The proximal internal carotid artery (ICA)

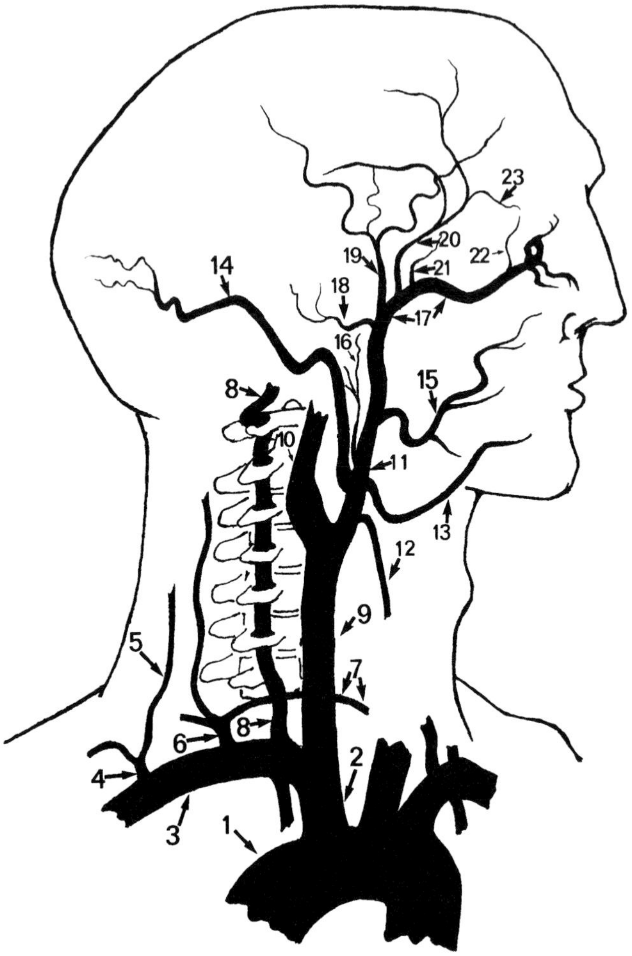

Figure 9-12 Origins of great vessels and major cranial arteries. Aortic arch (1). Innominate artery (2). Right subclavian artery (3). Costocervical trunk (4). Deep cervical artery (5). Thyrocervical trunk (6). Inferior thyroidal artery (7). Right vertebral artery (8). Right common carotid artery (9). Right internal carotid artery (10). Right external carotid artery (11). Superior thyroidal artery (12). Lingual artery (13). Occipital artery (14). Facial artery (15). Ascending pharyngeal artery (16). Internal maxillary artery (17). Posterior auricular artery (18). Superficial temporal artery (19). Middle meningeal artery (20). Accessory meningeal artery (21). Anterior deep temporal artery (22). Meningolacrimal branch (23).

usually runs posterolateral to the proximal external carotid artery (ECA) (Fig 9-12). The relatively dilated proximal portion of the ICA is referred to as the carotid sinus. There are no significant cervical ICA branches.

THE EXTERNAL CAROTID ARTERY

The most common branching order of the ECA is as follows: superior thyroidal (most proximal), ascending pharyngeal (which sometimes arises from a common trunk with the occipital artery), lingual, occipital, facial, posterior auricular, and internal maxillary. The superficial temporal, middle meningeal, accessory meningeal, and anterior deep temporal arteries are major branches of the internal maxillary artery (Fig. 9-12). The middle meningeal artery may occasionally arise from the ophthalmic artery, a branch of the ICA.

The superior thyroidal artery supplies the thyroid and larynx. The ascending pharyngeal artery mainly supplies the naso- and oropharynx and the tympanic cavity but may also provide blood supply to the lower cranial nerves, meninges, and tentorium via its neuromeningeal division. The lingual artery supplies the tongue, floor of the mouth, and submandibular gland. The occipital artery supplies the scalp and upper cervical musculature. A number of facial artery branches anastomose with other ECA vessels to provide vascular supply to the palate, pharynx, orbit, and face. The superficial temporal and posterior auricular arteries primarily supply scalp, buccal region, and ear structures. The internal maxillary artery gives vascular supply to the temporalis muscles, the meninges via (middle and accessory meningeal arteries), palatine and deep facial structures, turbinates and paranasal sinuses, mandible, and alveolar ridges.

One must be keenly aware of communications between the ECA and the intracranial circulation as well as the cranial nerves and ocular structures receiving vascular supply from ECA branches. Muscular branches from the distal occipital artery can communicate with the ipsilateral VA. The posterior auricular artery may communicate with the ICA via the stylomastoid artery. Facial nerve palsy is a concern during embolization of the occipital and posterior auricular arteries due to potential branches to the stylomastoid foramen. The odontoid arcade and neuromeningeal division of the ascending pharyngeal artery (entering the skull base through the jugular foramen) may communicate with the VA. The neuromeningeal division also provides vascular supply to CN IX to XII and sometimes the gasserian ganglion of the trigeminal nerve. The angular branch of the facial artery communicates with the ophthalmic artery via the infraorbital artery.

From the anterior division of the middle meningeal artery, a meningolacrimal branch giving retinal supply may arise. While traversing the foramen spinosum, the middle meningeal artery may supply a branch, through the petrous bone, to the facial nerve.

The ECA-to-ICA connections arising from the internal maxillary artery include the vidian artery (communicating with the petrous ICA through the vidian canal of the sphenoid bone), artery of the foramen rotundum (communicating with the inferolateral trunk/lateral mainstem artery of the cavernous ICA), and orbital branches of the anterior deep temporal artery (communicating with the intracranial circulation via the ophthalmic artery). The artery of the foramen rotundum may supply the V_2 division of the trigeminal nerve, which passes through the same foramen. The vidian artery may also collateralize with the ascending pharyngeal and accessory meningeal arteries.

INTERNAL CAROTID ARTERY

Petrous Portions of the Internal Carotid Artery There are relatively few branches arising from the petrous portion of the ICA traversing the carotid canal (anterior to the jugular foramen). These include the vidian artery (seen in 25 percent of angiograms), described above, as well as a persistent trigeminal artery (seen on less than 1 percent of angiograms), connecting the petrous ICA with the basilar artery (BA) of the posterior circulation. The latter is an embryonic vessel and is the most common type of carotid-vertebral anastomosis caudad to the circle of Willis.

The petrous ICA may take an aberrant course through the middle ear, where it may cause pulsatile tinnitus and a blue tympanic membrane. Obviously, biopsy of the tympanic membrane in this situation would be disastrous.

Cavernous Segment of the Internal Carotid Artery As the ICA exits the petrous bone, it enters the cavernous sinus, a confluence of venous drainage channels within the dura at the base of the brain. The paired cavernous sinuses, flanking the pituitary gland, are typically interconnected by circular sinuses. Other important structures traversing the cavernous sinus include CN III, IV, V_1, V_2, and VI. Within the cavernous sinus, the ICA assumes a sinusoidal shape. This portion plus the terminal ICA cephalad to the cavernous sinus (the supraclinoid portion) makes up the carotid siphon.

The typical branching order of angiographically visible vessels arising from the carotid siphon is as follows: meningohypophyseal trunk (most proximal), inferolateral trunk (lateral mainstem artery), ophthalmic artery, posterior communicating artery (PCOM), anterior choroidal artery, and anterior and middle cerebral arteries (terminal branches) (Fig. 9-13). In approximately 90 percent of patients, the ophthalmic artery is the first branch of the supraclinoid portion of the ICA and thus serves as a demarcation between the intracavernous and subarachnoid segments of the ICA.

The meningohypophyseal trunk supplies the tentorium (via the artery of Bernasconi and Cassinari), cavernous sinus dura, posterior pituitary, and at times cranial nerves III to VI. The inferolateral trunk provides vascular supply to the cavernous sinus dura as well as cranial nerves III to VII; it anastomoses with multiple ECA branches, including the artery of the foramen of rotundum. The ophthalmic artery supplies the globe, orbit and its contents (in conjunction with ECA branches), dura (via the anterior falx artery; rarely, the middle meningeal artery originates from the ophthalmic artery), and may serve as an important collateral pathway with flow received from orbital branches of the facial and internal maxillary arteries.

Posterior Communicating Artery The PCOM serves as a collateral pathway in the circle of Willis, connecting the internal carotid and vertebrobasilar circulations. It runs between the supraclinoid portion of the ICA and the P1 segment of the ipsilateral posterior cerebral artery (PCA) (Fig. 9-13). The PCOM supplies important minute perforating branches to the thalamus, hypothalamus, and optic chiasm. Some 30 to 35 percent of intracranial aneurysms occur within the ICA at the origin of the PCOM. A cone- or nipplelike dilation (less than 3 mm in greatest diameter), termed an infundibulum, may normally occur at the origin of the PCOM from the supraclinoid ICA. This must not be mistaken for an aneurysm.

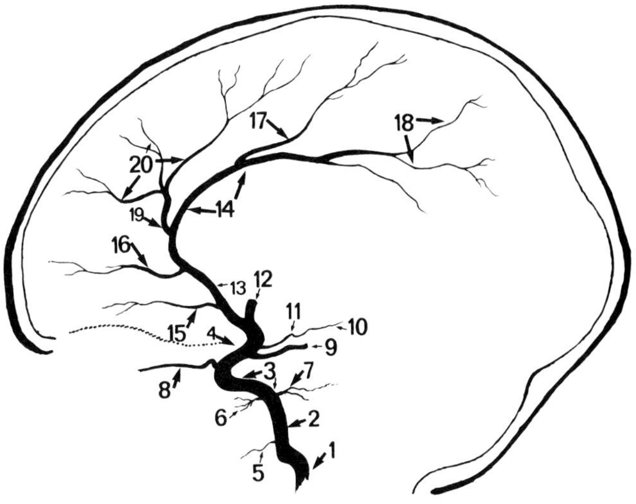

Figure 9-13 Interior carotid and anterior cerebral artery, lateral view. Cervical (1), petrous (2), cavernous (3), and supraclinoid (4) segments of the internal carotid artery. Vidian artery (5), Inferolateral trunk (6). Meningohypophyseal trunk (7). Ophthalmic artery (8). Posterior communicating artery (9). Anterior choroidal artery (10). Plexal point (11). Middle cerebral artery (12). A2 segment anterior cerebral artery (13). Pericallosal artery (14). Orbitofrontal artery (15). Frontopolar artery. (16). Paracentral artery (17). Internal parietal branches (18). Callosomarginal artery (19). Internal frontal branches (20).

Anterior Choroidal Artery The anterior choroidal artery usually originates from the ICA just distal to the PCOM and travels posteriorly in the crural cistern subjacent to the optic tract and medial to the uncus of the temporal lobe (Fig. 9-13). It then enters the choroidal fissure of the temporal horn of the lateral ventricle, where there is a slight kink in its contour called the plexal point. Distal to the plexal point, the anterior choroidal artery supplies the choroid plexus of the lateral ventricle and anastomoses with the lateral posterior choroidal artery. The anterior choroidal artery is quite strategic. Its occlusion may cause the devastating consequences of hemiplegia, hemiparesis, and/or homonymous hemianopsia due to thrombosis of minute perforators arising proximal to the plexal point serving the internal capsule, optic tract, thalamus, basal ganglia, a portion of the cerebral peduncle, and substantia nigra.

The Circle of Willis The circle of Willis is an important vascular collateral ring at the base of the brain surrounding the optic chiasm and pituitary stalk. It is composed of (from posterior to anterior) the basilar artery bifurcation (basilar tip), paired proximal P1 segments of the PCAs (PCA proximal to its junction with the PCOM), paired PCOMs, paired distal ICAs, paired proximal A1 segments of the ACAs, and the anterior communicating artery (ACOM) (linking both ACAs). This vascular ring is actually present in its complete form—i.e., no hypoplastic or absent segments—in only approximately 25 percent of persons. In about 20 percent, the PCA will arise directly from the supraclinoid ICA (fetal origin). The PCOM is hypoplastic in more than 30 percent of the population. Hypoplasia or absence may be seen in the A1 segment of the ACA. The ACOM may be multiple in up to 40 percent of cases.

Vital perforating vessels arising from the circle of Willis include branches to the thalamus, limbic system, reticular activating system, cerebral peduncles, posterior limb of the internal capsule, and oculomotor nerve nucleus from the basilar tip, P1 (most proximal PCA) segments, and the PCOMs. Branches to the optic chiasm and pituitary stalk may arise from the PCOMs and terminal ICA segments. Medial lenticulostriate arteries arise from the A1 segments and supply the internal capsule, hypothalamus, and basal ganglia (Fig. 9-14). Approximately 14 percent of the time, the recurrent artery of Heubner originates from the A1 segment (more commonly it arises from the ACA distal to the ACOM) to supply the anterior limb of the internal capsule, a portion of the globus pallidus, and the head of the caudate nucleus. Small perforators originate from the ACOM, supplying the limbic system and optic chiasm. Occlusion of these perforators risks akinetic mutism and bitemporal hemianopsia.

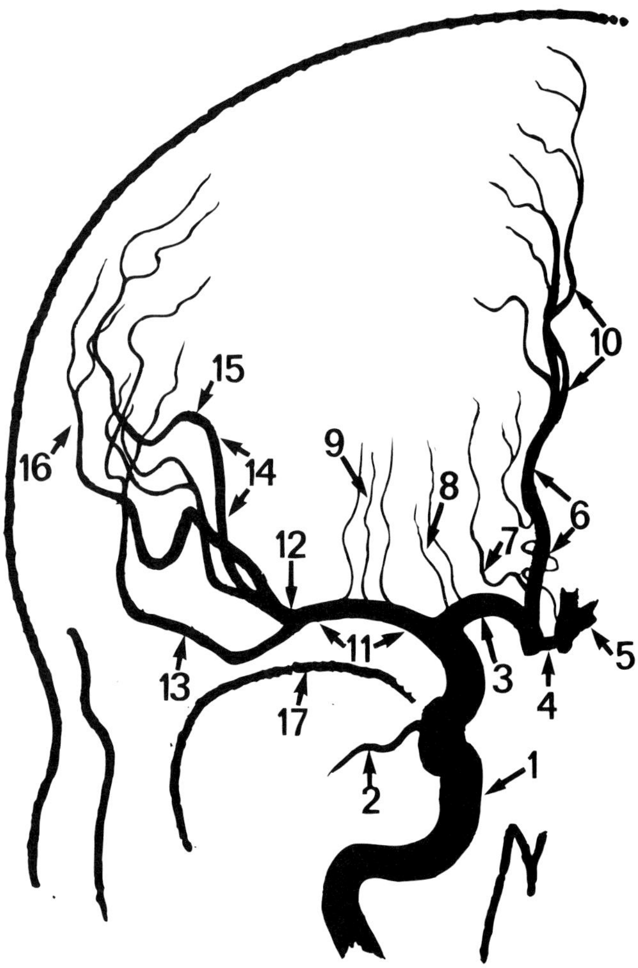

Figure 9-14 Right internal carotid artery and branches, frontal view. Right internal carotid artery (1). Ophthalmic artery (2). A1 segment of anterior cerebellar artery (3). Anterior communicating artery (4). Left anterior cerebellar artery (5). A2 segment (6). Recurrent artery of Heubner (7). Medial lenticulostriate arteries (8). Lateral lenticulostriate arteries (9). Callosomarginal and pericallosal branches of anterior cerebral artery (10). M1 segment of right middle cerebral artery (11). M1 trifurcation (12). Anterior temporal artery (13). M2 branches of right middle cerebral artery (14). Sylvian point (15). M3 and M4 branches of right middle cerebral artery (16). Roof of orbit (17).

The Anterior Cerebral Artery The initial portion of the ACA, between the terminal ICA and the ACOM, is termed the A1 segment. This segment passes anteromedially to enter the interhemispheric fissure, where it follows a generally cephalad curvilinear course around the genu and body of the corpus callosum (Fig. 9-13). The A2 segment of the ACA begins distal to the ACOM and extends to the distal ACA. The A2 segment supplies the head of caudate nucleus, portions of the globus pallidus and anterior limb of internal capsule (via the recurrent artery of Heubner), and the anterior two-thirds of the medial cerebral cortex (Fig. 9-13, 9-15, and 9-18).

The first two branches of the A2 segment are the orbitofrontal and frontopolar arteries, which provide vascular supply to the inferomedial frontal lobe cortex as well as the olfactory bulb and tract. Next, the ACA bifurcates into the pericallosal and callosomarginal arteries (Fig. 9-15). A well-defined callosomarginal artery is present in about 50 percent of cerebral arteriograms. This vessel roughly follows the course of the cingulate sulcus as it extends posterosuperiorly. Its three major branches are the anterior, middle, and posterior internal frontal arteries. When the callosomarginal artery is diminutive or absent, these three branches usually arise directly from the pericallosal artery.

The pericallosal artery runs between the corpus callosum and the cingulate gyrus. Its branches include the paracentral, superior internal parietal (precuneal), and inferior internal parietal arteries. Distally, the pericallosal artery courses around the splenium of the corpus callosum, where it anastomoses with the splenial artery of the PCA.

There is significant variability in the normal ACA, including varying degrees of A1-segment hypoplasia. The A1 segment may have a markedly attenuated caliber and

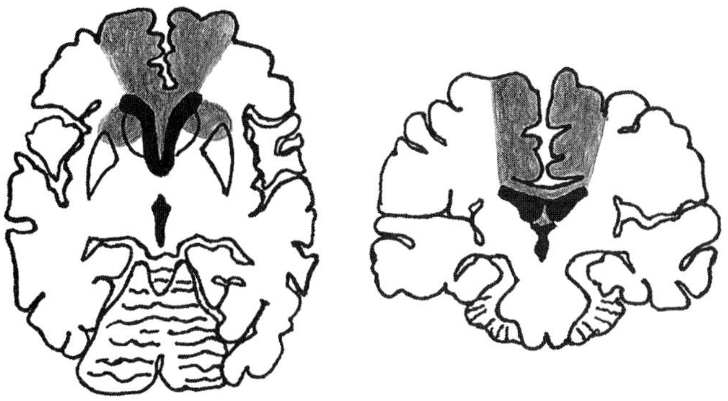

Figure 9-15 Vascular territories of the anterior cerebral artery. (*Adapted with permission from Berman et al.*[4])

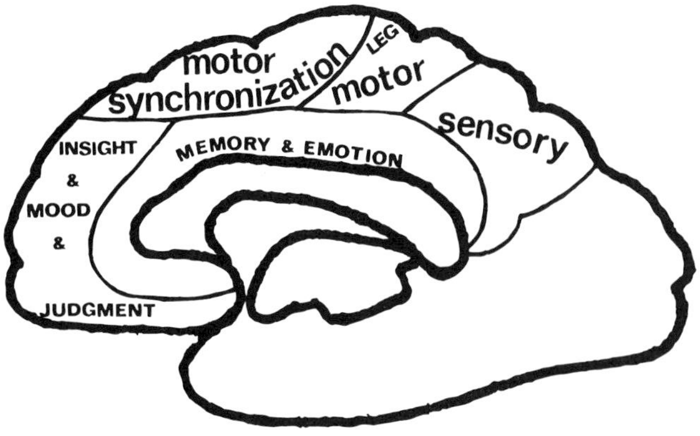

Figure 9-17 Functional territories of the anterior cerebral artery. (*Adapted with permission from Berman et al.*[4])

terminate in the orbitofrontal or frontopolar artery. It is not unusual to observe lack of opacification of the ACA during an ICA contrast injection and visualization of both ACAs during injection of the contralateral ICA. There may be one or more communicating vessels between the A2 segments distal to the ACOM. A single or azygous ACA supplying both cerebral hemispheres may occur uncommonly, arising in the midline from the confluence of the right and left A1 segments. A higher incidence of pericallosal artery aneurysms may be associated with this anomaly.

Occlusion of the ACA would affect cortical territories for motor and sensory functions of the contralateral lower extremity. Frontal lobe infarctions caused by deficient ACA blood flow may result in cognitive disorders, altered personality/initiative, disinhibited behavior and speech, incontinence, and akinetic mutism (in cases of bilateral frontal lobe infarctions) (Fig. 9-17).

The course of the ACA (as well as other intracranial vessels) can be altered and distorted as a result of intracranial masses, cerebral edema, and focal blood collections. However, as CT and MRI have largely replaced angiography in the diagnosis of intracranial masses, the angiographic localization of intracranial masses will not be broached in this chapter.

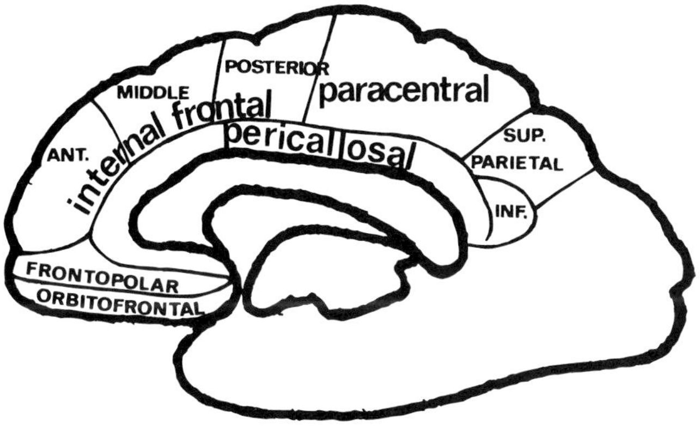

Figure 9-16 Cortical vascular territories of the anterior cerebral artery branches. (*Adapted with permission from Berman et al.*[4])

THE MIDDLE CEREBRAL ARTERY

The MCA follows a complex course and provides vascular supply to a wide expanse of both deep and cortical structures within the frontal, parietal, temporal, and sometimes lateral occipital lobes (Fig. 9-14). Great variability exists in MCA branching.

The most proximal portion of the MCA, termed the M1 segment, extends from the ICA bifurcation laterally and horizontally for 1 to 2 cm through the lateral cerebral fissure. Multiple lateral lenticulostriate arteries—which penetrate the inferior surface of the frontal lobe to supply portions of the basal ganglia, caudate nucleus, and internal capsule—originate from the M1 segment. The M1 segment may also give rise to anterior temporal branches (which may alternatively originate from the proximal M2 portions) supplying the temporal tip cortex. In its most distal portion, the M1 segment curves posterosuperiorly to the insular cortex (island of Reil) where it bifurcates into major anterior and posterior cortical branches. Approximately 20 percent of intracranial aneurysms occur at the M1 bifurcation.

The insular cortex is covered by the frontoparietal and temporal opercula, which coapt to form the Sylvian fissure. The MCA branches that course over the insular cortex and contours of the frontoparietal operculum (forming the M2 portion of the MCA) follow a complex, sinusoidal course as they travel posterosuperiorly to the superior margins of the insular cortex and then pass inferolaterally on the internal and inferior surfaces of the frontoparietal operculum. These multiple cortical branches then emerge from the sylvian fissure to again course superiorly over the frontoparietal cortex.

On frontal angiographic images, the most superior M2 arterial loop (usually formed by a branch of the angular artery) at the superior margin of the insula is called the Sylvian point. On lateral angiographic images, this complex array of MCA cortical branches, extending over the insular and opercular cortices, roughly forms a triangular shape (the sylvian triangle) with its base in the frontosellar region and apex in the parietal region. Intracranial mass lesions may cause distortions and displacements of the sylvian triangle.

A common branching order of the anterior cortical branches of the M2 portion would be as follows: lateral orbitofrontal, operculofrontal (also called ascending frontal or "candelabra" branch), and central sulcus arteries. The central sulcus arteries, usually called precentral (prerolandic) and central (rolandic) branches, supply the motor and sensory cortical strips. The posterior M2 cortical branches include the anterior and posterior parietal, angular, and posterior temporal arteries (Figs. 9-18, 9-19 and 9-20).

The M2 cortical branches provide vascular supply to cerebral centers of speech, comprehension, and calculating ability (dominant hemisphere) as well as the motor and sensory functions of the contralateral face, neck, upper extremities, thorax, and abdomen. Acute M1 occlusion results in contralateral hemiplegia, hemianesthesia, and hemianopsia; global aphasia (with dominant hemisphere involvement); and potentially coma or death. Ischemic injuries to the nondominant hemisphere are frequently associated with apraxia, problems with spatial orientation and dressing, and neglect of contralateral limbs (anosognosia). Ischemic injuries to the temporal lobe may be associated with cortical deafness, disturbances of short-term memory and learning, olfactory hallucinations, behavior changes, or damage to the optic radiations (Fig. 9-21).

Occlusion of a specific M2 branch is usually associated with characteristic neurologic deficits. Lateral occlusion of the orbitofrontal artery may result in expressive aphasia. Isolated precentral arterial blockage causes weakness in the contralateral lower face and tongue (and motor aphasia if occlusion is in the dominant hemisphere).

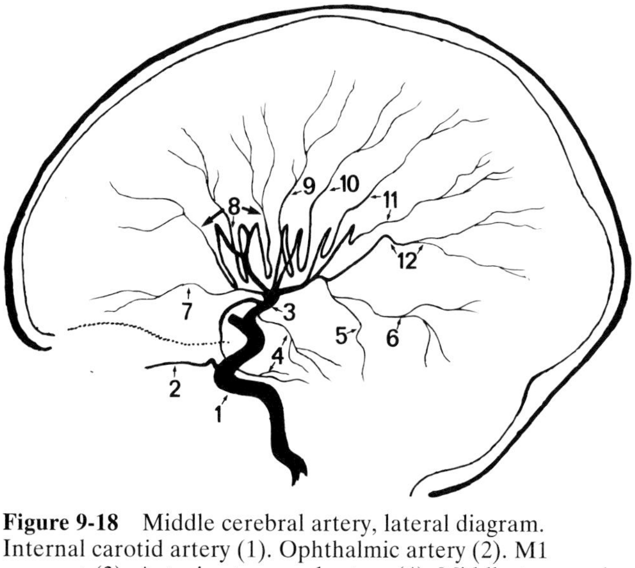

Figure 9-18 Middle cerebral artery, lateral diagram. Internal carotid artery (1). Ophthalmic artery (2). M1 segment (3). Anterior temporal artery (4). Middle temporal artery (5). Posterior temporal branches (6). Orbitofrontal artery (7). Operculofrontal artery (8). Precentral artery (9). Central artery (10). Parietal branches (11). Angular artery (12).

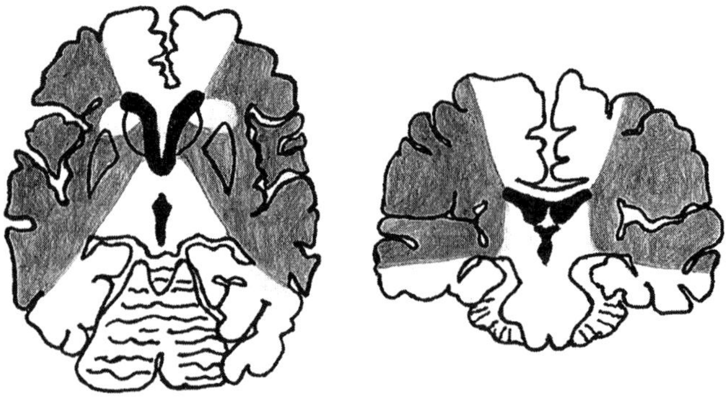

Figure 9-19 Vascular territory of the middle cerebral artery. (*Adapted with permission from Berman et al.*[2])

Occlusion of the rolandic artery leads to contralateral hemiplegia or hemiparesis (more prominent in the upper extremity). Occlusion of the anterior parietal artery frequently causes astereognosis of the contralateral side. Contralateral hemianopsia can occur with occlusion of the posterior parietal, angular, or posterior temporal arteries. Aphasia can result from blockage of the posterior temporal artery in the dominant hemisphere.

THE VERTEBROBASILAR CIRCULATION

The Vertebral Arteries The vertebral arteries (VAs) originate from the subclavian arteries adjacent to the origins of the internal maxillary arteries and just proximal to the thyrocervical and costocervical trunks (Fig. 9-12). In approximately 5 percent of cases, the VA (usually on the left) arises directly from the aortic arch. The thyrocervical and costocervical trunks may have anastomoses with the extracranial portion of the VA and provide branches to the anterior and posterolateral spinal arteries (along with the VA).

One of the two VAs may be dominant in size (usually left greater than right); sometimes one of the VAs may be so diminutive in diameter as to appear threadlike. A high-grade stenosis or segmental occlusion near the origin of the subclavian artery may result in retrograde flow

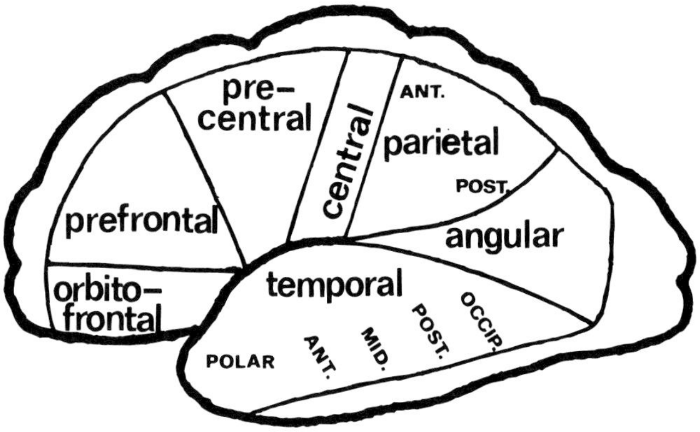

Figure 9-20 Cortical territories of the middle cerebral artery branches. (*Adapted with permission from Berman et al.*[2])

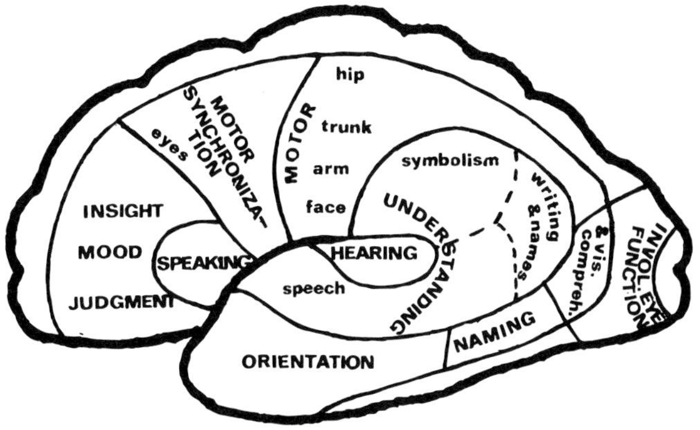

Figure 9-21 Functional territories of the middle cerebral artery. (*Adapted with permission from Berman et al.*[2])

within the ipsilateral VA. If vertebrobasilar insufficiency results, this is called subclavian steal syndrome.

As the vertebral artery ascends, it enters the transverse foramen of C6 and passes superiorly through the transverse foramina of C5-1. After emerging from the transverse foramen of C1, the VA courses posteriorly around the atlantooccipital joint and then ascends through the foramen magnum, penetrating the atlantooccipital membrane and dura. The origin of the posterior meningeal artery usually marks the dural penetration point of the VA. The intradural VA then travels superiorly around the lateral aspect of the medulla. In about 1 percent of angiograms, the VA may terminate in the posterior inferior cerebellar artery.

Posterior Inferior Cerebellar Artery The proximal posterior inferior cerebellar artery (PICA) assumes an inferiorly and then superiorly looping course (caudal and cranial loops, respectively) (Fig. 9-22). These loops are formed by the anterior, lateral, and posterior medullary segments of the proximal PICA. These proximal PICA segments, and at times the distal VA, provide crucial branches to the medulla, the occlusion of which can cause the lateral medullary syndrome (ipsilateral Horner's syndrome, facial pain/temperature sensory loss, and pharyngeal/laryngeal paralysis as well as contralateral pain and temperature sensory loss in the limbs and trunk) or occasional pyramidal tract ischemia (with resultant hemiparesis or hemiplegia).

The apex of the PICA's cranial loop (the choroidal point) roughly defines the floor of the fourth ventricle on lateral vertebral arteriograms and gives rise to fourth ventricular choroidal branches. Just distal to the choroidal point is the supratonsillar segment of the PICA, from which originate tonsillohemispheric and inferior vermian branches. The inferior vermian artery anastomoses distally with the superior vermian branch of the superior cerebellar artery (SCA), providing a major posterior fossa collateral pathway. Occlusion of the PICA's supratonsillar segment may present as dysarthria, ipsilateral limb ataxia, vertigo, and nystagmus.

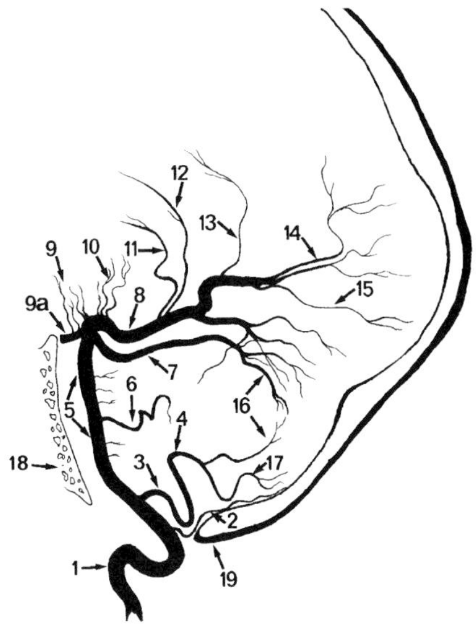

Figure 9-22 Vertebrobasilar vascular anatomy, lateral view. Vertebral artery (1). Posterior meningeal artery (2). Posterior inferior cerebellar artery (3). Choroidal point (4). Basilar artery (5). Anterior inferior cerebellar artery (6). Superior cerebellar artery (7). Posterior cerebral artery (8). Anterior thalamoperforators (9). Posterior communicating artery (9A). Posterior thalamoperforators (10). Medial posterior choroidal artery (11). Lateral posterior choroidal artery (12). Splenial artery (13). Parieto-occipital artery (14). Calcarine artery (15). Superior and inferior vermian branches (16). Hemispheric branches of posterior inferior cerebellar artery (17). Clivus (18). Basiocciput (19).

Anterior Spinal Arteries The anterior spinal arteries (ASA) originate from the VA just distal to the PICA origin; in approximately 50 percent of cases, they course inferomedially to join with their contralateral mate along the anterior cord (Fig. 9-23). There may normally be a variable degree of hypoplasia of the VA distal to the PICA origin.

Basilar Artery Near the pontomedullary junction, the two VAs coalesce to become the basilar artery (BA), which courses anterosuperiorly over the ventral pons (Fig. 9-23). Both the VAs and the BA may be fenestrated—i.e., they may divide into two parallel channels over short distances. Multiple small pontine perforating branches arise from the BA, supplying the pyramidal tracts, medial lemnisci, red nuclei, respiratory centers, and nuclei for CN III, VI, VII, and XII.

Prodromal symptoms of impending BA thrombosis may include visual defects, diplopia, paresthesias, paresis, ataxia, and vertigo. The clinical severity of BA occlusion varies depending on the extent of available collateral pathways. Acute thrombosis may lead to death, coma, respiratory arrest, cerebellar and cranial nerve signs, as well as bilateral motor and sensory dysfunction.

The first major branches of the BA distal to the joining of the VAs are the paired anterior inferior cerebellar arteries (AICAs), which course around the pons toward

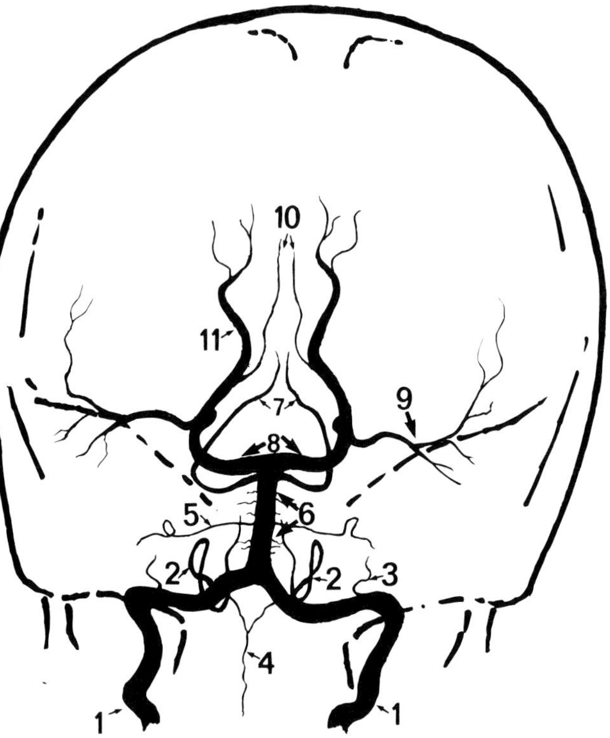

Figure 9-23 Vertebrobasilar arterial anatomy, Towne's view. Vertebral artery (1). Posterior interior cerebral artery (2). Posterior meningeal branch (3). Anterior spinal artery (4). Anterior inferior cerebral artery (5). Basilar artery (6). Superior cerebral artery (7). P1 segment of posterior cerebral artery (8). Temporal branches of PICA (9). Calcarine artery (10). Parietooccipital branches (11).

the cerebellopontine angle and the internal auditory canal to supply the anterior cerebellar hemispheres distally. The AICA also supplies lateral pontine structures and gives rise to the labyrinthine artery (which originates directly from the basilar artery 15 percent of the time). Occasionally, the PICA and AICA may originate from the BA as a common trunk. The labyrinthine artery travels with cranial nerve VIII through the internal auditory canal and supplies the inner ear. Besides ipsilateral hearing loss, occlusion of the AICA may result in ipsilateral limb ataxia, Horner's syndrome, facial pain/temperature sensory loss, dysfunction of CN X and XII, and contralateral pain/temperature sensory loss of the limbs and trunk.

Superior Cerebellar Artery The last infratentorial branches of the BA are the paired superior cerebellar arteries (SCAs). The SCA arises from the BA subjacent to the oculomotor motor nerve and travels above the trigeminal nerve in the perimesencephalic cistern around the brainstem. Proximally, it provides vascular supply to lateral pontine structures, including sympathetic and spinothalamic tracts. Distally, the SCA branches into cerebellar hemispheric branches (supplying portions of the cerebellar peduncles, the dentate nucleus, and superolateral aspects of the cerebellar hemispheres) and the superior vermian artery. Occlusion of the SCA may be accompanied by disturbed gait, limb ataxia, ipsilateral Horner's syndrome, and contralateral pain and temperature sensory loss.

Posterior Cerebral Artery The paired PCAs arise from the basilar tip at the level of the pontomesencephalic junction, superior to the oculomotor nerve and tentorium. The tentorium separates the proximal PCA and SCA on both frontal and lateral vertebral arteriograms. The proximal PCA is divided into P1 and P2 segments at the junction point of the PCA with the PCOM. A filling defect is frequently seen at the transition between P1 and P2 during frontal VA angiograms due to the inflow of unopacified blood from the ipsilateral PCOM. In approximately 20 percent of patients, the PCA arises directly from the ipsilateral ICA (fetal origin of the PCA), with absence or marked hypoplasia of the proximal P1 segment. Uni- or bilateral absence of the PCA during vertebral arteriography should prompt one to first consider fetal origin of the PCA rather than its occlusion.

The proximal P2 segment gives rise to posterior thalamoperforating and thalamogeniculate arteries (supplying portions of the thalamus, geniculate bodies, posterior limb of the internal capsule, and optic tract), as well as minute branches serving the cerebral peduncles. The PCA P2 segment also provides vascular supply to the choroid plexus of the third and lateral ventricles via the medial and lateral posterior choroidal arteries (which collateralize with the anterior choroidal artery) (Fig. 9-23).

The major branches of the P2 segment and more distal PCA include the splenial artery (coursing up and over the splenium of the corpus callosum and collateralizing with the distal ipsilateral pericallosal artery), anterior and posterior temporal branches (supplying the undersurface of the temporal lobe), parieto-occipital artery (supplying the inner posterior cerebrocortical surface), and calcarine artery (traveling within the calcarine sulcus and supplying the visual cortex). The PCA courses posteriorly around the brainstem in the ambient cistern, traveling more medially in the quadrigeminal plate cistern. The distal calcarine cortical branches of the two PCAs converge toward midline on a Towne's projection (with caudad angulation of the image intensifier) vertebral arteriogram, separated by the falx cerebri (Fig. 9-23).

Occlusions of the PCA's cortical branch may result in varying degrees of contralateral homonymous visual field defects, depending on the extent of pial collateral pathways. Occlusion of P1, resulting in blockage of perforating branches, or an aneurysm involving the P1 segment, with mass effect upon the adjacent cerebral peduncle and oculomotor nerve, may cause Weber's syndrome (ipsilateral third cranial nerve palsy together with contralateral hemiplegia). Occlusion of P1 perforators may also affect the reticular activating system and thus cause disturbances of consciousness and coma. Embolization or occlusion of the PCA may result in thalamic disorders, including chorea, hemiballismus, contralateral hemisensory deficits, and thalamic pain syndromes (Figs. 9-24, 9-25, and 9-26).

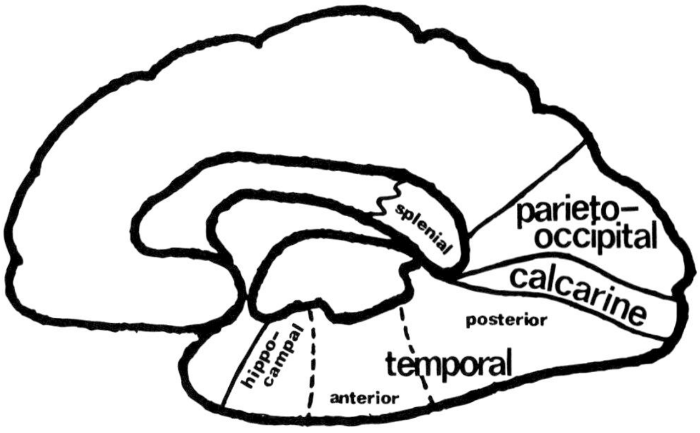

Figure 9-25 Cortical territories of the posterior cerebral artery branches. (*Adapted with permission from Hayman et al.*[3])

NORMAL VENOUS ANATOMY OF THE BRAIN

This brief overview will concentrate only on the most important venous pathways.

The Cerebral Cortical Veins These vessels run in highly variable superficial paths along the cortical sulci; they drain the cerebral cortex and some white matter. Multiple cortical veins drain superiorly toward the superior sagittal sinus (SSS) (Fig. 9-27). The superficial middle cerebral vein is located within the sylvian fissure and receives drainage from the surrounding opercular cortical regions. It frequently courses anteromedially around the temporal tip to empty into the sphenoparietal or cavernous sinus. It may have anastomotic communications with the deep cerebral venous system, the extracranial pterygoid venous plexus, and the facial veins.

Posteriorly, the superficial middle cerebral vein communicates with the veins of Trolard (draining superiorly toward the SSS) and Labbe (draining posteroinferiorly) toward the ipsilateral transverse sinus. Both the veins of Trolard and Labbe cross the subdural space to enter the dural sinuses. Accidental occlusion of the vein of Labbe or other cortical veins during endovascular or surgical procedures may result in cerebral venous infarction.

The Deep Cerebral Veins The paired septal veins run posteriorly near midline along the septum pellucidum. These veins drain the deep white matter of the anterior portions of the frontal lobes. The paired thalamostriate veins run in a subependymal course anteriorly and medially along the floor of the lateral ventricles, passing between the body of the caudate nucleus and the thalamus. They drain the caudate nucleus, deep white matter of the parietal and posterior frontal lobes, and internal capsule and pass anteriorly through the foramina of Monro, where they join with the septal veins to form the paired paramedian internal cerebral veins. The internal cerebral veins run posteriorly within the velum interpositum, defining the roof of the third ventricle (Fig. 9-27).

The paired basal veins of Rosenthal are formed by the confluence of the deep middle and anterior cerebral veins on the ventral surface of the brain and continue posteriorly around the cerebral peduncles. The basal veins also receive venous drainage from the insula and cerebral peduncles. The basal veins travel posteromedially and superiorly, coalescing with the internal cerebral veins (subjacent to the splenium of the corpus callosum) to form the vein of Galen. The midline vein of Galen travels posteriorly approximately 2 cm under the splenium of the corpus callosum within the quadrigeminal plate cistern. It receives the posterior pericallosal, posterior mesencephalic, internal occipital, and several posterior fossa veins before it joins with the inferior sagittal sinus to form the straight sinus at the junction of the falx and tentorial incisura.

The Posterior Fossa Veins The anterior pontomesencephalic vein, actually a network of multiple small veins along the ventral surface of the pons, provides drainage for this structure. Superiorly, it drains toward either the basal vein of Rosenthal or posterior mesencephalic vein. The precentral vein, providing drainage for a portion of the cerebellar hemispheres, runs just

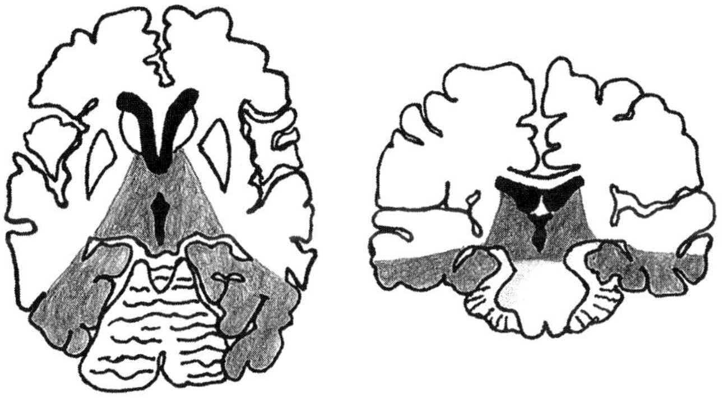

Figure 9-24 Vascular territory of the posterior cerebral artery. (*Adapted with permission from Berman et al.*[3])

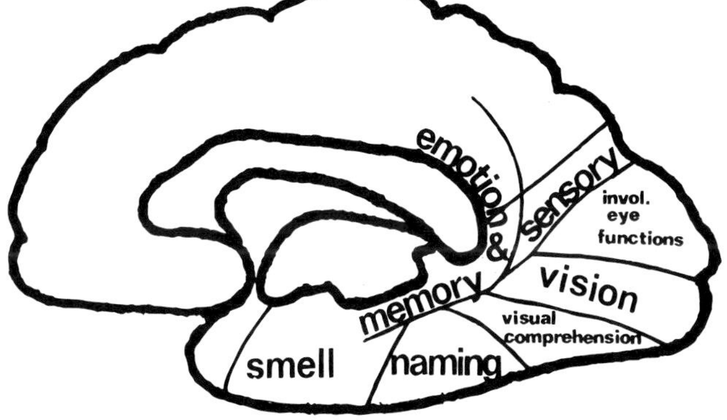

Figure 9-26 Functional territories of the posterior cerebral artery branches. (*Adapted with permission from Hayman et al.*[3])

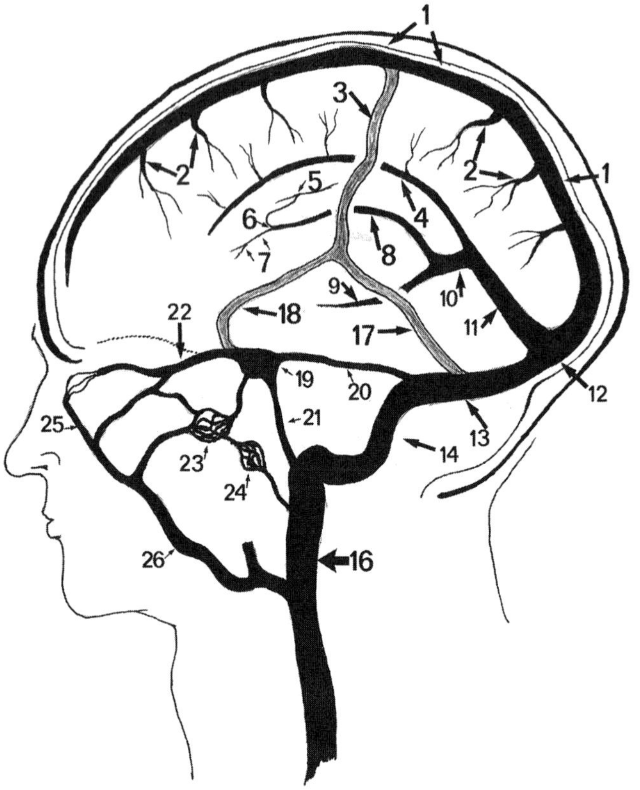

Figure 9-27 Venous anatomy of the head and neck, lateral view. Superior sagittal sinus (1). Cortical veins (2). Vein of Trolard (3). Inferior sagittal sinus (4). Thalamostriate vein (5). Venous angle (6). Anterior septal vein (7). Internal cerebral vein (8). Basal vein of Rosenthal (9). Vein of Galen (10). Straight sinus (11). Torcula (12). Transverse sinus (13). Sigmoid sinus (14). Jugular bulb (15). Internal jugular vein (16). Vein of Labbe (17). Superficial middle cerebral vein (18). Cavernous sinus (19). Superior petrosal sinus (20). Inferior petrosal sinus (21). Superior ophthalmic vein (22). Pterygoid plexus (23). Pharyngeal plexus (24). Angular vein (25). Facial vein (26).

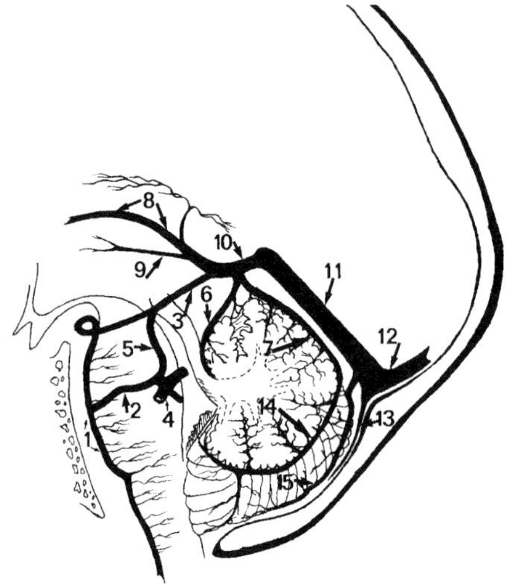

Figure 9-28 Venous drainage of the posterior fosa, lateral view. Anterior pontomesencephalic vein (1). Transverse pontine vein (2). Posterior mesencephalic vein (3). Petrosal vein (4). Lateral mesencephalic vein (5). Precentral cerebellar vein (6). Superior vermian vein (7). Internal cerebral vein (8). Superior thalamic vein (9). Vein of Galen (10). Straight sinus (11). Torcula (12). Occipital sinus (13). Inferior vermian vein (14). Hemispheric vein (15). (*Adapted with permission from Osborn.*[5])

posterior to the roof of the fourth ventricle. The precentral vein courses superiorly behind the inferior colliculi to drain into the vein of Galen.

The superior and inferior vermian veins run along the superior and inferior surfaces of the vermis, respectively, and provide drainage for the cerebellar vermis and hemispheres. The superior vermian vein drains anterosuperiorly toward the vein of Galen. The paramedian inferior vermian veins usually drain posteriorly into the straight sinus (Fig. 9-28).

The Dural Sinus Network The dura mater, which envelops the central nervous system, has two layers that form reflections known as the falx cerebri, tentorium, and falx cerebelli. These separate the cerebral hemispheres, cerebrum from cerebellum, and cerebellar hemispheres, respectively. The layers of the dura separate to form venous drainage channels or dural sinuses for the brain. Some of these dural sinuses communicate with veins in the scalp and diploic space of the calvarium via emissary veins. The superior sagittal sinus travels along the superior margin of the falx cerebri. It receives venous drainage from multiple cerebral cortical veins, the vein of Trolard, and emissary veins. At times, the anterior one-third of the superior sagittal sinus may not opacify during late-phase cerebral angiography or may be congenitally absent. This midline sinus carries blood flow posteriorly and inferiorly in a crescentic course to the posterior junction point between falx and tentorium containing the confluence of sinuses (also known as the torcular Herophili or torcula) near the occipital protuberance.

Multiple arachnoid invaginations, present along the superior sagittal as well as transverse sinuses, are known as arachnoid granulations; they serve as the sites of CSF resorption from the subarachnoid space. These structures may appear as filling defects during the venous phase of cerebral angiograms and should not be mistaken for intraluminal thrombi.

The inferior sagittal sinus is contained within the lower curvilinear edge of the falx, where it receives venous drainage from the falx and the cerebral hemispheres. This dural channel drains posteriorly in the midline to join with the vein of Galen, forming the straight sinus within the intersection between the falx cerebri and the tentorium. The straight sinus drains posteriorly toward the torcula. Occipital sinuses of variable caliber are frequently visualized during cerebral angiography, coursing superomedially within the dura of the posterior fossa, just lateral to the foramen magnum and draining toward the torcula.

The paired transverse sinuses follow a crescentic course within the periphery of the tentorium, laterally and anteriorly from the torcula. Usually the right transverse sinus is dominant or larger than the left. Occasionally, one may be extremely hypoplastic during cerebral angiography. The transverse sinuses receive drainage from the inferior cerebral veins and vein of Labbe and communicate with the cavernous sinuses via the superior petrosal sinuses, which run along the petrous ridges.

The transverse sinus, as it travels subjacent to the tentorium, becomes the sigmoid sinus. This sinus, contained within the dura of the posterior fossa, follows a curved course toward the jugular foramen, where it empties into the internal jugular vein (Fig. 9-29). A bend in contour at this junction point is called the jugular bulb. Other structures traversing the jugular foramen include CN IX through XI and small branches of the ascending pharyngeal and occipital arteries. The jugular bulbs communicate with the cavernous sinuses by means of the paired inferior petrosal sinuses, which ascend supramedially from the jugular foramen within the dura flanking the clivus. The inferior petrosal sinuses interconnect through a clival venous plexus.

The structure and contents of the paired cavernous sinuses have been discussed above. The cavernous sinuses receive venous drainage from the orbits and their contents via the superior and inferior ophthalmic veins (which, in turn, communicate with the angular, frontal scalp, and anterior facial veins). The cavernous sinuses may also communicate with the pterygoid venous plexus, situated between the temporalis and lateral pterygoid muscles and supplying drainage for the internal maxillary distribution. This venous drainage pattern may allow intracranial spread of central and deep facial infectious processes.

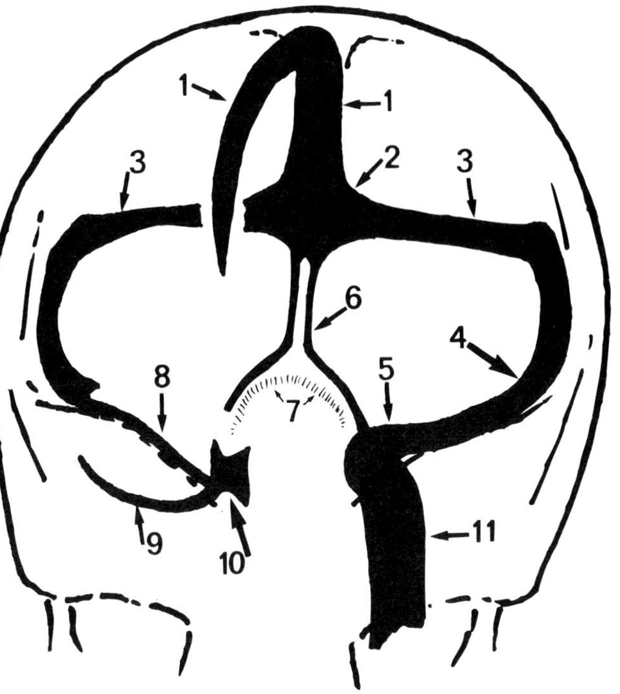

Figure 9-29 Major dural sinuses, oblique Towne's view. Superior sagittal sinus (1). Torcula (2). Transverse sinus (3). Sigmoid sinus (4). Jugular bulb (5). Occipital sinus (6). Foramen magnum (7). Superior petrosal sinus (8). Sphenoparietal sinus (9). Cavernous sinus (10). Internal jugular vein (11).

SUGGESTED READINGS

The Central Sulcus

1. Sobel DF et al: Locating the central sulcus: Comparison of MR anatomic and magnetoencephalographic functional methods. *AJNR* 14:915–925, 1993.

The Limbic System

1. Naidich TP et al: Hippocampal formation and related structures of the limbic lobe: anatomic–MR correlation Part I. Surface features and coronal sections. *Radiology* 162:747–754, 1987.

The Cranial Nerves and Skull Base

1. Harnsberger HR: *Head and Neck Imaging: A Year Book Handbook*, Chicago, Year Book, 1990.

Neuroanatomy

1. Carpenter MB: *Core Text of Neuroanatomy*, 4th ed. Baltimore, Williams & Wilkins, 1991.
2. De Groot J, Chusid JG: *Correlative Neuroanatomy*, 21st ed. Menlo Park, CA, Appleton & Lange, 1991.

Cerebrovascular Anatomy

1. Gilman S, Newman SW: *Manter and Gatz's Essentials of Clinical Neuroanatomy and Neurophysiology*, 7th ed. Philadelphia, Davis, 1987.
2. Lasjaunias P, Berenstein A: *Surgical Neuroangiography*, Vols. I–IV, 1st ed. New York, Springer-Verlag, 1987.
3. Osborn AG: *Introduction to Cerebral Angiography*. Philadelphia, Harper & Row, 1980.

Anatomical Illustrations

1. DeArmond SJ et al: *Structures of the Human Brain*, 3rd ed. Oxford, Oxford University Press, 1989.
2. Berman SA et al: Correlation of CT cerebral vascular territories with function: I. Anterior cerebral artery. *AJR* 135:253–257, 1980.
3. Hayman LA et al: Correlation of CT cerebral vascular territories with function: II, Posterior cerebral artery. *AJR* 137:13–19, 1981.
4. Berman SA et al: Correlation of CT cerebral vascular territories with function: III, middle cerebral artery. *AJR* 142:1035–1040, 1984.

Figure Legends

1. DeArmond SJ et al. *Structure of the Human Brain: A Photographic Atlas*, 3d ed. Oxford, England, Oxford University Press, 1989.
2. Berman SA et al: Correlation of CT cerebral vascular territories with function: 3. Middle cerebral artery. *AJR* 142:1035–1040, 1984.
3. Hayman LA et al: Correlation of CT cerebral vascular territories with function: II. Posterior cerebral artery. *AJR* 137:13–19, 1981.
4. Berman SA et al: Correlation of CT cerebral vascular territories with function: I. Anterior cerebral artery. *AJR* 135:253–257, 1980.
5. Osborn AG: Introduction to cerebral angiography. Philadelphia, Harper & Row, 1980, p 394.

☐ QUESTIONS

1. What artery provides blood supply to the lower cranial nerves (IX–XII)?

2. Name four external carotid-to-internal carotid collateral pathways.

3. Name two important collateral pathways between the external carotid and vertebral circulations.

4. What vessel must be examined for vascular supply to a tentorial meningioma?

5. The following structures traverse the cavernous sinus (T/F):
   1. The internal carotid artery
   2. Cranial nerves III and IV, divisions 1 and 2 of V and VI
   3. Optic nerve
   4. V_3

6. Regarding the central sulcus (T/F):
   1. The primary motor area is located between the precentral and central sulcus.
   2. The primary sensory area is located between central and postcentral sulcus.
   3. The central sulcus is the only major sulcus that extends from the surface of the brain to the midline.
   4. The central sulcus can be identified only on sagittal MRI images.
   5. The superior frontal sulcus forms a right angle with the central sulcus on axial CT.

7. Regarding the hippocampus (T/F):
   1. The white matter overlies the gray matter.
   2. A mesial temporal sclerosis is associated with partial complex seizures.
   3. The hippocampus is part of the limbic system.
   4. The hippocampus is connected to the fornix via the alveus.
   5. The hippocampus forms the uncus.

8. What part of the internal capsule do the corticospinal tract fibers pass through?

9. What part of the brain should one examine on MRI in a patient presenting with internuclear ophthalmoplegia?

10. What parts of the nervous system should be studied in a patient presenting with trigeminal neuralgia?

11. What parts of the body need to be studied in a patient with a recurrent laryngeal nerve palsy?

☐ ANSWERS

1. a. Ascending pharyngeal

2. a. Vidian artery
   b. Artery of the foramen rotundum
   c. Facial and anterior deep temporal collaterals to the ophthalmic artery
   d. Meningolacrimal branch off of the middle meningeal artery to the ophthalmic artery

3. a. Ascending pharyngeal neuromeningeal division to vertebral artery
   b. Muscular branches of occipital artery to distal vertebral artery

4. Meningohypophyseal trunk

5. a. T (1,2)
   b. F (3,4)

6. a. T (1,2,3)
   b. F (4,5)

7. a. T (1,2,3,4), F (5)

8. Posterior limb of internal capsule

9. The medial longitudinal fasciculus, located in the dorsal pons, immediately ventral to the fourth ventricle.

10. The thalamus, entire brainstem, and cervical cord down to the C5 level.

11. The imaging workup should include evaluation from the medulla down to the level of the aorticopulmonic window in the chest.

CHAPTER

10

Congenital Brain Malformations and the Phakomatoses

David G. Ashley
Marvin Nelson

☐ BRAIN DEVELOPMENT

As the anterior neuropore closes at approximately 25 days of gestation, three rostral neural tube vesicles have developed. These are the prosencephalon, mesencephalon, and rhombencephalon. The prosencephalon develops into the telencephalon and diencephalon. The telencephalon will eventually become the cerebral hemispheres, putamina, and caudate nuclei. The diencephalon eventually becomes the thalami, hypothalami, and globi pallidi. The mesencephalon becomes the midbrain. The rhombencephalon becomes the metencephalon (cerebellar hemispheres and vermis) and myelencephalon (medulla and pons). The germinal matrix lining the entire ventricular system reaches its peak at approximately 28 weeks. Most of the neurons that form the six-layer cerebral cortex migrate by way of the radial glial fibers. The order of migration of the nerve cell layers is layer 1 (molecular layer), followed by 6, 5, 4, 3, and, last, 2. Late-migrating neurons reach their position by approximately 20 weeks. Following this, cortical organization takes place. Glial scarring is thought not to occur before 20 weeks. Hemorrhage of the germinal matrix is unusual after 34 weeks, because the bulk of the germinal matrix has regressed.

☐ MYELINATION

Normal myelination begins in the fifth fetal month and continues into adulthood. In general, myelination occurs from caudad to cephalad, from central to peripheral, and from dorsal to ventral. There appears to be a window when delayed myelination may be detected. This is between the ages of 4 months and 2 years unless myelination delay is very severe. On magnetic resonance imaging (MRI), T1- as opposed to T2-weighted images are superior in assessing myelination in the first 6 months. After 6 months T2-weighted images are more useful.

Landmarks for normal myelination are as follows: there should be increased T1 signal in the anterior limbs of the internal capsules by 3 months, the splenium of the the corpus callosum by the fourth month, and the genu of the corpus callosum by 6 months. On T2, the genu of the corpus callosum should be of low signal by 8 months and the anterior limb of the internal capsule by 11 months. In normal infants, from 0 to 4 months, hemispheric white matter is hypointense relative to gray matter on T1 and bright on T2. Between 4 and 10 months, the white matter becomes relatively hyperintense on T1 but continues to have higher intensity on T2. After 10 months, the white matter normally appears hyperintense on T1 and hypointense on T2. There should be isointensity on T1 by about 4 months and isointensity on T2 by approximately 10 months.

☐ CLASSIFICATION OF CONGENITAL CNS ABNORMALITIES

A standardized classification of congenital malformations of the brain does not exist. Various classification systems have been attempted based upon morphology and embryologic stages of development. The developmental stages are dorsal induction, ventral induction, neuronal proliferation, migration, organization, and myelination. These classifications may be impractical to the radiologist because of the frequent multiplicity of anomalies, often occurring in different categories. An insult may result in defects of several structures, many of which may be forming at the same time. Also, a genetic abnormality may be displayed during development at different times. An important rule is to look closely for a second malformation after you have found the first.

DORSAL INDUCTION DEFECTS

These involve defects in neural tube closure which occur at around 4 weeks of gestation. They include anencephaly, cephalocele, myeloschisis, Chiari malformation, and hydromyelia.

Anencephaly Anencephaly is defined as absence of the calvarium (also called acrania), with the absence of most or all of the brain. The cranium is typically absent above the orbits. Some think that exencephaly (acrania with protrusion of the brain into the amnionic cavity) may eventually lead to anencephaly. Amniotic bands may be responsible for many cases of exencephalus, "nonanatomic" encephaloceles, and unusual facial clefts.

Cephalocele A cephalocele is a defect in the cranium and dura with extracranial herniation of intracranial structures. Cephaloceles are divided into four types: cranial meningoceles, cranial glioceles, cranial meningoencephaloceles, and atretic cephaloceles. The cranial meningoceles contain leptomeninges and cerebrospinal fluid (CSF). The glioceles contain only a glia-lined cyst containing CSF. The meningoencephaloceles contain leptomeninges, CSF, and brain. Some use the term *encephalocele* ("sac containing brain") to mean meningoencephalocele. Atretic cephaloceles (meningocele manque) are formes fruste of cephaloceles that usually appear as small, sparsely haired scalp lesions near the midline vertex or just above the external occipital protuberance. The significance of atretic cephaloceles is a high incidence of associated intracranial anomalies.

Cephaloceles are named for the location where they occur. In Caucasians, the occipital cephalocele, located at the midline between the foramen magnum and lambda, is the most common type (75 percent). They show a female predominance. Cephaloceles in other locations, associated with Chiari malformations and the Dandy-Walker malformation, show a male predominance. Most cephaloceles are not associated with syndromes. A notable exception is Meckel's syndrome, which includes occipital encephalocele, cystic dysplastic kidneys, orofacial clefting, and polydactyly.

The next location in frequency, although it is uncommon in the western hemisphere, is the parietal cephalocele (10 to 15 percent). These are located between the bregma and lambda. They are frequently associated with Dandy-Walker malformation, agenesis of the corpus callosum, and lobar holoprosencephaly.

Frontoethmoidal (sincipital) cephaloceles are most common in Southeast Asians. As opposed to occipital and parietal cephaloceles, they are not associated with other neural tube defects.

Imaging findings typically demonstrate microcephaly with cranium bifidum. The external sac may contain CSF, brain, neuroglial tissue, blood vessels, ventricles, and choroid plexus. Magnetic resonance imaging is most useful for evaluating the contents of the cephalocele sac and determining whether there is an associated dural venous sinus. Magnetic resonance angiography (MRA) may be helpful for this.

Chiari Malformations ***Chiari I Malformation*** Chiari I malformation represents a downward displacement of the cerebellar tonsils through the foramen magnum without low positioning of the fourth ventricle. Patients may present with a motor deficit (weakness, muscle atrophy, reflex changes), sensory loss, cranial nerve palsies, and pain. The motor deficits are usually bilateral.

In the first 15 years of life, cerebellar tonsillar protrusion below a line drawn from basion to opisthion up to 6 mm should be considered within normal limits. This distance decreases in subsequent decades. A protrusion of greater than 5 mm in adults is generally considered abnormal; however, 30 percent of adults with protrusions from 5 to 10 mm have been found to be asymptomatic. Herniations greater than 12 mm are invariably symptomatic. Asymmetrical tonsillar herniation is not considered significant. Frequently there is a tight appearance of the low posterior fossa contents with compression of the lower brainstem. Syringohydromyelia is common in about 25 to 40 percent. The syrinx may extend into the brainstem (syringobulbia) and uncommonly be isolated to the thoracic cord. There may be scoliosis and osseous abnormalities of the craniocervical junction with fused cervical vertebrae (Klippel-Feil syndrome). Chiari I malformations are not usually associated with other intracranial anomalies aside from occasional hydrocephalus.

Chiari II Malformation The incidence of the Chiari II malformation is approximately 2 per 1000. Females are affected 2:1. Chiari II malformation involves the hindbrain, mesodermal structures, and spine.

The findings of Chiari II malformation are as follows:

- A small posterior fossa with the hindbrain compressed inferiorly through the foramen magnum.
- A small, low-positioned, tubular fourth ventricle.
- Downward cord displacement to a point where the cord becomes fixed by the dentate ligaments, so that cervical roots ascend to the foramina.
- The medulla, which is not fixed by ligaments, may form a medullary kink.
- The cerebellum is indented inferiorly by a frequently enlarged foramen magnum.
- Frequently, a small or normal size of the posterior vertebral arch of C1.
- Low tentorial insertion.
- The cerebellum may protrude upward through a widened incisural notch.

- A cerebellar "peg" of tissue may extend inferiorly posterior to the cord.

Frequently associated findings are as follows:

- Hydrocephalus
- Lückenshädel skull
- Fenestration of the falx with gyral interdigitation
- Fused colliculli forming a tectal beak
- Callosal hypogenesis with absence of the splenium and rostrum
- Colpocephaly (prominent atria and occipital horns)
- Large massa intermedia
- Enlarged caudate heads with inferior pointing frontal horns on coronal imaging
- Posterior concavity of the clivus and petrous ridges
- Frequent association with syringohydromyelia
- Less frequent aqueductal stenosis and cerebral migrational abnormalities

The fourth ventricle may become trapped. If a "normal-sized" fourth ventricle is seen, then there should be heightened concern for concomitant hydrocephalus or syringohydromyelia.

Chiari III Malformation The Chiari III malformation, a rare condition with poor prognosis, involves herniation of the cerebellar contents through an upper cervical spina bifida or an occipitocervical meningomyeloencephalocele. Magnetic resonance imaging is useful to show the relationship with brainstem and venous structures.

VENTRAL INDUCTION DEFECTS (DISORDERS OF DIVERTICULATION)

Holoprosencephaly represents failure of cleavage of the prosencephalon into a discrete diencephalon and telencephalon. Common to holoprosencephaly types is the fusion of gray and white matter across the midline and absent septum pellucidum. Facial anomalies may be seen in the alobar and semilobar types but are absent or mild in the lobar type.

Alobar Holoprosencephaly Alobar holoprosencephaly represents the most severe form. Findings are as follows:

- Microcephaly
- Hypotelorism
- Absent interhemispheric fissure, falx, and sagittal sinus
- Fused thalami with absence of a third ventricle
- Horseshoe-shaped monoventricle
- Callosal agenesis
- Usually a large dorsal cyst
- Absent olfactory bulbs and tracts
- High torcula
- Azygous anterior cerebral artery

Semilobar Holoprosencephaly Semilobar holoprosencephaly has findings of:

- Partial formation of the posterior interhemispheric fissure and falx
- Rudimentary or absent corpus callosum
- Partial differentiation into temporal and occipital horns
- Rudimentary third ventricle
- Possible dorsal cyst

A unique finding is the presence of the callosal splenium with absence of the genu and body. This suggests the diagnosis of semilobar holoprosencephaly on a midline sagittal image. Holoprosencephaly with "middle interhemispheric fusion" of gray matter at the level of the body of the corpus callosum is considered an uncommon variant.

Lobar Holoprosencephaly Lobar holoprosencephaly demonstrates:

- A nearly complete interhemispheric fissure, although shallow anteriorly
- Gray matter crossing the midline at the inferior frontal lobes
- Relatively well formed ventricles with "squared off" fused frontal horns
- Possible callosal dysgenesis
- Absent septum pellucidum

Septooptic Dysplasia Septooptic dysplasia (DeMorsier's syndrome) is a group of disorders most commonly seen in females. It is possibly a mild form of holoprosencephaly. These patients have pituitary and hypothalamic-pituitary insufficiencies, anomalies of the septum pellucidum, and hypoplasia of the optic chiasm or nerves.

Findings are as follows:

- An absent or hypoplastic septum pellucidum with box-like frontal horns
- Hypoplastic optic chiasm and optic nerves (imaged in only 50 percent)
- Pituitary infundibular thinning or absence
- Schizencephaly in about 40 to 50 percent of cases

DISORDERS OF MIGRATION AND ORGANIZATION

Lissencephaly/Pachygyria The term *lissencephaly* means "smooth brain," *agyria* is synonymous. Pachygyria refers to a reduced number of thick, broad gyri with less than normal sulcal infolding. These differ only in degree.

The three diagnostic findings of lissencephaly are as follows:

- A smooth cortex
- Abnormal contour with shallow vertical sylvian fissures
- Abnormal gray/white matter distribution

Colpocephaly and callosal dysgenesis are commonly seen. Subcategories of lissencephaly are listed below.

Type I Lissencephaly (Agyria-Pachygyria Complex) This category represents a spectrum from the more common incomplete lissencephaly (agyria-pachygyria) to complete lissencephaly. Microscopically, there is a thin outer neuron layer, a cell-sparse zone, a thick inner neuron layer, and decreased thickness of the deep white matter layer. The symptoms are related to the severity of brain involvement. These patients may have one of several syndromes (Miller-Dieker, chromosome 17 deletion; Norman-Roberts, autosomal recessive; or Neu-Laxova, autosomal recessive), each of which has characteristic facies and microcephaly. Miller-Dieker syndrome is the most common.

The findings are a smooth cortex; abnormal cerebral contour with shallow vertical sylvian fissures; and abnormal gray/white matter distribution. There is a thin outer gray matter layer, a thin outer white matter layer (the cell-sparse zone), a very thick inner gray matter layer, and a thin inner white matter layer. More commonly, areas of pachygyria are present, usually in the frontal and temporal lobes. Remember that in imaging the early infant brain, the T1 and T2 relative intensities of gray and white matter on MRI are reversed as compared to the normal adult appearance.

Type II Lissencephaly These include three possibly related syndromes: Walker-Warburg syndrome, Fukuyama's congenital muscular dystrophy, and muscle-eye-brain disease. The latter two are similar but less severe, and these may represent a spectrum. The classic example is the lethal Walker-Warburg syndrome, which is characterized by lissencephaly, cerebellar and retinal malformations, and congenital muscular dystrophy. There is a thickened and severely disorganized unlayered cortex, sometimes with vertical neuron columns. On imaging, there is lissencephaly. As opposed to lissencephaly type I, there is not the thick, deep gray matter layer, and the thickness of white matter is relatively preserved. There may be a thin interrupted band of gray matter or irregular projections of gray matter just deep to the cortex. There is severe hypomyelination of the white matter, resulting in increased T2 signal. There may be obliteration of the interhemispheric fissure from leptomeningeal thickening, hydrocephalus, ocular abnormalities, cerebellar anomalies, Dandy-Walker malformation, and occipital cephalocele.

Types III to V Lissencephaly Type III lessencephaly, or microcephalia vera, is thought to be secondary to a depleted germinal zone at 26 weeks, with absence of layers 2 and 3. Pathology shows microcephaly, lissencephaly, and an extremely thin cortex. In type IV lissencephaly, or radial microbrain, pathology shows a normal cortical thickness and layering (1 to 6) but markedly reduced neuron number. Type V lissencephaly is a diffuse cortical dysplasia or polymicrogyria and is associated with congenital cytomegalovirus infection.

Polymicrogyria In polymicrogyria, the pathologic appearance of the brain demonstrates many small gyri externally and small interdigitations of the gray/white matter junction internally. Common to all polymicrogyrias is a derangement of the normal six-layered cortex. A "layered polymicrogyria" may be seen, with a cortical laminar necrosis of layer 5 and overlying normal layers 4, 3, and 2. This may result in different growth rates of inner and outer cortex, with subsequent polymicrogyria. As layer 2 is the last layer to arrive, this is a postmigratory event (after 20 weeks). Many authors believe that this condition stems from ischemic cortical damage, most commonly due to perfusion failures from cytomegalovirus. Toxoplasmosis and shock have also been implicated as causes. In "unlayered polymicrogyria," there is no cell sparse layer. This is thought to represent an earlier gestation event (early second trimester).

Like pachygyria, polymicrogyria usually demonstrates a thickened cortex. It may show multiple small gyri, or it may appear normal on routine imaging. The dysplastic cortex is usually isointense on MRI, most frequently near the sylvian fissure, and it may have deep cortical infolding with prominent draining veins. Bright T2 signal is seen in the subjacent white matter in approximately 20 percent of cases and calcification of the cortex in 5 percent. Inversion recovery sequences on MRI or volume three-dimensional gradient echo images with very thin slices may show multiple small gyri and subtle irregularities of the gray/white matter junction suggesting the presence of polymicrogyria.

Nonlissencephalic Cortical Dysplasia The term *nonlissencephalic cortical dysplasia* refers (1) to a general classification of an abnormally thickened cortex with diminished sulcal depth and an irregular, bumpy gyral pattern or (2) an abnormally deep infolding of thickened cortex, often with a high extension of the sylvian fissure. Bright T2 signal is seen in the white matter in 25 percent of cases. The term *cortical dysplasia* was used because of difficulty in distinguishing pachygyria and polymicrogyria on MRI. Many feel that most or all of these dysplasias represent polymicrogyria. Also in this category is congenital bilateral perisylvian syndrome or bilateral opercular cortical dysplasia. These patients have pseudobulbar paresis, dysarthria, seizures, and MRI findings of bilateral cortical malformations of the perisylvian regions. They are also thought to have polymicrogyria.

Schizencephaly The term *Schizencephaly* (agenetic porencephaly) refers to gray matter–lined clefts from the cerebral cortex to the lateral ventricle. The walls of the cleft may be apposed (closed-lip or type 1 schizencephaly)(Fig. 10-1*A*) or separated by CSF (open-lip or type 2 schizencephaly)(Fig. 10-1*B*). The gray matter at the cleft usually shows a "nonlayered polymicrogyria." The damages probably occurs during the first half of the second trimester. Clinical symptoms parallel the extent of cerebral involvement. The location is typically near the central sulcus. Bilaterality is present in 35 percent. The lateral ventricular wall may show an outward dimple where the cleft of the closed-lip type reaches the lateral ventricle. Multiplanar imaging may be necessary to demonstrate the dimple. Cortical dysplasia may be seen adjacent to the cleft and in the contralateral hemisphere. The septum pellucidum is usually absent. With the open-lip type, CSF pulsations may result in enlargement of the ipsilateral calvarium; this may respond to shunting.

Gray Matter Heterotopia A gray matter heterotopion represents a collection of nerve cells found in an abnormal location (Fig. 10-2). These may be isolated anomalies or associated with other malformations. Heterotopia may be subependymal, subcortical, or diffuse (band heterotopia). The latter appearance is similar to type I lissencephaly, with two gray matter layers separated by normally myelinated white matter. Heterotopia show isointensity on all MRI sequences, no surrounding edema, no enhancement, and absence of hemispheric enlargement with very large heterotopia. There may be CSF infolding into the outer brain surface, resulting in apparent increased T2 signal within the heterotopion, which can be confused for edema.

Unilateral Hemimegalencephaly Unilateral hemimegalencephaly represents hamartomatous overgrowth of all or part of a cerebral hemisphere. Findings are hemispheric enlargement, lateral ventricular dilation proportionate to the cerebral enlargement, normal gyral pattern to agyric, thickened cortex, and high T2 signal of the white matter. The border between gray and white matter may disappear. The cortex may be calcified. A straight, uplifted, anteriorly

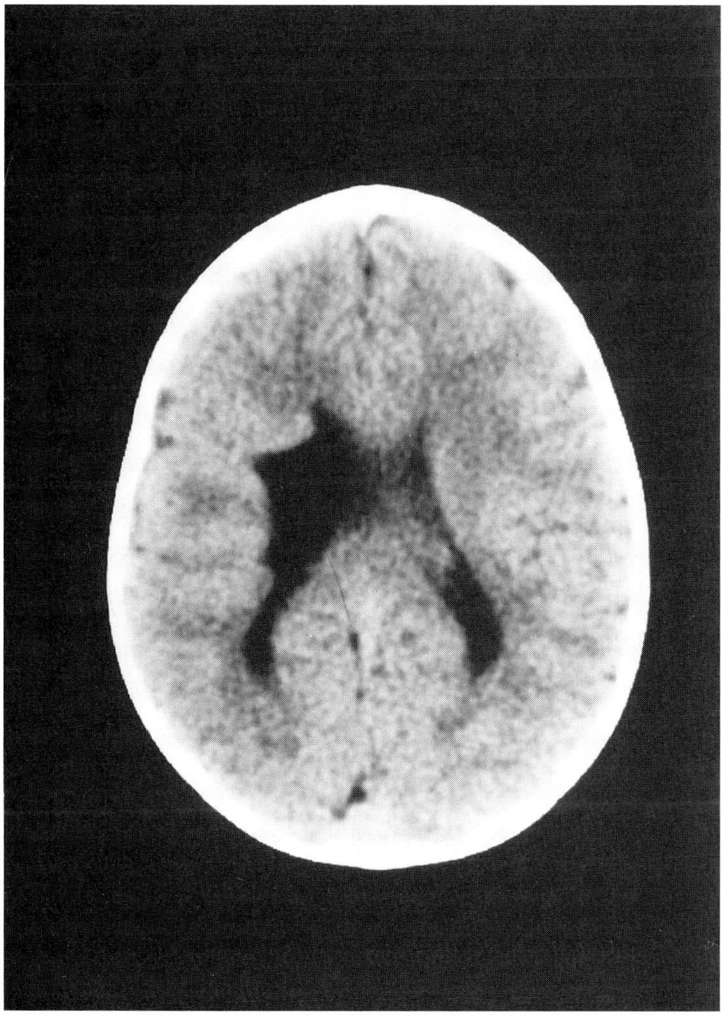

(A)

Figure 10-1 *A*. Closed-lip schizencephaly, axial CT. There are two ventricular dimples marking the clefts of closed-lip schizencephaly. The septum pellucidum is absent.

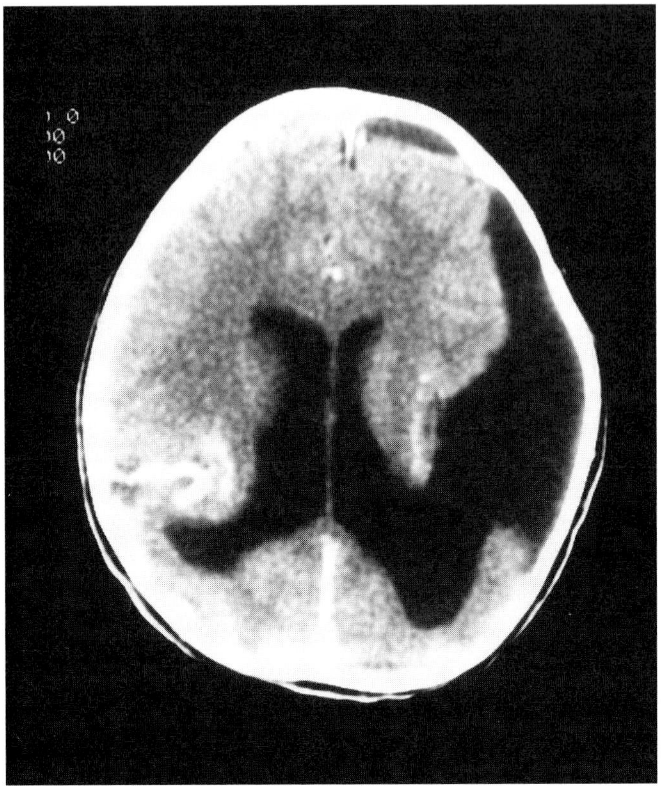

(B)

Figure 10-1 *B*. Open-lip schizencephaly, axial CT with contrast. A large open lip cleft is present with gray matter extending to the ventricular margin. Deep cortical infolding with an abnormal draining vein is seen in the contralateral hemisphere.

pointed anterior horn of the lateral ventricle is said to be characteristic. The age at diagnosis might be important, as a follow-up study on one patient with imaging findings of hemimegalencephaly has shown arrested interval growth and relative decreased size of the abnormal hemisphere.

☐ ABNORMALITIES OF THE CORPUS CALLOSUM

Corpus callosal development occurs between the eighth and sixteenth weeks. The genu, body and splenium of the corpus callosum form from anterior to posterior, with the rostrum forming last. Partial defects almost always affect the dorsal aspect.

Findings are as follows:

- Parallel lateral ventricles
- Colpocephaly
- A deep interhemispheric fissure that may extend to the third ventricle
- The roof of the third ventricle may be high, with possible midline cyst
- Crescentic or chalice-shaped frontal horns
- Radial orientation of gyri along medial hemispheres
- Longitudinal white matter tracts (Probst bundles) that indent superomedial lateral ventricles

Associated abnormalities are as follows:

- Chiari II malformation
- Lipomas
- Migrational disorders
- Dandy-Walker malformation
- Holoprosencephaly
- Cephaloceles
- Azygous anterior cerebral artery
- Aicardi syndrome

LIPOMA OF THE CORPUS CALLOSUM

Intracranial lipomas are believed to be secondary to abnormal differentiation of embryonic meningeal tissues, or the meninx primativa. Interhemispheric lipomas represent approximately 50 percent of intracranial lipomas. These are almost always associated with at least some callosal hypogenesis. The lipomas may calcify and vessels course through them. Intracranial lipomas are less frequently found at the quadrigeminal plate, supersellar cistern, cerebellopontine angles, and sylvian cisterns.

☐ HYDRANENCEPHALY

Hydranencephaly is considered a destructive process, possibly vascular or infectious. The brain has undergone liquefaction necrosis, and there are thin-walled sacs containing CSF. The sac is composed of leptomeningeal tissue and cerebral remnants. All that remains is the cerebellum, thalami, and occasionally the inferior aspects of the temporal and frontal lobes. The head may

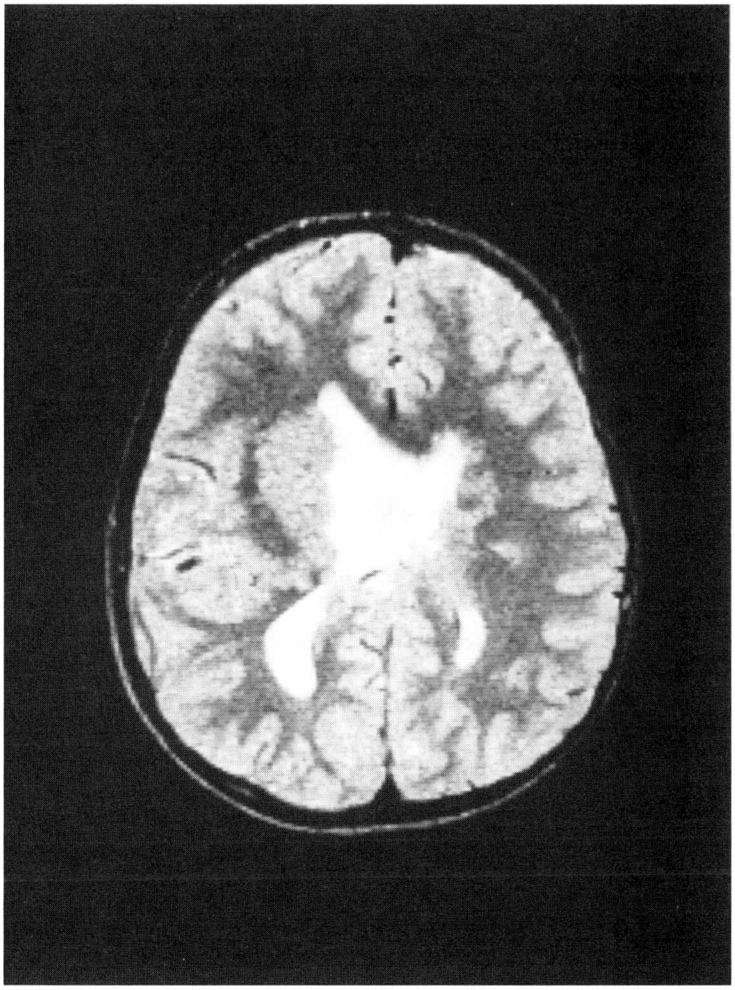

Figure 10-2 Gray matter heterotopia, axial T2-weighted MRI. Numerous subependymal gray matter nodules are seen bilaterally. There is deep cortical infolding near the sylvian fissure. The septum pellucidum is absent.

be microcephalic to macrocephalic, depending on the presence of hydrocephalus.

☐ POSTERIOR FOSSA MALFORMATIONS

DANDY-WALKER MALFORMATION

Dandy-Walker malformation involves a markedly enlarged fourth ventricular cyst expanding the posterior fossa and uplifting the tentorium and dural sinuses (torcular Herophili) in association with vermian hypoplasia or vermian absence. Hydrocephalus is present in over 80 percent of cases; however, it often does not present until after birth.

DANDY-WALKER VARIANT

The Dandy-Walker variant is more common, with a milder form of vermian hypogenesis, variably sized cyst, and no posterior fossa enlargement. Hydrocephalus may or may not be present. There is associated agenesis of the corpus callosum in 21 percent, migrational abnormalities, holoprosencephaly, and occipital cephaloceles.

MEGA CISTERNA MAGNA

Mega cisterna magna is a cystic malformation of the posterior fossa, with intact vermis, enlarged cisterna magna, and enlarged bony posterior fossa. There may be hydrocephalus and associated supratentorial anomalies.

There is a continuum of the above findings, with difficulty in categorization. This has prompted reclassification of the listed malformations as the "Dandy-Walker complex."

Small CSF collections are frequently seen posterior to the cerebellum in infants with a normal-sized posterior fossa and intact vermis. As long as there is no associated mass effect, hydrocephalus, or an associated congenital anomaly, these are considered incidental.

JOUBERT'S SYNDROME

Joubert's syndrome is an autosomal recessive disorder, more common in males, characterized by respiratory difficulties (episodic tachypnea and apnea), abnormal eye movements, psychomotor retardation, and ataxia. There is complete or almost complete absence of the vermis. Imaging demonstrates absence of the vermis with apposition

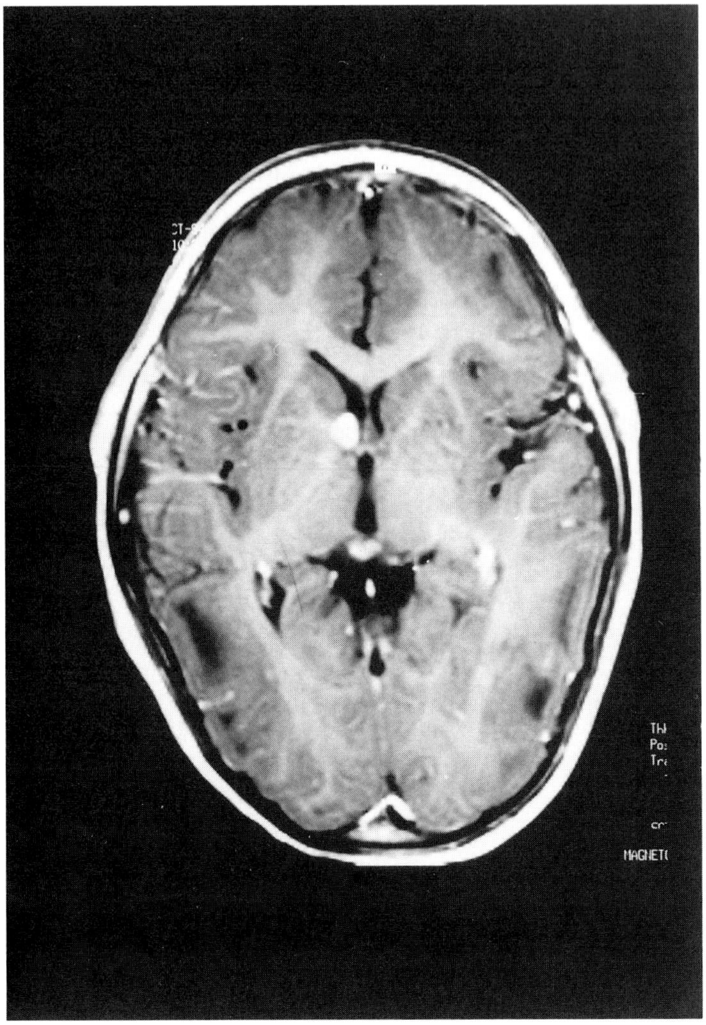

(A)
Figure 10-3 *A*. Tuberous sclerosis, axial T1-weighted MRI with contrast. An enhancing nodule is seen adjacent to the right foramen of Monro, consistent with a giant cell astrocytome.

of the cerebellar hemispheres. On axial imaging, the fourth ventricle has a characteristic "bat-wing" shape.

RHOMBENCEPHALOSYNAPSIS

Rhombencephalosynapsis is characterized by vermian agenesis or severe hypogenesis, fusion of the cerebellar hemispheres, and apposition or fusion of the dentate nuclei. This is associated with numerous infratentorial and supratentorial anomalies. The symptoms are generally related to the supratentorial abnormalites. The septum pellucidum is absent. There may be hydrocephalus, fusion of the inferior colliculi, and hypoplasia of the anterior commissure.

☐ DISORDERS OF HISTOGENESIS (PHAKOMATOSIS)

NEUROFIBROMATOSIS

As many as eight forms of neurofibromatosis have been described. The National Institutes of Health Consensus Development Conference has defined only two distinct types of neurofibromatosis: NF-1 and NF-2. These are distinctly different diseases with phenotypic similarities. Neurofibromatosis type I, which is about ten times more common than NF-2, shares some common features, such as that they are both autosomal dominant disorders without racial or sexual predilection and both may be aggravated by gestational hormones.

Neurofibromatosis Type 1 In neurofibromatosis type 1 (NF-1, also known as Von Recklinghausen's disease), a gene defect is present on chromosome 17. The incidence is about 1:3000. Approximately 50 percent of these patients represent spontaneous mutations. They may have seizures, macrocepaly, cutaneous neurofibromas, nerve sheath tumors (usually neurofibromas), vascular disease, and café au lait spots. There may be sarcomatous degeneration of the peripheral soft tissue neurofibromas as well as arterial occlusive disease with the moyamoya pattern or aneurysms. Plexiform neurofibromas commonly occur along the course of the orbital division of the fifth cranial nerve.

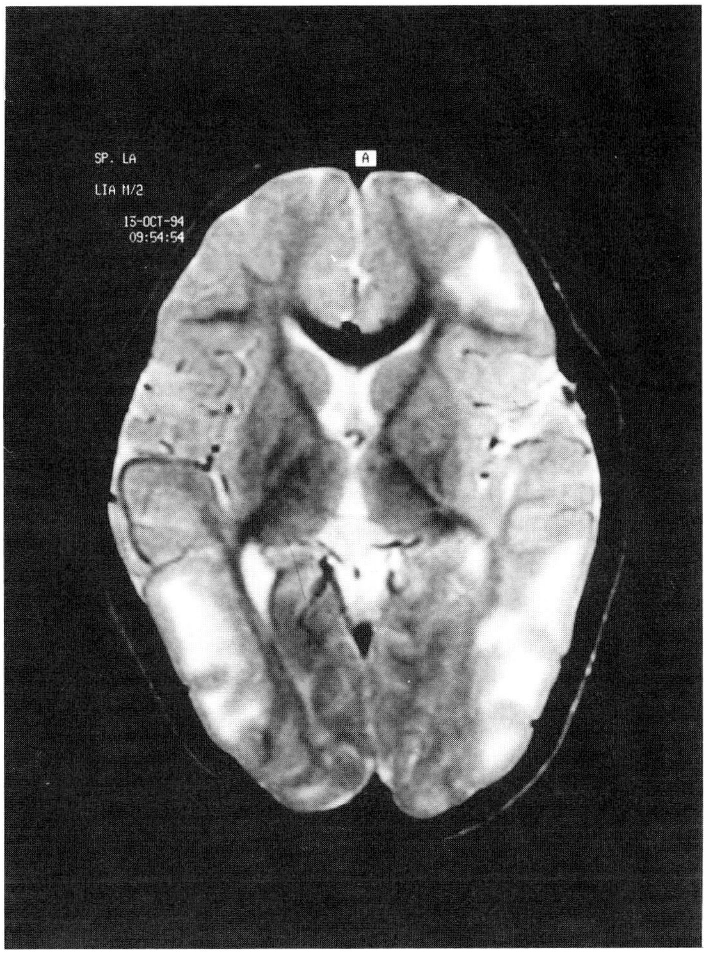

(B)
Figure 10-3 *B.* Tuberous sclerosis, axial T2-weighted MRI. Numerous cortical tubers are present. The tubers show bright T2 signal intensity. The nodule adjacent to the right foramen of Monro is difficult to see.

These patients may have numerous intracranial lesions, both hamartomas and neoplasias. Hamartomas are abnormal mixtures made up of tissue elements that are normally present at that site. Optic gliomas, mostly low-grade pilocytic astrocytomas, are the most common intracranial neoplasm, seen in 15 to 40 percent. These frequently affect the optic nerves and chiasm and infrequently the posterior optic pathways. The prognosis for optic chiasm and posterior optic pathway gliomas is poor compared to that for tumors confined to the optic nerves. Approximately 20 to 30 percent of optic gliomas become symptomatic before 10 years of age and rarely thereafter. Although the view is controversial, the NIH does not recommend routine neuroimaging of NF-1 unless the patient develops clinical symptoms. Screening of asymptomatic relatives may be helpful to establish the diagnosis and for genetic counseling. The majority of the intracranial neoplasms are astrocytomas, which may affect the basal ganglia, brainstem, and cerebellum. Neoplasms usually show edema, mass effect, and contrast enhancement.

Patients with NF-1 may have enlargement of the internal auditory canals from dural ectasia. Acoustic schwannomas are not a feature of NF-1. Patients may have "nonpulsatile proptosis" from a plexiform neurofibroma or "pulsatile proptosis" from congenital dysplasia of the sphenoid bone. The optic canal can be enlarged by an optic glioma or from optic canal dural ectasia, a distinction that cannot be made with computed tomography (CT). Hydrocephalus unrelated to tumor is not rare. Hydrocephalus, most commonly from narrowing at the aqueduct of Sylvius, may stem from a benign aqueductal stenosis or a tectal glioma. The presence of gadolinium enhancement and mass effect with a glioma can distinguish these findings on MRI. Lateral thoracic meningoceles, kyphoscoliosis, scalloping of posterior lumbar vertebral bodies, pseudoarthrosis of extremity fractures, and limb overgrowth are well-known manifestations of NF-1.

In over 60 percent of NF-1 patients, MRI demonstrates focal increased T2 abnormalities that lack mass effect or contrast enhancement. These involve the globus pallidus, putamen, cerebral peduncles, pons, midbrain, thalamus, cerebellar white matter, dentate nuclei, and, less commonly, the periventricular white matter. They are usually isointense on T1 but may be hyperintense, especially at the basal ganglia, with a frequent ring of increased T1 signal. The basal ganglia lesions will occasionally have mild mass effect. The globus pallidus lesions are seen as hypodense on CT in 30 percent of cases. The other lesions are not seen on CT. These T2 hyperintense foci are thought to be hamartomas or areas of abnormal myelination. The observation that they are transient and age-related suggests that they may not represent hamartomas. A follow-up MRI study with contrast may be helpful for the posterior fossa lesions in order to distinguish them from a glioma. Several studies have indicated that the bright T2 foci are unrelated to cognitive dysfunction. A recent study suggests an associated specific learning disability.

Neurofibromatosis Type 2 The genetic defect of neurofibromatosis type 2 (NF-2, or central neurofibromatosis) is deletion of chromosome 22. The neoplasms are often schwannomas, meningiomas, ependymomas, and, less commonly, neurofibromas. Cutaneous lesions are uncommon. The hallmark of the disease is acoustic schwannomas in the second or third decades as opposed to the non-NF-2 acoustic schwannomas seen typically in the fifth decade. Bilateral acoustic schwannomas are diagnostic of NF-2 by NIH criteria. Meningiomas and schwannomas in childhood are suspicious for NF-2.

TUBEROUS SCLEROSIS (BOURNEVILLE'S DISEASE)

Tuberous sclerosis (TS) is an autosomal dominate disease with classic clinical triad of epilepsy, mental retardation, and adenoma subaceum. This triad is actually seen in less than 30 percent of cases. The other features are occular hamartomas, bilateral renal angiolipomas and cysts, cardiac rhabdomyomas, shagreen patch, and hypopigmented macules. Inheritance is autosomal dominant. Mental disability and seizures at a young age are related to the extent of cerebral involvement. Seizures become more common with advancing age.

Characteristic subependymal nodules are seen in 95 percent of these patients. The nodules are located most frequently in the walls of the lateral ventricles at the foramen of Monro and the caudothalamic sulcus. They protrude into the lateral ventricles and tend not to calcify until after the first year of life. When calcified, they are more easily seen on CT. These do not enhance on CT; however, over half enhance on MRI at 1.5 T magnetic field strength. A lesser percent enhance at lower field strength. On MRI T2-weighted images best show the calcifications because of magnetic susceptibility differences.

A slow-growing, enhancing mass adjacent to the foramen of Monro indicates a subependymal giant-cell astrocytoma (SGCA), seen in 15 percent of TS patients. As noted above, subependymal nodules may enhance on MRI, so growth is the key to diagnosing subependymal giant cell tumor (Figure 10-3*A*). The SGCA may grow and obstruct the foramen of Monro, causing hydrocephalus. In fact, this is the most common cause of symptoms requiring surgery in TS.

Cortical tubers may be seen on MRI in 95 percent of patients. Most show a smooth, expanded outer cortical surface. Some show central cortical depressions. The MRI signal intensity of the peripheral component is isointense to gray matter on all sequences. The inner core is isointense to hypointense on T1 and hyperintense on T2 (Figure 10-3*B*). Some tubers that do not involve the white matter will not be seen on MRI. Cortical calcification of tubers is commonly seen in 50 percent of TS patients by the age of 10. These calcifications can at times be gyriform and confused with the gyriform calcifications of Sturge-Weber syndrome.

Four white matter patterns have been described. The white matter may show straight or curvilinear thin bands of increased T2 signal from the ventricle to the cortical tuber or cortex; this is seen in 88 percent of patients. Other white matter patterns are wedge-shaped (31 percent), tumefactive or conglomerate (14 percent), or of a cerebellar pattern involving a conglomerate focus with radial bands (12 percent). A small percentage of white matter lesions will enhance on contrast MRI and an even smaller percentage of the cortical lesions may enhance. These will usually be calcified.

STURGE-WEBER SYNDROME

Sturge-Weber syndrome (SWS), also known as encephalotrigeminal angiomatosis, is a congenital vascular disorder of the brain, meninges, and the face in a trigeminal distribution, often involving the eye. The intracranial lesion is an ipsilateral leptomeningeal vascular malformation (LVM) between the pia and the arachnoid membranes. Abnormal cerebral venous drainage is the primary abnormality, with resultant chronic venous hypertension leading to gradual cell death, progressive atrophy, and calcification of the cortex. Cortical calcification, which is not expected before age 2, occurs at the gray/white matter junction and layers 2 to 4. A parietal occipital location is most common. Angiomas may also involve the choroid plexus and eye.

Noncontrast CT best shows the "tram-track" calcifications, which may not be well appreciated on MRI. However, MRI is best for showing the leptomeningeal, gyral, and choroid enhancement. Abnormal deep draining veins may be seen as well as veins within the diploic spaces.

VON HIPPEL-LINDAU DISEASE

Von Hippel-Lindau disease (CNS angiomatosis, or cerebelloretinal hemangioblastomatosis) is an autosomal dominant disease with a chromosome 3 defect. Patients uncommonly present before puberty. They typically have retinal angiomas (50 percent), cerebellar hemangioblastomas (75 percent), spinal hemangioblastoma (25 percent), renal cell carcinomas (40 percent), pheochromocytomas (10 percent), and rare supratentorial hemangioblastomas.

Hemangioblastomas are most commonly located in the posterior fossa, usually in the cerebellum (90 percent). A cystic mass may be seen, associated with an intensely enhancing noncalcified mural nodule. These lesions are multifocal in 10 percent of cases; solid tumors occur in approximately 30 percent. The nodule may be associated with an MRI flow void from prominent vessels. Conventional angiography may still be performed to find a tumor nodule within a posterior fossa cyst and possible additional lesions. The rare supratentorial hemangioblastomas are more commonly solid. Spinal hemangioblastomas most commonly demonstrate a syringomyelia, an isointense nodule, and marked nodular enhancement.

ATAXIA TELANGIECTASIA

Ataxia telangiectasia is an autosomal recessive disease characterized by telangiectasias of the eye and skin, cerebellar ataxia, and immunodeficiencies. Death is usually the result of bronchiectasis and pulmonary failure. Imaging findings are those of progressive cerebellar volume loss.

☐ QUESTIONS (True or False)

1. Regarding brain development and myelination,
- **a.** The prosencephalon will become the cerebral hemispheres, basal ganglia, thalami, and hypothalami.
- **b.** The metencephalon will become the medulla and pons.
- **c.** The germinal matrix is most active between 8 and 28 weeks.
- **d.** The cerebral cortex normally has a four-layered cortex.
- **e.** In assessing myelination, T1-weighted MRI images are best from 6 to 12 months.

2. Regarding cephalocele,
- **a.** In the United States, frontal encephaloceles are the most common.
- **b.** Meckel's syndrome is associated with the occipital encephalocele.
- **c.** A dural venous sinus may extend into the cephalocele sac.
- **d.** There is a female predominance with occipital cephaloceles.
- **e.** Frontoethmoidal cephaloceles are most common in Southeast Asians.

3. Regarding Chiari I malformation,
- **a.** There are frequent associated intracranial malformations.
- **b.** In children, a 5-mm tonsilar protrusion is diagnostic of Chiari I malformation.
- **c.** Syringohydromyelia is frequently associated.
- **d.** Klippel-Feil syndrome is associated.
- **e.** Isolated asymmetrical tonsillar herniation is considered insignificant.

4. Regarding Chiari II malformation,
- **a.** The hindbrain, mesoderm, and spine are involved.
- **b.** Dilatation of the fourth ventricle may be associated with hydromyelia.
- **c.** There is exposure of neural tissues of the back through a spina bifida defect.
- **d.** There may be hypogenesis of the rostrum of the corpus callosum.
- **e.** The foramen magnum may be enlarged.

5. Regarding holoprosencephaly,
- **a.** Common to all types is the fusion of gray matter across the midline.
- **b.** Dorsal cysts are frequently seen with the lobar type.
- **c.** Facial anomalies are frequently associated with the lobar type.
- **d.** Semilobar holoprosencephaly may involve absence of the body and genu of the corpus callosum with an intact-appearing splenium.
- **e.** Septooptic dysplasia is thought to be a mild form of holoprosencephaly.

6. Regarding migrational abnomalities,
- **a.** Lissencephaly and pachygyria differ primarily in the degree of involvement.
- **b.** Type I lissencephaly is associated with the Miller-Dieker syndrome.
- **c.** Walker-Warburg syndrome is the classic example of type II lissencephaly.
- **d.** Type I lissencephaly typically shows a thick, deep gray matter band and decreased white matter thickness.
- **e.** Walker-Warburg syndrome typically shows severe hypomyelination of the deep white matter.

7. Regarding migrational abnormalities,
- **a.** A "layered polymicrogyria" reflects an event before 20 weeks.
- **b.** Pachygyria and polymicrogyria are easily distinguished with MRI.
- **c.** Schizencephaly must have gray matter lining the clefts.
- **d.** Schizencephaly is associated with "unlayered polymicrogyria."
- **e.** Polymicrogyria is most frequently located near the sylvian fissure.

8. Regarding the corpus callosum,
- **a.** Development is generally from front to back, except for the rostrum.

b. Corpus callosum lipomas are secondary to abnormal differentiation of the meninx primativa.
c. Callosal agenesis typically demonstrates colpocephaly.
d. With callosal agenesis there will be a radial orientation of the gyri along the medial hemispheres.
e. Partial agenesis is frequently seen with Chiari II malformation.

9. Regarding neurofibromatosis,
a. It is an autosomal recessive disorder.
b. Cutaneous manifestations are uncommon in NF-2.
c. Bilateral acoustic schwannomas are diagnostic of NF-2.
d. Optic glioma is the most common intracranial neoplasm in NF-1.
e. Globus pallidus CT hypodensity may be seen in 30 percent with NF-1.

10. Regarding tuberous sclerosis,
a. Epilepsy, mental retardation, and adenoma sebaceum are seen in most cases.
b. Characteristic subependymal nodules are seen in 95 percent.
c. Cortical tubers may be seen in 95 percent on MRI.
d. Cortical tubers may calcify.
e. A small percentage of cortical tubers may enhance on MRI.

☐ ANSWERS

1. a. T
b. F
c. T
d. F
e. F

2. a. F
b. T
c. T
d. T
e. T

3. a. F
b. F
c. T
d. T
e. T

4. a. T
b. T
c. T
d. T
e. T

5. a. T
b. F
c. T
d. T
e. T

6. a. T
b. T
c. T
d. T
e. T

7. a. F
b. F
c. T
d. T
e. T

8. a. T
b. T
c. T
d. T
e. T

9. a. F
b. T
c. T
d. T
e. T

10. a. F
b. T
c. T
d. T
e. T

SUGGESTED READINGS

Brain Development and Myelination

1. Barkovich AJ: Normal development, in *Pediatric Neuroimaging*, 2d ed. New York, Raven Press, 1995, pp 9–54.
2. Bird C et al: MR assessment of myelination in infants and children: Usefulness of marker sites. *Am J Neuroradiol* 9:69–76, 1989.

3. Van der Knaap MS, Valk J: Classification of congenital anomalies of the CNS. *Am J Neuroradiol* 9:315–326, 1988.

Congenital Brain Malformations

1. Ball WS: Pediatric neuroradiology: Part I, in Syllabus: Special Course in Neuroradiology, Clinical Approach and Management for Diagnostic Imaging, presented at RSNA 94, pp 113–126.
2. Barkovich AJ: Congenital brain malformations, in *Pediatric Neuroimaging*, 2d ed. New York, Raven Press, 1995, pp 177–276.
3. Barkovich AJ: Malformations of the brain, in Ramsey, RG: *American Society of Neuroradiology Core Curriculum Course in Neuroradiology 1994*. 1994, pp 15–21.
4. Barkovich AJ, Kjos BO: Nonlissencephalic cortical dysplasias: Correlation of imaging findings with clinical deficits. *Am J Neuroradiol* 13:95–103, 1992.
5. Barkovich AJ, Kjos BO: Gray matter heterotopias: MR characteristics and correlation with developmental and neurologic manifestations. *Radiology* 182:493–499, 1992.
6. Barkovich AJ, Kjos BO: Schizencephaly: Correlation of clinical findings with MR characteristics. *Am J Neuroradiol* 13:85–94, 1992.
7. Barkovich AJ et al: MR of neuronal migration anomalies. *Am J Neuroradiol* 8:1009–1017, 1987.
8. Barkovich AJ et al: Formation, maturation, and disorders of brain neocortex. *Am J Neuroradiol* 13:423–446, 1992.
9. Barkovich AJ et al: Formation, maturation and disorders of white matter. *Am J Neuroradiol* 13:447–461, 1992.
10. Barkovich AJ et al: Band heterotopias: A newly recognized neuronal migration anomaly. *Radiology* 171:455–458, 1989.
11. Barth PG: Commentary-schizencephaly and nonlissencephalic cortical dysplasias. *Am J Neuroradiol* 13:104–106, 1992.
12. Byrd SE et al: The CT and MR evaluation of migrational disorders of the brain: Part I. Lissencephaly and pachygyria. *Pediatr Radiol* 19:151–156, 1989.
13. Byrd SE et al: The CT and MR evaluation of migrational disorders of the brain: Part II. Schizencephaly, heterotopia and polymicrogyria. *Pediatr Radiol* 19:219–222, 1989.
14. Byrd SE et al: The CT and MR evaluation of lissencephaly. *Am J Neuroradiol* 9:923–927, 1988.
15. Castillo M et al: Radiologic-pathologic correlation of alobar holoprosencephaly. *Am J Neuroradiol* 14:1151–1156, 1993.
16. Dean B et al: MR imaging of pericallosal lipoma. *Am J Neuroradiol* 9:929–931, 1988.
17. Ferris NJ, Tien RD: Amnion rupture sequence with exencephaly: MR findings in a surviving infant. *Am J Neuroradiol* 15:1030–1033, 1994.
18. Flodmar O: Neuroradiology of selected disorders of the meninges, calvarium and venous sinuses. *Am J Neuroradiol* 13:483–491, 1992.
19. Gallucci M et al: MR imaging of incomplete band heterotopia. *Am J Neuroradiol* 12:701–702, 1991.
20. Kalifa GL et al: Hemimegalencephaly: MR imaging in five children. *Radiology* 165:29–33, 1987.
21. Kuban KCK et al: Septo-optic-dyslasia-schizencephaly: Radiographic and clinical features. *Pediatr Radiol* 19:145–150, 1989.
22. Kumar AJ et al: Chromosomal disorders: Background and neuroradiology. *Am J Neuroradiol* 13:577–593, 1992.
23. Kuzniecky R et al: The congenital bilateral perisylvian syndrome: Imaging findings in a multicenter study. *Am J Neuroradiol* 15:139–144, 1994.
24. Naidich TP et al: Cephaloceles and related malformations. *Am J Neuroradiol* 13:655–690, 1992.
25. Naidich TP, Zimmerman RA: Common diseases of the pediatric central nervous system, in Hardwood-Nash DC et al (eds): *Syllabus: A Categorical Course in Diagnostic Neuroradiology*. RSNA Division of Editorial and Publishing Services, 1987, pp 35–42.
26. Rhodes RE et al: Walker-Warburg syndrome. *Am J Neuroradiol* 13:123–126, 1991.
27. Scatliff JH, Bouldin TW: Supratentorial congenital abnormalities, in Taveras JM, Ferrucci JT (eds): *Radiology, Diagnosis, Imaging, Intervention*. Philadelphia, Lippincott 1992, pp 1–26.
28. Smith AS et al: Association of heterotopic gray matter with seizures: MR imaging. *Radiology* 168:195–198, 1988.
29. Wolpert SM et al: Hemimegalencephaly: A longitudinal MR study. *Am J Neuroradiol* 15:1479–1482, 1994.

Posterior Fossa Malformations

1. Altman NR et al: Posterior fossa malformations. *Am J Neuroradiol* 13:691–724, 1992.
2. Barkovich et al: Revised classification of posterior fossa cysts and cystlike malformation based on the results of multiplanar MR imaging. *Am J Neuroradiol* 10:977–988, 1989.
3. Castillo M et al: Chiari III malformation: Imaging features. *Am J Neuroradiol* 13:107–113, 1992.
4. Elster AD, Chen MYM: Chiari I malformations: Clinical and radiologic reappraisal. *Radiology* 183:347–353, 1992.
5. Kollias SS et al: Cystic malformations of the posterior fossa: Differential diagnosis clarified through embryologic analysis. *Radiographics* 13:1211–1231, 1993.
6. McLone DG, Naidich TP: Developmental morphology of the subarachnoid space, brain vasculature, and contiguous structures and the cause of the Chiari II malformation. *Am J Neuroradiol* 13:463–482, 1992.
7. Mikulis DJ et al: Variance of the cerebellar tonsils with age: Preliminary report. *Radiology* 173:725–728, 1992.
8. Naidich TP et al: Congenital malformations of the posterior fossa, in Taveras JM, Ferrucci JT (eds): *Radiology, Diagnosis, Imaging, Intervention*. Philadelphia, Lippincott, 1992, pp 1–17. 1992.
9. Oldfield EH et al: Pathophysiology of syringomyelia associated with Chiari I malformation of the cerebellar tonsils. *J Neurosurg* 80:3–15, 1994.

Phakomatoses

1. Balestrazzi P et al: Periaqueductal gliosis causing hydrocephalus in a patient with neurofibromatosis type I. *Neurofibromatosis* 2:322–325, 1989.
2. Barkovich, AJ: The phakomatoses, in *Pediatric Neuroimaging*, 2d ed. New York, Raven Press, 1995, pp 277–320.
3. Braffman BH et al: MR imaging of tuberous sclerosis: Pathogenesis of this phakomatosis, use of gadopentate dimeglumine, and literature review. *Radiology* 183:227–238, 1992.
4. Castillo M et al: Proton MR spectroscopy in patients with neurofibromatosis type 1: Evaluation of hamartomas and clinical correlation. *Am J Neuroradiol* 16:141–147, 1995.
5. Duffner PK et al: The significance of MRI abnormalities in children with neurofibromatosis. *Neurology* 39:373–378, 1989.
6. Dunn DW, Roos KL: Magnetic resonance imaging evaluation of learning difficulties and incoordination in neurofibromatosis. *Neurofibromatosis* 2:1–5, 1989.
7. Gean AD, Taveras JM: The phakomatoses, in Taveras JM, Ferrucci FT (eds): *Radiology, Diagnosis, Imaging, Intervention*. Philadelphia, Lippincott, 1992, pp 1–13.
8. Itoh T et al: Neurofibromatosis type I: The evolution of deep gray and white matter MR abnormalities. *Am J Neuroradiol* 15:1513–1519, 1994.

9. Menor F, Marti-Bonmati L: CT detection of basal ganglion lesions in neurofibromatosis type I: Correlation with MRI. *Neuroradiology* 34:305–307, 1992.
10. Menor F et al: Imaging considerations of central nervous system manifestations in pediatric patients with neurofibromatosis type I. *Pediatr Radiol* 21:389–394, 1991.
11. North K et al: Optic gliomas in neurofibromatosis type I: Role of visual evoked potentials. *Pediatr Radiol* 10:117–123, 1994.
12. North K et al: Specific learning disability in children with neurofibromatosis type I: Significance of MRI abnormalities. *Neurology* 44:878–883, 1994.
13. Pou-Serradell A, Ugarte-Elola AC: Hydrocephalus in neurofibromatosis contribution of MRI to its diagnosis control and treament. *Neurofibromatosis* 2:218–226, 1989.
14. Shepherd CW et al: MR findings in tuberous sclerosis complex and correlation with seizure development and mental impairment. *Am J Neuroradiol* 16:149–155, 1995.
15. Smirniotopoulos JG, Murphy FM: The phakomatoses: *Am J Neuroradiol* 13:725–746, 1992.
16. Truwit CL et al: MR imaging of rhombencephalosynapsis: Report of three cases and review of the literature. *Am J Neuroradiol* 12:957–965, 1991.

CHAPTER

11

Intraaxial and Mass Lesions in the Region of the Ventricular System

Chi S. Zee
George Pjura
Karen Ragland

In evaluating computed tomography (CT) or magnetic resonance imaging (MRI) for intraaxial neoplasms, the following characteristics of a mass lesion should be assessed: (1) location and extent, (2) mass effect and surrounding edema, (3) density on CT or signal intensity on MRI, and (4) pattern of contrast enhancement. By assessing these factors carefully, one may arrive at a reasonable differential diagnosis or probable diagnosis. Magnetic resonance imaging is superior to CT in detecting and localizing intracranial neoplasms. However, MRI is not as highly specific for diagnosing intracranial neoplasms as initially expected. Calcification is important in the differential diagnosis of intracranial neoplasms, and CT is superior to MRI in the detection of calcification. A noncontrast CT is sometimes required to aid in the differential diagnosis of an intracranial neoplasm.

Contrast enhancement of intracranial neoplasms is probably due to multiple factors. In general, tumors have a tendency to provoke the formation of new capillaries. Some of the tumor capillaries in gliomas may be near normal, while other capillaries in gliomas may be abnormal, with fenestrated endothelia—that is, breakdown of the blood-brain barrier (BBB). This is probably the basis for explaining why some gliomas enhance and others do not. Generally speaking, malignant gliomas are more likely to enhance than benign ones. However, there are many instances in which the opposite is true. Metastatic neoplasms contain non–central nervous system (CNS) capillaries (no BBB) that are similar to their tissue of origin; therefore, metastatic lesions always show contrast enhancement. Extraaxial neoplasms arise from tissues that contain capillaries without tight junction. This explains why extraaxial neoplasms always exhibit contrast enhancement. The correlation between MRI or CT contrast enhancement and hypervascularity on angiography is not good. Hypervascularity is not a prerequisite for contrast enhancement. The explanation of contrast enhancement is presumed to be related to the formation of tumor capillaries lacking BBB rather than to the destruction of existing BBB.

☐ SUPRATENTORIAL INTRAAXIAL TUMORS IN ADULTS

Brain tumors are uncommon lesions, accounting for 1.5 percent of all malignancies occurring in adults as well as children. The majority of the brain tumors in adults are supratentorial in location, whereas approximately half of the brain tumors in children are supratentorial. Supratentorial tumors are more common in neonates and children up to 3 years old, whereas infratentorial tumors are more common in children from 4 to 11 years old.

Approximately one-third of the intracranial neoplasms are gliomas, one-third are metastatic lesions, and one-third are of other primary origin (including extraaxial neoplasms)(Table 11-1). Gliomas have a slight male predominance of 3:2.

Gliomas can be divided into astrocytomas, ependymomas, and oligodendrogliomas. Since the choroid plexus contains modified ependymal cells, choroid plexus neoplasms are considered in the category of gliomas. They will be discussed under "Mass Lesions in the Region of Ventricular System," below. Three-quarters of gliomas are astrocytomas, which are traditionally divided into four grades according to Kernohan's grading system (Kernohan and Sayre, 1952) or according to the World Health Organization (WHO) grading system (Table 11-2). Grade 1 and 2 astrocytomas are considered low-grade

Table 11-1
INCIDENCE OF BRAIN TUMORS (100%)[a]

PRIMARY BRAIN TUMORS (66%)		
Glial Tumors (33%)	**Nonglial Tumors (33%)**	**Metastatic Tumors (33%)**
Astrocytomas 25%	Meningioma 15%	Lung carcinoma
Oligodendroglioma 4%	Primitive neuro-ectodermal tumor 5%	Breast carcinoma
Ependymoma 3%	Schwannoma 4%	Melanoma
Choroid plexus tumors 1%	Pituitary tumor 4%	Renal carcinoma
	Pineal region tumor 2%	Colon carcinoma
	Craniopharyngioma 2%	

[a]All percentages are approximations.

and associated with better prognosis. Grade 3 and 4 astrocytomas are anaplastic astrocytomas and glioblastoma multiforme, respectively, depending on their histologic features. Some 25 percent of astrocytomas are of low grade and 75 percent are of high grade (25 percent anaplastic astrocytoma and 50 percent glioblastoma multiforme). The majority of high-grade astrocytomas are glioblastoma multiforme.

LOW-GRADE ASTROCYTOMA

Incidence

- Astrocytomas (all grades) constitute almost 50 percent of the supratentorial brain tumors in all age groups and 30 percent of all infratentorial tumors in children.
- Low-grade astrocytomas constitute about 25 percent of all cerebral gliomas.
- Cerebral gliomas constitute approximately 33 percent of all intracranial neoplasms.

Table 11-2
CLASSIFICATION OF ASTROCYTOMA

	Kernohan	World Health Organization (WHO)
Pilocytic astrocytoma Subependymal giant-cell astrocytoma	Grade 1	Grade I
Low-grade astrocytoma	Grades 1 and 2	Grade II
Anaplastic astrocytoma	Grade 3	Grade III
Glioblastoma multiforme	Grade 4	Grade IV

Age

- Peak incidence for low-grade astrocytomas is between the ages of 20 and 40 years.
- Peak incidence for low-grade astrocytomas is generally 10 years below that for glioblastomas.

Location Astrocytomas may occur in any part of the cranial hemisphere with the exception of the occipital lobes. Deep structures, such as the corpus callosum and basal ganglia, are also involved.

Pathology This group of tumors has heterogeneous histopathologic features and variable clinical presentations. According to Kernohan, astrocytomas are divided into four grades, reflecting the tumor's degree of malignancy. Grade 1 and 2 astrocytomas (WHO grade II) are considered low-grade and correlate with a better survival rate than high-grade tumors.

The most common of these tumors in adults is the diffuse fibrillary astrocytoma. Although these tumors are usually low-grade, the incidence of anaplastic degeneration has been shown to be from 10 to 80 percent. Fibrillary astrocytomas are unencapsulated, infiltrating tumors. Microscopically, they are characterized by proliferation of well-differentiated fibrillary astrocytes that demonstrate only mild nuclear pleomorphism.

Imaging ***Computed Tomography*** Astrocytomas may show low density or occasionally isodensity on computed tomography (CT). Peritumoral edema is usually absent to minimal. Tumor calcification is detected in 20 percent of astrocytomas. In fact, the most common supratentorial tumor with calcification is astrocytoma, although oligodendrogliomas have the highest frequency of calcification. The pattern of contrast enhancement is quite variable, with 40 percent of low-grade astrocytomas exhibiting some degree of enhancement.

Magnetic Resonance Imaging On magnetic resonance imaging (MRI), astrocytomas are usually homogeneously hypointense or occasionally isointense on T1-weighted images and slightly hyperintense on T2-weighted images (Fig. 11-1*A* and *B*). A tumor margin can usually be defined. There is little associated edema or mass effect. Calcification is not well seen on spin-echo images but better visualized on gradient-echo images.

Contrast-enhanced MRI may show a wide variety of enhancing patterns; including no enhancement, inhomogeneous enhancement, or heterogeneous enhancement (Fig. 11-1*C*).

Low-grade astrocytomas may present as discrete masses with smooth margins, involving and expanding one or two gyri, mimicking the contour of an extraaxial mass. Another uncommon pattern of low-grade astrocytoma is that of a diffuse cortical and subcortical infiltrate, mimicking an infarct.

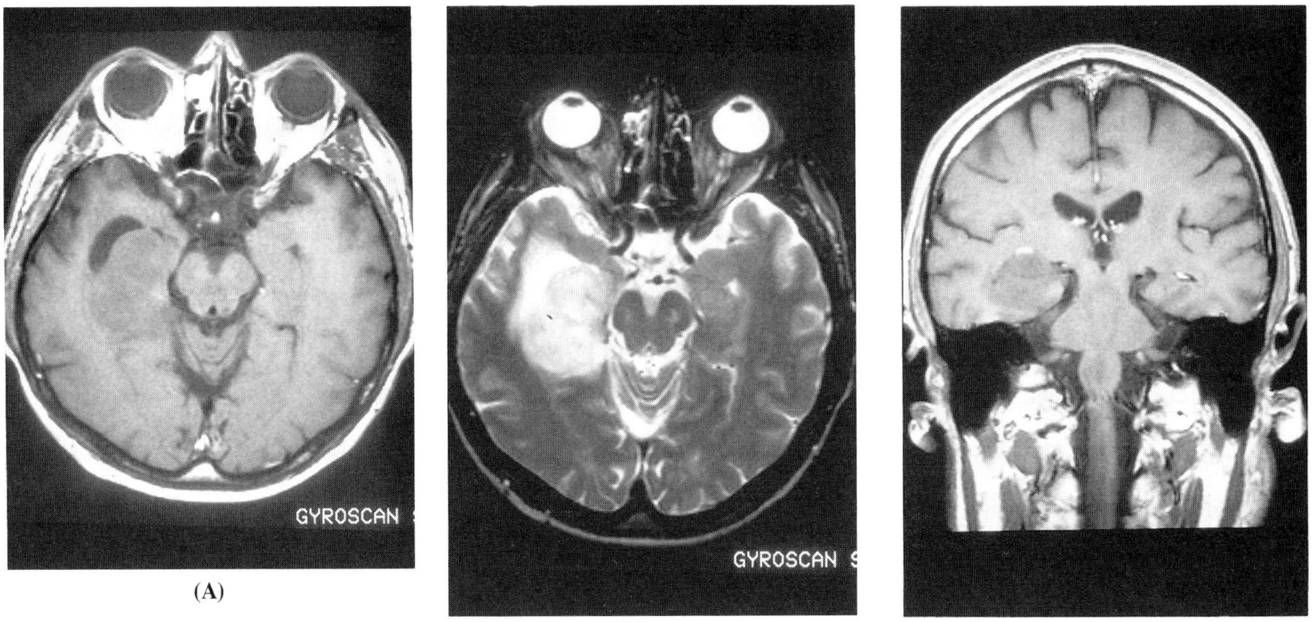

(A) (B) (C)

Figure 11-1 Low-grade astrocytoma. *A*. An axial T1-weighted image shows a slightly hypointense mass lesion involving the medial aspect of the right temporal lobe. Focal dilatation of the right temporal horn is due to trapping of the temporal horn by the tumor mass. *B*. An axial T2-weighted image shows the mass lesion to be hyperintense. Mild surrounding edema is seen. *C*. A Gd-enhanced coronal T1-weighted image demonstrates minimal enhancement of the mass lesion medially.

ANAPLASTIC ASTROCYTOMAS AND GLIOBLASTOMA MULTIFORME

Incidence

- These tumors represent 15 to 20 percent of all intracranial neoplasms.
- Glioblastoma multiforme constitutes 50 percent of all astrocytomas.
- Anaplastic astrocytoma constitutes 25 percent of all astrocytomas.
- Glioblastoma is the most common supratentorial neoplasm in an adult.

Age and Gender

- The age of onset is slightly older than low-grade astrocytomas.
- Patients present at 45 to 55 years of age in most cases.
- There is a slight male predominance of 3:2.

Location

- Glioblastoma tends to spread across the corpus callosum, forming the classic pattern of butterfly glioma.
- Glioblastoma has a predilection for white matter of the cerebral hemisphere, especially the frontal and temporal lobes. Invasion of the adjacent cortex, leptomeninges, and dura is often seen.

Pathology

- According to Kernohan's classification, grades 3 and 4 astrocytomas (WHO grades III and IV) are considered malignant (anaplastic astrocytoma corresponds to grade 3 astrocytoma and glioblastoma corresponds to grade 4 astrocytoma) (Table 11-3).
- The tumors are heterogeneous in appearance.
- Necrosis, hemorrhage, and cyst formation are often seen.

Table 11-3
ASTROCYTOMAS

Circumscribed Astrocytomas	Diffuse Fibrillary Astrocytoma
Pilocytic astrocytoma	Low-grade astrocytoma (Kernohan's grade 1 or 2) (WHO grade II)
Pleomorphic xanthoastrocytoma	Anaplastic astrocytoma (Kernohan's grade 3) (WHO grade III)
Subependymal giant-cell astrocytoma	Protoplasmic astrocytoma (Kernohan's grade 3) (WHO grade III)
Dysembryonic neuroepithelial tumor	Gemistocytic astrocytoma (Kernohan's grade 3 or 4) (WHO grades III, IV)
Optic glioma	Glioblastoma multiforme (Kernohan's grade 4) (WHO grade IV)
(All tumors Kernohan's grade 1 and WHO grade I)	Gliosarcoma (Kernohan's grade 4) (WHO grade IV)
	Gliomatosis cerebri (Kernohan's grade 2, 3, or 4) WHO grades II, III, IV)

- The tumor is composed of highly pleomorphic cells of astrocytic origin. The nuclei are bizarre, many cells are in mitotic division, and giant multinucleated cells are abundant. Bipolar spongioblasts tend to form pseudopalisades on the margins of the necrotic zones.
- Features of anaplasia, include vascular endothelial proliferation with doubling of basement membrane, resulting in large perivascular spaces.
- Partial incorporation of glial cells into the outer part of blood vessel walls results in occlusion of large arteries.
- Glioblastoma has a median survival of 6 months and anaplastic astrocytoma a median survival of 2 years.
- Gemistocytic astrocytomas consist of plump cells with an abundant eosinophilic cytoplasm. They are considered as malignant (high-grade) astrocytomas.
- Protoplasmic astrocytomas are seen at the cortex due to the presence of protoplasmic astrocytes in the cerebral cortex. They are considered anaplastic astrocytomas.

Imaging *Computed Tomography*

- Heterogeneous in density. Lesions may be of low density or high density or, more frequently, of mixed density.
- The margin of the neoplasm is usually not well defined.
- The contrast enhancement pattern is variable, including ringlike enhancement, nodular enhancement, heterogeneous enhancement, or occasionally no enhancement.
- Protoplasmic astrocytoma may present as a cortex-based, low-density mass lesion without significant contrast enhancement.

Magnetic Resonance Imaging

- Heterogeneous signal-intensity patterns on both T1- and T2-weighted images.
- Predominately low-signal-intensity mass lesion on T1-weighted images and predominately high-signal-intensity on T2-weighted images.
- Focal areas of necrosis and cystic changes are seen.
- Focal hemorrhage may be seen.
  High signal intensity on T1-weighted images and low signal intensity on T2-weighted images—intracellular methemoglobin.
  High signal intensity on both T1- and T2-weighted images—extracellular methemoglobin.
  Very low signal intensity on both T1- and T2-weighted images—hemosiderin. Hemosiderin is better shown on gradient-echo images.
- Protoplasmic astrocytoma (anaplastic) may present as a relatively homogeneous low-signal mass involving the cortex on T1-weighted images and a high-signal intensity mass on T2-weighted images.
- The contrast enhancement pattern is variable. Contrast enhancement does not reflect actual tumor margin. Tumor cells are frequently detected beyond the margin of contrast enhancement.

Cerebral Angiography

- Grades 1 and 2 astrocytomas are usually avascular or minimally vascular.
- Glioblastomas may present as highly vascular or avascular neoplasms. The majority of glioblastomas are hypervascular lesions (Fig. 11-2).
- Vascular tumors may show slightly dilated feeding arteries and early draining veins, which are not as prominent as in the case of arteriovenous malformation. Furthermore, the feeding arteries and draining veins in arteriovenous malformation show uniform dilatation, whereas the neovascularity of glioblastoma is irregular, with areas of dilatation and narrowing. A nidus of the vascular malformation is seen without intervening brain tissue. Tumor vascularity is seen within the tumor mass.
- Early draining, dilated, deep medullary veins leading to subependymal veins in a radiant pattern are characteristic for glioblastoma and not seen in vascular malformation or metastases.

OLIGODENDROGLIOMA

Incidence

- Oligodendroglioma constitutes 5 percent of all cerebral gliomas.

Age and Gender

- Young and middle-aged adults
- Slight male predominance of 3:2

Location

- These tumors typically involve the cerebral cortex and subcortical white matter in the cerebral hemisphere, especially in the frontal and frontotemporal region.
- They also occur in the cerebellum and spinal cord and occasionally in the ventricular wall.

Pathology

- Macroscopically, these tumors are usually solid, well-defined masses. Cystic degeneration or necrosis may be seen in large lesions. Calcification and hemorrhage are commonly seen.
- There is a wide range of grades within the category of oligodendroglioma due to the tumor's heterogeneity of histopathology.
- The tumor cell is identified by its round nucleus surrounded by a clear ring between the nuclear membrane and the cell wall. The cells are divided into lobules by vascularized connective tissue septa. The average oligodendroglioma has few cells in mitotic division.

Imaging *Plain X-ray*

- Oligodendrogliomas are among the few intracranial tumors that may be diagnosed on plain x-ray.

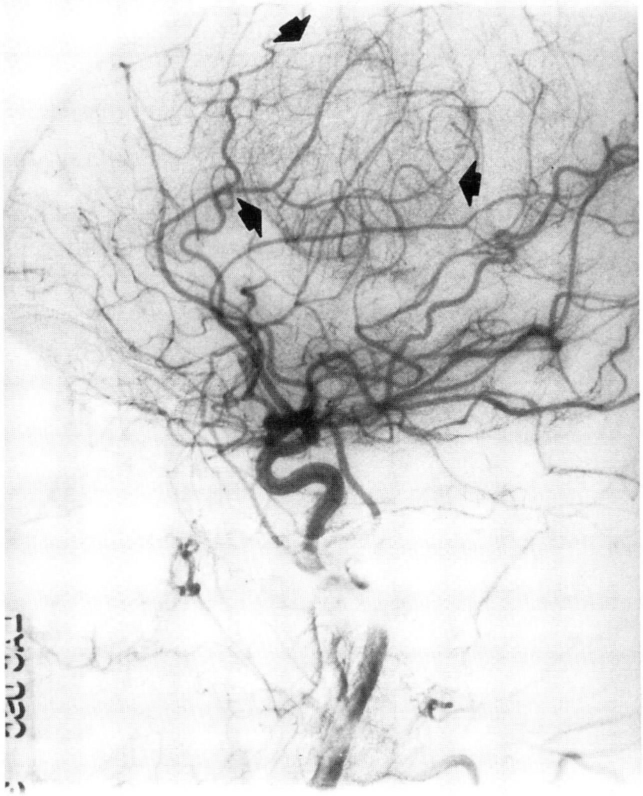

(A)

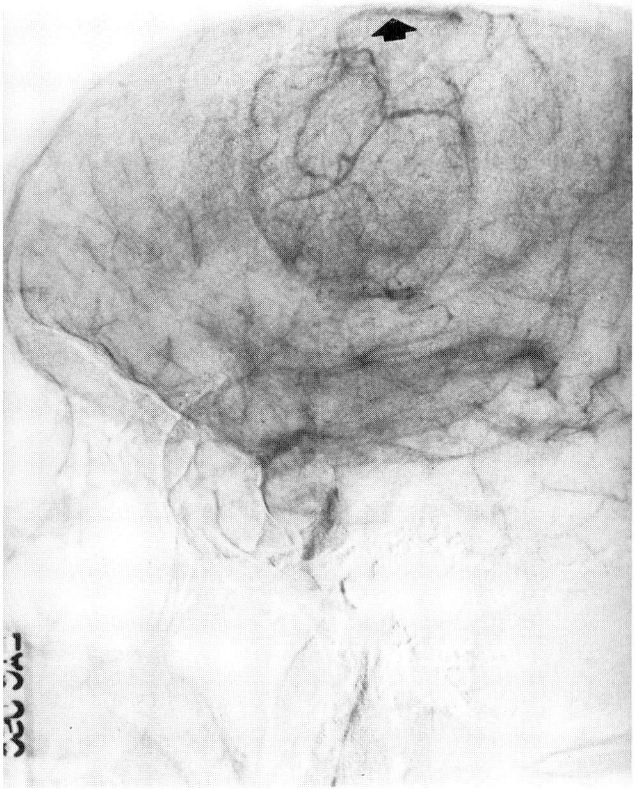

(B)

Figure 11-2 Glioblastoma. *A*. A lateral-view right common carotid angiogram (late arterial phase) shows a large, round area of tumor vascularity in the frontal lobe (*arrows*). *B*. A later view (capillary phase) shows a tumor stain as well as an early draining vein (*arrow*).

- Calcification is seen on 30 to 40 percent of cases on plain x-ray.
- Calcification has a popcornlike appearance.

Computed Tomography

- Calcification (linear or nodular) is demonstrated in 50 to 90 percent of cases on CT.
- The tumor is a hypodense to isodense mass with foci of calcification or hemorrhage.
- About half of the tumors will show contrast enhancement and the other half will not enhance.
- Cystic changes may be seen.
- Peritumoral edema is mild or absent.
- Occasionally, erosion of the adjacent bony calvarium may be observed.

Magnetic Resonance Imaging

- The signal intensity patterns are heterogeneous but predominately show isointensity to gray matter on T1-weighted images and hyperintensity on T2-weighted images.
- Cystic degeneration, hemorrhage, and calcification all contribute to the heterogeneous signal-intensity pattern seen on MRI.
- Peritumoral edema is minimal.
- Magnetic resonance imaging is more sensitive than CT in demonstrating contrast enhancement.

METASTASIS

The brain and its covering may be involved by neoplasms arising in extracranial tissues as a result of either direct extension of the primary tumor or hematogeneous spread. When hematogeneous spread is seen, it often occurs at the junction between the gray and white matter.

Incidence

- In autopsy series, 20 percent of patients with systemic cancer have intracranial metastases.
- Metastases represent 15 to 40 percent of all intracranial neoplasms.

Location

- Parenchymal lesions are typically seen at the corticomedullary junction.
- Uncommon sites include the choroid plexus, pineal body, and pituitary gland.
- Multiple lesions are seen in 70 to 80 percent of cases.

- Metastatic melanoma and breast carcinoma have a higher incidence of multiple lesions than metastatic lung carcinoma and renal cell carcinoma.
- Supratentorial location is seen in 60 to 80 percent of cases.
- Subependymal and intraventricular tumor spread occurs in lymphoma, melanoma, and occasionally breast carcinoma.
- Leptomeningeal and dural tumor spread may be seen from breast, lung, or prostate carcinoma.

Pathology

- Primary site in order of descending frequency: lung, breast, melanoma, kidney, colon.
- Primary site may be unknown in 10 to 15 percent of cases.
- Small parenchymal metastases frequently occur at the gray/white junction, where the arterioles show an abrupt reduction in their diameter, trapping tumor emboli.
- Metastatic lesions are usually spherical.
- Hemorrhage or cystic degeneration may be seen.

Imaging *Computed Tomography*

- Double-dose (up to 80 g of organically bound iodine) contrast-enhanced delayed (up to 45 min) scans are recommended for evaluation of metastatic disease. However, contrast-enhanced MRI is superior to contrast-enhanced CT for evaluation of metastatic disease.
- Metastatic lesions are of variable density on unenhanced CT. Certain lesions—including melanoma, colon carcinoma, choriocarcinoma, and osteosarcoma—show hyperdensity.
- Hemorrhage in metastatic lesions is seen in 15 percent of cases and may be seen in melanoma, choriocarcinoma, bronchogenic carcinoma, and hypernephroma.
- Calcification is extremely rare but may be seen in osteosarcoma and colon carcinoma.
- Contrast enhancement is typically seen. Lesions may show nodular enhancement or thick, irregular, ringlike enhancement.
- Marked vasogenic edema is commonly seen surrounding the lesion. Occasionally, an enhancing lesion may be seen without significant surrounding edema.

Magnetic Resonance Imaging

- The lesion is hypointense to isointense (to gray matter) on T1-weighted images.
- It is isointense to hyperintense on T2-weighted images.
- Hemorrhage in metastatic lesions can produce a complex signal intensity pattern.
- Edema presents as peritumoral areas of high signal in the white matter, which may vary from none to marked. Generally, marked edema is seen.
- Double- or triple-dose paramagnetic contrast agents (up to 0.3 mmol/kg) have been advocated by some.
- Contrast-enhanced MRI with magnetization transfer technique is the most sensitive to detect metastatic disease.
- The contrast enhancement pattern may be nodular, ringlike, or irregular (Fig. 11-3). Distinction from primary glioma or abscess may be difficult when the lesion is solitary.
- Subependymal or intraventricular spread of metastases is best shown on contrast-enhanced MRI.
- Skull base and dural involvement are best shown with gadolinium-enhanced, fat-suppressed MRI images.

LYMPHOMA

Incidence

- Primary lymphoma represents about 1 percent of all intracranial tumors.
- There has recently been an increase in incidence due to an increase in patients with acquired immunodeficiency syndrome (AIDS) and immunosuppression (renal transplant, chemotherapy, other malignancy).
- Primary CNS lymphoma is more common than secondary involvement by systemic lymphoma.

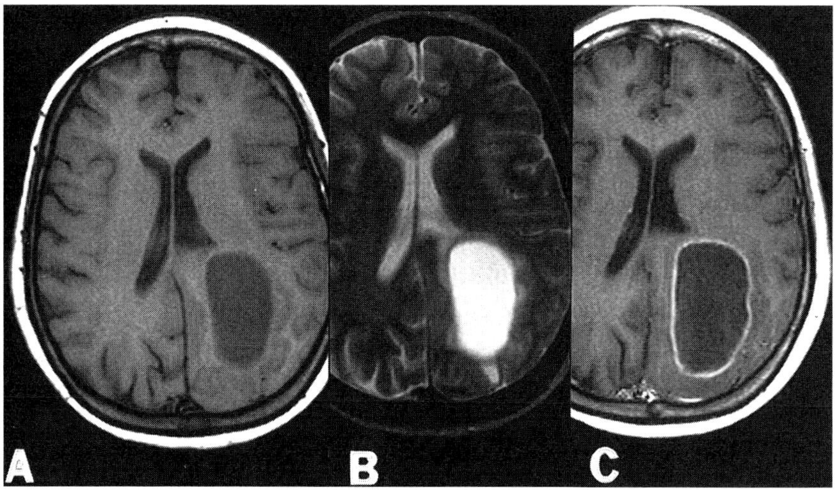

Figure 11-3 Metastatic lung carcinoma. *A*. An axial T1-weighted image shows a large, ovoid cystic mass lesion in the left parietooccipital region. The cyst fluid is of slightly higher signal intensity as compared to CSF. *B*. An axial T2-weighted image reveals the cyst fluid to be of higher signal intensity as compared to CSF secondary to increased protein content in the tumor cyst. A small amount of surrounding edema is seen. *C*. A gadolinium-enhanced T1-weighted image shows a smooth, ringlike enhancement.

- About 10 percent of the patients with systemic lymphoma develop CNS involvement on imaging studies, whereas CNS involvement is present in one-third of cases at autopsy.

Age
- All ages are affected.
- In patients with AIDS or immunosuppression, lymphoma is more common in the third or fourth decade.
- In other patients, it is more common in sixth decade.

Location
- Solitary or multiple intracranial lesion(s).
- Focal intraaxial lesions are the most common initial presentation of primary CNS lymphoma.
- Basal ganglia, periventricular white matter, corpus callosum, and septum pellucidum are often involved.
- Approximately 45 percent of lesions are multiple.
- Some 30 percent of patients with primary lymphoma develop leptomeningeal disease.
- Leptomeningeal disease is more common in patients with recurrent disease.

Pathology
- Primary CNS lymphomas are non-Hodgkin's lymphomas, usually of B-cell type.
- Grossly, parenchymal lesions are ill-defined masses with irregular borders.
- Relatively homogeneous—uniformly cellular neoplasm with some aggressive histologic features (in non-AIDS, nonimmunosuppressed patients).
- Heterogeneous masses with areas of necrosis (in AIDS or immunosuppressed patients).
- Leptomeningeal disease is a diffuse infiltrative process by tumor cells (lypophytes or large monocytes), which are seen in the perivascular spaces and in the subarachnoid space.

Imaging ***Computed Tomography***
- Typical lymphoma (in non-AIDS, nonimmunosuppressed patients) exhibits hyperdensity to isodensity to brain parenchyma.
- Uniform enhancement is seen.
- In immunosuppressed or AIDS patients, ringlike enhancing lesions with areas of necrosis may be seen.

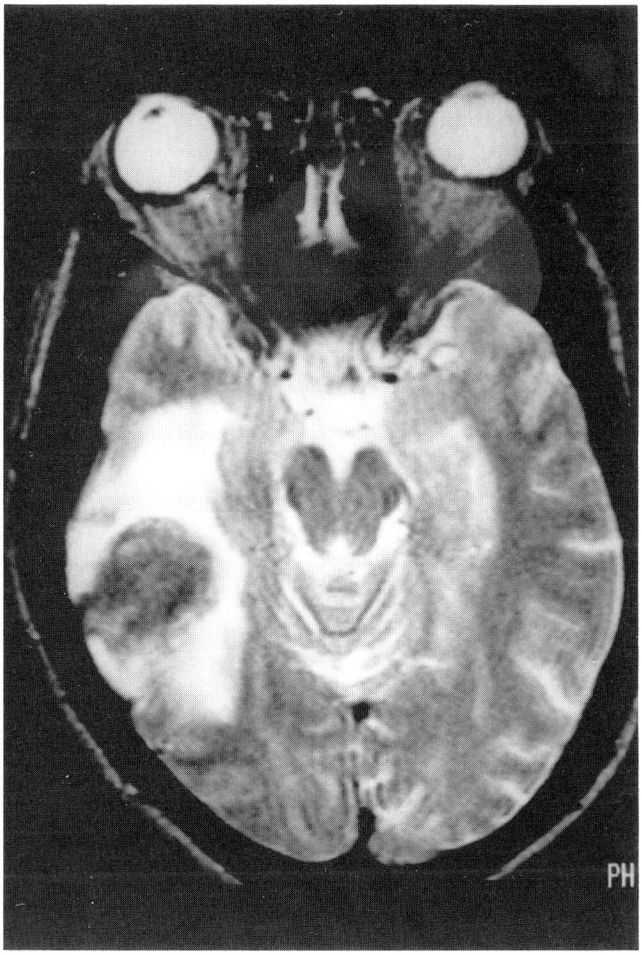

(A)

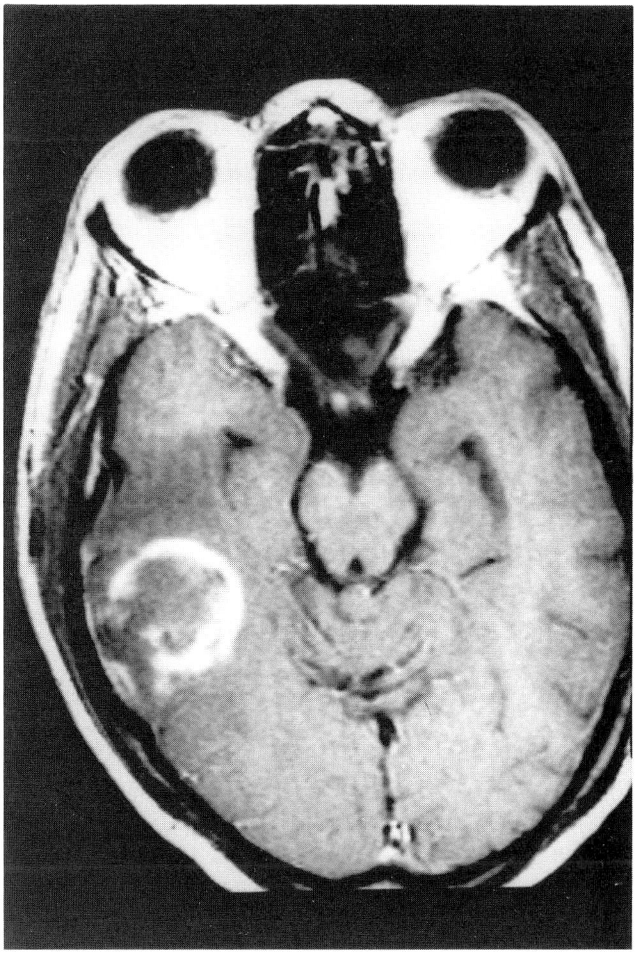

(B)

Figure 11-4 Primary lymphoma. *A*. An axial T2-weighted image demonstrates the low-intensity mass lesion with surrounding edema.

B A gadolinium-enhanced axial T1-weighted image shows an irregular ringlike enhancement.

- Calcification or hemorrhage is rare.

Magnetic Resonance Imaging

- Typically, lymphomas are solid masses that are hypointense to isointense on T1-weighted images and isointense to hyperintense on T2-weighted images. Occasionally, lymphoma can be hypointense on T2-weighted images (Fig. 11-4*A*).
- Contrast enhancement is intense and uniform in non-AIDS and non-immunosuppressed patients.
- In immunosuppressed or AIDS patients, lymphoma may present as ringlike enhancing lesions or irregular enhancing masses with areas of necrosis (Fig. 11-4*B*).
- Leptomeningeal seeding is better seen on contrast-enhanced MRI than on CT.

Whenever a single ringlike or irregular enhancing lesion with necrosis is seen, a glioma or an abscess should be considered, with lymphoma in the differential diagnosis. The solid component of the glioma usually shows low signal intensity on T1-weighted images and high signal intensity on T2-weighted images. Gliomas are less likely to show leptomeningeal or subependymal seeding, although such may be seen with anaplastic astrocytoma or glioblastoma. The tumor margin is poorly defined in glioma but can be seen in parenchymal lymphoma. Abscesses generally have a smooth, thin wall with ringlike enhancement and a moderate amount of surrounding edema. The abscess capsule tends to show slight hyperintensity on T1-weighted images and hypointensity on T2-weighted images. Abscesses can often be multiple or have small "daughter" abscesses adjacent to a large one.

Toxoplasmosis lesions can be difficult to differentiate from lymphoma in AIDS patients. A large single lesion is more likely to be lymphoma. Multiple small lesions in the deep gray matter and corticomedullary junction are more likely to be toxoplasmosis. Lesions located in the periventricular white matter or corpus callosum are more likely to be lymphoma.

☐ SUPRATENTORIAL INTRAAXIAL TUMORS IN CHILDREN

ASTROCYTOMAS

Incidence

- Constitute 30 to 40 percent of supratentorial brain tumors in childhood.
- Most common brain tumor in the pediatric age group.

Age and Gender

- Peak incidence at age 7 to 8 years
- Slightly higher peak age as compared to brainstem or cerebellar astrocytomas
- Slight male predominance

Classification

- Low-grade astrocytoma
  - Pilocytic astrocytoma
  - Fibrillary astrocytoma
- High-grade astrocytoma
  - Anaplastic astrocytoma
  - Glioblastoma multiforme

JUVENILE PILOCYTIC ASTROCYTOMA

Location

- Pilocytic astrocytomas in the supratentorial compartment tend to occur in the region of diencephalon, including the hypothalamus, visual pathway, optic chiasm, and basal ganglia. The most common location of pilocytic astrocytoma is in the region of diencephalon.
- The next most common location is the cerebellar vermis, hemispheres, and brainstem. The cerebral hemispheres and lateral ventricles are less common locations.

Pathology

- Pilocytic astrocytomas are cystic or multicystic, with a mural nodule in 55 percent; 45 percent are solid.
- Chiasmatic-hypothalamic pilocytic astrocytomas are usually solid infiltrating mass lesions and are often associated with neurofibromatosis.
- Calcification in a flecklike pattern may be seen.
- Pilocytic astrocytomas are well-circumscribed but unencapsulated masses of "hairlike" astrocytes and loosely aggregated protoplasmic astrocytes. Cysts are commonly seen.

Imaging *Computed Tomography*

- Cystic or solid mass.
- The cystic mass contains a mural nodule that enhances intensely. The cyst wall typically does not enhance.
- The solid mass is hypodense and shows variable contrast enhancement.
- Cyst fluid is generally of higher density than cerebrospinal fluid, owing to its higher protein content.
- Chiasmatic—hypothalamic pilocytic astrocytomas are usually solid mass lesion without a significant cystic component.

Magnetic Resonance Imaging

- The solid component of the mass is intense to hypointense on T1-weighted images and hyperintense on T2-weighted images (Fig. 11-5).
- Contrast enhancement of the mural nodule of the cystic mass is intense. Occasionally, enhancement of the cyst wall may be seen.
- Cyst fluid is generally of higher signal intensity than cerebrospinal fluid (CSF) due to its high protein content.
- Chiasmatic—hypothalamic pilocytic astrocytomas are usually solid mass lesions, whereas hemispheric pilocytic astrocytomas may be cystic mass lesions.

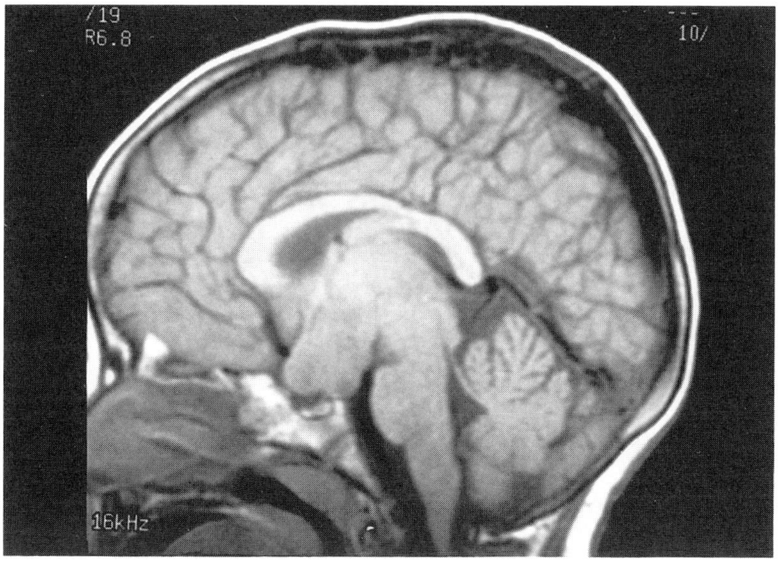

(A)

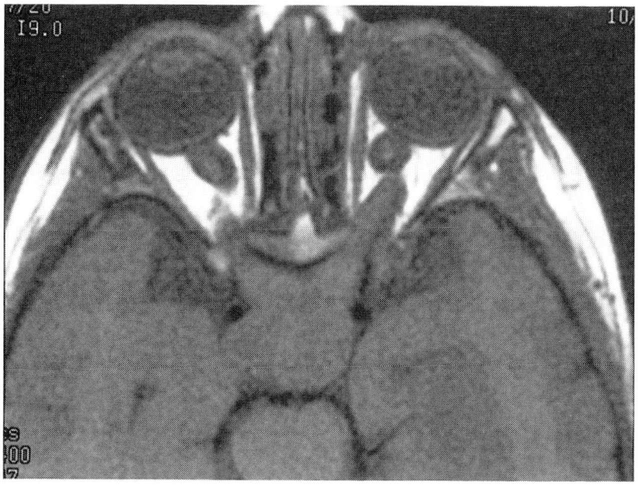

(B)

Figure 11-5 Hypothalamic/chiasmal pilocytic astrocytoma. *A*. A sagittal T1-weighted image demonstrates an isointense mass lesion involving the hypothalamus/chiasm. *B*. An axial T1-weighted image shows a suprasellar mass with extension into the proximal portion of optic nerves bilaterally.

LOW-GRADE FIBRILLARY ASTROCYTOMA

Location

- Any region may be involved, but these tumors most often appear in temporal and frontal lobes.

Pathology

- Cellular tumors that locally infiltrate the white matter of the cerebral hemisphere
- Less often cystic or calcified than pilocytic astrocytoma

Imaging ***Computed Tomography***

- A hypodense mass
- Usually does not enhance; occasionally, patchy enhancement

Magnetic Resonance Imaging

- A homogeneous mass that is hypointense on T1-weighted images and hyperintense on T2-weighted images.
- Occasionally, patchy, irregular contrast enhancement may be seen.

ANAPLASTIC ASTROCYTOMA AND GLIOBLASTOMA

Location

- They present as a mass in the white matter of cerebral hemisphere with ill-defined margins

Pathology

- Most malignant, aggressive histologic grades of astrocytoma.
- Tumor necrosis or hemorrhage is frequently seen.
- Calcification is rare.
- Poorly formed tumor vessels result in abnormal BBB with vasogenic edema and contrast enhancement.

Imaging ***Computed Tomography***

- Mixed but predominantly low-density mass with ill-defined margin and surrounding edema.

- Cystic, necrotic areas and foci of hemorrhage may be seen.
- Patchy irregular contrast enhancement.

Magnetic Resonance Imaging

- Ill-defined mass that shows hypointensity on T1-weighted images and hyperintensity on T2-weighted images.
- Heterogeneous signal-intensity pattern can be seen, due to areas of necrosis, hemorrhage, or tumor vessel.
- Patchy contrast enhancement.

PLEOMORPHIC XANTHOASTROCYTOMA

Incidence

- Rare, less than 1 percent of astrocytomas
- Age: children and young adults

Location

- The temporal lobe is the most common site.
- A superficially located cystic mass with a mural nodule abuts the leptomeninges.

Pathology

- They are well demarcated, partially cystic neoplasms with a mural nodule.
- A mixture of spindle-shaped cells, multinucleated giant cells, and foamy lipid-laden xanthomatous astrocytes is seen microscopically.

Imaging *Computed Tomography*

- Cystic mass with mural nodule located superficially
- Intense contrast enhancement of the mural nodule

Magnetic Resonance Imaging

- Well-demarcated cystic mass with mural nodule.
- Intense enhancement of the mural nodule.
- Occasionally, they can be solid, infiltrating neoplasms.

GANGLIONEUROMA AND GANGLIOGLIOMA

These rare tumors form a histologic spectrum ranging from the ganglioneuroma (which consists of well-differentiated, neoplastic gangliocytes with a scanty glial cell stroma) to tumors that may resemble a glioma.

Incidence

- They constitute about 4 percent of all pediatric CNS tumors.

Age and Gender

- They occur predominately in children and young adults but may be seen in any age group.
- There is a slight male predominance of 3:2.

Location

- These tumors have a predilection for the temporal, occipital, and frontal lobes.

Pathology

- The tumor is usually small, with well-defined margins.
- Cyst formation with partially calcified mural nodule is common.
- Calcification is seen in 30 to 40 percent of cases.
- Microscopically, the tumor varies from a predominantly neuronal proliferation to a lesion with dominant glial elements and only scanty ectopic ganglionic cells.
- Gangliocytomas are purely neuronal tumors that lack a glial component. They are probably brain malformations rather than neoplasia.

Imaging *Computed Tomography*

- A cystic component of these tumors can be identified in 50 percent of cases.
- The solid component shows hypodensity to isodensity; the cystic component shows CSF-like density.
- Contrast enhancement is seen in 50 percent of cases.
- Calcification is seen in 30 to 40 percent of cases.
- Surrounding edema is minimal.

Magnetic Resonance Imaging

- Well-circumscribed mass that is hypointense to isointense on T1-weighted images, hyperintense on T2-weighted images.
- Cystic components show signal intensity similar to CSF.
- Calcification is better seen on CT or gradient-echo images.

DESMOPLASTIC INFANTILE GANGLIOGLIOMA

Incidence

- Rare supratentorial neuroepithelial neoplasms

Age

- Typical age of onset is 4 months

Location

- Frontal and parietal lobes

Pathology

- Large cystic masses.
- Pleomorphic neuroepithelial cells that differentiate along astrocytic neuronal lines with an extensive desmoplastic component.

Imaging *Computed Tomography*

- A large, well-defined cystic mass with a smaller, solid component.
- The solid component is isodense to brain parenchyma.
- Cyst fluid is similar to CSF or slightly hyperdense.
- Calcification may be seen.
- Enhancement of the solid component and cyst wall is seen following the administration of contrast material.

Magnetic Resonance Imaging

- A large, well-defined cystic mass.
- Cyst fluid is similar to CSF or slightly hyperintense on both T1- and T2-weighted images.
- The solid component is isointense on T1-weighted images and heterogeneously hyperintense on T2-weighted images.

PRIMITIVE NEUROECTODERMAL TUMORS

Incidence

- Common CNS tumor in children, consisting of 25 percent of all intracranial tumors.
- Supratentorial primitive neuroectodermal tumors (PNET) are rare; 5 percent of all supratentorial tumor in children.
- Some authors now include medulloblastoma, primary cerebral neuroblastoma, ependymoblastoma, and pineoblastoma in the category of PNET. We shall discuss primary cerebral neuroblastoma only in this section; the other entities will be discussed separately.

Age and Gender

- The peak incidence is in the first decade. Majority present before the age of 5 years.
- Males and females are equally affected in the supratentorial compartment.

Location

- Most PNETs occur in the posterior fossa; supratentorial PNET are rare.
- Primary cerebral neuroblastomas are seen supratentorially.

Pathology

- Highly malignant and cellular neoplasms are made up of more than 90 percent of undifferentiated cells.
- Necrosis and cyst formation are seen in up to 60 percent of cases.
- Calcification is seen in up to 70 percent of cases.

Imaging *Computed Tomography*

- Large, irregular, heterogeneous mass deep in the cerebral white matter.
- The solid component of the mass is usually hyperdense.
- Necrosis, cyst formation, and calcification are frequently seen.
- Hemorrhage is occasionally seen.
- Enhancement is seen and may be heterogeneous or ringlike.

Magnetic Resonance Imaging

- Large, heterogeneous mass with necrosis, cyst formation, calcification, or hemorrhage.
- The solid component of the mass is slightly hypointense on T1-weighted images and slightly to moderately hyperintense on T2-weighted images.

EPENDYMOMA

Incidence

- Ependymomas constitute 2 to 6 percent of all gliomas.
- Only 40 percent of intracranial ependymomas occur in the supratentorial compartment.
- The reported incidence of parenchymal origin of the ependymomas varies from 55 to 85 percent. Parenchymal ependymomas are more commonly seen in the supratentorial compartment.

Age and Gender

- Ependymomas are four to six times more common in children than in the adult population.
- Infratentorial ependymomas occur predominantly in children, whereas supratentorial ependymomas are evenly distributed among all age groups.
- Both sexes are equally involved.

Location

- Supratentorial, 40 percent; Infratentorial, 60 percent.
- The most common site of origin is the fourth ventricle.
- In the supratentorial compartment, these tumors have a predilection for the frontal and parietal lobes.

Pathology

- Well-defined mass with cystic, necrotic degeneration and calcification.
- Hemorrhage is not common.
- Microscopically, the tumor cells are carrot-shaped, with their long polar processes pointing toward blood vessels in the form of rosettes. Calcium salt deposits are often seen.
- A higher proportion of supratentorial ependymomas tend to be malignant (ependymoblastoma); which may grow rapidly within the ventricular system and form a cast of tumor within the ventricular cavity.

Imaging *Computed Tomography*

- Hypodense to isodense to gray matter.
- Dense, punctate calcification is seen in 50 percent of cases. Intraparenchymal ependymomas are less frequently calcified; when uncalcified, they can mimic anaplastic astrocytoma or glioblastoma but occur at a younger age.
- Peritumoral edema is seen in about 50 percent of cases.
- Contrast enhancement is variable, from homogeneous to heterogeneous.

Magnetic Resonance Imaging

- Hypointense to isointense on T1-weighted images and hyperintense on T2-weighted images.

- A heterogeneous signal intensity pattern may be seen due to cystic degeneration, necrosis, calcification, or hemorrhage.
- Contrast enhancement pattern is variable from homogeneous to patchy heterogeneous.

☐ POSTERIOR FOSSA INTRAAXIAL TUMORS IN ADULTS (Table 11-4)

HEMANGIOBLASTOMA

Incidence

- These tumors represent approximately 1 to 2.5 percent of all primary CNS neoplasms and 8 to 12 percent of all primary posterior fossa neoplasms.
- They are the most common type of primary intraaxial posterior fossa neoplasm in adults.
- Between 4 to 40 percent of patients with hemangioblastoma have von Hippel-Lindau syndrome.
- Approximately 40 percent of patients with von Hippel-Lindau syndrome will eventually develop hemangioblastomas.

Age

- Peak age of presentation is 30 to 40 years.
- In von Hippel-Lindau syndrome, the tumors present in younger adults.

Location

- They are usually solitary lesions.
- Multiple lesions are seen in 10 percent of patients with von Hippel-Lindau syndrome.
- They are most frequently seen in the cerebellum (more than 90 percent), but can be found in the medulla or within the spinal cord.
- The lesions are usually located at the periphery of the cerebellum, with mural nodule at the pial surface.

Pathology

- Well-demarcated cystic masses with highly vascular solid nodules along the wall of the cyst. The cyst wall is not involved with tumor.
- Solid hemangioblastomas occur in 30 to 40 percent of cases.
- Microscopically, the tumor is not encapsulated and can invade the parenchyma.
- The mural nodule is a hypervascular mass of capillaries with intervening benign-appearing neoplastic stroma.
- On histopathology, the differentiation of hemangioblastoma from metastatic renal cell carcinoma may at times be difficult.
- Von Hippel-Lindau syndrome is autosomal dominant with variable penetrance.
- Microscopically, hemangioblastomas of the CNS are characterized by a fine hypervascular capillary mesh in a stroma composed of polygonal cells without mitotic activity.
- Cyst fluid may contain erythropoietin and patients may have polycythemia.

Imaging ***Computed Tomography***

- Some 60 percent are cystic masses and 40 percent predominantly solid masses.
- Cystic mass with an enhancing mural nodule.
- Solid enhancing mass.
- Beam-hardening artifacts in the posterior fossa limit sensitivity to CT.

Magnetic Resonance Imaging

- Most sensitive noninvasive imaging modality for evaluation of hemangioblastoma.
- A solid lesion presents as a heterogeneously low-signal-intensity mass on T1-weighted images and high-signal-intensity mass on T2-weighted images (Fig. 11-6*A* and *B*).
- Cystic lesion presents as a cyst with a pia-based mural nodule that enhances markedly. Solid mass also enhances markedly (Fig. 11-6*C*).
- Linear or curvilinear areas of signal void (vessels) are seen within or adjacent to the solid mass or mural nodule of the cystic mass.
- Cyst fluid has variable signal intensity, depending on the protein content—presence or absence of hemorrhage within the cyst fluid.

Angiography

- Intense tumor stains are seen involving the mural nodules.
- Superior to contrast-enhanced CT for detection of multiple lesions.
- Excellent for demonstration of cervical cord lesions.
- Solid tumors may show increased tumor vascularity with early draining vein, mimicking a vascular malformation (Fig. 11-6*D*).

ASTROCYTOMA

Incidence and Age

- The majority of cerebellar astrocytomas are of the pilocytic variety (75 percent), and they occur within the first two decades of life.
- The minority of cerebellar astrocytomas are of the fibrillary infiltrative type (25 percent), and they occur in young adults.

Pathology

- Fibrillary astrocytomas are infiltrative lesions. Microscopically, they are characterized by well-differentiated fibrillary astrocytes that demonstrate only mild nuclear pleomorphism. Mitoses are few and vascular proliferation is absent.

Table 11-4
POSTERIOR FOSSA INTRAAXIAL TUMORS

	Incidence	Peak Age	Location	CT	MRI	Other
Metastasis	Most common posterior fossa intraaxial neoplasm	50 years and over	Cerebellar	Density variable; nodular or ringlike enhancement with surrounding edema	Signal intensity variable; nodular or ringlike enhancement with surrounding edema.	Calcification—rare Hemorrhage—15%
Hemangioblastoma	Most common primary posterior fossa intraaxial neoplasm	30 to 40 years	Cerebellar medulla	60 to 70% cystic mass with enhancing mural nodule; 30% to 40% solid enhancing mass	Cystic mass with enhancing pia-based mural nodule. Solid enhancing mass. Linear or curvilinear areas of signal void (vessels) are seen within or adjacent to the solid mass or mural nodule.	Cerebral angiography shows intense tumor stain involving the solid mass or mural nodule
Cerebellar astrocytoma	Second most common posterior fossa neoplasm in children	5 to 20 years	Cerebellum	Cystic mass with enhancing mural nodule; solid mass with variable density and variable enhancing pattern	Cystic mass with enhancing mural nodule—may mimic hemangioblastoma. Solid mass that is hypointense on T1-weighted images and isointense to hyperintense on T2-weighted images; variable enhancing pattern.	
Medulloblastoma (primitive neuroectodermal tumor)	Most common posterior fossa neoplasm in children	1 to 10 years	Roof of fourth ventricle in children; cerebellum in young adults	Uniform high-density mass with homogeneous enhancement	Isointense on T1-weighted images and iso- to hyperintense on T2-weighted images. Contrast enhancement may be seen.	Intraventricular, subarachnoid seeding may be seen
Brainstem astrocytoma		5 to 15 years	Pons > medulla > midbrain	Hypodense to isodense lesion; contrast enhancement seen in 50% of cases	Hypointensity on T1-weighted images and hyperintensity on T2-weighted images. Contrast enhancement may be seen.	
Ependymoma	8% of brain tumor in children	5 to 10 years, but may be seen in any age group. Slight male predominance	60% infratentorial, 40% supratentorial. Fourth ventricle and lateral recess of fourth ventricle	Variable density; patchy contrast enhancement	Variable signal intensity; patchy contrast enhancement	Calcification—50%, cyst formation and necrosis—70%
Choroid plexus papilloma	0.5% of all intracranial neoplasms, less than 2% of gliomas	First decade, slight male predominance	Fourth ventricle—adults more common than children. Lateral ventricle—children	Variable density; intense contrast enhancement	Variable intensity; intense contrast enhancement	Calcification, hemorrhage

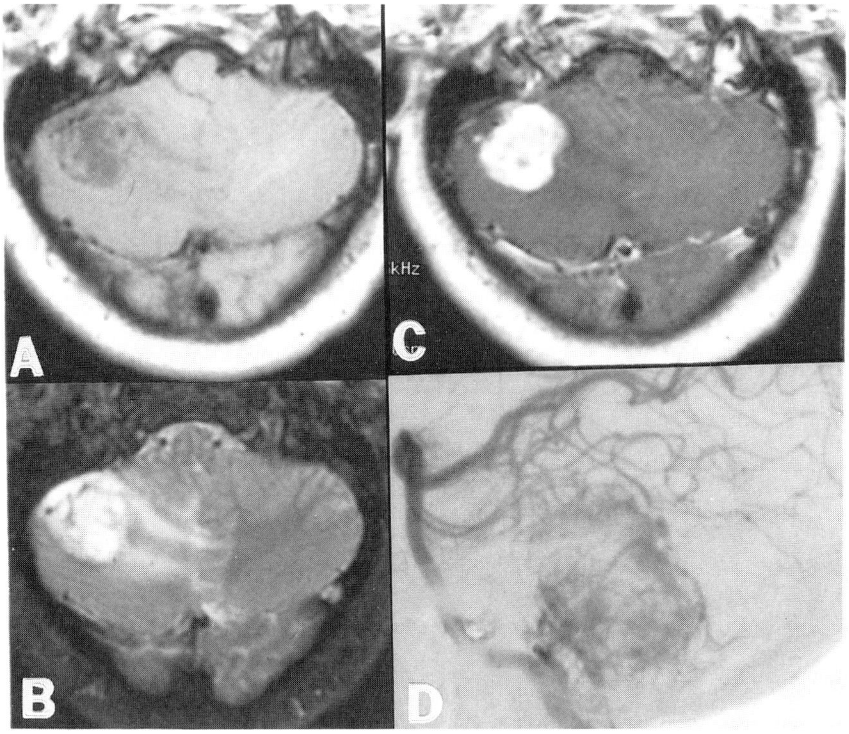

Figure 11-6 Hemangioblastoma. *A*. An axial T1-weighted image shows a right cerebellar mass of mixed iso- and low-signal intensity. *B*. An axial T2-weighted image reveals a predominantly hyperintense mass with areas of curvilinear hypointensity, consistent with tumor vascularity. *C*. A gadolinium-enhanced axial T1-weighted image shows intense enhancement of the mass lesion with small areas of signal void. *D*. A cerebral angiogram (in a different patient) shows tumor vascularity.

Imaging *Computed Tomography*

- Beam-hardening artifacts
- Low-density mass with ill-defined margin
- Patchy enhancement or no enhancement

Magnetic Resonance Imaging

- Hypointense to cerebellar parenchyma on T1-weighted images and hyperintense on T2-weighted images.
- Patchy enhancement or no enhancement on postcontrast images.

METASTASIS

Incidence and Location

- Supratentorial metastatic lesions are seen in 60 to 80 percent and infratentorial metastatic lesions are seen in 20 to 40 percent of cases.
- Multiple in 70 to 80 percent; solitary in 20 to 30 percent.
- Metastasis is the most common posterior fossa intraaxial tumor in adults.
- A single posterior fossa mass in a patient above 50 years of age is most likely a metastatic lesion.

Pathology

- Common origin of primary tumor in descending order of frequency: lung, breast, melanoma, kidney, and colon.

Imaging *Computed Tomography*

- Parenchymal lesions may show hypodensity, isodensity, or hyperdensity on noncontrast CT. Hyperdense lesions include melanoma, choriocarcinoma, colon carcinoma, osteosarcoma, and lymphoma.
- Contrast enhancement is typically seen.
- Necrosis and cavitation are common.
- Bone window images are essential in the evaluation of metastatic disease involving the bony calvarium.

Magnetic Resonance Imaging

- Contrast-enhanced MRI is the imaging modality of choice for the evaluation of metastatic disease.
- Leptomeningeal seeding and ependymal seeding are shown on contrast-enhanced MRI.
- Calvarial metastases are well shown on T1-weighted images without contrast. Contrast enhancement may obscure the visualization of bony metastases.

☐ POSTERIOR FOSSA INTRAAXIAL NEOPLASMS IN CHILDREN (Table 11-4)

PRIMITIVE NEUROECTODERMAL TUMOR (MEDULLOBLASTOMA)

Incidence

- Primitive neuroectodermal tumor (medulloblastoma) (PNET-MB) is the most common posterior fossa neoplasm in children (40 percent) in our series. Some authors have reported astrocytoma to be the most common posterior fossa neoplasm in children.

- Some 25 percent of all pediatric intracranial neoplasms are PNET-MB.

Age and Gender

- The peak incidence is in the first decade.
- Boys are two to four times more commonly affected.

Location

- Arising from the vermis, PNET-MB may extend to involve the cerebellar hemisphere, brainstem, or fourth ventricle.
- From the fourth ventricle, the tumor may extend into the cisterna magna via the foramen of Magendie, into the cerebellopontine angle cistern via the foramen of Luschka, or into the third ventricle via the aqueduct.

Pathology

- The PNET-MB originates from poorly differentiated germinative cells of the roof of the fourth ventricle that migrate superolaterally to the external granular layer of the cerebellar hemisphere. The medulloblastoma may arise anywhere along the path of migration.
- This concept is useful to explain the fact that medulloblastomas in childhood are usually in the midline along the roof of the fourth ventricle, whereas those in young adults are nearly always located more laterally in the cerebellar hemisphere.
- A relatively well-defined spherical mass arising from vermis.
- Microscopically, medulloblastomas are densely cellular tumors composed of immature cells with hyperchromatic nuclei and relatively scanty cytoplasm.

Imaging ***Computed Tomography***

- The medulloblastoma generally appears as a uniform, high-density lesion on noncontrast.
- These lesions tend to enhance homogeneously with sharp margins.
- Atypical features include small cystic or necrotic areas, calcification, hemorrhage, lack of contrast enhancement, eccentric location, and direct supratentorial extension.

Magnetic Resonance Imaging

- The PNET-MB is typically hypointense to isointense to brain parenchyma on T1-weighted images and isointense to hyperintense on T2-weighted images (Fig 11-7*A* through *C*).
- The pattern of contrast enhancement is similar to that of CT. However, the greater sensitivity of MRI often makes it possible to appreciate a slightly heterogeneous enhancing pattern. Occasionally, only minimal contrast enhancement is seen (Fig. 11-7*D*).

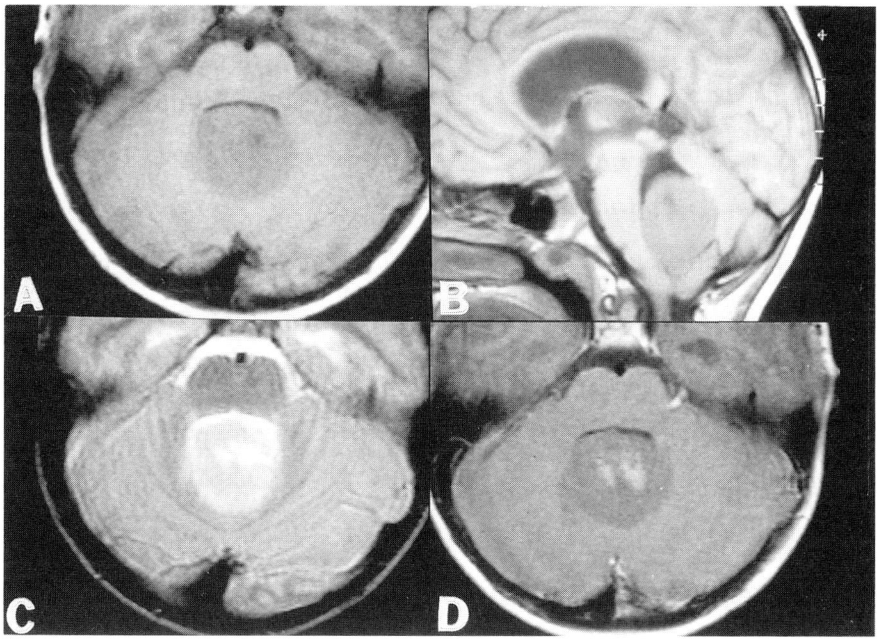

Figure 11-7 Primitive neuroectodermal tumor (medulloblastoma). *A*. An axial T1-weighted image shows a slightly hypointense mass with a small area of hypointensity in the midportion of the posterior fossa. A curvilinear, slitlike, low-signal-intensity area anterior to the mass is the compressed fourth ventricle. *B*. A sagittal T1-weighted image demonstrates a large, slightly hypointense mass arising from the posterior medullary velum and projecting into the fourth ventricle. *C*. An axial T2-weighted image shows a slightly hyperintense mass with focal areas of higher intensity. *D*. A gadolinium-enhanced axial T1-weighted image demonstrates minimal focal enhancement of the mass lesion.

- Subarachnoid seeding may be seen in up to 30 percent of newly diagnosed cases of PNET-MB.
- Subarachnoid seeding into the intracranial and spinal subarachnoid spaces and ependymal seeding along the ventricular wall occur more commonly with PNET-MB than with other pediatric posterior fossa neoplasms.

ASTROCYTOMA

Incidence

- Cerebellar astrocytoma is the second most common posterior fossa tumor in children, being slightly less common than PNET-MB. Some authors report astrocytoma to be the most common posterior fossa neoplasm in children.

Age and Gender

- Approximately 75 percent of cerebellar astrocytomas are benign juvenile pilocytic astrocytomas, which have a peak incidence in the first decade of life.
- The remaining 25 percent are diffuse, infiltrative, fibrillary astrocytomas, which have a peak incidence in adolescents and young adults.

Location *Pilocytic Astrocytoma*

- About 50 percent appear in the chiasmatic-hypothalamic region.
- About 30 percent appear in the cerebellar vermis and hemisphere.
- Less common locations include brainstem, basal ganglia, cerebral hemisphere, and intraventricular.
- Cerebellar astrocytomas may compress and displace the fourth ventricle.

Fibrillary Astrocytoma

- Low-grade fibrillary astrocytomas are more commonly seen in the cerebral hemispheres. Less common locations are brainstem and cerebellum.
- High-grade fibrillary astrocytomas are uncommon in the posterior fossa, especially in children.

Pathology *Pilocytic Astrocytoma*

- Benign juvenile pilocytic astrocytoma of cerebellum has a 94 percent 25-year survival rate.
- Cerebellar pilocytic astrocytomas are well-circumscribed masses that are cystic with a small, reddish-tan mural nodule.
- Chiasmatic-hypothalamic pilocytic astrocytomas are lobulated, solid masses that are infiltrating in the floor or wall of the third ventricle microscopically.
- Brainstem pilocytic astrocytomas are uniform, diffuse infiltrating neoplasms involving the medulla or pons.
- Microscopically, densely compact regions of elongated cells with hairlike processes and prominent Rosenthal fibers are seen.
- Cerebellar astrocytomas are generally large at the time of presentation due to their benign nature and slow growth.

Low-Grade Fibrillary Astrocytoma

- Infiltrating fibrillary astrocytoma has a 40 percent 25-year survival rate.
- These are unencapsulated tumors that infiltrate diffusely.
- There are well-differentiated fibrillary astrocytes that show only mild nuclear pleomorphism.

Imaging Since the majority of cerebellar astrocytomas in children are pilocytic, we will discuss the imaging findings of cerebellar pilocytic astrocytomas only in this section. Imaging findings of low-grade fibrillary astrocytomas are similar to their supratentorial counterparts.

Computed Tomography

- Sharply marginated cystic mass with mural nodule, which enhances intensely with contrast.
- Cyst fluid density may be similar to or higher than that of CSF, owing to increased protein content in the fluid.
- Cystic walls usually do not enhance and merely represent compressed brain. Occasionally, tumor involvement of the cyst wall with enhancement may be seen.

Magnetic Resonance Imaging

- Well-demarcated cystic mass with mural nodule, which enhances intensely with contrast.
- Cyst fluid may be of slightly higher signal intensity than CSF due to its high protein content.
- Cyst walls usually do not enhance and merely represent compressed brain tissue. Occasionally, tumor involvement of the cyst wall with enhancement may be seen.
- The appearance of cerebellar astrocytoma may resemble that of hemangioblastoma. However, hemangioblastomas are rare in children. The mural nodule of the hemangioblastoma tends to be pia-based, and curvilinear areas of signal void vessels are seen within or adjacent to the mural nodule.

EPENDYMOMA

Incidence

- Ependymomas make up 2 to 8 percent of primary intracranial brain tumors.
- Intracranial ependymomas are more frequently found in children, whereas intraspinal ependymomas are more frequently seen in adults.
- The majority (60 percent) of intracranial ependymomas are infratentorial in location, particularly in the fourth ventricle. They may also originate in or extend into the cerebellopontine angle (CPA) cistern, vallecula or medulla.

Age and Gender

- Ependymomas have a bimodal age distribution: the larger peak occurs in children and adolescents. The second, much smaller peak occurs in adults (40 to 50 years of age). They are four to six times more common in children than in adults.
- Both sexes are equally involved.
- Infratentorial ependymomas occur predominantly in children, whereas supratentorial ependymomas are evenly distributed among all age groups.

Pathology

- Ependymomas are gliomas arising from the ependymal cells, usually within the ventricles of the brain or central canal of the spinal cord.
- Ependymal rests in the white matter supratentorially may be the origin of parenchymal ependymomas.
- Infratentorial ependymomas usually arise from fourth ventricle and its lateral recesses.
- An especially malignant variant (ependymoblastoma) may grow rapidly within the ventricular system and form a cast of tumor within the ventricular cavity.

Ependymomas are slow-growing, firm, often lobulated, well-circumscribed white to grayish avascular masses that arise from ependymal cells lining the walls of ventricles or from ependymal rests in paraventricular white matter. They most commonly arise from the floor of the fourth ventricle and may protrude through foramina into adjacent cisterns (plastic ependymoma). About 50 percent calcify (two-thirds infratentorial, one-third supratentorial). Cyst formation is common. Hemorrhage is uncommon (less than 14 percent). Larger tumors (4 to 5 cm) more frequently demonstrate cysts, calcification, or hemorrhage.

Microscopically, ependymomas are sparsely cellular neoplasms with prominent fibrillary background. They are classified as cellular (most common), epithelial, papillary (uncommon), and myxopapillary (conus medullaris or filum terminale only). Malignancy is rare and they grow by expansion toward the ventricle, in contrast to gliomas that infiltrate surrounding tissue as they grow. Recurrence is common, resulting in a relatively poor prognosis (25 to 50 percent 5-year survival).

Imaging ***Computed Tomography***

- Hypodense to isodense mass with variable contrast enhancement.
- Intratumoral cysts are common.
- Approximately 50 percent are calcified, with the incidence of calcification increased in residual tumor after surgery and/or radiation therapy.
- Intraparenchymal ependymomas are less frequently calcified; when uncalcified, they can mimic anaplastic astrocytoma or glioblastoma, but ependymomas occur at a younger age.
- Intraventricular ependymomas may mimic choroid plexus papilloma on CT.

Magnetic Resonance Imaging

- Solid components are uniformly (homogeneously) hypo- to isointense to brain and cystic portions are slightly hyperintense to CSF on T1-weighted images (Fig 11-8*A*).
- Solid portions hyperintense to brain and cystic portions isointense to CSF on T2-weighted images (Fig. 11-8*B*).
- Ependymomas are somewhat lobulated soft tissue masses that may display heterogeneous intratumoral signal due to the presence of necrosis, calcification, tumor vascularity, blood degradation products, and intratumoral cysts.
- These lesions have a distinctive tendency to expand within ventricles and extrude through the foramina (e.g., Magendie and Lushka) into surrounding cisterns, the "plastic" configuration (Fig. 11-8*A*).
- Contrast enhancement pattern is heterogeneous (Fig. 11-8*C*).

Angiography Angiographic characteristics range from hypovascular mass to extremely hypervascular lesion with intense vascular staining, contrast stasis, irregular tumor vessels, and arteriovenous shunting.

BRAINSTEM GLIOMA

Incidence

- Brainstem glioma represents approximately 10 percent of all childhood and adolescent brain tumors.
- Brainstem glioma constitutes approximately 15 percent of all posterior fossa neoplasms in children.

Age and Gender

- They commonly occur before the age of 10 years.
- Slight male predominance is seen, 2.5:1.

Location

- The tumors usually arise within the pons and less frequently originate in the midbrain and the medulla.

Pathology

- Most brainstem gliomas (80 percent) arise from the pons and are fibrillary astrocytomas, which consist of low-grade astrocytomas, anaplastic astrocytomas, and glioblastomas.
- There is a tendency for low-grade fibrillary astrocytoma to show malignant degeneration.
- A smaller percentage (20 percent) of brainstem gliomas arise in the medulla or midbrain and are pilocytic astrocytomas.
- Some 55 percent of brainstem gliomas are low-grade fibrillary astrocytomas or pilocytic astrocytomas.
- About 45 percent of brainstem gliomas are anaplastic astrocytomas or glioblastomas.

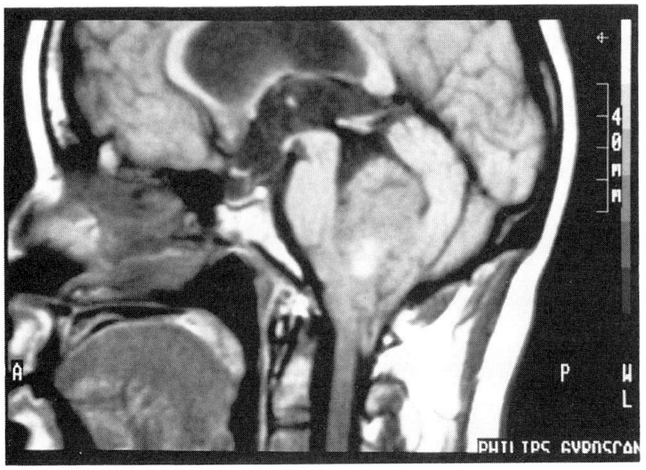

(A)

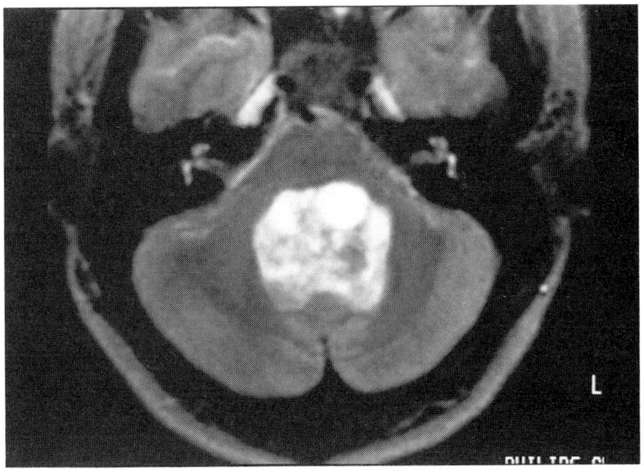

(B)

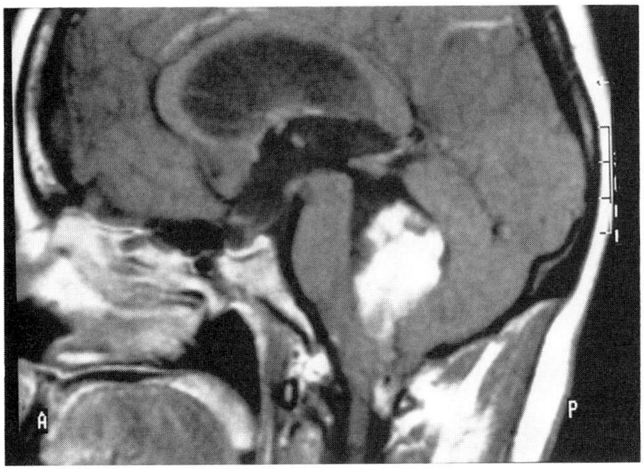

(C)

Figure 11-8 Posterior fossa ependymoma. *A*. A sagittal; T1-weighted image demonstrates a mass lesion in the fourth ventricle with a tonguelike tumor tissue extending through the foramen of Magendie. A focal area of hyperintensity seen at the inferior portion of the tumor is secondary to hemorrhage. *B*. An axial T2-weighted image reveals a heterogeneously high-signal-intensity mass lesion. *C*. A gadolinium-enhanced sagittal T1-weighted image shows heterogeneous enhancement of the mass.

Imaging ***Computed Tomography***

- Hypodense to occasional isodense lesion with enlargement of the brainstem.
- Contrast enhancement is seen in more than 50 percent of cases.
- Exophytic extension of the tumor occurs in 60 percent of cases.

Magnetic Resonance Imaging

- Magnetic resonance imaging is superior to CT in evaluating brainstem tumors owing to the availability of direct sagittal imaging, high-contrast resolution, and lack of bone artifacts.
- Brainstem tumors show hypointensity on T1-weighted images and hyperintensity on T2-weighted images.
- Contrast enhancement is more sensitive than CT. Only a small portion of the tumor may enhance.
- Pilocytic astrocytomas are usually cystic with mural nodules.
- Pilocytic astrocytoma is more likely to show contrast enhancement than fibrillary astrocytoma.
- There is a tendency for low-grade fibrillary astrocytoma to undergo malignant degeneration with cystic necrosis, hemorrhage, and contrast enhancement.

PINEAL REGION NEOPLASMS

Although pineal region tumors (Table 11-5) constitute only 0.3 to 2.7 percent of all intracranial tumors, they are considered an important clinical entity due to their strategic location. Pineal region neoplasms can be classified into three major groups according to their cell origin: tumors of germ cell origin, tumors of pineal cell origin, and tumors of other cell origin. Tumors of germ cell origin include germinoma, mature teratoma, malignant teratoma, embryonal cell carcinoma, endodermal sinus tumor, choriocarcinoma, and mixed germ-cell tumors. Tumors of pineal cell origin include pineocytoma and pineoblastoma. Tumors originating from other cells include astrocytoma, metastasis, hemangiopericytoma, meningioma, ganglioneuroma, and ganglioglioma.

GERMINOMA

Incidence

- This is the most common pineal region neoplasm, constituting more than 50 percent of the cases.

Table 11-5
PINEAL REGION NEOPLASMS

	Germinoma	Teratoma	Pineoblastoma	Pineocytoma	Glioma	Meningioma
Age	First and second decades	First decade	First and second decades	Adult	First and second decades	Adult
Sex predilection	Male	Male	None	None	None	None
Signal on T1-weighted images	Isointense	Mixed, contains fat	Hypo- to isointense	Mixed	Hypo- to isointense	Iso- to hypointense
Signal on T2-weighted images	Iso- to mildly hyperintense	Mixed	Hyperintense	Mixed	Hyperintense	Iso- to hyperintense
Contrast enhancement	Homogeneous	Yes	Yes	Homogeneous	Yes	Homogeneous
Calcificants	Rare	Typical	Common	Common	Uncommon	Common
Cystic changes	Uncommon	Yes	No	Uncommon	Yes	Rare
Hemorrhage	Uncommon	Uncommon	Yes	No	Uncommon	Rare
Metastatic seeding	Yes	Variable: benign—no malignant—yes	Yes	No	Variable	No

Age and Gender
- First and second decades
- Predominately male, 9:1 male-to-female ratio

Pathology
- Occasionally a pineal region mass may be seen in association with a suprasellar mass.
- The tumors arise from the germ cell rests within the pineal gland.
- Densely cellular tumor.
- They consist of large polygonal cells of a distinctive appearance alternating with islands of small round cells.

Imaging *Computed Tomography*
- Hyperdense on precontrast CT.
- Homogeneous contrast enhancement is usually seen.
- Tumor calcification is usually not seen, although the tumor may engulf a prominent calcified pineal gland.

Magnetic Resonance Imaging
- Isointense on both T1-weighted and T2-weighted images. Occasionally, slightly hyperintense on T2-weighted images (Fig. 11-9*A* and *B*).
- Intense contrast enhancement is seen on postcontrast images (Fig. 11-9*C* and *D*).
- Cystic areas may be seen.
- Invasion of the posterior thalamus by the tumor is frequently seen.
- Gadolinium-enhanced MRI is an excellent modality in the detection of subarachnoid and spinal seeding of germinoma.

TERATOMA

Incidence
- The pineal region is the most common site of intracranial teratoma.
- About 8 percent of pineal region neoplasms.

Age and Gender
- Occurs exclusively in males.
- Is seen in the first decade.

Pathology
- All three germinal layers are seen.
- Fat, calcification, or tooth is identified in all cases.
- Histologically, teratomas can vary from benign to malignant.

Imaging *Computed Tomography*
- Well-demarcated mass with focal fat (low density) and calcification (high density).
- Patchy contrast enhancement is seen.

Magnetic Resonance Imaging
- Mixed isointense and low-signal-intensity lesions on T1-weighted images and mixed high-signal-intensity lesions on T2-weighted images.
- Focal fatty tissue can be identified as focal high signal intensity within the lesion on T1-weighted images.
- Calcification may not be well shown on the spin-echo sequences but is better seen on gradient-echo images.

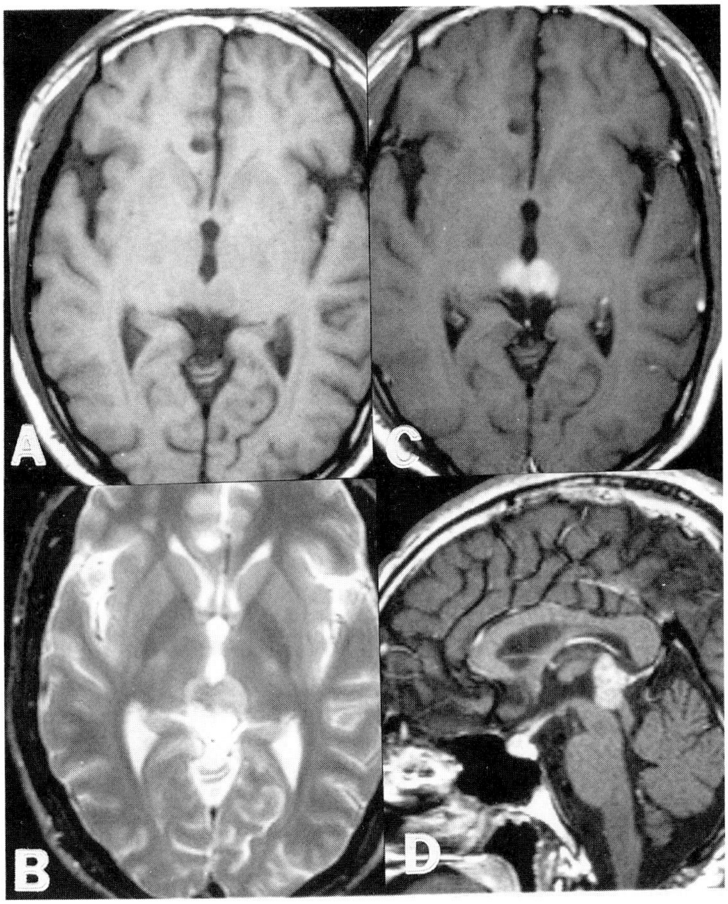

Figure 11-9 Pineal germinoma. *A*. An axial T1-weighted image reveals an isointense mass in the region of pineal and posterior third ventricle. *B*. An axial T2-weighted image shows a predominantly isointense (to gray matter) mass lesion with a central focus of lower signal intensity. *C*. A gadolinium-enhanced axial T1-weighted image shows homogeneous enhancement of the mass lesion. Invasion of the neoplasm into both thalami is seen. *D*. A gadolinium-enhanced sagittal T1-weighted image demonstrates the enhancing mass compression of the quadrigeminal plate, partially obstructing the cerebral aqueduct.

OTHER GERM-CELL TUMORS

Teratocarcinoma, choriocarcinoma, embryonal cell carcinoma, endodermal sinus tumor, and mixed germ-cell tumors are all rare tumors. They tend to occur in the first or second decade of life. There is a male predominance. They tend to show variable but often mixed signal intensity on both T1- and T2-weighted images. The marker profile in CSF or serum may be helpful in the differential diagnosis of germ-cell tumors in the pineal region. Choriocarcinoma produces beta-HCG; endodermal sinus tumor, alpha-fetoprotein; embryonal cell carcinoma, alpha-fetoprotein and beta-HCG. Intratumoral hemorrhage may be seen in choriocarcinoma.

Imaging ***Computed Tomography***

- Well-circumscribed, noninvasive, slowly growing masses that are isodense or hyperdense on noncontrast CT.
- Homogeneous enhancement is seen.
- Calcification may be seen.

Magnetic Resonance Imaging

- Low, iso-, or mixed signal intensity on T1-weighted images.
- High signal intensity on T2-weighted images.
- Homogeneous contrast enhancement.
- Tumor calcification is better seen on gradient-echo images.

PINEOCYTOMA

Incidence

- About 2 percent of all pineal region neoplasms.

Age and Gender

- Male and female incidence is equal.
- Any age group.

Pathology

- Arising from mature pineal parenchymal cells.

PINEOBLASTOMA

Incidence

- These tumors represent some 12 percent of all pineal region neoplasms.
- They are about six times more common than the benign pineocytoma.

Age and Gender

- Male-to-female ratio is equal.
- Predominately seen in first and second decades.

Pathology

- Pineoblastoma is a form of PNET.
- Histologically, the tumor is densely cellular, invasive, and highly malignant.
- Cystic changes may be seen.
- There is an increased incidence of pineoblastoma in association with congenital bilateral retinoblastoma.

Imaging ***Computed Tomography***

- Isodense or hyperdense on noncontrast CT.
- Inhomogeneous or homogeneous contrast enhancement.
- Calcification may be seen.
- Invasive tumor with involvement of thalami and tectum.

Magnetic Resonance Imaging

- Isointense to hypointense on T1-weighted images and isointense to hyperintense on T2-weighted images.
- Contrast enhancement is seen.
- Invasive tumor with involvement of thalami and tectum.

ASTROCYTOMA

Incidence

- The second most common pineal region neoplasm after germinoma.
- Constitutes approximately 25 percent of all cases.

Age and Gender

- The same as astrocytomas in other locations.

Pathology

- Since the normal pineal gland contains fibrillary astrocytes, an astrocytoma may arise from the pineal gland.
- The majority of pineal region astrocytomas arise from the quadrigeminal plate or wall of the third ventricle.

Imaging ***Computed Tomography***

- Hypodense mass on noncontrast CT.
- Contrast enhancement is seen but may occasionally be absent.
- Tumor mass may be cystic.
- Tumor calcification may be seen.

Magnetic Resonance Imaging

- Isointense to low signal intensity on T1-weighted images and high signal intensity on T2-weighted images.
- Contrast enhancement is seen.
- Cystic mass is well shown on postcontrast studies.

MENINGIOMA

Incidence

- Rare tumors in the pineal region

Age and Gender

- No gender predilection in pineal region meningioma, in contrast to the female predominance in other locations.
- Seen in middle age.

Pathology

- Arise from the velum interposition or from the free edge of the tentorium.
- Rarely arise from arachnoid cell inclusion in the pineal.

Imaging ***Computed Tomography***

- Hyperdense mass on noncontrast CT.
- Homogeneous enhancement.

Magnetic Resonance Imaging

- Iso- to hypointense mass on T1-weighted images and iso- to hyperintense mass on T2-weighted images (Fig. 11-10*A* and *B*).
- Homogeneous contrast enhancement (Fig. 11-10*C*).
- Dural attachment is better shown on coronal postcontrast images.

PINEAL CYSTS

Incidence

- Common incidental finding at MRI or autopsy.
- Approximately 5 percent on MRI.

Age and Gender

- The incidence of pineal cysts decreases with age, with peak incidence seen in young females.

Pathology

- May be a residual ependyma-lined space of the pineal diverticulum from the third ventricle.
- May be a degenerative process.
- Large pineal cysts may show compression of midbrain, but the majority of cases are asymptomatic.

Imaging ***Computed Tomography***

- Smoothly marginated cyst that may be a portion of the pineal gland or may replace the entire pineal gland.
- Cyst fluid may be slightly hyperdense as compared to CSF (high protein content, old hemorrhage).

Magnetic Resonance Imaging

- Smoothly marginated cyst with thin wall.
- Cyst fluid may be isointense to hyperintense to CSF (high protein content, old hemorrhage).
- Cyst wall does not show contrast enhancement, but normal pineal tissue may enhance.

☐ MASS LESIONS IN THE REGION OF THE VENTRICULAR SYSTEM

Approximately 10 percent of CNS neoplasms are partly or completely intraventricular (Table 11-6). The most

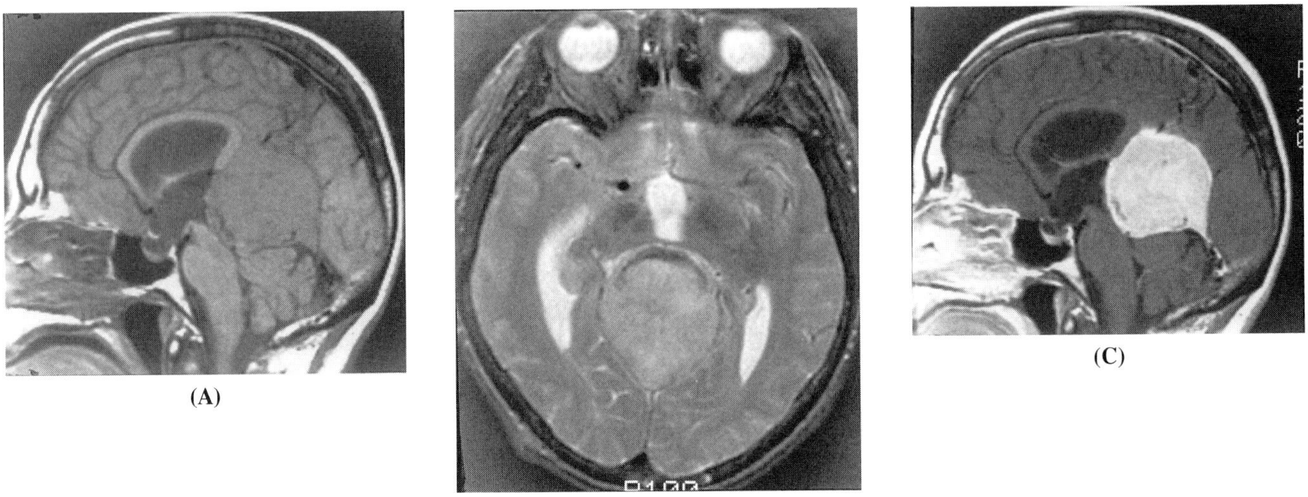

(A) (B) (C)

Figure 11-10 Pineal region meningioma. *A*. A sagittal T1-weighted image shows a large, isointense mass lesion in the pineal region. *B*. An axial T2-weighted image shows a large, isointense mass lesion with attachment to the tentorial incisura bilaterally. A curvilinear hypointensity at the anterior aspect of the mass lesion is due to calcification. *C*. A gadolinium-enhanced sagittal T1-weighted image demonstrates homogeneous enhancement of the mass lesion. Extension of contrast enhancement along the tentorium is seen in a "dural tail"-like appearance.

common lateral ventricular masses, in descending order of frequency, are choroid plexus papillomas, meningiomas, ependymomas, subependymomas, subependymal giant-cell astrocytomas, and metastases or lymphomas. The most common third-ventricular masses are colloid cysts, subependymal giant cell astrocytomas, choroid plexus papillomas, ependymomas, and craniopharyngiomas.

The most common fourth ventricular masses are ependymomas, astrocytomas, choroid plexus papillomas, medulloblastomas, dermoids, epidermoids, subependymomas, and metastases. Cysticercosis cysts, a parasitic disease, can be seen anywhere in the ventricular system.

COLLOID CYST

Incidence

- Colloid cysts make up 15 to 20 percent of intraventricular masses and 0.5 to 1 percent of intracranial tumors.

Age and Gender

- Colloid cysts are congenital in origin, but only 1 to 2 percent present before 10 years of age.
- Most become symptomatic between the third and fifth decades, occurring equally in males and females.

Location

- Colloid cysts occur most frequently in the anterior third ventricle, originating from the roof near the foramen of Monro.
- Less frequently, they may arise from, and subsequently widen, the septum pellucidum.

Pathology Colloid cysts are smooth, spherical, well-circumscribed cystic lesions ranging from a few millimeters to 3 to 4 cm in diameter; they originate from the ependyma (neuroepithelium) of the roof of the anterior third ventricle near the foramen of Monro. They are composed of a dense, fibrous capsule lined by simple or pseudostratified flattened, cuboidal, or columnar epithelium and are filled by epithelial secretory and breakdown products of variable viscosity, including blood degradation products, foamy cells, cholesterol crystals, mucin, and clear fluid (e.g., CSF). Colloid cysts are usually homogeneous, round to ovoid, well-circumscribed masses. They do not calcify. Moderate, symmetrical hydrocephalus of the lateral ventricles and splaying of the posterior frontal horns around a mass at the foramen of Monro are frequent accompanying findings.

Imaging ***Computed Tomography***

- These lesions are homogeneously hyperdense as compared to brain parenchyma in two-thirds of the cases and isodense to hypodense in one-third.
- They are usually nonenhancing except that occasionally there is a thin rim of peripheral (wall) enhancement.

Magnetic Resonance Imaging

- These lesions are most often hyperintense but variable with cyst content on T1-weighted images.
- They are most often hyperintense but rarely circumferentially hyperintense with a profoundly hypointense center on T2-weighted images.
- Hyperintensity on T1-weighted images correlates with high cholesterol content, as does the inverse on T2-weighted images.
- There is occasional peripheral (capsule) enhancement.

Table 11-6
INTRAVENTRICULAR MASS LESIONS

Mass Lesion	Location	Age	Imaging Features
Colloid cyst	Foramen of Monro Anterior third ventricle	3rd to 5th decades	CT—hyperdense (2/3), isodense to hypodense (1/3). Usually no enhancement. Occasionally rim enhancement. MR—hyperintense on both T1- and T2-weighted images. Infrequently, hyperintense rim with very hypointense center on T2-weighted images. Usually no enhancement.
Subependymal giant cell astrocytoma	Foramen of Monro Anterior third ventricle	Under 20 years of age	CT—heterogeneous density with calcification. Inhomogeneous enhancement. MR—heterogeneous signal intensity with inhomogeneous enhancement.
Ependymoma	(1) Fourth ventricle and its lateral recesses (2)Trigone and body of lateral ventricle (3) Third ventricle	Two peaks: (1) Under 5 years (larger peak) (2) 4th to 5th decade	CT—heterogeneous mass with variable contrast enhancement. Calcification and cystic changes are common. MR—heterogeneous mass with heterogeneous contrast enhancement. Heterogeneous signal pattern is due to cystic changes, hemorrhage, and calcification.
Choroid plexus papilloma (carcinoma)	(1) Trigone and atrium of lateral ventricle (2) Fourth ventricle and its lateral recesses (3) Body of lateral ventricle	(1) Trigone and atrium of lateral ventricle in children (2) Fourth ventricle in adults	CT—isodense to hyperdense mass with intense enhancement. MR—isointense on T1-weighted images and isointense to slightly hyperintense in T2-weighted images. Intense contrast enhancement.
Meningioma	Trigone and atrium	4th to 6th decade	CT—iso- to hypderdense mass with homogeneous enhancement. Calcification. MR—isointense to gray matter on both T1- and T2-weighted images. Homogeneous enhancement.
Astrocytoma	(1) Frontal horn and body of lateral ventricle (2) Third ventricle (3) Fourth ventricle	Variable	CT—hypodense mass with variable enhancement. MR—hypointense on T1-weighted images and hyperintense on T2-weighted images. Variable contrast enhancement.
Subependymoma	(1) Fourth ventricle (2) Frontal horn and body of lateral ventricle	3rd to 5th decade	CT—lobulated mass with faint enhancement. Calcification is less common than ependymoma. MR—lobulated mass with mild heterogeneity and mild enhancement.
Central neurocytoma	Body of lateral ventricle near foramen of Monro	Young adults	CT—intraventricular mass with cystic, necrotic changes and calcification. Contrast enhancement is heterogeneous. MR—heterogeneous, but predominantly isointense on T1-weighted images and isointense to hyperintense on T2-weighted images. Heterogeneous enhancement.

NEUROEPITHELIAL CYSTS

Neuroepithelial cysts are small, generally asymptomatic inclusion cysts most commonly found in the choroid plexus.

Incidence

- Neuroepithelial cysts occur anywhere along the neuraxis—they may be intraparenchymal, intraventricular, extraaxial, or occasionally intraosseous.
- They most commonly occur in the choroid plexus, particularly in the lateral ventricles, and are found in 50 percent of autopsies.

Age and Gender

- Neuroepithelial cysts occur at any age but most are identified in older adults (mean age, 33 years).
- There is a moderate male predominance in symptomatic ependymal cysts.

Location Neuroepithelial cysts occur throughout the neuraxis, including the choroid plexus, ventricles, and occasionally brain parenchyma. Most symptomatic neuroepithelial cysts occur in the lateral ventricles near the trigone, where they can cause hydrocephalus. Choroid plexus cysts are frequently bilateral. Intraventricular and posterior fossa cysts are relatively uncommon.

Pathology Neuroepithelial cysts are well-circumscribed lesions lined by cells which, morphologically, resemble epithelium. Choroid plexus cysts are thought to arise from sequestrations of developing neuroectoderm and choroid fissure cysts from infolding of vascular pia mater.

Imaging ***Computed Tomography***
- Homogeneous, sharply marginated, round to ovoid cysts isodense to CSF. Large cyst may mimic a dilated third ventricle.
- They usually do not calcify or enhance.

Magnetic Resonance Imaging
- The signal intensity is similar to that of CSF (hypointense on T1-weighted images and hyperintense on T2-weighted images).
- No contrast enhancement is seen.

EPENDYMOMA

Incidence Ependymomas represent 2 to 8 percent of primary intracranial brain tumors overall but are the third most common intracranial neoplasm in children, accounting for 15 percent of posterior fossa neoplasms in this group.

Age and Gender
- Ependymomas have a bimodal age distribution: the larger peak occurs in children and adolescents; the second, much smaller peak occurs in adults (40 to 50 years).
- They are four to six times more common in children than in adults.
- Infratentorial ependymomas occur predominantly in children, whereas supratentorial ependymomas are evenly distributed with respect to age.

Location Approximately 40 percent of intracranial ependymomas are supratentorial. Of these, between two-thirds and three-quarters are extraventricular (most near the trigones of the lateral ventricles) and 15 percent are within the third ventricle. Ependymomas adjacent to the lateral ventricle may have an intraventricular component.

Pathology Ependymomas are slow-growing, firm, often lobulated, well-circumscribed white to grayish avascular masses that arise from ependymal cells lining the walls of ventricles or from ependymal rests in paraventricular white matter. About 50 percent calcify (two-thirds infratentorial, one-third supratentorial). Cyst formation is common. Hemorrhage is uncommon (less than 14 percent). Larger tumors (4 to 5 cm in diameter) more frequently demonstrate cysts, calcification, or hemorrhage.

Microscopically, ependymomas are sparsely cellular neoplasms with prominent fibrillary background. Malignancy is rare and they grow by expansion toward the ventricle, in contrast to gliomas, which infiltrate surrounding tissue as they grow.

Imaging ***Computed Tomography***
- The lesion is seen as a hypodense to isodense mass with variable contrast enhancement.
- Intratumoral cysts are common.
- Approximately 50 percent are calcified.
- Intraventricular ependymomas may mimic choroid plexus papilloma on CT.

Magnetic Resonance Imaging
- Solid components are uniformly (homogeneously) hypo- to isointense to brain and cystic portions slightly hyperintense to CSF on T1-weighted images.
- Solid portions are hyperintense to brain and cystic portions isointense to CSF on T2-weighted images.
- Ependymomas are somewhat lobulated soft tissue masses that may display heterogeneous intratumoral signal due to the presence of necrosis, calcification, tumor vascularity, blood degradation products, and intratumoral cysts.
- Intraventricular ependymomas may mimic choroid plexus papillomas.
- The contrast enhancement pattern is heterogeneous.

SUBEPENDYMOMA

Incidence
- Subependymomas are relatively rare tumors found primarily in the middle-aged and elderly.

Age and Gender
- Symptomatic subependymomas, those that cause obstructive hydrocephalus by occluding CSF pathways, present at an average age of 40 years.
- Asymptomatic subependymomas are usually discovered incidentally at an average age of 60 years.

Location Subependymomas most frequently arise from the lower medulla and project into the fourth ventricle. They have also been found in the frontal horns of the lateral ventricles and along the septum pellucidum (about 5 percent) and, less frequently, along the midbody of the lateral ventricles.

Pathology Subependymomas are benign, well-circumscribed, lobulated tumors that grow by expanding toward ventricles, in contrast to gliomas, which grow by infiltrating surrounding structures. They also incite less edema. Larger tumors (4 to 5 cm in diameter) frequently demonstrate cysts, focal calcification, and hemorrhage. Microscopically, a sparsely cellular neoplasm with a prominent fibrillary background is seen.

Imaging *Computed Tomography*

- Subependymomas are well-circumscribed, lobulated tumors that resemble ependymomas but are less frequently calcified.
- Enhancement, when present, is rather homogeneous and typically not intense.
- Occasionally, these lesions may be associated with extensive hemorrhage.

Magnetic Resonance Imaging

- Subependymomas are typically less heterogeneous, less intense on T2-weighted images, and less likely to enhance than ependymomas. Heterogeneity arises primarily from multiple small intratumoral cysts.

Angiography

- Subependymomas have no neovascularity. Their principal angiographic presentation is displacement of adjacent arteries and stretching of subependymal veins.

ASTROCYTOMA

Incidence Gliomas account for 40 to 50 percent of primary CNS neoplasms; of these, 75 percent are astrocytomas. Astrocytomas are further subdivided into three subtypes on the basis of malignant potential: low-grade astrocytoma (25 to 30 percent), anaplastic astrocytoma (25 to 30 percent), and glioblastoma (about 50 percent).

Age and Gender There is a general correlation between the patient's age and malignancy: the older the patient, the more malignant the tumor and the worse the prognosis.

Location

- Gliomas involving the roof of the third ventricle usually extend from a point of origin in the corpus callosum.
- Gliomas represent 10 to 25 percent of masses in the region of the pineal and posterior third ventricle; these include astrocytomas and glioblastomas. Most gliomas of the pineal region arise from parapineal structures such as the corpora quadrigemina and posterior thalamus.
- Intraventricular astrocytomas usually arise from the anterior column of the fornix and may be attached to the ependyma by a pedicle. The frontal horn is the most common intraventricular location.

Pathology

- Focal or diffuse calcifications occur in 15 to 20 percent of low-grade astrocytomas.
- Glioblastoma multiforme characteristically demonstrates necrosis and hemorrhage.
- Anaplastic astrocytomas exhibit mitosis, vascular proliferation, and cyst formation, particularly microcysts with significant surrounding edema.

Imaging *Computed Tomography* LOW GRADE

- Seen as a well-circumscribed, hypodense mass.
- Calcification in 15 percent.
- Mild to no enhancement.

ANAPLASTIC

- Inhomogeneous, hypo-, iso-, or hyperdense.
- Calcification rare.
- Sharply outlined cysts.
- Variable enhancement pattern.

GLIOBLASTOMA MULTIFORME

- Inhomogeneous, mixed-density, irregular thick-walled rings are common.
- Calcification is rare.
- Irregular ringlike enhancement.

Magnetic Resonance Imaging LOW GRADE

- Hypointense on T1-weighted images and hyperintense on T2-weighted images.
- Mild to no enhancement.

ANAPLASTIC

- Heterogeneous and hypointense on T1-weighted images; heterogeneous and hyperintense on T2-weighted images.
- Variable pattern of contrast enhancement.

GLIOBLASTOMA MULTIFORME

- Heterogeneous and hypointense on T1-weighted images; heterogeneous and hyperintense on T2-weighted images. Areas of hemorrhage, as well as cystic or necrotic changes may be seen.
- Enhancement is ringlike, with irregular walls and central necrosis.

SUBEPENDYMAL GIANT CELL ASTROCYTOMA

Incidence Subependymal giant cell astrocytomas (SGCA) are found in 10 to 15 percent of patients with tuberous sclerosis.

Age and Gender Subependymal giant cell astrocytomas usually occur in patients below 20 years of age.

Location Subependymal giant cell astrocytomas usually occur in the walls of the lateral ventricles after malignant degenerations of hamartomas associated with tuberous sclerosis. The roof of the third ventricle is involved if the tumor grows inferiorly. In such cases, it may obstruct the foramen of Monro.

Pathology Subependymal giant-cell astrocytomas most frequently are associated with degeneration of hamartomas in tuberous sclerosis. They are characterized by large bi- and multinucleated astrocytes. Cysts are common but mitosis and necrosis rare. They are classified as grade I astrocytoma by the WHO. Giant-cell astrocytomas occurring in isolation may be hard to differentiate from calcified ependymomas.

Imaging *Computed Tomography*

- Heterogeneous with mixed hypo- and isodense regions.
- Calcification and cysts are common.
- Strong, inhomogeneous enhancement.
- Cortical tubers are not well seen on CT.
- Subependymal heterotopic nodules are frequently calcified and well demonstrated on CT.

Magnetic Resonance Imaging

- Heterogeneous and hypointense on T1-weighted images.
- Heterogeneous and hyperintense on T2-weighted images.
- Strong but inhomogeneous enhancement.
- Cortical tubers are better seen on MRI as areas of high signal intensity on T2-weighted images.

Angiography Subependymal giant-cell astrocytomas have variable vascular patterns. A typical finding is elongated, stretched subependymal veins around dilated lateral ventricles.

CHOROID PLEXUS PAPILLOMA

Incidence

- Choroid plexus papillomas make up less than 1 percent of all primary intracranial neoplasms, between 0.5 and 0.6 percent of intracranial neoplasms in adults, and 2 to 5 percent of intracranial neoplasms in children.
- They account for 2 to 3 percent of intracranial gliomas.

Age and Gender

- Choroid plexus papillomas are among the most common brain tumors in children below 2 years of age.
- Some 40 percent occur in the first year of life and between 50 and 80 percent by 5 years of age.
- Malignant degeneration of benign papillomas in children occurs in approximately 20 percent of cases.

Location Choroid plexus papillomas occur in locations distributed in rough proportion to the normal distribution of choroid plexus: trigone (atrium) of the lateral ventricle (50 percent), fourth ventricle (40 percent), third ventricle and cerebellopontine angle (CPA) cisterns (10 percent). In children, 70 percent occur in the atria of the lateral ventricles and 10 percent in the third ventricle. In adults, most occur in the fourth ventricle. Bilateral sites are rare for primaries (3 to 4 percent). Extraventricular primaries (e.g., in choroid projecting through the foramen of Lushka) are very rare. Seeding along CSF pathways occurs with both benign and malignant tumors, often to the CPA cisterns but also to the suprasellar cistern and pineal region.

Pathology Choroid plexus papillomas present grossly as reddish-tan globular to cauliflowerlike masses of frondlike papillar tissue resembling normal choroid. They are composed of a single layer of cuboid or columnar epithelium surrounding a thin fibrovascular core. Calcification (microscopic more frequently than gross), hemorrhage, and cystic degeneration are common. Choroid plexus papillomas are histologically benign in 90 percent of cases. Both benign and malignant forms seed along CSF pathways and may demonstrate focal parenchymal invasion.

Hydrocephalus and basal cistern enlargement in the absence of obstruction are characteristic and most often attributed to a four- to fivefold overproduction of CSF and/or impairment of CSF resorption at the convexities secondary to intermittent hemorrhage. Supratentorial papillomas may produce asymmetrical hydrocephalus. A fourth-ventricle papilloma may cause obstructive hydrocephalus with headaches and ataxia. Tumors of the CPA may cause cranial nerve palsies. A large third ventricle may obstruct the foramen of Monro.

Imaging *Computed Tomography*

- About 75 percent are iso- to hyperdense with respect to brain and 25 percent are hypodense or mixed.
- Virtually all enhance intensely, most homogeneously, and some slightly heterogeneously.

Choroid plexus papillomas are predominately well-circumscribed, smooth or lobulated masses that may display frondlike margins.

Magnetic Resonance Imaging

- Isointense to brain on T1-weighted images
- Iso- to slightly hyperintense to brain on T2-weighted images.
- Homogeneous contrast enhancement (Fig. 11-11).
- Calcification and hemorrhage are common and may produce signal voids or focal heterogeneities within the tumors. Occasionally a signal void may result from a vascular pedicle.

Angiography Angiography is important in defining the vascular pedicle prior to excision. Choroid plexus papillomas demonstrate enlarged arterial feeders and a persistent vascular blush similar to that of meningiomas, whereas normal choroid plexus demonstrates a vascular tangle and small-capillary blush. Elevation and distortion of the internal cerebral vein is a common sign of a third ventricular mass. Choroid plexus papilloma in the atrium of the lateral ventricle is supplied by the anterior choroidal artery; that of the third ventricle, by the posterior medial choroidal artery; and that of the fourth ventricle, by the posterior inferior cerebellar artery (choroidal branch).

CHOROID PLEXUS CARCINOMA

Incidence

- Choroid plexus carcinoma represents 10 to 20 percent of choroid plexus neoplasms.

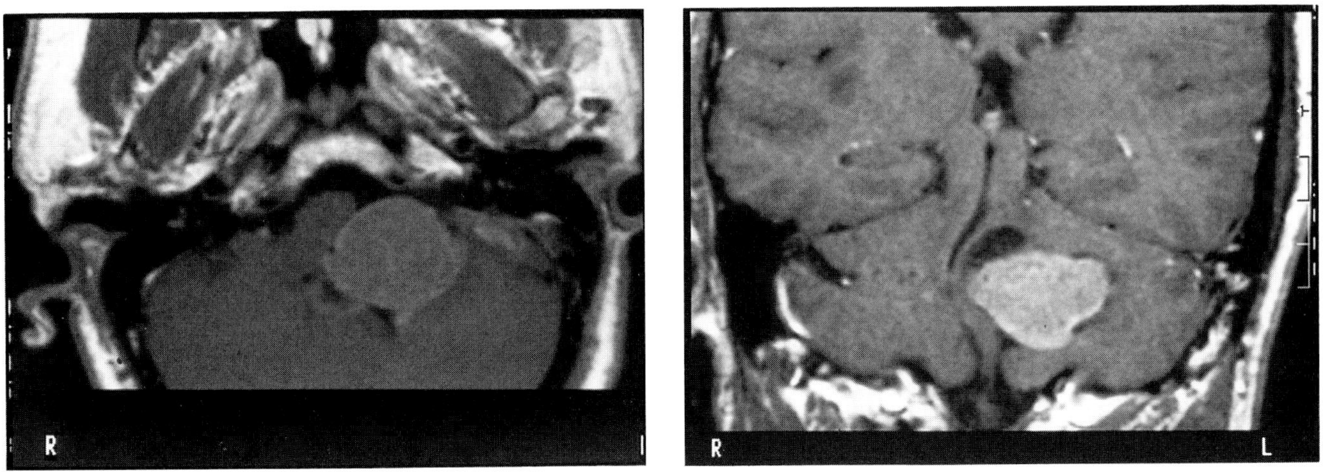

(A) (B)

Figure 11-11 Choroid plexus papilloma. *A* and *B*. Gadolinium-enhanced axial and coronal T1-weighted images show a mildly, homogeneously enhancing mass in the left lateral recess of the fourth ventricle.

Age and Gender

- Choroid plexus carcinomas are malignancies of the pediatric age group, the majority presenting between 2 and 4 years of age (median age, 26 months).

Location

- The distribution of choroid plexus carcinomas parallels that of papillomas.
- Both are seen within the CSF.

Pathology Choroid plexus carcinomas resemble choroid plexus papillomas generally in their gross characteristics. Cystic and hemorrhagic components are more common in the malignant lesions.

Imaging

- Choroid plexus carcinomas cannot be reliably distinguished from choroid plexus papillomas on the basis of imaging characteristics. Both may show local parenchymal invasion and CSF dissemination.

Angiography Choroid plexus carcinomas share the principal angiographic findings of choroid plexus papillomas. Additionally, they display neovascularity and arteriovenous shunting.

CRANIOPHARYNGIOMA

Incidence

- Craniopharyngiomas represent 3 to 5 percent of all primary intracranial neoplasms, 5 to 10 percent of all pediatric intracranial neoplasms, 50 percent of suprasellar tumors in children, and 15 percent of supratentorial tumors in children.

Age and Gender

- Craniopharyngiomas have a bimodal age distribution: more than half occur in children and young adults. A second, smaller peak occurs in the fifth and sixth decades.
- They are the most common neoplasm to calcify in children (70 to 90 percent calcify); the incidence of calcification decreases with age.
- Males and females are equally affected.
- Some 40 percent of craniopharyngiomas in children occur between 8 and 12 years of age.

Location

- Craniopharyngiomas are both intra- and suprasellar in about 70 percent of cases. They are suprasellar in only about 20 percent and intrasellar in nearly 10 percent of cases.
- Less than 1 percent arise within an anterior third ventricle.

Craniopharyngiomas arising from the infundibulum typically present with diabetes insipidus and visual symptoms, while those arising in the third ventricle may present with obstructive hydrocephalus and hypothalamic dysfunction.

Pathology Craniopharyngiomas arise from squamous epithelial rests along an involuted hypophyseal Rathke's duct. They are typically well-circumscribed, lobulated masses, 85 percent of which are totally or partially cystic. Calcification is common in children (90 percent) but less common in adults (50 percent). The lesions can enlarge the sella and erode the dorsum sellae. They may form epithelial fronds that insinuate themselves into and around the brain, 25 percent extending into the anterior, middle, or posterior fossa.

The cystic portions consist of an outer epithelial cell layer on a collagenous basement membrane. Cyst contents range from straw-colored fluid to a mixture of keratin, cholesterol, necrotic debris and blood products resembling crankcase oil. Contents spilled into the subarachnoid space may cause arachnoiditis.

Although they are histologically benign, craniopharyngiomas may become so large that they are impossible to excise. Recurrence is common.

Imaging *Computed Tomography*

- Craniopharyngiomas are well-circumscribed, multilobulated masses, 90 percent of which have both cystic and solid components. The cystic portions typically have a density approximating CSF but may be hypodense in proportion to cholesterol content or hyperdense in proportion to proteinaceous content. Both enhancement and calcification are more common in pediatric patients.
- Solid portions, or nodules, enhance in 66 percent of cases.
- Calcification is present in 90 percent of pediatric cases and 50 percent of adult cases.
- Intraventricular craniopharyngiomas typically lack calcification and enhance homogeneously.

Magnetic Resonance Imaging

- The signal characteristics of the cystic component of a craniopharyngioma are highly variable: hyperintensity correlates with high cholesterol or methemoglobin content on T1-weighted images; T2-weighted images are more typically hyperintense. Layering or intermingling of differing cyst components adds to heterogeneity, making craniopharyngiomas the most heterogeneous of sellar-region masses.
- There is strong but heterogeneous enhancement of the solid component.

MENINGIOMA

Incidence

- Meningioma is the most common nonglial primary brain tumor and most common intracranial, extraaxial neoplasm, making up 15 percent of primary brain tumors.

Age and Gender The peak incidence of meningiomas occurs between 40 and 70 years; they are rare in children without accompanying neurofibromatosis, making up 1 to 3 percent of pediatric intracranial tumors, which often occur in unusual locations such as the posterior fossa and lateral ventricles.

The female-to-male ratio is 2:1.

Location

- Meningiomas arise from meningothelial cells of arachnoid villi; consequently, they occur along dural venous sinuses, at sutural confluences, and in other arachnoid rests such as the choroid plexus.
- Intraventricular meningiomas represent 1 percent of meningiomas.
- The most common location of an intraventricular meningioma is the atrium of the lateral ventricle.
- Intraventricular meningiomas in the third ventricle are extremely rare and occur near the foramen of Monro, where they may cause obstruction and mimic colloid cyst.
- Extraventricular meningiomas of the planum sphenoidale, olfactory groove, medial sphenoid ridge diaphragma sellae, and tuberculum sellae can extend superiorly to deform the anterior third ventricle.
- Meningiomas of the diaphragma sellae , chiasm, or tentorial incisura can grow into the posterior suprasellar and prepontine cistern.
- Pineal region meningiomas can arise from the pineal, velum interpositum, or falx-tentorium junction.

Pathology The WHO classification subdivides meningiomas into three types: benign (88 to 94 percent), atypical (5 to 7 percent), and anaplastic or malignant (1 to 2 percent). Malignant meningiomas tend to invade the brain. Both benign and malignant forms can (rarely) metastasize extracranially. Between 20 and 30 percent of seemingly completely excised meningiomas recur.

Imaging *Computed Tomography*

- Meningiomas are sharply circumscribed extraaxial tumors.
- Calcification (20 to 50 percent) may be diffuse or focal, appearing in psammomatous, sunburst, globular, or ringlike patterns.
- Hemorrhage is uncommon. A higher incidence of hemorrhage is seen in intraventricular meningioma.

Intense enhancement is characteristically seen.

- An intraventricular meningioma may mimic choroid plexus papilloma or ependymoma, but meningiomas are seen in an older age group unless the patient has neurofibromatosis.

Magnetic Resonance Imaging

- Intraventricular meningiomas are well-delineated, round masses that are more typically isointense to gray matter on all sequences.
- Intense contrast enhancement is seen (Fig. 11-12).
- Choroid plexus papillomas and ependymomas may have an appearance similar to that of intraventricular meningioma.

Angiography Meningiomas have characteristic vascular supplies, determined by their location. Intraventricular tumors are served by regional choroidal arteries; meningiomas of the lateral ventricle derive from anterior

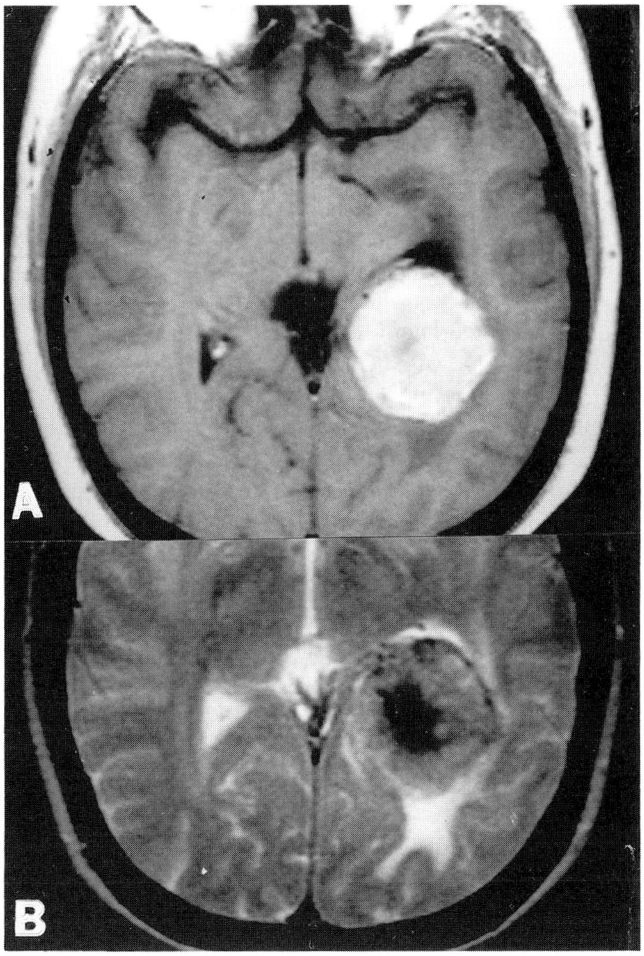

Figure 11-12 Intraventricular meningioma. *A*. A gadolinium-enhanced axial T1-weighted image shows a round, enhancing mass in the region of atrium of left lateral ventricle. *B*. An axial T2-weighted image reveals a round mass lesion of isointensity to gray matter with a central irregular area of low signal intensity (calcification).

choroidal arteries; meningiomas of the anterior third ventricle derive from the distal medial posterior choroidal artery (MPChA). Meningiomas of the tuberculum sellae are supplied principally by meningeal branches of the cavernous ICA and may elevate the A1 segment of the anterior cerebral artery (ACA). Meningiomas of the planum sphenoidale elevate the septal vein and close the carotid siphon. They may also elevate the septal vein and displace the anterior internal cerebral vein posteriorly. Diaphragma sellae meningiomas elevate the A1 segment of the ACA and, together with tentorial incisura meningiomas, may derive blood supply from the meningohypophyseal artery. In all of these situations, supplying arteries may become noticeably enlarged.

CENTRAL NEUROCYTOMA

Incidence
- Approximately 0.5 percent of primary brain tumors.

Age and Gender
- Young adults
- No preference as to gender

Location
- Most common location is the lateral ventricle adjacent to foramen of Monro.

Pathology
- Well-circumscribed, lobulated mass.
- Necrotic, cystic changes are common.
- Hemorrhage can occur but is uncommon.
- Light microscopy shows similar features to oligodendroglioma.
- Electron microscopy confirms the neuronal origin of the tumor.

Imaging ***Computed Tomography***
- Mass lesion in the body of lateral ventricle with cystic, necrotic change and broad-based attachment to the superolateral ventricular wall.
- Tumor calcification is common.
- Contrast enhancement is heterogeneous.

Magnetic Resonance Imaging
- Heterogeneously isointense on T1-weighted images and isointense to hyperintense on T2-weighted images.
- Heterogeneous contrast enhancement.
- Differential diagnosis includes oligodendroglioma, subependymal giant-cell astrocytoma, low-grade astrocytoma and ependymoma.

☐ QUESTIONS (True or False)

1. Regarding tumor calcification,
   a. Calcification is seen in 50 percent of intracranial ependymomas.
   b. Calcification is frequently seen in brainstem astrocytomas.
   c. Calcification is seen in 70 percent of oligodendrogliomas.
   d. Calcification is seen in 60 percent of diffuse fibrillary astrocytomas.
   e. Choroid plexus papillomas do not contain any calcification.

2. Regarding incidence of intracranial gliomas,

a. Astrocytomas are the most common supratentorial tumors in children.
b. Pilocytic astrocytoma is more common than fibrillary astrocytoma in the posterior fossa in children.
c. Subependymal giant cell astrocytoma is found in up to 10 percent of patients with tuberous sclerosis.
d. Infratentorial tumors are more common in neonates and children under 3 years of age.
e. Ependymomas are less common than astrocytomas in the posterior fossa in children.

3. Regarding pilocytic astrocytomas,
a. They tend to occur in the region of the diencephalon when they are seen in the supratentorial compartment.
b. Pilocytic astrocytomas are cystic or multicystic with a mural nodule in 55 percent; they are solid in 45 percent.
c. High-grade fibrillary astrocytomas in the posterior fossa are common in children.
d. Nearly 50 percent of cerebellar astrocytomas are grossly cystic with a mural nodule within the cell wall.
e. The cyst fluid shows iso- to slightly hyperdensity or iso- to slightly hyperintensity as CSF on CT or MRI respectively.

4. Regarding tuberous sclerosis,
a. Subependymal giant cell astrocytomas are seen at the foramina of Monro in children and young adults with tuberous sclerosis.
b. Intracranial lesions include hamartomatous cortical tubers and subependymal heterotopic nodules in addition to giant-cell astrocytomas.
c. Cortical tubers are usually well seen on CT.
d. Subependymal heterotopic nodules may enhance on gadolinium-enhanced MRI.
e. Giant-cell astrocytomas commonly demonstrate calcification.

5. Regarding oligodendrogliomas,
a. Typically, they involve the cerebral cortex and subcortical white matter in the frontotemporal region.
b. Calcifications and hemorrhage are commonly seen.
c. Erosion of the adjacent bony calvarium excludes the possibility of oligodendroglioma.
d. Extensive peritumoral edema is commonly seen.
e. Cystic degeneration, hemorrhage, and calcification all contribute to the heterogeneous signal intensity pattern seen on MRI.

6. Regarding ependymomas,
a. Intracranial ependymomas are more common in adults than in children.
b. The majority of the supratentorial ependymomas are parenchymal in location rather than intraventricular.
c. These tumors have a predilection for frontal and parietal lobes.
d. Dense, punctate calcifications are seen in 50 percent of cases on CT.
e. Contrast-enhancing pattern on CT or MRI is quite variable.

7. Regarding infratentorial ependymomas,
a. The majority of the intracranial ependymomas are infratentorial in location.
b. Ependymomas are seen predominantly in females.
c. Occasionally, ependymomas may extend into upper cervical canal.
d. Ependymomas in the posterior fossa occur more commonly during the first 5 years of life.
e. Calcifications are seen in approximately 50 percent of pediatric posterior fossa ependymomas.

8. Regarding choroid plexus papillomas,
a. They consist of less than 1 percent of all intracranial neoplasms.
b. They are seen in lateral ventricles, more on the left side, in children.
c. In adults, they are seen in the fourth ventricle.
d. Approximately 50 percent of these tumors are malignant.
e. Hydrocephalus is due to obstruction of the ventricular system.

9. Regarding ganglioglioma,
a. They occur predominantly in elderly patients.
b. They may be associated with congenital CNS anomalies.
c. Calcification is not seen.
d. Clinically, these patients usually present with epilepsy.
e. These tumors have a predilection for temporal lobes and the third ventricle.

10. Regarding lymphoma,
a. Primary CNS lymphoma is more common than secondary involvement by systemic lymphoma.
b. Focal intraaxial lesions are the most common initial presentation of primary CNS lymphoma.
c. Leptomeningeal disease is more common in patients with recurrent disease.
d. Ringlike enhancing lesions are seen in non-AIDS patients only.
e. Leptomeningeal disease is better seen on contrast-enhanced MRI than on CT.

11. Regarding hemangioblastoma,
a. They are the most common primary intraaxial posterior fossa neoplasms in adults.
b. Multiple lesions are seen in patients with von Hippel-Lindau syndrome.
c. They occur exclusively in the cerebellum in the intracranial compartment.
d. Solid hemangioblastomas occur in 30 to 40 percent of cases.
e. Linear or curvilinear areas of signal void (vessels) are seen within or adjacent to the solid mass or mural nodule on MRI.

12. Regarding germinomas,
a. They are the most common pineal region neoplasm.
b. Both males and females are equally affected.
c. Tumor can invade into the posterior thalamus.
d. They are isointense on both T1- and T2-weighted images. Occasionally, they are slightly hyperintense on T2-weighted images.
e. Occasionally, a pineal region mass may be seen in association with a suprasellar mass.

13. Regarding teratoma,
a. The pineal region is the most common site of intracranial teratoma.
b. Teratomas occur exclusively in males.
c. Histologically, teratomas can vary from benign to malignant.
d. Fat can be identified as focal high signal intensity on T1-weighted images.
e. Calcification is usually absent.

14. Regarding colloid cyst,
a. Colloid cysts occur most frequently in the anterior third ventricle, originating from the roof near the foramen of Monro.
b. They are frequently calcified.
c. Hyperdense to brain parenchyma in two-thirds of the cases and isodense in one-third of cases on CT.
d. Occasionally, peripheral capsular enhancement may be seen.
e. Moderate symmetrical hydrocephalus of the lateral ventricles is seen.

15. Regarding intraventricular mass lesions,
a. Approximately 10 percent of CNS neoplasms are partly or completely intraventricular.
b. The most common lateral ventricular mass is choroid plexus papilloma.
c. The most common third-ventricular mass is colloid cyst.
d. The most common fourth-ventricular mass is ependymoma.
e. Cysticercosis cysts are seen only in the lateral ventricle.

☐ ANSWERS

1. **a.** T
b. F
c. T
d. F
e. F

2. **a.** T
b. T
c. T
d. F
e. T

3. **a.** T
b. T
c. F
d. T
e. T

4. **a.** T
b. T
c. F
d. T
e. T

5. **a.** T
b. T
c. F
d. F
e. T

6. **a.** F
b. T
c. T
d. T
e. T

7. **a.** T
b. F
c. T
d. T
e. T

8. **a.** T
b. T
c. T
d. F
e. F

9. **a.** F
b. T
c. F
d. T
e. T

10. **a.** T
b. T
c. T
d. F
e. T

11. **a.** T
b. T
c. T
d. T
e. T

12. **a.** T
b. F
c. T
d. T
e. T

13. **a.** T
b. T
c. T
d. T
e. F

14. **a.** T
b. F
c. T
d. T
e. T

15. **a.** T
b. T
c. T
d. T
e. F

SUGGESTED READINGS

Astrocytoma

1. Atlas SW: Adult supratentorial tumors. *Semin Roentgenol* 25:130–154, 1990.
2. Burger PC et al: Glioblastoma multiforme and anaplastic astrocytoma: Pathologic criteria and prognostic implication. *Cancer* 56:1106–1111, 1985.
3. Castillo M et al: Radiologic-pathologic correlation: Intracranial astrocytoma, *AJNR* 13:1609–1616, 1992.
4. Dean BL et al: Gliomas: Classification with MR imaging. *Radiology* 174:411–415, 1990
5. Earnest F IV et al: Cerebral astrocytomas: Histopathological correlation of MR and CT contrast enhancement with sterotactic biopsy. *Radiology* 166:823–827, 1988.
6. Epstein FJ, Farmer J-P: Brain stem glioma growth patterns. *J Neurosurg* 78:408–412, 1993.
7. Hoshino T et al: Prognostic implication of the proliferative potential of low-grade astrocytomas. *J Neurosurg* 69:839–842, 1988.
8. Kleihues P et al: The new WHO classification of brain tumors. *Brain Pathol* 3:255–268, 1993.
9. Latchaw RE et al: Primary intracranial tumors: Neuroepithelial tumors, sarcomas, and lymphoma, in Latchaw R (ed): *MR and CT Imaging of the Head, Neck, and Spine*. St Louis, Mosby, 1991.
10. Osborn AG: *Diagnostic Neuroradiology*. St. Louis, Mosby-Year Book, 1994.
11. Philippon JH et al: Supratentorial low-grade astrocytomas in adults. *Neurosurgery* 32:554–559, 1993.
12. Radkowshi MA et al: Neonatal brain tumors: CT and MR findings. *J Comput Assist Tomogr*, 12:10–20, 1988.
13. Segall HD et al: Computed tomography of neoplasms of the posterior fossa in children. *Radiol Clin North Am* 20:237–253, 1982.
14. Tervonen O et al: Diffuse "fibrillary" astrocytomas: Correlation of MRI features with histopathologic parameters and tumor grade. *Neuroradiology* 34:173–178, 1992.
15. Tien RD et al: Pleomorphic xanthoastrocytoma of the brain: MR findings in six patients. *AJR* 159:1287–1290, 1992.
16. Watanabe M et al: Magnetic resonance imaging and histopathology of cerebral gliomas. *Neuroradiology* 35:463–469, 1992.
17. Yoshino MT, Lucio R: Pleomorphic xanthoastrocytoma. *AJNR* 13:1330–1332, 1992.
18. Zimmerman RA: Pediatric supratentorial tumors. *Semin Roentgenol* 25:225–248, 1990.
19. Zulch KJ: *Histological Typing of Tumors of the Central Nervous System, International Histological Classification of Tumors*, No. 21. Geneva, World Health Organization, 1979.

Gliomatosis Cerebri

1. Dickson DW et al: Gliomatosis cerebri presenting with hydrocephalus and dementia. *AJNR* 9:200–202, 1988.
2. Rippe DJ et al: Gadopentetate dimeglumin-enhanced MR imaging of gliomatosis cerebri: Appearance mimicking leptomeningeal tumor dissemination. *AJNR* 11:800–801, 1990.
3. Ross IB et al: Diagnosis and management of gliomatosis cerebri: Recent trends, *Surg Neurol* 36:431–440, 1991.
4. Yanaka K et al: MR imaging of diffuse glioma. *AJNR* 13:349–351, 1992.

Oligodendroglioma

1. Dolinskas CA, Simeone FA: CT characteristics of intraventricular oligodendrogliomas. *AJNR* 8:1077–1082, 1987.
2. Lee Y-Y, Van Tassel P: Intracranial oligodendrogliomas: Imaging findings in 39 untreated cases. *AJNR* 10:119–127, 1989.
3. Mork SJ et al: Oligodendroglioma: Incidence and biologic behavior in a defined population. *J Neurosurg* 63:881–889, 1985.
4. Shaw EG et al: Oligodendrogliomas: the Mayo Clinic experience. *J Neurosurg* 76:428–434, 1992.
5. Shimizu KT et al: Management of oligodendrogliomas. *Radiology* 186:569–972, 1993.

Metastasis

1. Pots DG et al: NCI study: Evaluation of CT on the diagnosis of intracranial neoplasms: III. Metastatic tumors. *Imaging* 136:664–675, 1980.
2. Russell EJ et al: Multiple cerebral metastases: Detectability with Gd-DPTA-enhanced MR imaging. *Imaging* 165:609–617, 1987.
3. Sze G et al: Detection of brain metastases: Comparison of contrast-enhanced MR with unenhanced MR and enhanced CT. *AJNR* 11:785–791, 1990.
4. Taphoorn MJB et al: Imaging of brain metastases. *NeuroImaging* 31:391–395, 1989.
5. West MS et al: Calvarial and skull base metastases: Comparison of nonenhanced and Gd-DTPA-enhanced MR images. *Imaging* 174:85–91, 1990.

Lymphoma

1. Cordoliana Y-S et al: Primary cerebral lymphoma in patients with AIDS: MR findings: 17 cases. *AJR* 159:841–847, 1992.
2. Dumas J-L et al: MRI and neurological complications of adult T-cell leukemia/lymphoma. *J Comput Assist Tomogr* 16:820–823, 1992.
3. Knorr JR et al: Cerebellar T-cell lymphoma: An unusual primary intracranial neoplasm. *Neuroradiology* 35:79–81, 1992.
4. Roman-Goldstein SM et al: MR in primary CNS lymphoma in immunologically normal patients. *AJNR* 13:1207–1213, 1992.
5. Watanabe M et al: Correlation of computed tomography with the histopathology of primary malignant lymphoma of the brain. *Neuroradiology* 34:36–42, 1992.

Gangliocytoma, Ganglioneuroma, and Ganglioglioma

1. Altman NR: MR and CT characteristics of gangliocytoma: A rare cause of epilepsy in children. *AJNR* 9:917–921, 1988.
2. Benitez WI et al: MR findings in childhood gangliogliomas. *J Comput Assist Tomogr* 14:712–716, 1990.
3. Castillo C et al: Intracranial gangliogliomas: MR, CT, and clinical findings in 18 patients. *AJNR* 11:109–114, 1990.
4. Haddad SF et al: Ganglioglioma: 13 years of experience. *Neurosurgery* 31:171–178, 1992.
5. Hashimoto M et al: Magnetic resonance imaging of ganglion cell tumors. *Neuroradiology* 35:181–184, 1993.
6. Silver JM et al: Ganglioglioma: A clinical study with long-term follow-up. *Surg Neurol* 35:206–266, 1991.
7. Tampieri D et al: Intracerebral gangliogliomas in patients with partial complex seizures, CT and MR findings. *AJNR* 12:749–755, 1991.
8. Tien R et al: Ganglioglioma with leptomeningeal and subarachnoid spread: Results of CT, MR and PET imaging. *AJR* 159:391–393, 1992.
9. Townsend JJ et al: Unilateral megalencephaly: Hamartoma or neoplasm? *Neurology* 25:448–453, 1975.

Supratentorial PNET (Cerebral Neuroblastoma)

1. David R et al: The many faces of neuroblastoma. *RadioGraphics* 9:859–882, 1989.
2. Davis PC et al: Primary cerebral neuroblastoma: CT and MR findings in 12 cases. *AJNR* 11:115–120, 1990.
3. Wiegel B et al: MR of intracranial neuroblastoma with dural sinus invasion and distant metastases. *AJNR* 12:1198–1200, 1991.

Desmoplastic Infantile Ganglioglioma

1. Martin DS et al: Desmoplastic infantile ganglioglioma: CT and MR features. *AJNR* 12:1195–1197, 1991.
2. VandenBerg SR et al: Desmoplastic supratentorial neuroepithelial tumors of infancy with divergent differentiation potential ("desmoplastic infantile gangliogliomas"). *J Neurosurg* 66:58–71, 1987.

Hemangioblastoma

1. Elster AD, Arthur DW: Intracranial hemangioblastomas: CT and MR findings. *J Comput Assist Tomogr* 12:736–739, 1988.
2. Ho VB et al: Radiologic-pathologic correlation: Hemangioblastoma. *AJNR* 13:1343–1352, 1992.
3. Lee SR et al: Posterior fossa hemangioblastomas: MR imaging. *Radiology* 171:463–468, 1989.
4. Neumann HH et al: Central nervous system lesion in von Hippel-Lindau syndrome. *J Neurol Neurosurg Psychiatry* 55:898–901, 1992.
5. Smirniotopoulos JG et al: Pineal region masses: Differential diagnosis. *RadioGraphics* 12:577–596, 1992.

PNET (Medulloblastoma)

1. kCi TM et al: Adult cerebellar medulloblastoma: Imaging features with emphasis on MR. *AJNR* 14:929–939, 1993.
2. Lizak PF, Woodruff WW: Posterior fossa neoplasms: Multiplanar imaging. *Semin Ultrasound, CT, MRI* 13:182–206, 1992.
3. Meyers SP et al: MR imaging features of medulloblastomas. *AJR* 158:865–895, 1992.
4. Mueller DP et al: MR spectrum of medulloblastoma. *Clin Imaging* 16:250–255, 1992.

Cerebellar Astrocytoma

1. Favre J et al: Pilocytic cerebellar astrocytoma in adults: Case report. *Surg Neurol* 39:360–364, 1993.
2. Lee Y-Y et al: Juvenile pilocytic astrocytomas: CT and MR characteristics. *AJNR* 10:363–370, 1989.
3. Mishima K et al: Leptomeningeal dissemination of cerebellar pilocytic astrocytoma. *J Neurosurg* 77:788–791, 1992.
4. Obana WG et al: Metastatic juvenile pilocytic astrocytoma. *J Neurosurg* 75:972–975, 1991.
5. Strong JA et al: Pilocytic astrocytoma: Correlation between the initial imaging features and clinical aggressiveness. *AJR* 161:369–372, 1993.

Ependymoma

1. Armington WG et al: Supratentorial ependymoma: CT appearance. *Radiology* 157:367–372, 1985.
2. Lobato RD et al: Symptomatic subependymoma: Report of four new cases studied with computed tomography and review of the literature. *Neurosurgery* 19:594–598, 1986.
3. Lyons MK, Kelly PJ: Posterior fossa ependymoma: Report of 30 cases and review of the literature. *Neurosurgery* 28:659–672, 1991.
4. Palma L et al: Supratentorial ependymomas of the first two decades of life: Long-term follow-up of 20 cases (including two subependymoma). *Neurosurgery* 32:169–175, 1993.
5. Spoto GP et al: Intracranial ependymoma and subependymoma: MR manifestations. *AJNR* 11:83–91, 1990.
6. Zee CS et al: Computed tomography of posterior fossa ependymomas in childhood. *Surg Neurol* 20:221, 1983.

Brainstem Glioma

1. Epstein FJ, Farmer J-P: Brain stem glioma growth patterns. *J Neurosurg* 78:408–412, 1993.
2. Kane AG et al: Diffuse pontine astrocytoma. *AJNR* 14:941–945, 1993.
3. Stroink AR et al: Diagnosis and management of pediatric brain-stem gliomas. *J Neurosurg* 65:745–750, 1986.
4. Vandertop WP et al: Focal midbrain tumors in children. *Neurosurgery* 31:186–194, 1992.

Pineal Region Neoplasm and Cyst

1. Chang T et al: CT of pineal tumors and intracranial germ-cell tumors. *AJNR* 10:1039–1044, 1989.
2. Hoffman HJ et al: Intracranial germ cell tumors in children. *J Neurosurg* 74:545–551, 1991.

3. Nakagawa H et al: MR imaging of pineocytoma: Report of two cases. *AJNR* 11:195–198, 1990.
4. Robles HA et al: Understanding the imaging of intracranial primitive neuroectodermal tumors from a pathological perspective: A review. *Semin Ultrasound, CT, MRI* 13:170–181, 1992.
5. Tien RD et al: MR imaging of pineal tumors. *AJNR* 11:557–565, 1990.
6. Zee CS et al: MR imaging of pineal region neoplasms. *J CAT* 15(1):56–63, 1990.

Intraventricular Mass Lesions

1. Coates TL et al: Pediatric choroid plexus neoplasms: MR, CT, and pathologic correlation. *Radiology* 173:81–88, 1989.
2. Goergen SK et al: Intraventricular neurocytoma: Radiologic features and review of the literature. *Radiology* 182:787–792, 1992.
3. Hassoun J et al: Central neurocytoma: A synopsis of clinical and histological features. *Brain Pathol* 3:297–306, 1993.
4. Jelinek J et al: Lateral ventricular neoplasms of the brain: Differential diagnosis based on clinical, CT, and MR findings. *AJR* 155:365–372, 1990.
5. Ken JG et al: Choroid plexus papillomas of the foramen of Luschka: MR appearance. *AJNR* 12:1201–1202, 1991.
6. Packer RJ et al: Choroid plexus carcinoma of childhood. *Cancer* 69:580–585, 1992.
7. Shoemaker EI, Romano AS, Gado M: Neuroimaging—case of the day: choroid plexus papilloma, third ventricle. *AJR* 152:1333–1338, 1989.

CHAPTER 12

Extraaxial Mass Lesions

Chi S. Zee

It is important to determine whether an intracranial mass lesion is intraaxial or extraaxial in location. Magnetic resonance imaging (MRI) permits the separation of an extraaxial mass from the brain surface by demonstrating the presence of cerebrospinal fluid (CSF), pial blood vessels, and dura. Normal gray and white matter can be readily identified on MRI images, which permit the demonstration of white matter buckling secondary to an extraaxial mass lesion. The multiplanar imaging capability of MRI also permits the demonstration of broad-based attachment of the mass lesion to the dura. Many extraaxial masses are situated in the posterior fossa, where lesions are often obscured on computed tomography (CT) images by beam-hardening artifacts due to dense bone surrounding the posterior fossa. Contrast-enhanced MRI usually demonstrates homogeneous, intense enhancement of the extraaxial mass lesions. The anatomic boundaries of the mass lesions are better delineated with contrast-enhanced MRI. Sometimes, enhancement of the adjacent dura may be seen with an extraaxial mass lesion, which could represent reactive change in the adjacent dura or infiltration of the neoplasm into the adjacent dura. This so-called "dural-tail" sign was initially thought to be associated exclusively with meningiomas. However, it has been found to be associated with any intracranial mass lesion that has invaded the dura or caused reactive change in the dura.

☐ NEOPLASMS AND MASS LESIONS BASED IN THE MENINGES (Tables 12-1 and 12-2)

MENINGIOMA

Incidence Meningiomas are the most common nonglial primary neoplasm of the central nervous system. They constitute approximately 15 percent of all operative intracranial tumors. Their incidence in the general population is undoubtedly higher, because many asymptomatic meningiomas are found at the autopsy and on imaging studies. The incidence of meningioma in postmortem series is 1 to 2 percent.

Age and Gender Meningiomas tend to occur more often in females between the ages of 40 to 70 years. Women are preferentially affected by a ratio of 2:1. These tumors are rare in childhood, accounting for less than 2 percent of intracranial tumors. There is a strong association of neurofibromatosis with meningioma in the pediatric age group. When meningiomas occur in children, they are found in unusual locations, such as the posterior fossa or lateral ventricles.

Location There is a close relationship between the location of the arachnoid granulation and the prevalent sites of origin for meningioma. The common sites of meningiomas, in order of decreasing frequency, are as follows:

1. Parasagittal
2. Convexity
3. Sphenoid wing
4. Planum sphenoidale and olfactory groove

Table 12-1
DURA-BASED MASSES AND NEOPLASMS—FINDINGS BY COMPUTED TOMOGRAPHY

	Unenhanced	Enhanced	Bony Changes	Calcification	Other
Meningioma	Isodense to hyperdense	Homogeneous	Hyperostosis Destruction—unusual	Yes	Commonly seen in areas where arachnoid granulations are located
Lymphoma	Isodense to hyperdense	Homogeneous; ringlike or heterogeneous in AIDS or immunosuppressed patients	Destruction less common than metastasis	No, unless post-radiation treatment	Extension of dura-based lesion through skull to involve scalp; often multifocal
Sarcoidosis (nonneoplastic)	Isodense to hyperdense	Homogeneous	No	No	Lesions are thin and show broad-based attachment to dura; often multifocal
Metastasis	Hypodense	Variable	Destruction common	No	Dura-based lesions often secondary to skull lesions, also often multifocal
Myeloma	Hypodense	Variable	Destruction common	No	Dura-based lesions often secondary to skull lessions, also often multifocal

5. Parasellar and cavernous sinus
6. Posterior fossa (CPA cistern, foramen magnum)
7. Intraventricular
8. Orbital
9. Pineal

An association of neurofibromatosis with multiple meningiomas also exists. Multiple meningiomas may also be seen in patients with previous radiation therapy, or they may be idiopathic in nature. Multiple meningiomas in the same patient may represent the same histologic type or different histologic types.

Pathology Classically, benign meningiomas are subdivided into four basic subtypes: fibroblastic, transitional, meningothelial, and angioblastic. "Angioblastic" meningiomas include angiomatous meningiomas, hemangioblastoma, and hemangiopericytomas. Hemangiopericytomas are now considered as a separate entity, as they do not arise from meningothelial cells.

Histologic variations can occur. Mixed forms are not uncommon. Xanthomatous changes, melanin deposits, lipoblastic changes, and myxomatous changes may occur. Malignant meningiomas are rare. Invasion of brain parenchyma is generally considered to be evidence of

Table 12-2
DURA-BASED MASSES AND NEOPLASMS—FINDINGS ON MRI

	T1-Weighted	T2-Weighted	Gadolinium-Enhanced	Others
Meningioma	Isointense to hypointense	Isointense to hyperintense, occasionally hypointense	Intensely homogeneous to inhomogeneous	Hyperostosis, bone destruction unusual, single lesion
Lymphoma	Hypointense to isointense	Isointense to hyperintense—some hypointense lesions are seen	Homogeneous; heterogeneous or ringlike in AIDS or immunosuppressed patients	Infiltration through the bone to produce extracalvarial mass; associated leptomeningeal disease; lesions often multiple
Sarcoidosis (nonneoplastic)	Isointense to hypointense	Hypointense to variable	Homogeneous	Thin, widespread, broad-based attachment to dura; associated leptomeningeal disease
Metastasis	Hypointense	Hyperintense to variable	Variable; nodular or ringlike	Bone destruction; lesions often multiple
Myeloma	Isointense	Hypointense to variable	Homogeneous	Bone destruction; lesions often multiple

malignancy. However, local invasion of dura, paranasal sinus, regional muscle, or bone may be seen in histologically benign meningiomas. Aggressive histologic features seen in malignant meningiomas are anaplasia, increased mitotic figures, and necrosis. Distant metastasis may occur in malignant meningiomas.

Grossly, most of the meningiomas are of the globular type, which is a well-demarcated mass with lobulated appearance and attachment to dura. A less common form, meningioma en plaque, has a flattened appearance and follows the contour of the bony calvarium. A rare form, intraosseous meningioma, is seen arising from the diploic space. Bony destruction, bony sclerosis, and hyperostosis are more commonly associated with intraosseous meningioma (Fig. 12-1). The annual growth rate of meningioma has been reported to range from 0.5 to 21 percent, with a median rate of 3.6 percent. Meningioma that occurs following radiation treatment of other intracranial neoplasms tends to have a higher growth rate.

The World Health Organization (WHO) classification subdivides meningiomas into three types: benign (88 to 94 percent), atypical (5 to 7 percent) and anaplastic or malignant (1 to 2 percent). Malignant meningiomas tend to invade the brain. Both benign and malignant forms can (rarely) metastasize extracranially. Between 20 and 30 percent of seemingly completely excised meningiomas recur.

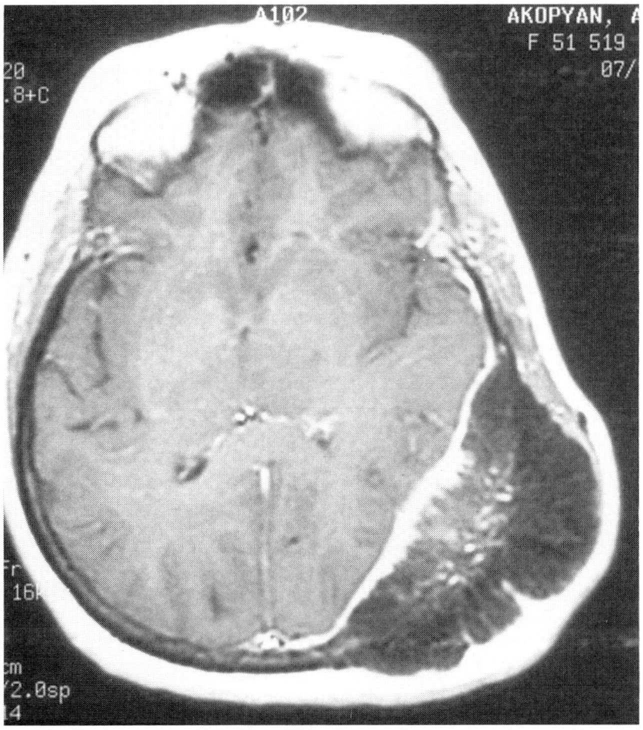

Figure 12-1 Intraosseous meningioma. A gadolinium-enhanced axial T1-weighted image shows enhancement of the predominantly medial aspect of the mass. Note the extension of the enhancement into the adjacent dura.

Imaging *Skull X-ray*

- Bony hyperostosis
- Calcification—10 percent
- Prominent middle meningeal grooves
- Blistering–upward bulging of the bony cortex of the posterior boundary of the ethmoid sinus and anterior portion of the sphenoid sinus
- Enlargement of the foramen spinosum

The diagnosis of meningioma can be made on plain x-ray of the skull if one sees a prominent middle meningeal artery groove leading into the focus of hyperostosis with adjacent calcification. Enlargement of foramen spinosum may be seen in meningioma or dural arteriovenous malformation.

Computed Tomography

- Hyperdense or isodense mass lesion with well-delineated margin.
- Broad-based attachment to dura.
- Tumor can be globular or en plaque. En plaque meningiomas, which may be difficult to detect on CT, are more frequently seen at the sphenoid ridge or convexity and are more likely to be associated with hyperostosis.
- Calcification—20 to 50 percent. The extent of calcification varies markedly radiologically. Calcification may be psammomatous (diffuse) or globular (focal) in nature.
- Hyperostosis—20 percent.
- Bone destruction is rare. Bone destruction is more commonly seen in intraosseous types of meningioma, which arise from the ectopic inclusion of meningeal cells during the formation of the calvarium. When destruction is seen, differential diagnosis from lymphoma, myeloma, or metastasis may be difficult.
- Bone erosion is rare. Bone erosion may also be seen in slow-growing intraaxial neoplasms such as low-grade gliomas or oligodendrogliomas.
- The amount of surrounding edema is variable and does not correlate with malignancy, lesion size, or location. Edema is seen in up to 75 percent of meningiomas. In some cases, there is a large amount of edema associated with meningioma; in other cases, there is little or no edema.

The cause of peritumoral edema in meningioma is controversial. Some theories suggest active fluid production by the tumor, others imply that the tumors produce injuries to the brain by mechanical compression. Still others imply that tumor compression or invasion of the adjacent cortical veins and dural sinuses may produce peritumoral edema.

- White matter buckling indicates extraaxial location.
- Uniform contrast enhancement.
- Hemorrhage (3 percent), cystic changes, or necrosis (10 percent) are uncommon.

- An unusual lipoblastic meningioma may show very low density, like fat within the lesion.

Magnetic Resonance Imaging The typical meningiomas are isointense (60 percent) or mildly hypointense (30 percent) to gray matter on T1-weighted images. On T2-weighted images, the tumors are isointense (50 percent) or mildly to moderately hyperintense (40 percent) to gray matter. The remaining 10 percent of meningiomas have varied features with regard to signal intensity. In half of these cases, diffuse calcification within the tumor may produce hypointensity on both T1- and T2-weighted images. Cystic meningiomas may exhibit areas of low signal intensity on T1-weighted images and high signal intensity on T2-weighted images. Calcification is less well detected on MRI than on CT. Gradient-echo imaging may improve the detection of tumor calcification. However, the dramatic hypointensity on gradient-echo imaging is not sufficient to warrant a conclusive diagnosis of calcification, because other substances such as acute or old hemorrhage can exhibit similar signal losses. Hemorrhage, cystic changes, and necrotic changes are better demonstrated on MRI than on CT. Extraaxial location of the mass lesion is better demonstrated on MRI. A low-signal rim around the tumor margin (CSF cleft, vascular rim, dura) and buckling of the gray/white interface are signs of extraaxial location.

Tumors can be globular or en plaque. En plaque meningiomas may be hard to detect on noncontrast T1- and T2-weighted images due to their small size, isointensity to brain parenchyma, and lack of surrounding edema. Gadolinium enhancement is extremely useful to demonstrate an en plaque meningioma.

Extension of meningioma enhancement into the adjacent dura may be seen in 60 percent of patients. This "dural-tail" sign does not necessarily mean tumor infiltration into the adjacent dura, and it may represent a reactive change of the adjacent dura. Furthermore, the dural-tail sign is not specific for meningioma and may be seen in lymphoma, sarcoid, metastasis, and any neoplasm that involves the dura.

Lymphoma, myeloma, and sarcoidosis may exhibit similar intensity features—namely, isointense to gray matter on T1-weighted and iso- or hyperintense on T2-weighted images, similar to meningiomas. Due to the compact cellular nature of these lesions, they can occasionally be hypointense on T2-weighted images, which could also be seen in certain meningiomas, especially those with psammomatous calcification. The majority of metastatic lesions exhibit low signal intensity on T1-weighted images and high signal intensity on T2-weighted images. Certain metastatic lesions—such as those from breast, prostate, and GI tract—may show hypointensity or isointensity on T1-weighted images and mild hypointensity to hyperintensity on T2-weighted images. Melanomas may show hyperintensity on T1-weighted images and hypointensity on T2-weighted images. Bone destruction is common in metastasis and lymphoma, rare in meningioma, and not seen in sarcoidosis. Breast cancer in females and prostate cancer in males are commonly seen dural-based metastatic lesions.

The detection and characterization of meningiomas is markedly enhanced with the administration of gadolinium. The majority of meningiomas exhibit intense, uniform enhancement. Densely calcified and cystic meningiomas may show inhomogeneous or heterogeneous enhancement. Small tumors that might otherwise be missed are readily shown with gadolinium enhancement, especially those of the en plaque type.

Vasogenic edema within the white matter of the brain is seen around meningiomas in up to 75 percent of cases. The degree of paratumoral edema in meningiomas has little correlation with tumor size. Some authors have reported increased edema in angioblastic and meningothelial meningiomas as compared with fibroblastic and transitional types.

Cerebral Angiography Meningiomas are very vascular tumors and are supplied by enlarged external carotid artery branches or meningeal branches of the internal carotid artery. The internal maxillary artery, one of the branches of the external carotid artery, gives rise to the middle meningeal artery. From its origin, the middle meningeal artery courses laterally in the base of the skull to enter the intracranial compartment through the foramen spinosum. The vessel then turns laterally to lie within the middle meningeal groove. The middle meningeal artery then bifurcates into anterior and posterior branches. The anterior branch ascends in a groove near the coronal suture. The posterior branch runs posteriorly and slightly superiorly.

Meningiomas derive their primary vascular supply from regional dural vessels at the site of dural attachment. Tumor-feeding vessels typically "radiate" from the base into the tumor, which shows an intense homogeneous blush beginning in the late arterial phase and persisting throughout the venous phase. Early venous drainage is unusual. Mid- and late-venous-phase images reveal dural sinus occlusion. Large tumors may parasitize pial vessels.

Whenever a tumor derives a significant amount of its blood supply from the external carotid circulation or meningeal branches of the internal carotid artery, it is more likely to be a meningioma. However, an occasional metastatic lesion or glioma may mimic a meningioma by deriving some of its blood supply from the external carotid circulation. One important differential point is that a large meningioma is supplied by external carotid branches (meningeal vessels) at its center and internal carotid branches (pial vessels) at its periphery, whereas the opposite is true for gliomas. Furthermore, the meningeal vascular supply to meningiomas is almost always more prominent than the meningeal vascular supply to gliomas or metastases. In patients with metastatic disease, bone destruction is usually seen.

Depending on its location, a meningioma derives its blood supply from various meningeal branches of the external carotid artery and internal carotid artery. A typical parasagittal or convexity meningioma is usually supplied by an enlarged middle meningeal artery. Sometimes, a superficial temporal artery may participate in its blood supply by penetrating through the skull.

A frontal falx meningioma may be supplied by an anterior meningeal branch of the ophthalmic artery. A subfrontal meningioma is usually supplied by the ethmoidal branches of the ophthalmic artery.

A sphenoid meningioma, cavernous meningioma, or tentorial meningioma derives its blood supply from the meningohypophyseal trunk of the internal carotid artery. Posterior fossa meningiomas may be supplied by anterior or posterior meningeal branches of the vertebral artery or accessory meningeal arteries.

A tumor stain in meningioma is usually homogeneous and sharply marginated, and persists into the late venous phase. Classically, it has a sunburst appearance. Early draining vein is not common but may be seen in 15 percent of cases.

MENINGEAL HEMANGIOPERICYTOMA

- Hemangiopericytoma of the meninges is an aggressive, highly vascular neoplasm that is commonly grouped with "angioblastic meningiomas."
- Hemangiopericytoma of the meninges is a distinct entity that arises from the vascular pericytes rather than from meningothelial cells.
- Macroscopically, hemangiopericytomas resemble meningioma. They are well-circumscribed masses with numerous penetrating vessels.
- Microscopically, they have a dense, pervasive reticular network with lobules of neoplastic cells.
- Imaging features are similar to those of "angioblastic" or malignant meningiomas, with a heterogeneous appearance caused by cystic, necrotic areas and prominent vascular channels.

LYMPHOMA

Incidence Until recently, primary central nervous system (CNS) lymphomas were considered to be rare. They constitute about 1 percent of all intracranial tumors. However, with the increased number of patients with AIDS and immunosuppression (renal transplant, chemotherapy, other malignancy) there has been an increased incidence of these lesions. Up to 6 percent of immunocompromised patients may have CNS disease.

- About 10 percent of the patients with systemic lymphoma develop CNS involvement in clinical series. In autopsy series, secondary CNS involvement by lymphoma may be found in up to 26 percent of cases.
- Primary CNS lymphomas are more common than secondary involvement by systemic lymphoma.

Age All ages are affected. Patients with immunosuppression or AIDS present in the third or fourth decade, other patients in the sixth decade.

Location Solitary or multicentric location is frequently seen in primary brain lymphoma. Focal intraaxial lesions are the most common initial presentation of primary CNS lymphoma. Basal ganglia, periventricular white matter, corpus callosum, cerebellar vermis and septum pellucidum are often involved. Approximately 20 to 40 percent of lesions are multiple. Some 30 percent of patients with primary lymphoma develop leptomeningeal disease. Leptomeningeal disease is more common in patients with recurrent disease. Leptomeningeal involvement is also common in secondary CNS lymphoma. Secondary invasion of the brain may occur through the Virchow-Robin spaces, producing parenchymal lesions. Secondary invasion of the dura produces dural-based mass lesion.

Pathology Primary CNS lymphomas are non-Hodgkins lymphomas, usually of B-cell type with demonstrable cytoplasmic immunoglobulin production. They have a wider spectrum of morphologic cell types than lymphoma outside the CNS. Grossly, parenchymal lesions are ill-defined masses with irregular borders. Dura-based lesions often spread via the Virchow-Robin spaces and invade the brain.

Secondary CNS lymphomas are also non-Hodgkin's lymphomas. Diffuse varieties of non-Hodgkin's lymphoma affect the CNS more frequently, especially diffuse histiocytic lymphoma. Secondary CNS lymphoma may involve brain parenchyma, leptomeninges, dura, and epidural tissue.

Imaging ***Computed Tomography*** Both primary and secondary lymphoma have similar imaging findings. The typical lymphoma (in non-AIDS, nonimmunosuppressed patients) exhibits hyperdensity to isodensity to brain parenchyma. Uniform enhancement is seen following the intravenous injection of contrast material. The CT appearance of a dura-based lymphoma may be difficult to differentiate from a meningioma. Leptomeningeal involvement is not well identified with CT.

Magnetic Resonance Imaging Typically, lymphomas are solid masses that are hypointense to isointense on T1-weighted images and isointense to slightly hyperintense on T2-weighted images. Some cases of lymphoma show hypointensity on T2-weighted images. These signal intensity features make dura-based lymphoma similar to meningioma. However, lymphoma is often multi-focal, and lymphoma may infiltrate the bone to produce an extracalvarial mass. Furthermore, leptomeningeal and subependymal seeding is often detected on contrast-enhanced MRI.

SARCOIDOSIS

Incidence The intracranial compartment is involved in 15 percent of patients with sarcoidosis.

Age and Gender Sarcoidosis is more prevalent in the third and fourth decades of life. Incidence is equal among males and females.

Location Sarcoidosis may present as leptomeningitis or intracerebral granulomas. Granulomatous meningitis frequently involves the suprasellar cistern in the region of the optic chiasm and hypothalamic pituitary axis. Solitary or multiple lesions based in the meninges may be seen.

Pathology A chronic multisystem inflammatory disease. The lungs, hilar lymph nodes, skin, and eyes are the organs commonly involved. Involvement of the meninges and brain by noncaseating granulomas constitutes CNS disease.

Imaging ***Computed Tomography*** The granulomatous lesions are hyperdense or isodense to brain with minimal surrounding edema. On contrast-enhanced CT, they show homogeneous enhancement. A meninges-based sarcoid lesion may mimic meningioma. Diffuse meningeal enhancement may be seen. Parenchymal lesions may be solitary or multiple. Secondary hydrocephalus due to leptomeningeal disease may be seen.

Magnetic Resonance Imaging The sarcoid granulomatous lesions are usually isointense to hypointense on T1-weighted images and variable but predominantly hypointense on T2-weighted images. Parenchymal lesions may be solitary and large or multiple and small. Leptomeningeal disease may be diffuse or focal. Diffuse periventricular lesions of the white matter with high-signal-intensity on T2-weighted images are common but nonspecific.

Contrast-enhanced MRI usually show homogeneous enhancement of the granulomatous lesions. Enhancement of thickened pituitary infundibulum as well as enhancement of cranial nerves, especially the optic nerve and facial nerve, may be seen. A focal, enhancing, sarcoid lesion based in the meninges may be difficult to differentiate from meningioma, lymphoma, or certain metastatic lesions (Fig. 12-2). Although a small group of meningiomas may exhibit low signal intensity on T2-weighted images, the majority of meningiomas show iso- or hyperintensity on T2-weighted images. Sarcoid lesions tend to be thinner and more spread out in a broad-based fashion than meningioma. Diffuse or localized leptomeningeal enhancement may be seen in sarcoid or lymphoma. Lymphomas often involve the skull by infiltration, demonstrating low signal in the marrow. Metastatic lesions are often accompanied by bone destruction.

METASTASIS

Incidence Variable, depending on the primary site of the neoplasm. About 20 percent of patients with systemic cancer show evidence of intracranial metastasis at postmortem studies. Common primary sources for dura-based metastases include breast, prostate, melanoma, and lung

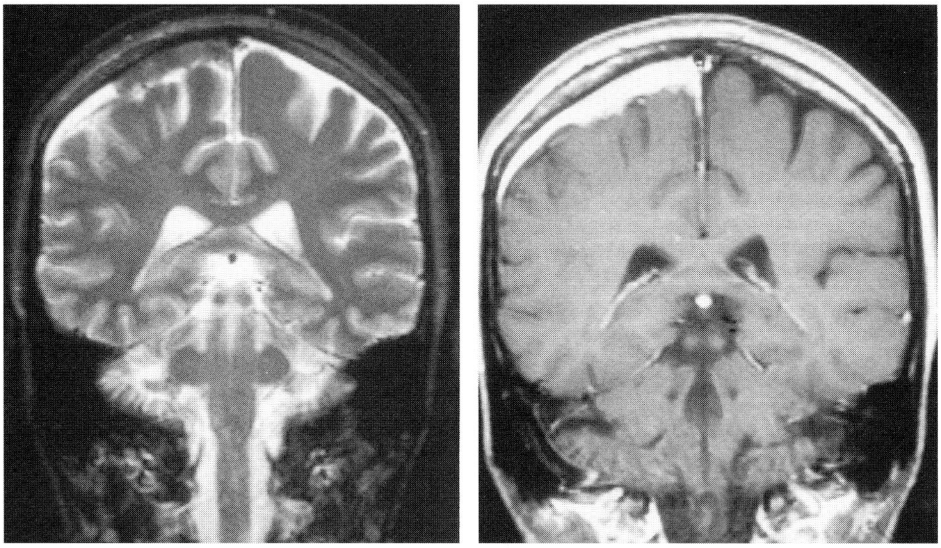

(A) (B)

Figure 12-2 Extraaxial sarcoidosis. *A*. A coronal T2-weighted image demonstrates an extraaxial mass of low signal intensity secondary to its dense cellularity. The adjacent peripheral high-signal-intensity area is probably due to the masking of dural changes by CSF. *B*. A gadolinium-enhanced coronal T1-weighted image shows intense enhancement of the extraaxial mass. Note that enhancement involves the low-signal area as well as the adjacent high-signal area.

in adults and neuroblastoma of the adrenal in children. Some 60 percent of metastases are seen supratentorially and 40 percent infratentorially. Metastasis is the most common intraaxial cerebellar tumor in adults. Metastasis is the most likely diagnosis for intraaxial cerebellar mass seen in a patient over 50 years of age.

Age Peak incidence is in the sixth and seventh decades.

Location Metastatic disease typically exhibits multiple enhancing lesions in the brain parenchyma at the gray/white junction. Dura-based metastatic lesions are less common and often associated with adjacent bone destruction.

Imaging ***Computed Tomography*** Computed tomography has a distinct disadvantage for detecting dura-based metastasis. A thin layer of enhancing tumor along the bony calvarium may be obscured by the high density of the skull. Expanding the window to the proper setting (wide window width) is essential in separating the enhancing neoplasm from dense bony calvarium. Furthermore the majority of the metastatic lesions are associated with bone destruction. They are readily detected on bone window images but could be easily missed on standard soft tissue window images. When intravenous contrast is given to the patient, the enhancing tumor may further mask the bone defect. Approximately 10 percent of patients with leptomeningeal metastasis exhibit hydrocephalus. A metastatic lesion in the posterior fossa frequently causes obstructive hydrocephalus.

Magnetic Resonance Imaging Magnetic resonance imaging is superior to CT in demonstrating dura-based metastatic disease. Gadolinium-enhanced MRI demonstrated broad-based enhancing lesion along the calvarium. Associated bone destruction can easily be detected. The high signal intensity of normal bone marrow seen on T1-weighted images is replaced by tumor cells, which show low to isointense signal to adjacent muscle on T1-weighted images. On gadolinium-enhanced T1-weighted images, enhancement of the tumor may show similar signal intensity to fatty marrow. A calvarial metastatic lesion may actually be obscured on gadolinium-enhanced T1-weighted images. Fat-suppression technique is necessary to demonstrate the enhancing lesion. Particularly, in the skull base and orbit, gadolinium-enhanced MRI with fat suppression can better demonstrate the enhancing metastatic lesion. The signal intensity patterns of metastatic lesions on T1- and T2-weighted images are variable depending on the primary origin of the neoplasm, but are generally low on T1-weighted images and high on T2-weighted images.

MYELOMA (PLASMACYTOMA)

Incidence Primary plasmacytoma of the skull is rare. Secondary involvement of the bony calvarium due to myeloma is more common.

Age and Gender Peak incidence is in the sixth and seventh decades, as in metastatic disease. Myeloma occurs more frequently in males than in females.

Location A dura-based mass lesion is usually an extension of a bony lesion. Clivus, skull base, and bony calvarium may be involved.

Pathology A plasma-cell tumor.

Imaging ***Skull X-ray***

- Multiple lucencies involving the bony calvarium.
- Destructive lesion involving the clivus or skull base.

Computed Tomography

- Well-defined lucencies in the skull with or without epidural mass.
- Destructive lesion involving the clivus and skull base with adjacent soft tissue mass.

Magnetic Resonance Imaging

- Plasmacytoma exhibits isointensity to surrounding brain parenchyma on T1-weighted images and hypointensity on T2-weighted images.
- The epidural component of the lesion is better seen on MRI, especially following intravenous injection of gadolinium (Fig. 12-3).
- Mass lesions involving the clivus and skull base are better seen with gadolinium-enhanced, fat-suppressed images.

☐ NONNEOPLASTIC EXTRAAXIAL MASSES (TABLE 12-3)

ARACHNOID CYST

Incidence One percent of intracranial masses.

Age and Gender

- Any age group, but 75 percent in children.
- Male predominance, with a 3:1 ratio.

Location ***Supratentorial, 90 percent***

- Middle cranial fossa
- Suprasellar cistern and quadrigeminal cistern
- Convexity

Infratentorial, 10 percent

- Retrocerebellar
- Cerebellopontine angle cistern

Pathology Duplication of arachnoid membrane containing CSF

Imaging ***Computed Tomography***

- Focal bony erosion and expansion involving the calvarium.

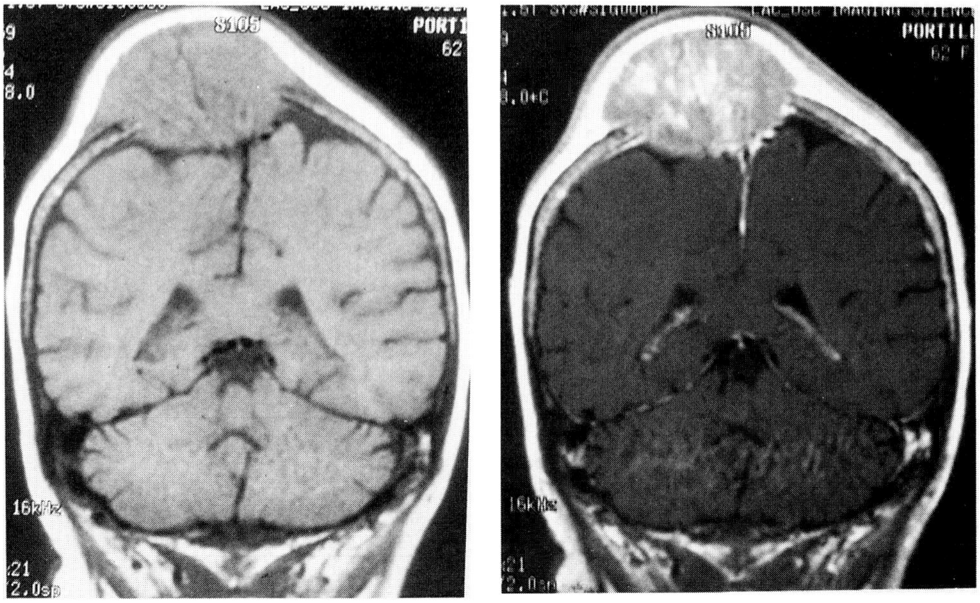

(A) (B)

Figure 12-3 Plasmacytoma. *A*. A coronal T1-weighted image demonstrates a large extraaxial mass with destruction of the bony calvarium and extension into the subcutaneous soft tissue. The mass shows isointensity to brain parenchyma. *B*. A gadolinium-enhanced coronal T1-weighted image reveals moderate, slightly inhomogeneous enhancement.

- Cerebrospinal fluid density.
- No contrast enhancement.
- Hemorrhage may occur within the cyst, especially after minor head trauma.
- Hydrocephalus may be associated with posterior fossa arachnoid cyst.

Magnetic Resonance Imaging

- Focal bony erosion and expansion can also be seen.
- Similar signal intensity to CSF on T1-weighted, proton-density-weighted, and T2-weighted images.
- Sharply marginated.
- A middle fossa cyst may have a straight posterior margin with hypoplasia of the temporal lobe.

A suprasellar cyst shows the oval or square appearance of the suprasellar cistern, splaying of cerebral peduncles,

Table 12-3
NONNEOPLASTIC EXTRAAXIAL MASSES

	COMPUTED TOMOGRAPHY		MAGNETIC RESONANCE IMAGING		
	Unenhanced	**Enhanced**	**T1-Weighted**	**T2-Weighted**	**Gadolinium-Enhanced**
Arachnoid cyst	CSF density	No enhancement	Low signal intensity, same as CSF	High signal intensity, same as CSF	No enhancement
Epidermoid	CSF density with internal stranded density. Calcification seen occasionally	Usually no enhancement unless there is adjacent inflammation	Low signal intensity with internal intensity; dirty CSF	High signal intensity	Usually no enhancement unless there is adjacent inflammation
Lipoma	Very low density; lower than CSF similar to fat	No enhancement	High signal intensity	Relatively low signal intensity	No enhancement
Dermoid	Mixed density; very low density; fat; calcification; thick wall	Usually no enhancement	Mixed intensity: high signal—fat, low signal—calcification. May rupture into subarachnoid space or lateral ventricles	Mixed signal intensity	Usually no enhancement

and anterior displacement of optic chiasm. A suprasellar arachnoid cyst should be differentiated from an enlarged anterior third ventricle due to hydrocephalus.

An arachnoid cyst in the retrocerebellar region may be difficult to differentiate from a Dandy-Walker cyst or giant cisterna magna. Complete or partial agenesis of the vermis is seen in Dandy-Walker cyst but not arachnoid cyst. Dandy-Walker cyst is contiguous with the fourth ventricle, but arachnoid cyst is separate from fourth ventricle.

A retrocerebellar arachnoid cyst can be associated with hydrocephalus, whereas a giant cisterna magna will not cause hydrocephalus.

Computed Tomography Cisternography A nonionic-contrast CT cisternogram is often useful in differentiating an arachnoid cyst from epidermoid or dermoid. If there is free communication between the subarachnoid space and the arachnoid cyst, contrast opacification of the cyst may be seen immediately following the intrathecal injection of non-ionic contrast material.

In most cases of arachnoid cyst, there is no communication between the cyst and the subarachnoid space. A delayed CT study 4 to 6 h following intrathecal injection of contrast commonly demonstrates opacification of the arachnoid cyst due to diffusion of the contrast through the cyst wall.

EPIDERMOID (Table 12-4)

Incidence Less than 1 percent of intracranial masses.

Age Congenital tumor, but clinical presentation usually in the third or fourth decade.

Location Predominately located in basal cisterns and lateral in position.

Table 12-4
COMPARISON OF EPIDERMOID AND DERMOID CYSTS

	Epidermoid	Dermoid
Incidence	0.5 to 1.58% of all intracranial neoplasms	One-fifth as common as epidermoid
Age	25 to 60 years	30 to 50 years; may be discovered in pediatric age group
Location	Paramedian, cerebellopontine angle cistern, parasellar	Midline; fourth ventricle, vermis, parasellar, and subfrontal
Pathology	Ectodermal inclusion cyst, squamous epithelium, keratinaceous debris, cholesterol crystals	Ectodermal inclusion cyst, squamous epithelium, keratinaceous debris, liquid cholesterol
Dermal appendage	No	Yes; contains hair follicles, sebaceous glands, and sweat glands
Rokitansky nodule	No	Yes; "hairball"
Wall	Thin	Thick
Calcification	Uncommon	Common
CT		
Density	Low (similar to CSF)	Very low (similar to fat)
Cyst wall	Thin	Thick
Calcification	Uncommon	Common
Enhancement of wall	Usually no enhancement unless there is adjacent inflammatory response	May be seen
Rupture of cyst	No	Yes, subarachnoid fat droplets; fat-fluid level in ventricles
Rokitansky nodule	No	Yes, floating "hairball"
MRI		
Signal intensity	Low on T1-weighted images and high on T2-weighted images (similar to CSF or "dirty" CSF)	Hyperintense on T1-weighted images and hypointense on T2-weighted images (similar to fat); may have variable intensity on T2-weighted images
Cyst wall and enhancement	Thin wall that usually does not enhance unless there is adjacent inflammatory response	Thick wall that may show enhancement
Rupture of cyst	No	Yes; high-signal-intensity fat droplets in subarachnoid space and fat-CSF level in ventricles on T1-weighted images

Intradural

- Cerebellopontine angle
- Middle fossa
- Suprasellar
- Fourth ventricle

Extradural

- Diploic space of calvarium
- Petrous bone

Pathology These tumors are composed of ectodermal elements and are lined with stratified squamous epithelium containing epithelial keratinaceous debris and cholesterol crystals. Grossly, epidermoids have a lobulated, grayish-white appearance—"pearly tumors."

Imaging *Computed Tomography*

- Low-density lesion conforming to the shape of adjacent brain. The density of an epidermoid on CT is similar to that of CSF.
- Occasionally, a high-density lesion (10 percent) may be seen due to saponification of the fat within the tumor.
- Occasionally, calcification may be seen with epidermoid.
- Epidermoids usually do not show contrast enhancement unless there is an adjacent inflammatory reaction.

Magnetic Resonance Imaging

- Epidermoids have signal intensity features similar to those of CSF on T1- and T2-weighted images.
- Sometimes, an internal stranded appearance can be seen, giving a "dirty CSF" appearance (Fig. 12-4).
- Proton-density-weighted sequences can sometimes be useful in differentiating an epidermoid from an arachnoid cyst. Most of the time, epidermoids exhibit higher signal intensity than CSF on proton-density-weighted images. However, there are instances when an epidermoid is indistinguishable from an arachnoid cyst, even on proton-density-weighted images.

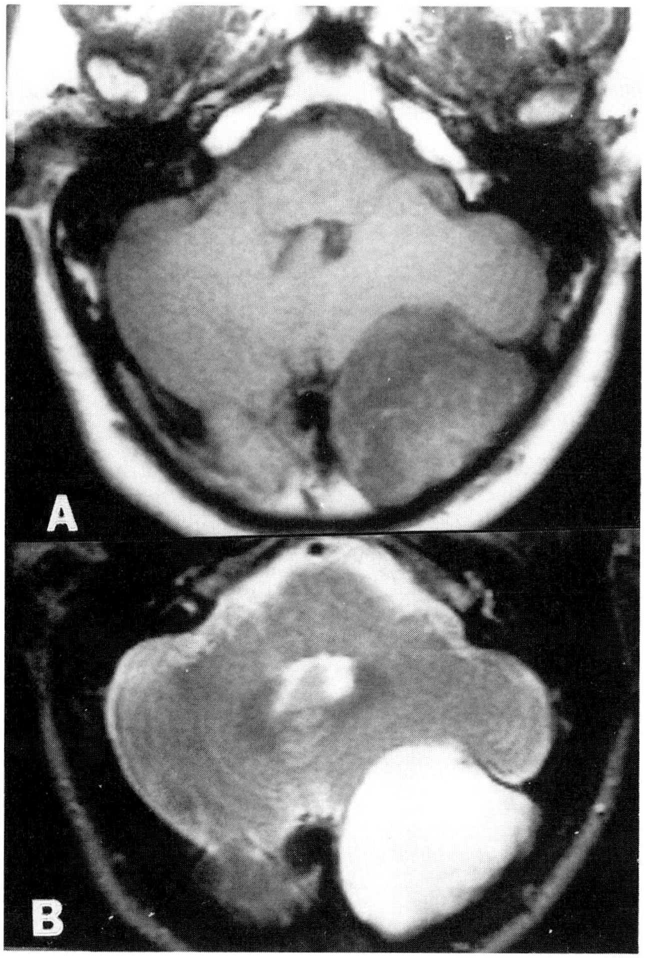

Figure 12-4 Epidermoid. *A*. An axial T1-weighted image shows an extraaxial mass of low signal intensity in the left posterior fossa. Slight inhomogeneity of the signal-intensity pattern is seen; otherwise the signal intensity is similar to that of CSF. *B*. An axial T2-weighted image demonstrates a high-signal-intensity (similar to that of CSF) extraaxial mass.

DERMOID (TABLE 12-4)

Incidence

- Intracranial dermoids are rare lesions.
- They are approximately one-fifth as common as epidermoids.

Age and Gender

- Congenital tumor, but intracranial lesions become symptomatic during the third decade due to their slow growth.
- Slight male predominance.

Location Usually midline lesions

- Fourth ventricle, vermian
- Suprasellar, juxtasellar
- Subfrontal
- Pineal region

Pathology Dermoids are composed of ectodermal elements and are lined with stratified squamous epithelium with skin appendages such as hair follicles and sebaceous and sweat glands. Desquamative debris containing cholesterol and keratin is common to both epidermoids and dermoid cysts.

Dermoids characteristically show slow, expansile growth and a tendency to insinuate themselves within and around adjacent neural structures. If the cyst has ruptured, its fatty contents can spread into the ventricles and subarachnoid spaces, inciting a chemical meningitis.

Posterior fossa and spinal dermoids are frequently associated with a dermal sinus tract.

Imaging *Computed Tomography*

- Low-density mass with sharp margin due to cholesterol within the tumor (Fig. 12-5*A*).
- A distinguishing feature of dermoid is the presence of an inhomogeneous density (hair ball) within the lesion.

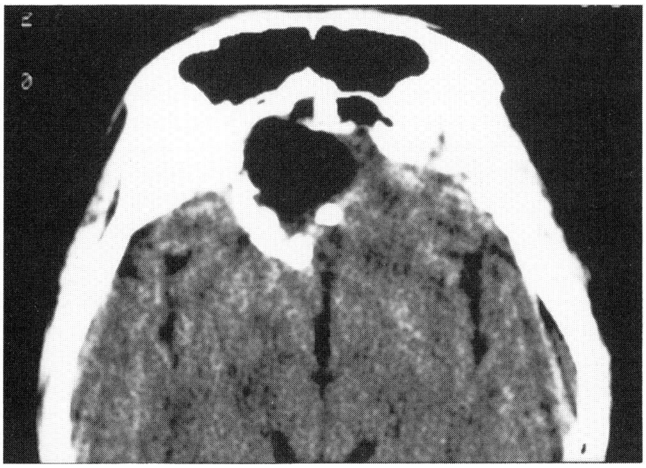

(A)

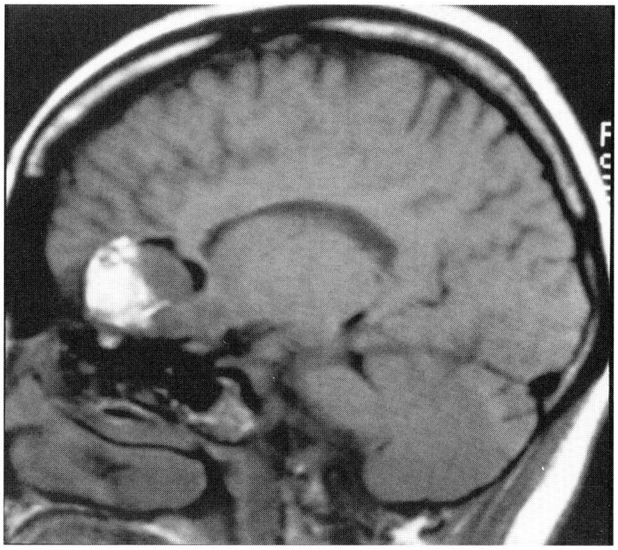

(B)

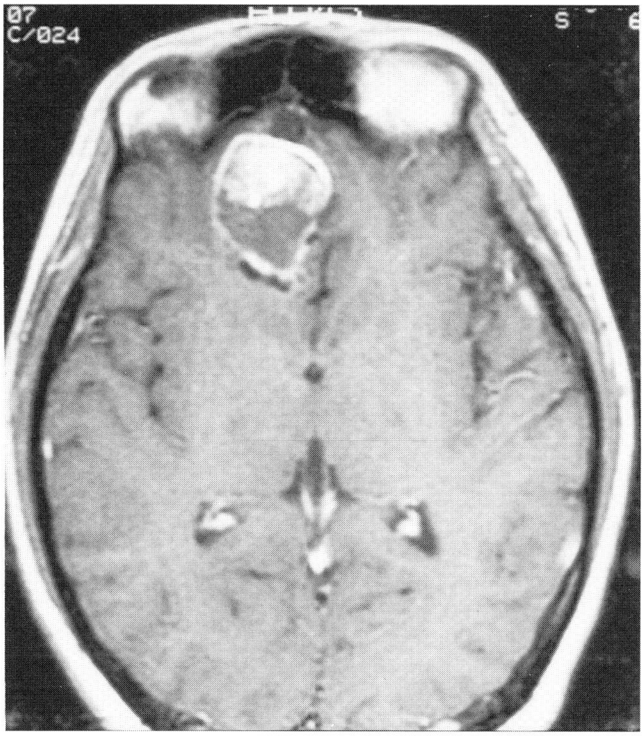

(C)

Figure 12-5 Dermoid cyst. *A*. An axial CT scan reveals a frontal mass of very low density (fat) with a rim of high density (calcification) seen posteriorly. *B*. A sagittal T1-weighted image shows a subfrontal mass of mixed signal intensity. High signal intensity fat is seen anteriorly, intermediate signal tissue in the middle and low signal calcification posteriorly. *C*. A gadolinium-enhanced axial T1-weighted image demonstrates a rim of contrast enhancement surrounding the mass.

- Calcification is more common in dermoid than in epidermoid.
- Capsule is thicker than epidermoid.
- Enhancement of the capsule is infrequent.
- A bone defect with dermal sinus may be seen in a posterior fossa dermoid.

Magnetic Resonance Imaging

- High-signal-intensity lesion with focal heterogeneous area (hair ball) on T1-weighted images (Fig. 12-5*B*).
- In posterior fossa dermoid, a high-signal sinus tract may be seen connecting the lesion with the skin surface on T2-weighted images.
- The cyst wall is thicker than that of epidermoid and may show contrast enhancement (Fig. 12-5*C*).
- Dermoids tend to rupture and cause fat droplets to spread out in the basal cisterns, subarachnoid space, and the ventricles. T1-weighted images are exquisitely sensitive to this, exhibiting multiple small high-signal-intensity areas in the basal cistern and subarachnoid space. A fat-fluid level may be seen in lateral ventricles.

LIPOMA

Location

- Dorsal pericallosal (45 percent)
- Quadrigeminal cistern, Superior vermian cistern (25 percent)
- Suprasellar cistern (14 percent)

- Cerebellopontine angle cistern (9 percent)
- Sylvian fissure (5 percent)

Pathology Congenital malformations. Lipomas are believed to result from maldifferentiation of the meninx primitiva during the formation of the subarachnoid cistern and are associated with dysgenesis of adjacent cerebral tissue in 55 percent of cases. Lipoma of the dorsal callosal area may be associated with dysgenesis of the corpus callosum in 50 percent of cases. Intracranial nerves and vessels course through these masses rather than being displaced by them. Lipomas are associated with midline facial clefts and frontonasal, frontoethmoidal encephaloceles.

Imaging ***Computed Tomography***
- Low-density mass with smooth margin (−10 HU or below).
- May be associated with rims of calcification.

Magnetic Resonance Imaging
- High signal intensity on T1-weighted images.
- Magnetic resonance imaging is useful in demonstrating associated anomalies such as dysgenesis of corpus callosum.
- The presence of chemical shift artifact at the boundary between fat and soft tissue can help to differentiate lipoma from subacute hematoma (methemoglobin). Chemical shift artifact occurs in the frequency-encoding direction. The frequency or spectral difference between fat and water is about 3.5 ppm or approximately 230 Hz at 1.5 Tesla. A fat-suppression technique may be used to confirm the diagnosis.

☐ NEOPLASMS IN THE REGION OF THE CLIVUS (Table 12-5 and 12-6)

CHORDOMA

Incidence Rare, slow-growing bone tumors. Chordomas represent 1 percent of all intracranial neoplasms and 4 percent of all primary bone tumors.

Age and Gender Peak incidence at age 20 to 40 years. Male predominance with a male:female ratio of 2:1.

Location Common locations of chordoma:

- Sacrococcygeal, 50 percent
- Clivus, 35 percent
- Vertebral body, 15 percent
- Clival chordomas tend to occur near sphenooccipital synchondrosis.

Pathology Chordomas arise from the remnants of primitive notochord, which extends from Rathke's pouch to the clivus, continuing caudally to the vertebral bodies.
Grossly, chordomas are soft, gelatinous tumors that frequently result in bone destruction.

Imaging ***Computed Tomography***
- Bone destruction involving the clivus associated with a soft tissue mass.
- Calcification, 50 percent.
- Extension of the soft tissue mass through dura posteriorly into the posterior fossa, laterally to the middle fossa, and anteriorly into nasopharynx.

Table 12-5
COMPUTED TOMOGRAPHY FINDINGS IN NEOPLASMS IN THE REGION OF CLIVUS

	Unenhanced	Enhanced
Chordoma	Bone destruction, calcification, soft tissue mass	Intense enhancement
Chondrosarcoma	Bone destruction, calcification, soft tissue mass, frequently seen at petrooccipital suture	Inhomogeneous enhancement
Metastasis	Soft tissue mass, bone destruction	Enhancement pattern may vary depending on primary site of neoplasm
Plasmacytoma	Bone destruction, soft tissue mass	Intense enhancement
Cancer of Sphenoid Sinus	Bone destruction, soft tissue mass extending from sphenoid sinus	Intense enhancement
Nasopharyngeal Carcinoma	Bone destruction, soft tissue mass extending from nasopharynx	Enhancement
Lymphoma	Soft tissue mass along the clivus, bone destruction may or may not be seen, abnormal signal within fatty marrow of clivus	Enhancement
Meningioma	Usually no bone destruction, hyperostosis may be seen, soft tissue mass along the clivus, calcification	Intense enhancement

Table 12-6
MAGNETIC RESONANCE IMAGING FINDINGS IN NEOPLASMS IN THE REGION OF CLIVUS

	T1-Weighted	T2-Weighted	Gadolinium Enhancement	Others
Chordoma	Hypointense to isointense	Heterogeneous, hyperintense	Intense enhancement	Bone destruction; calcification may be seen as signal voids
Chondrosarcoma	Hypointense to isointense	Heterogeneous, hyperintense	Heterogeneous	Bone destruction; calcification may be seen as signal voids
Metastasis	Variable but predominantly hypointense	Predominately hyperintense	Variable enhancement	Bone destruction; other metastatic foci.
Plasmacytoma	Hypointense	Variable to hypointense	Enhancement	Bone destruction; other sites of lesions in myeloma
Cancer of sphenoid sinus	Hypointense	Mildly hyperintense; relatively hypointense to mucosal disease	Enhancement	Bone destruction; extensive sphenoid sinus lesion
Nasopharyngeal carcinoma	Hypointense	Mildly hyperintense	Enhancement	Bone destruction; extensive nasopharyngeal mass lesion
Lymphoma	Hypointense to isointense	Isointense to hyperintense; some cases show hypointensity	Homogeneous enhancement	Bone infiltration with abnormal signal seen in the fatty marrow
Meningioma	Isointense to hypointense	Isointense to hyperintense	Intense enhancement	Bone hyperostosis; bone destruction rare; calcification

- Contrast enhancement is seen on postcontrast examinations.

Magnetic Resonance Imaging

- Hypointense mass lesion involving the clivus that replaces the normal hyperintense fatty marrow on T1-weighted images.
- Heterogeneous, hyperintense mass lesion on T2-weighted images. Heterogeneity may be secondary to calcification, vascularity, hemorrhage, or variation in cellular histology.
- Contrast-enhanced MRI shows intense enhancement. The enhancing mass may have high signal intensity similar to that of the adjacent normal fatty marrows. A fat-suppressed, contrast-enhanced image better delineates the mass lesion as well as the adjacent meningeal involvement and intracranial extension.
- Differential diagnosis includes chondrosarcoma, plasmacytoma, metastasis, nasopharyngeal carcinoma, sphenoid sinus carcinoma, lymphoma, and meningioma.
- To evaluate chordoma, MRI is superior to CT due to the availability of a sagittal sequence.

Cerebral Angiography

- Posterior displacement of the basilar artery and anterior pontomesencephalic vein.
- Chordomas are not very vascular tumors; however, they may be supplied by anterior meningeal branches of the vertebral artery and ascending pharyngeal artery.
- Lateral displacement of internal carotid arteries may be seen.

CHONDROSARCOMA

Incidence

- Approximately 20 percent of primary bone tumors.
- Approximately 10 percent of chondrosarcoma occur in the bones of the face and skull base.

Age and Gender

- They occur predominantly in patients between 20 and 50 years of age.
- Male:female ratio is 2:1.

Location

- Chondrosarcomas arise in different locations associated with sutures, such as the petrooccipital suture.
- Parasellar, retrosellar.
- Cerebellopontine angle.
- Paranasal sinuses.

Pathology The neoplastic tissue of this malignant tumor is fully developed cartilage with secondary myxoid changes, calcification, and ossification. Bluish-white, pearly, translucent masses with lobulated appearance.

Imaging *Computed Tomography*

- Calcification in chondroid type.
- More often lateral than midline.
- Bony destruction and soft tissue mass.
- Contrast-enhancement of the mass is inhomogeneous.

Magnetic Resonance Imaging

- Bony destruction and soft tissue mass.

- Calcification may be seen as signal voids.
- Hypointensity on T1-weighted images and heterogeneous hyperintensity on T2-weighted images.
- Gadolinium-enhanced MRI may show intense but inhomogeneous enhancement.

METASTASIS

- Metastatic disease to clivus is not uncommon.
- Primary sites include breast, prostate, melanoma, and lung.
- Bone destruction is associated with replacement of normal fatty marrow within the clivus.
- T1-weighted sagittal MRI is excellent for demonstrating metastatic disease involving the clivus by exhibiting a low-signal-intensity mass replacing the high-signal fatty marrow.
- Fat-suppression technique in conjunction with gadolinium-enhancement is superior to CT in the detection of intracranial extension of metastatic disease.

PLASMACYTOMA

- Plasmacytoma involving the clivus has radiologic findings similar to those of metastatic disease.

LYMPHOMA

- Lymphoma involving the clivus may or may not demonstrate bone destruction.
- Lymphomatous infiltration of the clivus with replacement of the normal fatty marrow may be seen on T1-weighted MRI without discrete bone destruction.
- Fat-suppression technique in conjunction with gadolinium-enhancement is a superb method for demonstrating enhancing infiltrative tumor in the clivus without definite bone destruction.

NASOPHARYNGEAL CARCINOMA

- Posterior extension of nasopharyngeal carcinoma to involve the clivus and invade the dura with intracranial extension is not uncommon.
- Frequently, a recurrent nasopharyngeal carcinoma may present with lesions involving the skull base and clivus with intracranial extension, whereas the primary site at the nasopharynx may be normal, following previous radiation therapy and chemotherapy.
- The tumor is isointense to muscle on T1-weighted images and heterogeneously hyperintense on T2-weighted images.
- Contrast enhancement is inhomogeneous.

CARCINOMA OF THE SPHENOID SINUS

- Extension of the carcinoma of the sphenoid sinus to involve the clivus is not common.
- Neoplasms involving the paranasal sinuses tend to show low to intermediate signal intensity, in contrast to the high-signal intensity mucosal disease on T2-weighted images.
- Intense enhancement is seen following the intravenous injection of contrast material (Fig. 12-6).

☐ POSTERIOR FOSSA EXTRAAXIAL MASS LESIONS (Table 12-7)

☐ NEOPLASMS (SEE CHAPTER 8)

VESTIBULAR SCHWANNOMA

Incidence Most common neoplasm of the cerebellopontine angle (80 percent).

Age The peak incidence is from 40 to 60 years.

Pathology Vestibular schwannoma arises from Schwann cells that envelop the eighth cranial nerve, particularly its peripheral superior vestibular division.

Imaging
- Unenhanced CT shows isodense lesion to brain.
- Enhanced CT shows marked contrast enhancement.
- Enlargement of internal auditory canal can be seen on bone window images.
- On MRI, schwannomas show hypointensity on T1-weighted images and marked hyperintensity on T2-weighted images.
- Gadolinium-enhanced MRI shows intense enhancement.
- Tumor may show cystic or necrotic changes.
- The four components of the seventh- and eighth-nerve complex can be visualized on MRI. The seventh (anterior, superior), superior vestibular (posterior, superior), inferior vestibular (posterior, inferior), and cochlear (anterior, inferior) nerves can be identified individually on high resolution MRI.

FACIAL-NERVE SCHWANNOMA

- Much less common than eighth-nerve schwannoma.
- Seen along the entire course of the facial nerve.
- Imaging features are similar to those of vestibular schwannoma.

FIFTH-NERVE SCHWANNOMA

- Occurs along the course of the fifth nerve.
- Tumor may extend from the ambient cistern in the posterior fossa into Meckel's cave and cavernous sinus in the middle fossa.
- Bone erosion of the petrous apex may be seen.

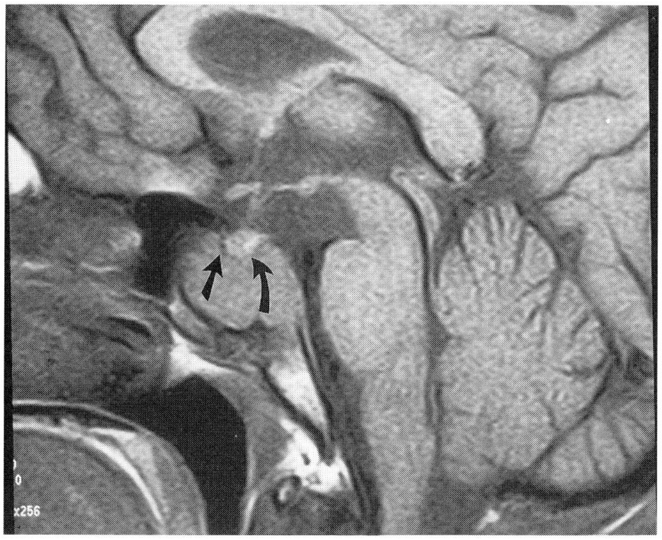

(A)

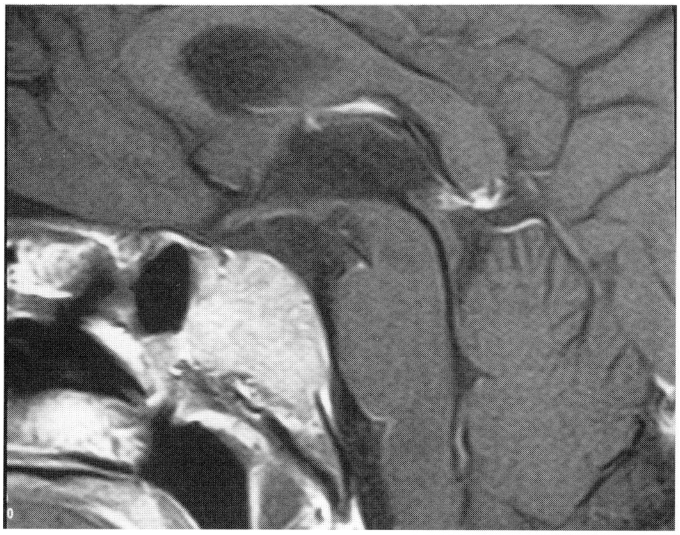

(B)

Figure 12-6 Sphenoid sinus carcinoma. *A*. A sagittal T1-weighted image shows a mass lesion (isointense to brain) in the region of the sphenoid sinus with involvement and destruction of the upper clivus and bony sella turcica. The pituitary gland (*arrows*) is seen at the top of the mass. *B*. A gadolinium-enhanced sagittal T1-weighted image demonstrates an enhancing mass involving the sphenoid sinus, upper clivus, and bony sella turcica. The enhancing mass extends beyond the dural margin posteriorly and is not separable from the enhancing pituitary gland.

- Imaging features are similar to eighth nerve schwannoma.

MENINGIOMA

- Some 10 percent of meningiomas occur in the posterior fossa.
- Meningioma is the most common benign extraaxial tumor of the foramen magnum.
- It has imaging features similar to those of supratentorial meningioma.
- Broad-based attachment to dura.

GLOMUS JUGULARE PARAGANGLIOMA

- Arise in the lateral portion of the jugular foramen.
- Irregular destruction of the jugular foramen.
- Unenhanced CT shows hyperdense mass.

Table 12-7
INCIDENCE OF CEREBELLOPONTINE ANGLE LESIONS

Pathology	Incidence
Vestibular schwannoma (acoustic neurinoma)	80%
Meningioma	10%
Epidermoid	5%
Primary malignancy	2%
Metastasis	2%
Arachnoid cyst, lipoma, glomus tumor, vascular lesion	1%

- Enhanced CT shows intense homogeneous enhancement.
- On MRI, there is a heterogeneous, mixed-intensity lesion with a "salt-and-pepper" appearance on both T1- and T2-weighted images. These small signal voids represent tumor vascularity.
- Gadolinium-enhanced MRI shows intense contrast enhancement.
- Cerebral angiographic findings include dense vascular stain that persists into the capillary phase and arteriovenous shunting with early filling of the jugular vein.
- Arterial supply is usually from ascending pharyngeal artery.

METASTASES

- Metastatic disease can involve the entire skull base.
- Osteoblastic metastases are usually caused by prostate, breast or colon carcinoma and Hodgkin's disease.
- Osteolytic metastases are usually produced by thyroid, renal, and lung carcinoma.

☐ NONNEOPLASTIC LESIONS

ARACHNOID CYST

- About 10 percent of arachnoid cysts are infratentorial in location.
- The most common location for arachnoid cyst in the posterior fossa is retrocerebellar.
- Hydrocephalus may be associated with posterior fossa arachnoid cysts.

EPIDERMOID

- Posterior fossa epidermoid may be seen in cerebellopontine angle, cisterna magna, fourth ventricle.
- Third most common lesion of the cerebellopontine angle, following "acoustic" schwannoma and meningioma.
- Posterior fossa epidermoid may extend supratentorially.

LIPOMA

- Posterior fossa lipomas are commonly seen at cerebellopontine angle cisterns.
- Chemical shift artifact is seen on MRI, especially when low bandwidth is used.
- Less than 1 percent of cerebellopontine angle mass.

VERTEBROBASILAR DOLICHOECTASIA

- Unenhanced CT shows curvilinear high density with peripheral calcification.
- Enhanced CT shows intense enhancement.
- Partial thrombosis may be seen.
- On MRI, there is signal void due to flow or calcification on both T1-weighted and T2-weighted images.
- Partial thrombosis or slow flow may exhibit high signal intensity on T1-weighted images.

☐ QUESTIONS (True or False)

1. Regarding meningioma,
   a. Calcification is seen in 20 to 50 percent of meningiomas on CT.
   b. Tumor vessels usually arise from branches of the external carotid artery.
   c. Parenchymal invasion is a sign of malignant meningioma.
   d. Hemorrhage is common in meningioma
   e. Hyperostosis is seen more commonly in en plaque meningioma.

2. Regarding meningioma,
   a. The surrounding edema correlates with tumor size.
   b. Multiple meningiomas in the same patient may be of the same histological type or different histological type.
   c. Cystic changes are seen in 60 percent of cases.
   d. Parasagittal location is the most common.
   e. "Dural tail" sign is specific for meningioma.

3. Regarding primary CNS lymphoma,
   a. It is frequently multifocal.
   b. Basal ganglia is a common location.
   c. Ringlike enhancement may be seen in patients with AIDS or immunosuppression.
   d. May show hypointensity on T2-weighted images.
   e. Usually show heterogeneous contrast enhancement on CT or MRI.

4. Regarding epidermoids,
   a. They may arise from the intradiploic space, petrous bone, or cerebellopontine angle cistern.
   b. Differentiation from arachnoid cyst may be difficult on imaging studies (CT or MRI).
   c. They show intense contrast enhancement on MRI.
   d. Calcification is very common.
   e. High-density lesions are seen in 10 percent of cases.

5. Regarding arachnoid cyst,
   a. The most common site in the posterior fossa is the cerebellopontine angle cistern.

b. A suprasellar arachnoid cyst should be differentiated from an enlarged anterior third ventricle.
c. Supratentorial arachnoid cysts are more common than infratentorial ones.
d. Erosion of bone adjacent to an arachnoid cyst is commonly seen.
e. Contrast enhancement is common on CT or MRI.

6. Regarding dermoids,
a. Calcification is commonly seen on CT.
b. They are composed of elements of one germ layer.
c. Posterior fossa and spinal dermoids are frequently associated with a dermal sinus tract.
d. Rupture of a dermoid is demonstrated by fat particles in subarachnoid space and fat-fluid level in ventricle.
e. They have a thinner capsule than epidermoids.

7. Regarding meningiomas,
a. They are the most common benign intracranial neoplasms.
b. They are the most common extraaxial tumor in adults.
c. Blistering is seen at the convexity.
d. Cerebral edema is less common in the en plaque type of meningioma.
e. Meningiomas in childhood are frequently associated with neurofibromatosis.

8. Regarding primary CNS lymphoma,
a. The incidence of primary CNS lymphoma is increasing due to the increase in patients with AIDS and immunosuppression.
b. Leptomeningeal involvement is not seen in primary lymphoma.
c. Multiple lesions are seen in about 20 to 40 percent of the cases.
d. A dura-based lesion may mimic meningioma.
e. Up to about one-third of the patients with systemic lymphoma develop CNS disease.

9. Regarding lipoma,
a. The cerebellopontine angle cistern is the most common location.
b. Dysgenesis of adjacent tissue is seen in 55 percent of cases.
c. Intracranial nerves and vessels are frequently displaced by lipoma.
d. Chemical-shift artifact occurs because there is a resonance frequency difference between fat and water.
e. There is maldifferentiation of the meninx primitiva.

10. Regarding mass lesions in the region of the clivus,
a. Calcification is seen in 50 percent of chordomas.
b. The petrooccipital suture is a common location for clivus chondrosarcoma.
c. Meningioma in the clivus region is commonly associated with bone destruction.
d. Plasmacytoma does not involve the clivus.
e. The clivus is the most common site for chordoma.

☐ ANSWERS

1. a. T
b. T
c. T
d. F
e. T

2. a. F
b. T
c. F
d. T
e. F

3. a. T
b. T
c. T
d. T
e. F

4. a. T
b. T
c. F
d. F
e. T

5. a. F
b. T
c. T
d. T
e. F

6. a. T
b. T
c. T
d. T
e. F

7. a. T
b. T
c. F
d. T
e. T

8. a. T
b. F
c. T
d. T
e. T

9. **a.** F
b. T
c. F
d. T
e. T

10. **a.** T
b. T
c. F
d. F
e. F

SUGGESTED READINGS

Meningioma

1. Bird CR et al: Meningiomas and skull base neoplasms. *Top Magn Reson Imaging* 1:52–68, 1989.
2. Elster AD et al: Meningiomas: MR and histopathologic features. *Radiology* 170:857–862, 1989.
3. Geoffray A et al: Extracranial meningiomas of the head and neck. *AJNR* 5:599–604, 1984.
4. Rosenbaum AE, Rosenbloom SB: Meningiomas revisited. *Semin Roengenol* 29:8–26, 1984.
5. Russell EJ et al: Atypical computed tomographic features of intracranial meningioma: Radiological-pathological correlation in a series of 131 consecutive cases. *Radiology* 135:673–682, 1980.
6. Schubeus P et al: Intracranial meningiomas: Comparison of plain and contrast-enhanced examinations in CT and MR. *Neuroradiology* 32:12–18, 1990.
7. Spagnoli MV et al: Intracranial meningiomas: High-field MR imaging. *Radiology* 161:369–375, 1986.
8. Vassilouthis J, Ambrose J: Computerized tomography scanning appearances of intracranial meningiomas: An attempt to predict histological features. *J Neurosurg* 50:320–327, 1979.
9. Zee CS et al: Magnetic resonance imaging of meningiomas. *Semin Ultrasound CT MRI* 13:154–169, 1992.
10. Zimmerman RD et al: Magnetic resonance imaging of meningiomas. *AJNR* 6:149–157, 1985.

Lymphoma

1. Berry I et al: Gd-DTPA in clinical MR of the brain: 2. Extra-axial lesions and normal structures. *AJR* 147:1231, 1986.
2. Jack CR et al: Central nervous system lymphoma: Histological types and CT appearance. *Radiology* 167:211–215, 1988.
3. Lee Y et al: Primary central nervous system lymphoma: CT and pathologic correlation. *AJR* 147:747–752, 1986.
4. Roman-Goldstein SM et al: MR of primary CNS lymphoma in immunologically normal patients. *AJNR* 13:1207–1213, 1992.
5. Schwaighofer BW et al: Primary intracranial lymphoma: MR manifestations. *AJNR* 11:785–791, 1990.
6. Sze G et al: Detection of brain metastases: Comparison of contrast-enhanced MR with unenhanced MR and CT. *AJNR* 11:785–791, 1990.
7. Weingarten KL et al: Spontaneous regression of intracerebral lymphoma. *Radiology* 149:721, 1983.
8. Zimmerman RA: Central nervous system lymphoma. *Radiol Clin North Am* 28:697–721, 1990.

Sarcoidosis

1. Atlas SE (ed): *Magnetic Resonance Imaging of the Brain and Spine*. New York, Raven Press, 1991.
2. Bahr AL et al: Neuroradiological manifestations of intracranial sarcoidosis. *Radiology* 127:713–717, 1978.
3. Brooks BS et al: Radiologic evaluation of neurosarcoidosis: Role of computerized tomography. *AJNR 3:513–521, 1982.*
4. Kumpe DA et al: Intracranial neurosarcoidosis. *Comput Assist Tomogr* 3:324–339, 1979.
5. Lee BCP, Deck MDF: Sellar and juxtasellar lesion detection with MR. *Radiology* 157:143, 1985.
6. Post MJD et al: Demonstration of sarcoidosis of the optic nerve, frontal lobes, and falx cerebri: Case report and literature review. *AJNR* 3:523–526, 1982.

Metastasis

1. Atlas SW et al: MR imaging of intracranial metastatic melanoma. *J Comput Assist Tomogr* 11:577, 1987.
2. Bradley WG et al: Initial clinical experience with Gd-DPTA in North America: MR contrast enhancement of brain tumors. *Radiology* 157:125, 1985.
3. Davis PC et al: Leptomeningeal metastasis: MR imaging. *Radiology* 163:449, 1987.
4. Davis JM et al: Metastases to the central nervous system. *Radiol Clin North Am* 20:417, 1982.
5. Ginaldi S et al: Cranial computed tomography of malignant melanoma. *AJR* 136:145, 1981.
6. Rao KCVG, Williams JP: Intracranial tumors: Metastatic, in Lee SH, Rao KCVG (eds): *Clinical Computed Tomography*. New York, McGraw-Hill, 1983.
7. Yuh WT et al: Experience with high dose gadolinium MR imaging in the evaluation of brain metastases. *AJNR* 13:335–345, 1992.

Arachnoid Cyst

1. Crisi G et al: Metrizamide-enhanced computed tomography of intracranial arachnoid cysts. *J Comput Assist Tomogr* 8:928–935, 1984.
2. Leo JS et al: Computed tomography of arachnoid cysts. *Radiology* 130:675–680, 1979.
3. Little JR et al: Infratentorial arachnoid cysts. *J Neurosurg* 39:380–386, 1973.
4. Rengachary SS: Intracranial arachnoid and ependymal cysts, in Wilkins RH, Rengachary SS (eds): *Neurosurgery*. New York, McGraw-Hill, 1985, pp 2160–2172.
5. Robertson SJ et al: MR imaging of middle cranial fossa arachnoid cysts: Temporal lobe agenesis syndrome revisited. *AJNR* 10:1007–1010, 1989.
6. Rock JP et al: Arachnoid cysts of the posterior fossa. *Neurosurgery* 18:176–179, 1986.
7. Weiner SN et al: MR imaging of intracranial arachnoid cysts. *J Comput Assist Tomogr* 11:236–241, 1987.

Epidermoid and Dermoid

1. Braun IF et al: Dense intracranial epidermoid tumors: Computed tomographic observations. *Radiology* 122:717–719, 1977.
2. Chambers AA et al: Cranial epidermoid tumors: Diagnosis by computed tomography. *Neurosurgery* 1:276–280, 1977.

3. Davis KR et al: Diagnosis of epidermoid tumor by computer assisted tomography: Analysis and evaluation of findings. *Radiology* 119:347–353, 1976.
4. Hiratsuka H et al: Diagnosis of epidermoid cysts by metrizamide CT cisternography. *Neuroradiology* 26:153–155, 1984.
5. Smith AS et al: Diagnosis of ruptured intracranial dermoid cyst: Value of MR over CT. *AJNR* 12:175–180, 1991.
6. Steffey D et al: MR imaging of primary epidermoid cysts. *AJNR* 10:351–356, 1989.
7. Tampieri D et al: MR imaging of epidermoid cysts. *AJNR* 10:351–356, 1989.
8. Wilms G et al: CT and MRI of ruptured intracranial dermoids. *Neuroradiology* 33:149–151, 1991.
9. Yuh W et al: MR of fourth-ventricular epidermoid tumors. *AJNR* 9:794–796, 1988.

Lipoma

1. Eghwrudjakpor PO et al: Intracranial lipomas: Current perspectives in their diagnosis and treatment. *Br J Neurosurg* 6:139–144, 1992.
2. Kazner E et al: Intracranial lipoma: Diagnostic and therapeutic considerations. *J Neurosurg* 52:234–245, 1980.
3. Maiuri F, Cirillo S: Intracranial lipomas. *Acta Neurol* 10:29–82, 1988.
4. Maiuri F et al: Lipoma of the sylvian region. *Clin Neurol Neurosurg* 91:321–323, 1989.
5. Rubio G et al: MR and CT diagnosis of intracranial lipoma. *AJR* 157:887–888, 1991.
6. Truwit CL, Barkovich AJ: Pathogenesis of intracranial lipoma: An MR study in 42 patients. *AJR* 155:855–864, 1990.
7. Wilberger JE et al: Lipoma of the septum pellucidum: Case report. *J Comput Assist Tomogr* 11:79–82, 1987.

Chordoma and Chondrosarcoma

1. Heffelfinger MJ et al: Chordomas and cartilaginous tumors at the skull base. *Cancer* 32:410–420, 1973.
2. Kendall BE, Lee BCP: Cranial chordomas. *Br J Radiol* 50:687–698, 1977.
3. Lee YY, Van Tassel P: Craniofacial chondrosarcoma: Imaging findings in 15 untreated cases. *AJNR* 10:165, 1989.
4. Lee YY et al: Craniofacial osteosarcomas: Plain film, CT and MR findings in 46 cases. *AJNR* 9:379, 1988.
5. Meyers SP et al: Chondrosarcomas of the skull base: MR imaging features. *Radiology* 184:103, 1992.
6. Oot RF et al: The role of MR and CT in evaluating clival chordomas and chondrosarcomas. *AJR* 151:567–575, 1989.
7. Sze G et al: Chordomas: MR imaging. *Radiology* 166:187–191, 1988.

Nasopharyngeal Carcinoma and Carcinoma of the Sphenoid Sinus

1. Sham JST et al: Nasopharyngeal carcinoma: CT evaluation of patterns of tumor spread. *AJNR* 12:265, 1991.
2. Som PM et al: Benign and malignant sinonasal lesions with intracranial extension: Differentiation with MR imaging. *Radiology* 172:763, 1989.

Vestibular Schwannoma (Acoustic Neurinoma)

1. Atlas SW: *Magnetic Resonance Imaging of the Brain and Spine*. New York, Raven Press, 1991.
2. Bilaniuk LT: Adult infratentorial tumors. *Semin Roentgenol* 25:155–173, 1990.
3. Daniels DL et al: MR detection of tumor in the internal auditory canal. *AJNR* 8:249–252, 1987.
4. Lee BCP et al: Posterior fossa lesions: Magnetic resonance imaging. *Radiology* 153:137–143, 1984.
5. Mafee MF: Acoustic neuroma and other acoustic nerve disorders: Role of MRI and CT: An analysis of 238 cases. *Semin Ultrasound CT MRI* 8:256–283, 1987.
6. New PFJ et al: MR imaging of the acoustic nerves and small acoustic neuromas at 0.6T: Prospective study. *AJNR* 6:165–170, 1985.
7. Pinto RS, Kricheff II: Neuroradiology of intracranial neuromas. *Semin Roentgenol* 19:44–52, 1984.
8. Press GA, Hesselink JR: MR imaging of cerebellopontine angle and internal auditory canal lesions at 1.5 T. *AJNR* 9:241–251, 1988.
9. Young IR et al: The role of NMR imaging in the diagnosis and management of acoustic neuroma. *AJNR* 4:223–224, 1983.

Glomus Tumor

1. Brown JS: Glomus jugulare tumors revisited: A ten year statistical follow-up of 231 cases. *Laryngoscope* 95:284–288, 1985.
2. Jackson CG et al: Glomus tumors: Diagnosis, classification and management of large lesions. *Arch Otolaryngol* 108:401–406, 1982.
3. Olsen WI et al. MR imaging of paragangliomas. *AJNR* 7:1039, 1986.
4. Vogl T et al: Paragangliomas of the jugular bulb and carotid body: MR imaging with short sequences and Gd-DTPA enhancement. *AJNR* 10:823–827, 1989.

CHAPTER 13

Sellar and Parasellar Lesions

Jamshid Ahmadi

Modern imaging of the sellar region combined with hormonal immunoassay has greatly improved the diagnosis of pituitary disorders. Magnetic resonance imaging (MRI) is particularly important in providing detailed information about the extent of a pituitary tumor and its anatomic relationship to adjacent structures. This information, in turn, guides management planning. In addition to MRI, hormonal assay is also important in follow-up studies.

NORMAL ANATOMY

ANATOMY OF SELLAR REGION

For practical diagnostic purposes, the sellar region may be divided into three parts: the pituitary fossa, cavernous sinuses, and suprasellar cisterns. Many disorders may originate in more than one compartment or extend from one part to another or beyond.

The pituitary fossa is situated in the sella turcica; it is confined anteriorly by the tuberculum sellae and posteriorly by the dorsum sellae. An extension of the dura mater lines the pituitary fossa, encapsulates the pituitary glands, and forms an incomplete covering for the sella turcica known as the diaphragma sellae. The pituitary gland occupies almost all of the pituitary fossa.

The cavernous sinus is a paired duroperiosteal space lying on either side of the pituitary; it contains a trabeculated network of venous channels surrounding the juxtasellar segment of the internal carotid artery and its dural branches (meningohypophyseal trunk). The internal carotid artery and cranial nerve VI (Abducens) lie deep within the cavernous sinus, whereas cranial nerves III (oculomotor), IV (trochlear), V_1 (ophthalmic) and V_2 (maxillary) divisions of the trigeminal nerve traverse the cavernous sinus close to its lateral margin. The ophthalmic nerve enters the orbit via the superior orbital fissure and the maxillary nerve passes through the foramen rotundum. The mandibular division (V_3) is the largest of the three; it remains mainly external to the cavernous sinus and exits through the foramen ovale (along with the motor root of the trigeminal nerve) into the infratemporal fossa.

The trigeminal ganglion (gasserian ganglion) is situated in Meckel's cave. The sensory root fibers of the trigeminal nerve traverse the porus trigeminus of the petrous apex. They enter posteriorly into the concave margin of the ganglion, and the three sensory divisions exit from its anterior convex side. The motor root passes beneath the ganglia and exits through the foramen ovale without merging with the sensory root or ganglia. The foramen ovale is a vertically oriented canal beneath Meckel's cave and is readily identified on computed tomography (CT) or MRI (the coronal plane is better).

The suprasellar cisterns contain vascular and neural structures such as components of the circle of Willis, the optic nerves and optic chiasm, the hypothalamus, the infundibular stalk, and the anterior recess of third ventricle.

ANATOMY OF PITUITARY GLAND

The pituitary gland in the adult is a bean-shaped, fairly symmetrical organ and has two major anatomic divisions, the anterior lobe or adenohypophysis (making up three-quarters of the total gland) and the posterior lobe or neurohypophysis. The adenohypophysis consists of the pars distalis, pars intermedia, and pars tuberalis, which is an upward extension forming a cuff around the inferior portion of the infundibular stalk. The neurohypophysis consists of the pars nervosa, the infundibular stalks, and the infundibula proper. The neurohypophysis is supplied directly by multiple small branches of the meningohypophyseal trunk, which, in turn, arises from each internal carotid artery. The major blood supply to the adenohypophysis is derived from the hypophyseal portal system. The neurovascular connections between the pituitary gland and hypothalamus play a crucial role in regulating the secretion of hormones. The neurohypophysis is directly connected to the hypothalamus by axons of neurons that originate in the supraoptic and paraventricular nuclei and traverse the infundibular stalk. Vasopressin and oxytocin are synthesized within the supraoptic and paraventricular nuclei of hypothalamus, attached to a specific carrier protein, and then transported down the axons of the hypothalamohypophyseal tract to the posterior lobe of the pituitary gland and stored for subsequent release into the bloodstream. As normally seen on T1-weighted MRI, these secretory granules appear as a bright spot on the posterior lobe of the pituitary. As a rule, hyperintensity of the posterior pituitary lobe is observed in 90 to 100 percent of healthy subjects.

The pathway connecting the adenohypophyses to the hypothalamus has two components: the tuberohypophyseal neural tract and the hypophyseal portal system. The tuberohypophyseal tract originates from neurons in the hypothalamus and terminates in the infundibulum, adjacent to the primary capillary beds of the hypophyseal portal system. Releasing and inhibiting factors that are synthesized in the cell bodies of hypothalamus are transported along their axons; they are deposited at the capillaries of the infundibulum and then carried down to the adenohypophysis by way of the pituitary portal system.

□ PITUITARY DISORDERS

DEVELOPMENTAL ANOMALIES

A background knowledge of the embryologic development of the pituitary gland can help one to understand and recognize anomalies in the sellar region.

The pituitary gland consists of two distinct lobes: the anterior lobe or adenohypophysis and the posterior lobe or neurohypophysis. Traditional embryology holds that the adenohypophysis arises from the primitive foregut (the stomodeum), whereas the neurohypophysis derives from neuroectoderm. More recent studies, however, suggest that the adenohypophysis may be of neuroectodermal origin as well. According to traditional views, the adenohypophysis develops from a midline evagination of Rathke's pouch, the primitive buccal cavity or the stomodeum. Rathke's pouch grows upward, loses its connection with the roof of the pharynx, and comes to lie within the developing sphenoid bone. The proliferation of cells from Rathke's pouch forms the adenohypophysis, and the lumen of the pouch is eventually obliterated. Occasionally, however, remnants of Rathke's pouch persist, and these may lead to the formation of congenital pituitary cysts. The pars distalis of the adenohypophysis develops from the anterior distal wall of Rathke's pouch and executes anterior pituitary functions. The pars intermedia develops from the posterior wall of Rathke's pouch and is usually vestigial. The pars tuberalis normally forms a cuff around the infundibular stalk and is thought to be the moderator of certain functions of the pars distalis.

The neurohypophysis is formed from a downgrowth of tissue from the floor of the developing diencephalon. The upward growth of developing adenohypophysis and downward growth of the developing neurohypophysis meet and join early in embryonic life to form the pituitary gland. Normally, the neurohypophysis permanently retains direct communication with the brain by the infundibular stalk. The posterior pituitary lobe, infundibular stalk, and supraoptic and paraventricular hypothalamic nuclei are generally considered parts of the neurohypophysis.

AGENESIS

Agenesis of the entire pituitary gland is rare and has been described in association with gross malformation of the neural tube and axial skeleton, such as cyclopia.

Agenesis of the adenohypophysis in normocephalic infants is rare. Hypoplasia of the pituitary gland is frequently seen in association with anencephaly, but it is quite uncommon in normocephalic infants. Affected individuals present with clinical signs of panhypopituitarism. In such cases, the sella turcica may be smaller than normal and the craniopharyngeal canal may be persistent. Absence of stimulating hormones results in hypoplastic adrenals, thyroid, and gonads.

MALPOSITION

Ectopic Neurohypophysis The neurohypophysis may lie between the hypothalamus and the sella turcica. On noncontrast T1-weighted MRI, a focal "bright spot" is frequently observed in the suprasellar region. In addition, the infundibular stalk is difficult to identify. Congenital ectopic neurohypophysis is rare and the ectopic bright spot is more commonly caused by acquired processes such as tumors or trauma that had caused disturbances of transport or releasing of hormones from the hypothalamus to the neurohypophysis.

Ectopic adenohypophysis may be identified in the pharynx or in the suprasellar region. The pituitary function, however, remains normal. Hypophysectomy is occasionally performed to relieve symptoms of metastatic breast cancer, particularly bone pain. In some of these patients, activation of ectopic pharyngeal pituitary may compensate for the absence of pituitary hormones. Ectopic pituitary adenoma with normal intrasellar pituitary has also been reported.

"EMPTY SELLA"

A subarachnoid space of variable size may extend into the pituitary fossa due to an incompetent diaphragma sellae or prior pituitary surgery. It is commonly observed on routine CT or MRI. With a few exceptions, the "empty sella" has no clinical significance. Coexistence of pituitary microadenoma and empty sella has occasionally been reported. The diagnosis of empty sella is easily made on CT or MRI. The pituitary gland is flattening and displacement toward the posteroinferior aspect of pituitary fossa without causing impairment of pituitary functions. The sella turcica is often larger than normal and filled with variable amounts of CSF. The infundibular stalk follows its normal course and inserts in the midline of thinned and flattened pituitary gland. Intrasellar herniation of the optic nerve, optic tract, or anteroinferior portion of the third ventricle may occasionally occur within a primary or postoperative empty sella. Rarely, it may result in a visual field defect.

Necrosis and shrinkage of the pituitary gland secondary to adenohypophysis or Sheehan's syndrome can eventually result in an acquired empty sella.

PITUITARY HYPERPLASIA

1. *Physiologic*: Diffuse enlargement of the adenohypophysis occurs during pregnancy and lactation, predominantly due to hypertrophy of prolactin cells. On CT or MRI, the pituitary gland appears spherical with an upward convexity; it may reach up to 12 mm in height. In addition, the adenohypophysis may appear hyperintense relative to brain parenchyma on T1-weighted MRI. Diffuse enlargement of the pituitary may also be seen during adolescence. However, involution of the physiologically hypertrophic gland occurs subsequently.
2. *Secondary to end-organ failure*: Hypofunction of the thyroid, adrenals, or gonads may result in nodular or diffuse hyperplasia of the anterior pituitary lobe due to lack of negative feedback.
3. *Addison's disease*: Diffuse or nodular hyperplasia of the pituitary may occur secondary to bilateral adrenalectomy or idiopathic atrophy of the adrenal gland. The extent of hyperplasia correlates with the duration of disease. Idiopathic atrophy of the adrenals is frequently associated with atrophy of the thyroid, presumably on an autoimmune basis. This association is known as Schmidt's syndrome.
4. *Primary hyperplasia*: Nodular or diffuse primary hyperplasia of corticotroph cells is one of the uncommon but established causes of Cushing's disease.

Nonneoplastic Sellar Cysts Small cysts (seen microscopically) have been reported in 20 percent of unselected autopsies. Some 2 to 5 percent of surgical specimens are nonneoplastic pituitary cysts.

RATHKE'S CLEFT CYSTS

Rathke's cleft cysts are lined by columnar or cuboidal epithelium. Cystic fluid within the Rathke's cleft cysts varies from serous to mucoid; therefore, MRI signal intensities on T1- and T2-weighted images are variable and related to cyst contents. A cystic mass with low protein content (less than 9000 mg/dL) appears hypodense on CT; it appears hypointense on T1- and hyperintense on T2-weighted MR images compared to brain. Cystic fluid containing free methemoglobin or high protein concentration is hyperintense on both T1- and T2-weighted MR images. The hemorrhagic cystic fluid (at the phase with free methemoglobin and without high protein content) is hypodense on CT. A cystic mass with a very high protein content appears hyperdense on CT; it is hyperintense on T1- and hypointense on T2-weighted MR images. A mild rimlike enhancement is occasionally seen following administration of contrast.

- In surgical specimens, 25 percent of Rathke's cleft cysts are intrasellar, 70 percent are both intra- and suprasellar, and 5 percent are completely suprasellar.

ARACHNOID CYSTS

Approximately 10 percent of intracranial arachnoid cysts occur in the sellar region (mostly in the suprasellar compartment). Arachnoid cysts are smoothly marginated, nonenhanced masses that may displace or compress the third ventricle or infundibular stalk. The imaging characteristics of arachnoid cysts on CT and on all MRI sequences are similar to those of CSF.

ISCHEMIA

Microscopic foci of coagulative necrosis have been reported in 1 to 3 percent of unselected autopsies. In most of these cases, pituitary infarcts occurred in the terminal stage of severe systemic illness; therefore they are of little clinical significance. Acute infarct in pituitary adenoma is discussed elsewhere in this chapter.

Postpartum Pituitary Necrosis (Sheehan's Syndrome) Obstetric shock (hemorrhagic or septic) may lead to an insufficiency of the hypophyseal portal system and result in infarction and necrosis of the adenohypophysis. The degree of postpartum pituitary insufficiency depends on the extent of destruction of the anterior lobe of the pituitary. The involved pituitary gradually shrivels to a thin scar tissue. The pituitary fossa is subsequently filled in by intrasellar herniation of the subarachnoid space.

□ PITUITARY NEOPLASMS

Many types of tumors and tumorlike conditions occur in the sellar region. Some are found incidentally (they are often of no clinical importance), while others are of considerable clinical significance (Table 13-1).

PITUITARY ADENOMAS

The incidence of pituitary microadenomas in unselected autopsies is approximately 25 percent. The early diagnosis and hence occurrence of symptomatic pituitary adenomas have risen sharply in the past two decades, mainly due to advances in neuroimaging, clinical immunochemistry, and microsurgery. Improved clinical diagnosis of pituitary adenomas and hence early transsphenoid surgery without any disturbance of pituitary function have revolutionized the management of pituitary adenomas.

In adults, pituitary adenoma is the most common lesion originating within the pituitary fossa. Such adenomas may present clinically with evidence of abnormal (hypersecretion or hyposecretion) production of trophic hormones and/or visual field defects due to compression of the optic nerve and chiasm. Occasionally, pituitary adenoma may be discovered incidentally on MRI performed for other reasons. There are several classifications of pituitary adenomas based on their anatomic changes, endocrine function, and biologic behavior.

Table 13-1
CLASSIFICATION OF PITUITARY LESIONS

Pituitary adenomas	80%
Other lesions of the sellar region	20%
Rathke's cleft cyst	
Craniopharyngioma	
Meningioma	
Germinoma	
Metastasis	
Dermoid	
Arachnoid and paracystic cysts	
Paraganglioma	
Inflammatory	
Lymphocytic adenohypophysitis	
Sarcoidosis	
Giant-cell granulomas	
Tuberculosis/fungal infection	
Aneurysms	
Lipoma	

CLASSIFICATION ACCORDING TO MORPHOLOGIC FEATURES

Sophisticated imaging techniques (particularly MRI) provide detailed anatomic information about the size, extent, and sometimes consistency of sellar tumors. If a pituitary adenoma is equal to or less than 10 mm in its largest diameter and hence is confined to the pituitary fossa, it is called a microadenoma. Typically, a microadenoma is hypointense on T1-weighted MRI relative to the remaining normal pituitary tissue, and it often (immediately after administration of contrast) enhances to a lesser degree than normal pituitary gland. Occasionally, on the basis of their imaging characteristics, it may be difficult to differentiate pituitary microadenomas from cysts of the pars intermedia, Rathke's pouch cyst, or focal pituitary infarct. On the other hand, in approximately 20 percent of cases, a pituitary microadenoma may not be identified on MRI. Therefore, pituitary microadenoma cannot be excluded on the basis of a normal MRI. Correlation between pituitary hormone assay and MRI findings is very important for accurate diagnosis.

If a pituitary tumor is larger than 10 mm in diameter and hence extends beyond the pituitary fossa, it is called a macroadenoma. The majority of pituitary macroadenomas are solid. However, hemorrhage, infarction, necrosis, or cystic changes may occur in approximately 10 percent of pituitary adenomas. Typically uncomplicated, macroadenomas are isointense relative to gray matter on both T1- and T2-weighted MRI and homogeneously enhance with contrast. However, the occurrence of hemorrhage, infarction, and necrosis within the pituitary adenoma may alter the MRI signals of pituitary adenomas.

CLASSIFICATION ACCORDING TO ENDOCRINE FUNCTION AND CYTOGENESIS

The old classification of pituitary adenomas into acidophilic, basophilic, and chromophobes has been replaced by a modern functional classification based on electron microscopic and immunohistochemical studies, in which each cell is named according to its secretory activity (Table 13-2).

Approximately 75 percent of pituitary adenomas are accompanied by clinical and biochemical evidence of excessive hormone production. These tumors may secrete prolactin (PRL), growth hormone (GH), adrenocorticotropic hormone (ACTH), thyrotropin or thyroid-stimulating hormone (TSH), follicle-stimulating hormone (FSH), luteinizing hormone (LH), and subunits of the glycoprotein hormones. In a small group of patients, pituitary adenomas may produce more than one hormone.

Serum prolactin levels over 200 ng/mL are almost always due to prolactin-secreting adenomas; however, values under 200 ng/mL are nonspecific. Such a mild-to-moderate

Table 13-2
FUNCTIONAL CLASSIFICATION OF PITUITARY ADENOMAS

Type	Clinical	Prevalence	Remarks
Prolactin-cell adenoma	Amenorrhea, galactorrhea	30%	Microscopic calcification is common Serum prolactin σ 200
Growth-hormone-cell adenoma Densely granulated Sparsely granulated	Acromegaly or gigantism	16%	Mild to moderately elevated prolactin may be seen in many conditions due to compression of hypothalamus, pituitary Slow-growing, high surgical rate Frequently invasive; less favorable surgical cure rate
Corticotropic-cell adenoma Biochemically active Biochemically silent	Cushing's disease or Nelson's syndrome	14%	Normal serum ACTH, but positive immunostaging for ACTH Aggressive tumor, hemorrhage infarct is common
Thyrotropic-cell adenoma		0.5%	Mostly associated with pituitary primary hypothyroidism
Gonadotropic cell adenoma	No specific syndrome	3%	
Plurihormonal adenoma Mixed growth-hormone cell–prolactin-cell adenoma Acidophil: stem-cell adenoma Mammosomatotropic cell adenoma	Acromegaly or gigantism	10%	More separate hormones PACL is moderately elevated; GH is normal
Null cell adenoma		20%	Lack immunocytochemical or fine structural markers Seen more commonly in ages over 40 Serum prolactin may be mildly elevated due to compression of hypothalamic hypophyseal axis
Onocytoma		6.5%	Hormonally inactive but tumor cells contain abundant mitochondria

elevated prolactin may be due to pituitary adenoma or due to other causes including compression of pituitary-hypophyseal axis. Compression of hypothalamus or pituitary stalk may interfere with production, release, or transport of prolactin-inhibiting factors to the adenohypophysis, and thus cause hyperprolactinemia.

The remaining 25 percent of pituitary adenomas are inactive clinically and biochemically. However, these functionally silent tumors may contain cytoplasmic secretory granules.

BIOLOGIC CLASSIFICATION

On the basis of their biologic behavior, pituitary neoplasms may be subdivided into expanding adenomas, invasive adenomas, and carcinomas.

Expanding Adenomas Most pituitary adenomas are slow-growing and tend to grow in an upward direction into the suprasellar cisterns. Intrasellar expansion of these adenomas may erode the sella turcica and compress the cavernous sinus laterally. The dura mater forming the medial walls of the cavernous sinus remains intact but is displaced somewhat because of pressure from the expanding pituitary adenoma. Most expanding adenomas demonstrate a globular configuration. The diaphragma sellae, however, may impose a waistline indentation between the intrasellar and suprasellar components of large adenomas, resulting in an "hourglass" configuration. Occasionally, more rapid nodular outgrowths of one part of an adenoma may burst focally (like a bud perforating the skin of a potato) through the thin mesodermal envelope (pituitary adenomas do not have a capsule) encasing the adenoma. In some cases, nodular outgrowths that originate from suprasellar component of the tumors result in a multilobulated adenoma that can further extend in a subfrontal, middle cranial fossa (without invasion into cavernous sinus), or retrosellar direction.

Invading Adenomas Nodular outgrowths arising from the intrasellar component of the adenoma may destroy adjacent structures by invading them. Those pituitary adenomas that invade directly into the cavernous sinus and/or adjacent skull base are often referred to as "invasive" pituitary adenomas. There is no rule enabling one to predict when invasion of the surrounding structures will begin. Invasion of the cavernous sinus may occur when the tumor is small and limited to the pituitary fossa (Fig. 13-1). On the other hand, some patients may have had very long histories of pituitary adenoma

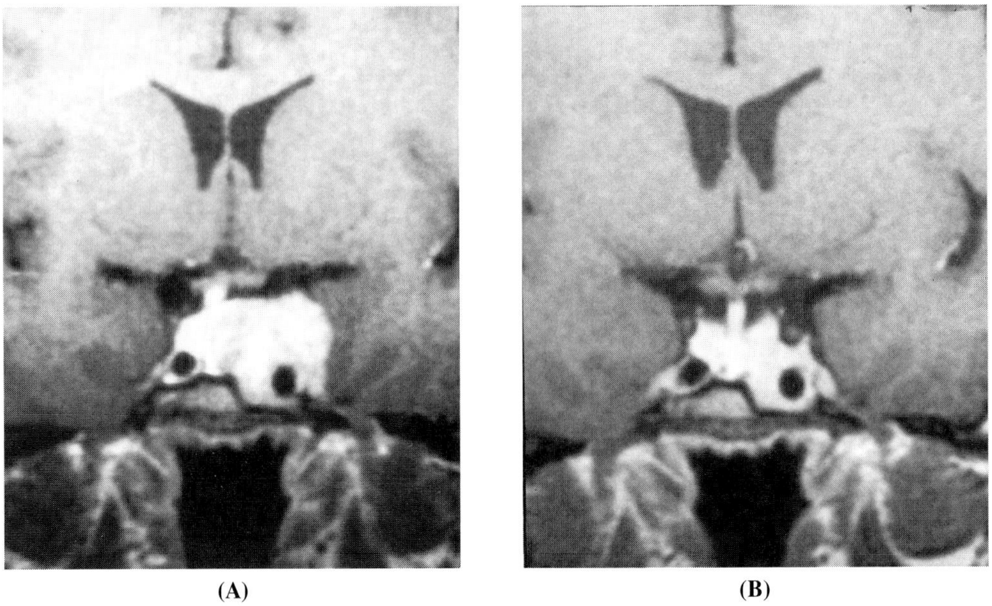

Figure 13-1 Pituitary adenoma (prolactinoma) extending into the left cavernous sinus. *A*. Postcontrast T1-weighted MRI shows mild expansion of the left cavernous sinus by the mass. Engulfment of the intracavernous internal carotid artery is readily visible. *B*. Postcontrast T1-weighted MRI 3 months after bromocriptine therapy shows marked reduction in the size of tumor.

before a diagnosis of cavernous sinus invasion is made. Most of the invasive pituitary adenomas have a benign microscopic appearance, which demonstrates the poor correlation between biologically aggressive behavior and histopathologic features.

Pituitary Carcinoma A review of the literature reveals a diversity of opinion with regard to nomenclature in connection with pituitary carcinomas. Several authors have indicated that such characteristics as increased cellularity, cellular pleomorphism, and the presence of mitotic features are not necessarily proof of malignancy. They believe that the diagnosis of pituitary carcinoma can be considered conclusive only when distant metastases occur. Other researchers consider anaplastic histopathologic features to be sufficient for the diagnosis of carcinoma.

Hemorrhage within Pituitary Adenomas Hemorrhage and/or infarction occurs in approximately 7 percent of pituitary adenomas. In half of these cases, the event is minor, without clinical presentation. In some instances, it may cause mild symptoms such as headaches. The hemorrhage is easily discovered with MRI (Fig. 13-2). In other cases, the clinical presentation of acute hemorrhage or infarct within the pituitary tumor is severe and characterized by headaches, ophthalmoplegia, meningismus, and alterations of mental status. Such a fulminating presentation is known as pituitary apoplexy. In a few of these patients, pituitary apoplexy may be the first manifestation of a pituitary adenoma. Pituitary apoplexy is an emergency situation. Compression of the optic nerves or chiasm may result in visual impairment, and impaction of the remaining functioning pituitary tissue may result in acute pituitary failure.

☐ INFLAMMATORY DISEASE OF THE PITUITARY

ACUTE

Pituitary Abscesses Purulent acute adenohypophysis is rare. Predisposing symptoms include sepsis, sinusitis, sphenoid osteomyelitis, cavernous sinus thrombophlebitis, meningitis, and the postoperative state after pituitary removal. Symptoms relating to pituitary abscess are often of much longer duration (compared with other types of intracranial abscesses). Such a relatively slow pathogenesis may allow for remodeling of the sella to occur. Computed tomography or MRI may show a sellar mass with a rim of enhancement. The clinical radiologic diagnosis of pituitary abscess may be quite difficult, and differential diagnosis includes a wide variety of intrasellar cysts and tumors.

CHRONIC

A variety of inflammatory processes such as sarcoidosis, fungal infections, tuberculosis, lymphocytic adenohypophysitis, and giant-cell granulomas may involve the

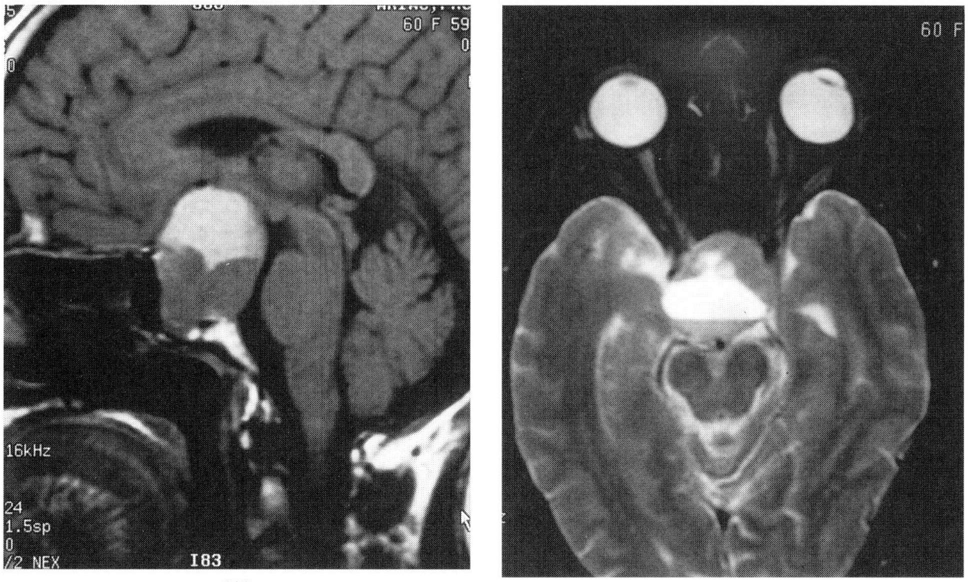

(A) (B)

Figure 13-2 Hemorrhagic pituitary adenoma. *A* and *B*. Sagittal T1- and axial T2-weighted images demonstrate a partially cystic sellar/suprasellar mass compressing the optic chiasm. The fluid-fluid level is best appreciated on T2-weighted MRI images. The supernatant contained free methemoglobin. The lower portion contained many red blood cells and cellular debris.

pituitary gland. Symptoms of pituitary insufficiency occur when 70 percent or more of the pituitary gland is destroyed.

- *Sarcoidosis of the CNS* has a predilection for the leptomeninges, although other areas such as the hypothalamus, optic chiasm, and pituitary gland may be involved. Histologically, noncaseating granulomas are composed of epithelial cells, lymphocytes, and reinstate Langerhans' giant cells, which may contain characteristic asteroid and Schaumann's bodies.
- *Giant-cell granuloma* of the pituitary is a rare disease that usually occurs in middle-aged women. Histologically, it is fairly similar to Boeck's sarcoidosis; unlike sarcoid, however, it is not a multiorgan disease.
- *Lymphocytic adenohypophysitis* is presumably an autoimmune disorder; it has been diagnosed primarily in women who were or had recently been pregnant. Lymphocytic adenohypophysitis may also present in women with no recent history of pregnancy, in postmenopausal women, and in men. Histologic study of the involved gland reveals a varying degree of infiltration by lymphocytes and other inflammatory cells as well as associated fibrotic changes. Multinucleated giant cells are absent in lymphocytic adenohypophysis. Similar inflammatory changes may also occur within pituitary adenomas secondary to necrosis, infarction, or hemorrhage inside the tumor. Such reactive changes may occasionally be so intense that it becomes difficult to differentiate complicated pituitary adenomas from adenohypophysitis even histopathologically.
- *Tuberculosis and fungal infections* of the pituitary gland are rare and may be spread either by the hematogenous route or by direct extension from tuberculous meningitis.

Imaging Findings of Lymphocytic Adenohypophysitis
Contrast-enhanced imaging is the best modality. Various combinations of findings may be seen:

1. The involved pituitary gland is usually isointense or minimally hyperintense relative to gray matter on precontrast T1-weighted images.
2. The posterior pituitary "bright spot" may be preserved.
3. Intense enhancement of a pituitary mass, which may be homogenous or heterogenous.
4. A dural tail—consisting of strips of abnormal enhancing tissue adjacent to the sella turcica—is often seen.
5. Abnormal enhancement along the posterior aspect of the infundibulum extending to the floor of the hypothalamus is commonly seen.
6. Extrapituitary components such as subarachnoid enhancing nodules, focal submucosal sphenoid sinus enhancement, or involvement of the cavernous sinus may be observed.

The MRI findings described above are not entirely specific and may be seen in complicated pituitary adenomas, metastasis to the pituitary, sarcoidosis, and various pituitary inflammations. Involvement of the cavernous sinus may result in narrowing of the cavernous portion of the internal carotid artery, mimicking, on MRI, features of Tolosa-Hunt syndrome.

☐ SUPRASELLAR LESIONS

Pituitary adenomas with suprasellar extension (discussed earlier in this chapter) are the most common suprasellar tumors in adults. Meningiomas are the second and craniopharyngiomas are the third most common suprasellar tumors. In children, craniopharyngiomas and hypothalamic/chiasmal gliomas are the two most common tumors in this location.

CRANIOPHARYNGIOMAS

Craniopharyngiomas are benign, but locally progressive tumors. They originate from remnants of Rathke's pouch. Some 70 percent of craniopharyngiomas are located in both intra- and suprasellar sites, 20 percent are suprasellar only, and 10 percent are found only in the intrasellar compartment. Rarely, occurrences within the sphenoid bone or the third ventricle have been reported. Craniopharyngiomas most commonly occur in children, representing 50 percent of all suprasellar tumors in children, but they may be seen in adults as well. Craniopharyngiomas are encapsulated tumors but are often adherent to adjacent structures (optic nerves and chiasm, hypothalamus, pituitary gland, and circle of Willis), which often makes their total resection difficult. Cystic changes and/or calcification within craniopharyngiomas are a very common occurrence (85 to 90 percent). Microscopically, the solid components of the tumor contain well-differentiated stratified squamous epithelium set in a stroma of connective tissue. On MRI, the solid component is inhomogeneous and shows variable contrast enhancement, whereas the cystic component may be lined by similar epithelial cells containing desquamated keratin, cellular debris, cholesterol crystals, lipids in solution, blood products, and protein. Various combinations of signal intensity patterns on T1- and T2-weighted MRI of craniopharyngiomas have been attributed to the composition of the cystic fluid. Correlation of MRI signal intensities and quantitative analysis of the cystic contents have shown that the increased signal intensity of cystic fluid on T1-weighted MRI can be caused by a high protein concentration, the presence of free methemoglobin, or both, whereas cholesterol and other lipids have no significant effect on MRI signal.

Hemorrhage within the cystic component of craniopharyngioma occasionally occurs. In the acute phase, the cystic tumor is fairly isointense on T1- and markedly hypointense on T2-weighted MRI relative to brain. Gradually, within several weeks after hemorrhage, the lysis of red blood cells occurs, releasing free methemoglobin into the cystic fluid and resulting in marked shortening of the cystic fluid on T1-weighted MRI. In addition to the effect of free methemoglobin on T2-weighted images, the release of the protein and water content of lysed red blood cells leads to T2 prolongation of hemorrhagic cyst fluid. Therefore, cyst fluid containing free methemoglobin becomes markedly hyperintense on both T1- and T2-weighted images.

In the absence of free methemoglobin and with protein concentrations of less than 9000 mg/dL, a cystic tumor is hypointense on T1- and hyperintense on T2-weighted images relative to brain. The protein concentrations of approximately 9000 to 10,000 mg/dL seem to be a turning point for significantly altering the T1 signal intensity from hypointensity to isointensity. Higher protein concentrations in the range of 10 to 30 percent in cyst fluid result in hyperintensity of signal on both T1- and T2-weighted images relative to brain.

At ultrahigh protein concentrations (over 30 percent), there is significant cross-linking between protein molecules; therefore, the consistency of the cyst fluid becomes more jellylike. T2 relaxation time is more sensitive than T1 relaxation time to these macromolecular changes. As a result, there are much more abrupt changes in the T2 signals. At ultra high protein concentration, cystic lesions with markedly reduced free water, the contents become markedly hypointense on T2-weighted images. The effect of lipids (in solution or crystal) on signal intensities, however, seems to be either minimal or insignificant (Fig. 13-3).

ASTROCYTOMA

Astrocytomas arising from the hypothalamus, optic nerve, chiasm, or optic tract account for 30 percent of suprasellar neoplasms in childhood. Approximately one-third of cases are associated with neurofibromatosis type I. Hypothalamic/chiasmal glioma is much less common in adults. Suprasellar astrocytomas are usually low-grade and most of them are of the juvenile pilocytic variety. Hypothalamic/chiasmal gliomas are often hypo- to isodense on CT, hypointense on T1-weighted and hyperintense on T2-weighted images. Enhancement of the tumor is frequently noted (on CT or MRI) following the administration of contrast. The differential diagnosis of hypothalamic/chiasmal gliomas includes Langerhans-cell histiocytosis; sarcoid involving the infundibular stalk; tuber cinereum, optic nerve, and chiasm; germinoma; and lymphoma. Biopsy may be necessary to establish the correct diagnosis.

MENINGIOMAS

Meningiomas arise from the tuberculum or diaphragma sellae and may grow downward into the pituitary fossa, or grow upward into suprasellar cisterns. On MRI, a depressed diaphragma sellae is seen in association with an enhancing mass or thickened diaphragma sellae.

On MRI, an enhancing suprasellar mass associated with thickened and/or depressed diaphragma sellae is suggestive of the diagnosis of meningioma; however, this sign is not always present. A truly intrasellar meningioma is rare.

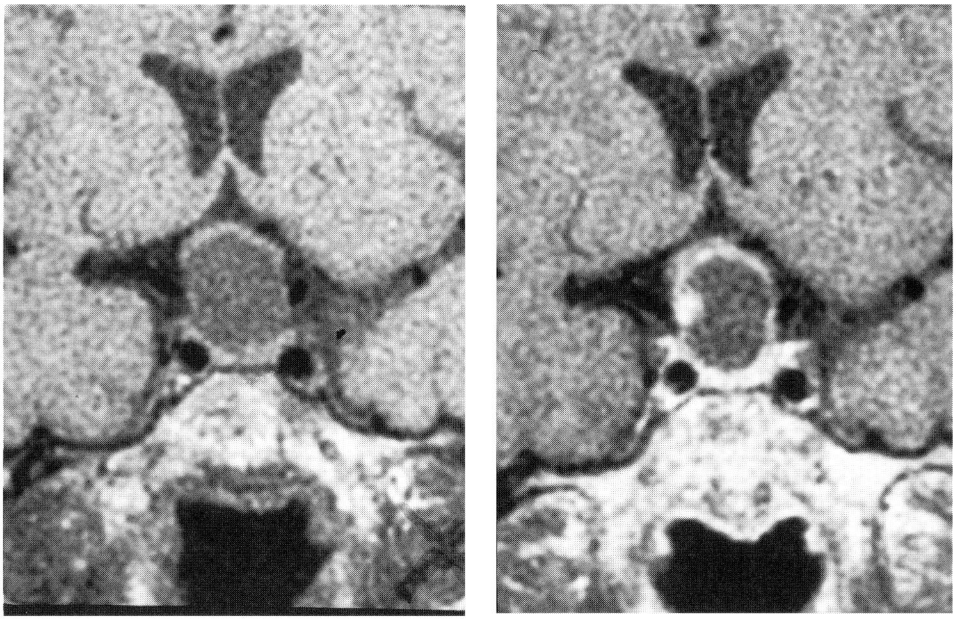

(A) (B)

Figure 13-3 Craniopharyngioma. *A* and *B*. Pre- and post-contrast coronal T1-weighted images (550/18) show a suprasellar cystic tumor compressing the optic chiasm. The mass is hypointense relative to the white matter, and its periphery enhances following contrast administration. Note that the mass can be distinguished from the pituitary gland, which is seen inferiorly within the sella turcica. Biochemical analysis of the cystic fluid revealed protein, 6800 mg/dL, and cholesterol, 805 mg/dL. Note that despite a high cholesterol level, the cystic mass remains hypointense relative to brain on the T1-weighted image.

ANEURYSMS

An aneurysm may arise from circle of Willis or cavernous internal carotid and then may project completely into the suprasellar cisterns and (rarely) into the sella turcica. On MRI or CT, most aneurysms in this region appear as well circumscribed sellar/suprasellar masses. The MRI signal intensity of aneurysms is variable and depends on the flow rate and the presence or absence of blood clots. A nonthrombosed aneurysm is readily diagnosed on MRI as a typical "flow void" mass. Heterogenous "rings inside rings" may be seen in thrombosed aneurysms.

SUPRASELLAR GERMINOMA AND TERATOMA

The sellar/suprasellar region is the second common site of intracranial germ-cell tumors. In 10 percent of such tumors, synchronous pineal and suprasellar foci are seen. Purely intrasellar germinoma is rare. In contrast with pineal germinoma, which is predominant in males, sellar/suprasellar germinoma is seen with equal frequency in males and females, usually before age 30. Diabetes insipidus, visual disturbances, and pituitary dysfunction are the common clinical presentations. Diabetes insipidus may precede other signs and symptoms by several years. Germinomas are isodense or slightly hyperdense on CT. On MRI, they often appear as a somewhat inhomogeneous sellar/suprasellar mass that is predominantly isointense with adjacent brain on T1-weighted and isointense or moderately hyperintense on T2-weighted images and they show strong contrast enhancement. Diagnosis of germinoma is usually confirmed by biopsy. Germinomas are very sensitive to radiotherapy and some of them rapidly disappear on follow-up CT or MRI.

EPIDERMOID

These lesions are developmental epithelial lesions resembling inclusion cysts. They are occasionally seen in the suprasellar cisterns, uncommon in the cavernous sinus, and rarely discovered in the pituitary fossa on imaging studies. In the suprasellar region, epidermoids are lobulated, frondlike, nonenhancing masses that are heterogenously hypointense on T1-weighted images and hyperintense on T2-weighted images relative to brain. The MRI signal intensity of epidermoid by comparison to that of CSF appears heterogenous (like a "dirty" CSF) on T1- and T2-weighted images. On CT, the density of epidermoid and CSF is similar.

HAMARTOMA OF THE TUBER CINEREUM

It is a rare developmental anomaly (heterotopia), usually discovered in childhood. Affected children present with clinical signs and symptoms of precocious puberty or, less commonly, with seizures. Other congenital anomalies such as callosal agenesis, optic malformations, and hemispheric heterotopias may be seen in association with hamartomas of the tuber cinereum.

Imaging Findings

- Pedunculated or sessile suprasellar mass involving the hypothalamus.
- On CT, a nonenhancing isodense mass.
- On MRI, an isointense mass on T1-weighted images, usually hyperintense on T2-weighted images relative to gray matter and nonenhancing.
- The posterior bright spot is usually preserved.

Differential Diagnosis Hypothalamic glioma. (Some hypothalamic gliomas do not enhance.)

INFUNDIBULAR LESIONS

The pituitary stalk (infundibulum) is a funnel-shaped structure that is normally 3 to 3.5 mm wide superiorly near the medial eminence and 2 mm wide inferiorly near its insertion on the pituitary gland. The infundibulum normally enhances strongly following intravenous administration of contrast. The infundibulum may be involved in a variety of inflammatory and neoplastic processes. In children, Langerhans'-cell histiocytosis, germinomas, and chronic meningiomas are the common causes of a thickened, abnormal infundibulum. In adults, sarcoidosis, germinoma, and metastasis are common. The underlying pathology is outlined in Table 13-3.

METASTASES

Metastases to the pituitary-hypothalamic axis are uncommon. They represent approximately 1 percent of sellar/suprasellar masses.

☐ CAVERNOUS SINUS NEOPLASMS

INVASIVE PITUITARY ADENOMA

Occasionally, a pituitary adenoma grows into the cavernous sinus by penetrating a thin dural wall that separates the pituitary gland from the cavernous sinus. In adults, invasive pituitary adenoma is the most common tumor seen in the cavernous sinus.

Incidence

- About 10 percent of all pituitary adenomas.

Pathology Most often shows benign histologic features.

Radiology

- Isodense on CT, isointense on T1- and T2-weighted MRI; modest but uniform enhancement.
- Combination of these findings may be seen on CT or MRI.

1. Continuity of tumor in the sella and cavernous sinus.
2. Cavernous sinus expansion.
3. Engulfment (but not encasement) of intracavernous internal carotid artery.
4. Partial obliteration of cavernous portion of gasserian ganglion.
5. Destruction of central skull base.

Table 13-3
CAUSES OF THICKENED PITUITARY STALK

Langerhans'-cell histiocytosis
Neurosarcoidosis
Germinoma
Lymphoma
Tuberculosis
Infiltration by adjacent neoplasms (pituitary adenomas, hypophyseal microgliomas)
Metastasis
Craniopharyngioma/Rathke's cleft cyst

MENINGIOMA

These tumors arise directly from the dural wall of the cavernous sinus or extend to the cavernous sinus from Meckel's cave. Meningiomas also may arise in the sphenoid bone, orbital apex, clinoid processes, clivus, or middle cranial fossa. In adults, meningioma is the second most common neoplasm of the cavernous sinus.

Incidence

- About 5 to 10 percent of intracranial meningiomas.

Radiology Any combinations of the following findings may be seen:

1. Hyperostosis and bony erosion are fairly common, but destructive changes are less common (better seen on CT).
2. Calcification in 20 to 25 percent (better seen on CT).
3. Most often hyperdense on CT, with strong, uniform enhancement.
4. Most often isointense with gray matter on both T1- and T2-weighted MRI with strong enhancement.
5. Narrowing and encasement of cavernous internal carotid artery (a feature distinguishing meningiomas from invasive pituitary adenomas).
6. Expansion of the involved cavernous sinus with extension along dural base and particularly along the medial tentorial edge (a distinctive feature).
7. Extension to orbits, Meckel's cave, and the perimesencephalic cistern.

SCHWANNOMA

Nerve sheath tumors comprise the third most common tumor in the cavernous sinus. Most schwannomas arise from the trigeminal ganglion, or trigeminal nerve affecting the cavernous sinus and Meckel's cave. Schwannomas of cranial nerves III, IV, and VI are rare. Plexiform neurofibromas are also rare and often infiltrate along cranial nerves V_1, V_2, and V_3.

Imaging

- Expansion of cavernous sinus.
- Erosion of adjacent bone.
- Compression and displacement of cavernous internal carotid (most often medially); encasement is uncommon.
- Iso- to hyperdense on CT with uniform enhancement.
- Most often mildly hypointense on T1-weighted images and hyperintense on T2-weighted images relative to brain and strongly enhance with contrast (Fig. 13-4).
- Hemorrhage or necrosis plus cystic changes and calcification within the tumor may occur, although these are fairly uncommon.
- Often, on MRI, the lateral dural wall of the cavernous sinus can be distinguished as a hypointense band from that of the tumor (a distinctive feature in differentiating the enhancement of schwannomas from that of meningiomas).

JUVENILE ANGIOFIBROMA

This is a highly vascular, markedly enhancing tumor that occurs in adolescent males. The tumor originates near the sphenopontine foramen and may extend to the cavernous sinus and orbits.

OSTEOCARTILAGINOUS TUMORS

Chordomas, osteochondroma, and chondrosarcoma may involve the cavernous sinus, but they are less common.

Radiologic Features

- Expansion of cavernous sinus.
- Calcification is very common.
- Erosion or destruction of adjacent bone is common.
- Mixed density on CT, heterogenous enhancement.
- Mixed intensity signal on T1- and T2-weighted MRI, with heterogenous enhancement.
- Encasement or displacement of the cavernous carotid may occur.

METASTASIS

Metastasis to the cavernous sinus may occur in two forms: via the hematogenous route or the perineural route. The third (mandibular) division of the trigeminal nerve, passing through the foramen ovale, is a common route of perineural spread of head and neck malignancies. Smooth thickening of cranial nerve V_3, concentric expansion of the foramen ovale, enlargement of the cavernous sinus, and atrophy of the masticator muscles are imaging findings that are commonly observed in perineural tumor extension to the cavernous sinus and into the middle cranial fossa.

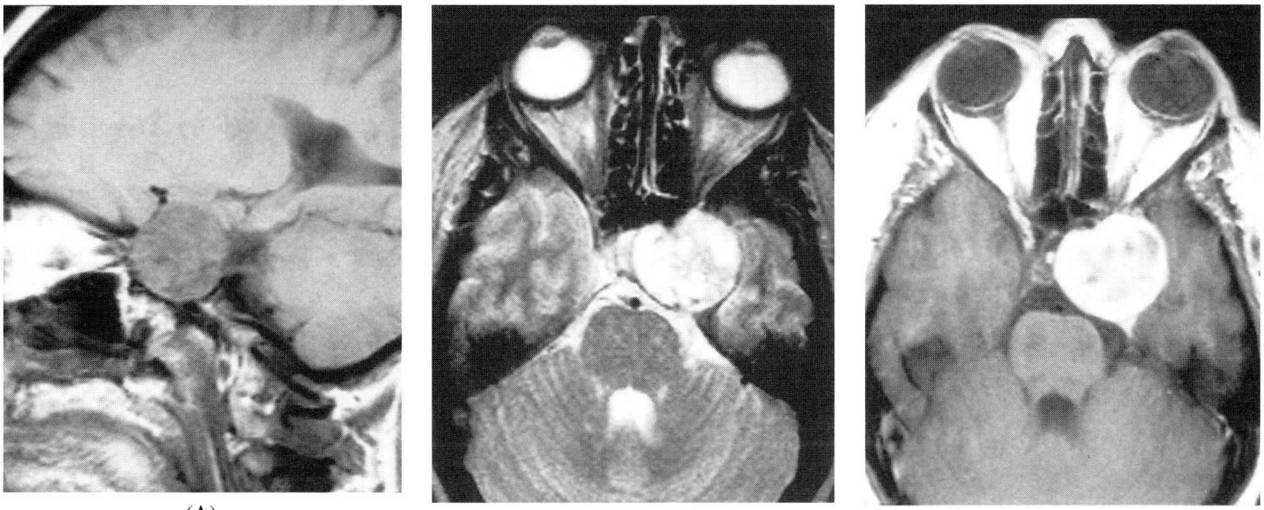

(A) (B) (C)

Figure 13-4 Schwannoma (trigeminal). On MRI, sagittal precontrast T1-weighted image (*A*), axial T2-weighted image (*B*), and axial postcontrast T-weighted image (*C*) show a mass in the left cavernous sinus. The tumor is hypointense relative to brain on T1-weighted images, heterogeneously hyperintense on T2-weighted images, and strongly enhanced following administration of contrast.

LYMPHOPROLIFERATIVE DISORDERS

Occurrence of lymphoma in the sellar/parasellar region is rare. Granulocytic sarcoma (chloroma) is associated with acute myeloid leukemia. Lymphoproliferative disorders are essentially isointense with brain on both T1- and T2-weighted images on MRI. They show some degree of contrast enhancement.

PARASELLAR CAVERNOUS HEMANGIOMAS

Parasellar cavernous hemangiomas may appear as a hyperdense masses on CT and may enhance markedly, simulating meningiomas. Cerebral angiography may not help to differentiate a parasellar cavernous hemangioma from a meningioma. It is very difficult to remove these tumors totally because they tend to be adherent to the cavernous sinus and may also bleed profusely.

☐ VASCULAR LESIONS OF CAVERNOUS SINUS

CAVERNOUS CAROTID ANEURYSMS

Approximately 3 to 5 percent of intracranial aneurysms occur in the cavernous portion of the internal carotid artery. They are more common in elderly women and frequently accompany ophthalmoplegia caused by compression of cranial nerves passing through the cavernous sinus. Rarely, they may rupture, leading to subarachnoid hemorrhage (SAH), carotid cavernous fistula, or fatal epistaxis. Intracavernous aneurysms less than 6 mm in diameter are often asymptomatic. Cavernous internal carotid aneurysms larger than 10 mm may extend into the cavernous sinus but are generally not associated with enlargement of the superior ophthalmic vein (a hallmark of carotid-cavernous fistula). On CT, partial or complete thrombosis of an intracavernous carotid artery aneurysm may demonstrate abnormal low-attenuation values within the enhancing cavernous sinus. The signal intensity of partially or completely thrombosed aneurysm is variable, depending on age of the thrombus. Magnetic resonance imaging of an unthrombosed aneurysm shows high-velocity signal loss within the lumen of the aneurysm (Fig. 13-5).

CAROTID-CAVERNOUS FISTULA

Carotid-cavernous fistula is an uncommon disorder. Spontaneous or traumatic rupture of the wall of the intracavernous segment of the internal carotid artery or its dural branches results in sudden shunting of the arterial blood into the cavernous sinus and hence into the orbital veins and other venous connections. Its dramatic ocular/orbital manifestations are principally due to altered regional hemodynamics and orbital venous hypertension. The eyes are at risk because of the potential development of ocular necrosis.

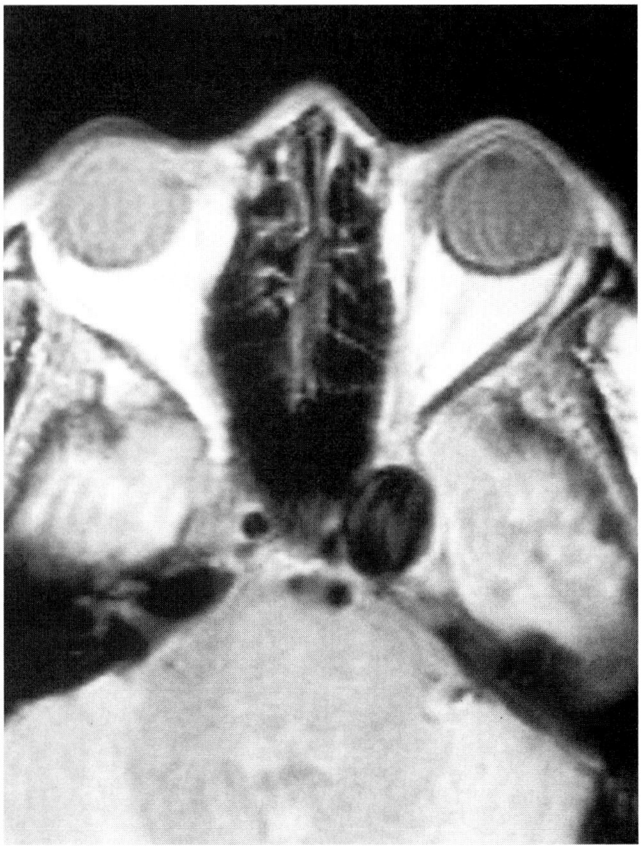

Figure 13-5 Intracavernous internal carotid artery aneurysm. High-velocity signal loss is seen within the lumen of the aneurysm. Some signal heterogeneity is seen due to turbulent blood flow in the aneurysm.

There is a rich venous network in the orbit. These venous channels are without valves and drain into the cavernous sinus. The superior ophthalmic vein is the major intraorbital vein, which interconnects with all other intraorbital veins. The diameter of the superior ophthalmic vein varies considerably in normal individuals, measuring 1 to 4 mm in diameter on CT or MRI. Under the continuous load of shunted or arterial blood (as in carotid cavernous fistula), the intraorbital veins dilate tremendously and their media thicken considerably. Tortuousity and dilation of the intraorbital veins are the hallmarks of CT and MRI findings in carotid-cavernous fistulas. Exophthalmos, periorbital swelling, and enlargement of the extraocular muscles due to congestion and edema of the intraorbital soft tissues are also frequently seen in CT and MRI studies of carotid cavernous fistula. Orbital findings on CT or MRI are nonspecific and may be seen in other conditions such as cellulitis, orbital varices, Graves' ophthalmopathy, acute orbital pseudotumors, and cavernous sinus thrombophlebitis. Focal bulging or distention of the cavernous sinus (as a result of altered hemodynamics) is another radiologic sign of carotid-cavernous fistula (Fig. 13-6*A*). This sign alone may also be seen in intracavernous internal carotid aneurysm, the tortuous cavernous portion of the internal

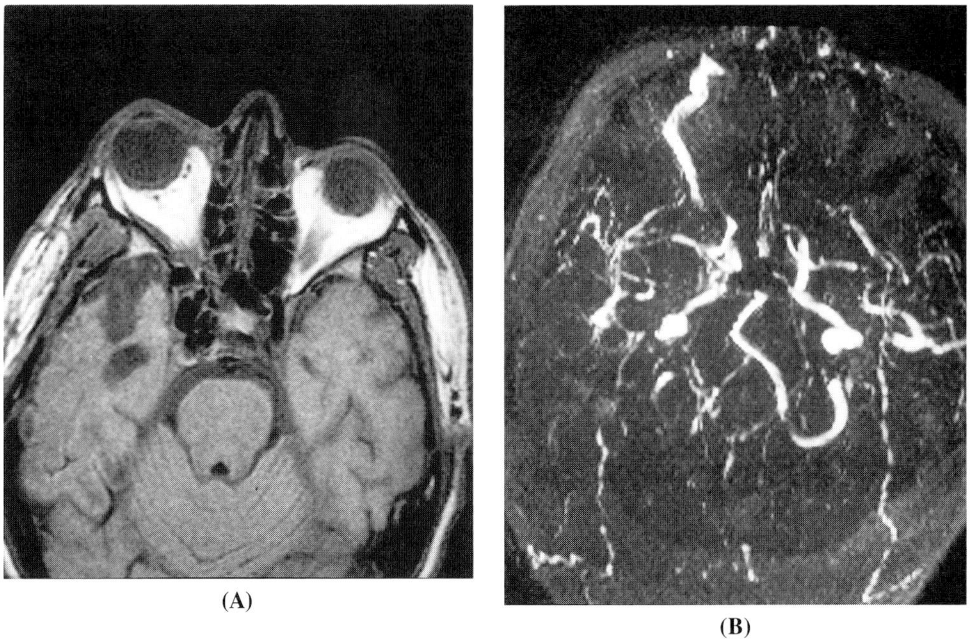

Figure 13-6 Carotid cavernous fistula. *A*. The right cavernous sinus is minimally larger than the left; it contains multiple foci of signal voids. *B*. Note high-velocity signal flow in the enlarged superior ophthalmic vein and right cavernous sinus as demonstrated by MR angiogram.

carotid artery, pituitary adenoma extending into the cavernous sinus, and primary or metastatic neoplasm involving the cavernous sinus. In this regard, MRI is superior to CT and can easily differentiate vascular lesions from solid tumors in the cavernous sinus by showing flow void in the expanded cavernous sinus and the superior ophthalmic vein. Magnetic resonance angiography readily establishes the diagnosis of carotid cavernous fistula (Fig. 13-6*B*). Selective cerebral catheter angiography (at the time of endovascular therapy) furnishes the details of circulatory status before embolization of the fistula.

Several factors alone or in combination may affect the CT or MRI manifestations of carotid-cavernous fistula: (1) time interval between trauma and commencement of fistula, (2) CT/MRI pattern of venous drainage, and (3) type of fistula. Since there is usually a delay of weeks or months between the traumatic incident and the clinical manifestation of carotid-cavernous fistula, it is likely that the development of the orbital and cavernous changes secondary to fistula is either slow or delayed. This would account for the occasional paucity of CT/MRI findings within the first few days after head trauma. If, in the presence of fistula, the intercommunicating venous channels are large enough to allow free flow of blood into the opposite side, both cavernous sinuses may expand and both eyes may become involved.

In most instances, the clinical picture of pulsating exophthalmos and chemosis with a distressing persistent bruit in the head is so striking that a confident diagnosis of carotid-cavernous fistula is made on the basis of the clinical manifestations alone. Occasionally, however, only part of the symptom complex is manifest, such as proptosis without bruit, presenting a diagnostic problem from a clinical standpoint. Either MRI or CT may play a useful role in the evaluation of unilateral or bilateral proptosis. When the superior ophthalmic vein is noted to be prominent, with focal bulging or distention of the cavernous sinus, carotid-cavernous sinus fistula must be considered. Magnetic resonance angiography often establishes the diagnosis. However, the definitive diagnostic test is catheter angiography.

CAVERNOUS SINUS THROMBOSIS

Spontaneous aseptic thrombosis of the cavernous sinus and/or its tributaries (particularly the superior ophthalmic vein) may occur in a preexisting carotid-cavernous sinus fistula (with or without cavernous sinus expansion). Such a development may cause abrupt proptosis, chemosis, and periorbital swelling, or it may exacerbate existing symptoms. If the underlying carotid-cavernous fistula has not been diagnosed previously, it would be difficult to differentiate it from septic cavernous sinus thrombosis. Clinically, the absence of fever and the signs and symptoms of meningeal irritation (commonly associated with septic cavernous sinus thrombosis) are useful clues. Cerebral angiography in this instance can establish the correct diagnosis by showing changes associated with the carotid-cavernous fistula.

☐ INFLAMMATORY DISEASES OF CAVERNOUS SINUS

CAVERNOUS SINUS THROMBOPHLEBITIS

Since the introduction of antibiotics, septic cavernous sinus thrombosis (thrombophlebitis) has become a rare disease. Pathologically in septic cavernous sinus thrombosis, infection of the orbital tissue, infiltration of the extraocular muscles with inflammatory cells, septic thrombi in the cavernous sinus and the superior ophthalmic veins, and meningitis have been reported. Contrast-enhanced CT can directly reveal thrombosis in the cavernous sinus as well as the associated orbital changes and will permit earlier diagnosis and vigorous treatment. Currently, experience with MRI is very limited. On CT, findings in patients with septic cavernous sinus thrombosis include multiple irregular filling defects (low attenuation) in enhancing cavernous sinuses. There may also be heterogenous enhancement of an enlarged superior ophthalmic vein, proptosis, and periorbital swelling. Narrowing or occlusion of the cavernous internal carotid artery and cerebral infarction associated with cavernous sinus thrombophlebitis also have been reported. Because of the rarity of this entity, MRI experience is currently very limited. However, early experience suggests that MRI is at least equal to contrast-enhanced CT in the diagnosis of cavernous sinus thrombosis.

TOLOSA-HUNT SYNDROME

This is a painful ophthalmoplegia caused by nonspecific cavernous sinus inflammation; it is responsive to steroid treatment. In some instances, patients with the clinical diagnosis of Tolosa-Hunt syndrome may have a normal CT or MRI study of the orbit and cavernous sinuses. However, in most cases, abnormal signal and/or mild enlargement of the affected cavernous sinus and/or intense enhancement is seen. A dural tail consisting of enhancing strips of dura is seen emanating from the affected cavernous sinus. Extension into the orbital apex may occur. Narrowing of the cavernous internal carotid artery may also be seen within enhancing cavernous sinus. The differential diagnosis includes meningioma, lymphoma, and sarcoidosis.

SUGGESTED READINGS

Anatomy and Physiology

1. Atwell WJ: The development of the hypophysis cerebre in men with special reference to the pars tuberalis. *Am J Anat* 37:159–193, 1926.
2. Colombo N, Berry I, Kucharczyk J et al: Posterior pituitary gland: appearance on MR imaging in normal and pathological states. *Radiology* 165:481–485, 1987.
3. Elster AD, Chen MY, Williams DW, Ley LL: Pituitary gland: MR imaging of physiologic hypertrophy in adolescence. *Radiology* 174:681–685, 1990.
4. Kucharczyk W, Leninski RE, Kucharczyk J, Henkelman RM: The effect of phospholipid vesicles on the NMR relaxation of water: An explanation for the MR appearance of the neurohypophysis? *AJNR* 11:693–700, 1990.
5. Mark LP, Haughton VM, Hendrix LE et al: High-intensity signals within the posterior pituitary fossa: a study with fat-suppression MR techniques. *AJNR* 12:929–932, 1991.
6. Page RB: Hypothalamic control of anterior pituitary function: surgical implications, in Wilkins RH, Rengachary SS (eds): *Neurosurgery.* New York, McGraw-Hill, pp 791–804, 1995.
7. Pearse AGE, Takor TT: Neuroendocrine and the APUD concept. *Clin Endocrinol* 5:229s-244s, 1976.

Pituitary Anomalies

1. Armstrong EA, Harwood-Nash DC, Hoffman et al: Benign suprasellar cysts: The CT approach. *AJNR* 4:163–166, 1983.
2. Crenshaw WB, Chew FS: Rathke's cleft cyst. *AJR* 158:1312, 1992.
3. Itoh J, Usui K: An entirely suprasellar symptomatic Rathke's cleft cyst: case report. *Neurosurgery* 30:581–585, 1992.
4. Kuroiwa, Okabe Y, Hasuo K et al: MR imaging of pituitary hypertrophy due to juvenile primary hyperthyroidism: A case report. *Clin Imaging* 15:202–205, 1991.
5. Lloyd RV: Non-neoplastic pituitary lesions, including hyperplasia. In Lloyd RV (ed): *Surgical Pathology of the Pituitary Gland.* Philadelphia, Saunders pp 25–33, 1993.
6. Miki Y, Asato R, Okumura R, et al: Anterior pituitary gland in pregnancy: Hyperintensity at MR. *Radiology* 187:229–231, 1993.
7. Ross DA, Norman D, Wilson CB: Radiologic characteristics and results of surgical management of Rathke's cleft cysts in 43 patients.
8. Voelker JL, Campbell RL, Muller J: Clinical, radiographic, and pathologic features of symptomatic Rathke's cleft cysts. *J Neurosurg* 74:535–544, 1991.
9. Warner NE: Pituitary gland. In Kissane JM (ed): Anderson's Pathology. St Louis, Mosby-Yearbook, pp 1517–1543, 19??.

Pituitary Neoplasms

1. Ahmadi J, North C, Segall HD, Zee CS, Weiss MH: Cavernous sinus invasion by pituitary adenomas. *AJNR* 6:893–898, 1985.
2. Kovacs K, Horvath E, Asa SL: Classification and pathology of pituitary tumors in neurosurgery. In Wilkins RH, Rengachary (eds): *Neurosurgery.* New York, McGraw-Hill, pp 795–804, 1995.
3. Loes DJ, Barloon TJ, Yuh WTC, et al: MR anatomy and pathology of the hypothalamus. *AJR* 156:579–585, 1991.

4. Okazaki H. Neoplastic and related conditions. In *Fundamentals of Neuropathology,* 2d ed. Tokyo, Igaku-Shoin, 203–274, 1989.
5. Rausching W, Osborn AG: Sellar/suprasellar masses. In Osborn AG (ed): *Diagnostic Neuroradiology.* St. Louis, Mosby-Yearbook, pp 461–528.
6. Shucart WA, Jackson IMD: Anatomy and physiology of the neurohypophysis. In Wilkins RH, Rengachary, (eds): *Neurosurgery* New York, McGraw-Hill, pp 805–811, 1995.
7. Sugiyama K, Uozumi T, Kiya K et al: Intracranial germ-cell tumor with synchronous lesions in the pineal and suprasellar regions: Report of six cases and review of the literature. *Surg Neurol* 38:114–120, 1993.
8. Tindall GT, Kovacs K, Horvath E, Thorner MO: Human prolactin-producing adenomas and bromocriptine: A histological, immunocytochemical, ultrastructural, and morphometric study. *J Clin Endocrinol Metab* 55:1178–1183, 1982.
9. Wakai S, Fukushima T, Teratomo A, Sano K: Pituitary apoplexy: Its incidence and clinical significance. *J Neurosurg* 55:187–193, 1981.

Pituitary Inflammations

1. Ahmadi J, North C, Segall HD, Sharma C, Hinton D: Lymphocytic adenohypophysitis: contrast enhanced MR imaging in five cases. *Radiology* 195:30–34, 1995.
2. Cosman F, Post KD, Holub DA, Wardlaw SL: Lymphocytic hypophysitis: Report of 3 new cases and review of the literature. *Medicine* 68:240–256, 1989.
3. Enzman DR et al: CT of pituitary abscesses. *AJNR* 4:79–80, 1983.
4. Hashimoto M, Yanaki T, Nakara N, Masuzawa T: Lymphocytic adenohypophysitis: an immunohistochemical study. Surg Neurol 36:137–144, 1991.
5. Higuchi M, Arita N, Mori S et al: Pituitary granuloma and chronic inflammation of hypophysis: Clinical and immunohistochemical studies. *Acta Neurochir* 121:152–158, 1993.
6. Levine SN, Benzel EC, Fowler MR, Shroyer JV, Mirfakhraee M: Lymphocytic adenohypophysitis: Clinical, radiological, and magnetic resonance imaging characterization. *Neurosurgery* 22:937–941, 1988.
7. Scott TF: Neurosarcoidosis: progress and clinical aspects. *Neurology* 43:8–12, 1993.
8. Seltzer S, Mark AS, Atlas SW: CNS sarcoidosis: Evaluation with contrast enhanced MR imaging. *AJNR* 12:1227–1233, 1991.
9. Sherman JL, Stern BJ: Sarcoidosis of the CNS: Comparison of unenhanced and enhanced MR imaged. *AJNR* 11:915–923, 1990.

Suprasellar Lesions

1. Ahmadi J, Destian S, Apuzzo MLJ et al: Cystic fluid in craniopharyngiomas: MR imaging and quantitative analysis. *Radiology* 182:783–785, 1992.
2. Ahmadi J, Savabi F, Apuzzo MLJ, Hinton D, Segall HD: Magnetic resonance imaging and quantitative analysis of intracranial cystic lesions; surgical implications. *Neurosurgery* 35:199–207, 1994.
3. Boyko OB, Curnes JT, Oakes WJ, Burger PC: Hamartomas of the tuber cinereum: CT, MR, and pathologic findings. *AJNR* 12:309–314, 1991.
4. Fujisawa I, Asato R, Okumura R et al: Magnetic resonance imaging of neurohypophyseal germinomas. *Cancer* 68: 1009–1014, 1991.
5. Maghnie M, Arico M, Villa A et al: MR of the hypothalamic pituitary axis in Langerhans cell histiocytosis. *AJNR* 13:1365–1371, 1993.
6. Michael AS, Paige ML: MR imaging of intrasellar meningioma stimulating pituitary adenomas. *JCAT* 12:949–956, 1988.
7. Rosenfield NS, Abrahams J, Komp D: Brain MR in patients with Langerhans cell histiocytosis: Findings and enhancement with Gd-DTPA. *Pediatric Radiol* 20:433–436, 1990.
8. Schubiger O, Haller D: Metastases to the pituitary-hypothalamic axis. *Neuroradiology* 34:131–134, 1992.
9. Simmons GE, Suchnicki JE, Rak KM, Damiano TR: MR imaging of the pituitary stalk: Size, shape, and enhancement pattern. *AJR* 159:375–377, 1992.
10. Stull MA, Kransdorf MJ, Devaney KO: Langerhans cell histiocytosis of bone. *RadioGraphics* 12:801–823, 1992.
11. Takeuhi J, Handa H, Nagata I: Suprasellar germinoma. *J Neurosurg* 49:41–48, 1978.
12. Taylor SL, Barakos JA, Harsh R IV, Wilson CB: Magnetic resonance imaging of tuberculum sellae meningiomas: preventing preoperative misdiagnosis as pituitary adenomas. *Neurosurgery* 31:621–627, 1992.
13. Tien RD, Newton TH, McDermott MW et al: Thickened pituitary stalk on MR images in patients with diabetes insipidus and Langerhans cell histiocytosis. *AJNR* 11:703–708, 1990.
14. Tien RD, Kucharczyk J, Kuchaczyk W: MR imaging of the brain in patients with diabetes insipidus. *AJNR* 12:533–542, 1991
15. Zimmerman RA: Imaging of intrasellar, suprasellar, and parasellar tumors. *Semin Roentgenol* 25:174–197, 1990.

Cavernous Sinus

1. Ahmadi J, Teal JS, Segall HD, Zee CS, Han JS, Becker TS: Computed tomography of carotid cavernous fistula. *AJNR* 4(2):131–135, 1983.
2. Ahmadi J, Keane JR, Segall HD, Zee CS: CT observations pertinent to septic cavernous sinus thrombosis. *Am J Neuroradiol* 5:755–758, 1985.
3. Ahmadi J, Miller CA, Segall HD, Park S, Zee CS: CT patterns in histopathologically complex cavernous hemangiomas. *Am J Neuroradiol* 6:389–393, 1985.
4. Celli P, Ferrante L, Acqui M et al: Neuromas of the third, fourth, and sixth cranial nerves: a survey and report of a new fourth nerve case. *Surg Neurol* 38:216–224, 1992.
5. Ellie E, Houang B, Lovall C et al: CT and high field MRI in septic thrombosis of the cavernous sinuses. *Neuroradiology* 34:22–24, 1992.
6. Laine FJ, Braun IF, Jensen ME et al: Perineural tumor extension through the foramen ovale: evaluation with MR imaging. *Radiology* 174:65–71, 1980.
7. Parker GD, Harnsberger HR: Clinical-radiologic issues in perineural tumor spread of malignant disease of the extracranial head and neck. *RadioGraphics* 11:383–399, 1991.
8. Sham JST, Cheung YK, Choy D et al: Nasopharyngeal carcinoma: CT evaluation of patterns of tumor spread. *AJNR* 12:265–270, 1991.
9. Youssem DM, Atlas SW, Grossman RI, Sergott RC, Savino PJ, Bosley TM: MR imaging of Tolosa-Hunt syndrome. *AJNR* 10:1181–1184, 1989.
10. Yuh WTC, Wright DC, Barlan TJ et al: MR imaging of primary tumor of trigeminal nerve and Meckel's cave. *AJNR* 9:665–670, 1988.
11. Freedy RM, Miller KD, Jr. Granulocytic sarcoma (chloroma): Sphenoidal sinus and paraspinal involvement as evaluated by CT and MR. *AJNR* 12:259–262, 1991.
12. Fukisawa I, Asato R, Okumura R et al: Magnetic resonance imaging of neurohypophyseal germinomas. *Cancer* 68:1009–1014, 1991.

☐ QUESTIONS (True or False)

1. Regarding "empty sella,"
   a. Empty sella generally has no clinical significance, but exceptions do exist.
   b. Coexistence of pituitary microadenoma and empty sella has occasionally been reported.
   c. The sella turcica is usually normal in size.
   d. The infundibulum stalk follows its normal course.
   e. It may be due to incompetent diaphragm sella or prior surgery.

2. Regarding Rathke's cleft cysts,
   a. They are lined by columnar or cuboidal epithelium.
   b. Cyst fluid within the Rathke's cleft cyst is similar to CSF.
   c. Hemorrhage may occur in the cyst.
   d. A thin rim of contrast enhancement of the cyst wall may be seen.
   e. The majority of Rathke's cleft cysts are both intra- and suprasellar in location.

3. Regarding microadenoma,
   a. Pituitary microadenomas are less than 15 mm in diameter.
   b. The majority of pituitary microadenomas are solid.
   c. Hemorrhage, necrosis, or cystic changes may occur in approximately 10 percent of pituitary adenomas.
   d. Typically, microadenomas enhance homogeneously with contrast.
   e. Calcification is uncommon.

4. Regarding craniopharyngiomas,
   a. They originate from remnants of Rathke's pouch.
   b. The majority of craniopharyngiomas are located in both intra- and suprasellar regions.
   c. Craniopharyngioma is never seen in the third ventricle.
   d. Cystic changes and/or calcification are commonly seen.
   e. Hemorrhage is occasionally seen within craniopharyngiomas.

5. Regarding suprasellar germinoma,
   a. In 10 percent of intracranial germ-cell tumors, synchronous pineal and suprasellar foci are seen.
   b. Purely intrasellar germinoma is rare.
   c. There is no sex predilection for suprasellar germinoma.
   d. Diabetes insipidus, visual disturbances, and pituitary dysfunction are common clinical presentations.
   e. Germinomas are usually radiotherapy-resistant.

☐ ANSWERS

1. a. T
   b. T
   c. F
   d. T
   e. T

2. a. T
   b. F
   c. T
   d. T
   e. T

3. a. F
   b. T
   c. T
   d. T
   e. T

4. a. T
   b. T
   c. F
   d. T
   e. T

5. a. T
   b. T
   c. T
   d. T
   e. F

CHAPTER

14 Intracranial Infection

Sylvie Destian

Intracranial infection occurs as a result of either hematogenous dissemination from a remote focus or from direct extension (e.g., from the paranasal sinuses, the temporal bone, or trauma).

The role of radiologic imaging in the evaluation of intracranial infection is to identify the location—leptomeningeal, parenchymal, or both—and extent of infection, to determine what if any complications or sequelae of infection are present, and to follow patients during treatment.

☐ MENINGITIS

Meningitis is an inflammation of the leptomeninges and subarachnoid space. It can be caused by a number of factors, including bacterial and fungal organisms, viruses, neoplasm, blood, granulomatous processes, or chemical irritants. The diagnosis is usually made clinically. Morbidity and mortality are high, most likely because of the nonspecificity of signs and symptoms as well as the relative lack of radiologic findings in the early stages. Mortality can be as high as 30 percent and morbidity following meningitis caused by certain organisms such as *Haemophilus influenzae* has been reported at between 30 and 50 percent. Therefore it is important for the neuroradiologist to recognize the earliest signs of infection as well as the sequelae.

The clinical presentation is similar in acute pyogenic, acute lymphocytic, and chronic meningitis. The most common signs and symptoms include fever, headache, nuchal rigidity, photophobia, seizures, cranial nerve palsies, and altered level of consciousness.

Computed tomography (CT) and magnetic resonance imaging (MRI) will initially demonstrate no abnormality of the subarachnoid spaces. Subacute findings include leptomeningeal enhancement and areas of low density in the parenchyma, which may or may not enhance. Pathologically, these areas of low density represent areas of infarction and subsequent necrosis secondary to focal vasculitis. They rarely represent cerebritis.

Complications of meningitis include hydrocephalus, atrophy, subdural empyema (more common in children, secondary to necrosis of the arachnoid), ventriculitis, infarction (secondary to leptomeningeal vessel congestion, cortical vein thrombosis, or vasculitis), and encephalomalacia (secondary to infarction).

ACUTE PYOGENIC MENINGITIS

Most cases of acute pyogenic meningitis are caused by *H. influenzae*, *Neisseria meningitidis*, and *Streptococcus pneumoniae*. *Haemophilus influenzae* is most frequently seen in children under the age of 7 who have a concurrent otitis media or pharyngitis. It is currently the most common cause of meningitis in the United States. *Neisseria meningitidis* is seen in children and young adults, while *S. pneumoniae* is the most common cause of bacterial meningitis in adults. The source can be otitis media, pneumonia, mastoiditis, sinusitis, or endocarditis. *Streptococcus pneumoniae* is the most common cause of meningitis following head trauma even in the absence of a cerebrospinal fluid (CSF) leak. Gram-negative meningitis caused by *Klebsiella*, *Escherichia coli*, or *Pseudomonas aeruginosa* can be seen in immunosuppressed patients, patients who have had head trauma or neurosurgery, and neonates. The CSF is cloudy and demonstrates a high neutrophil count, elevated protein, and decreased glucose.

Imaging studies are usually normal, but diffuse meningeal enhancement, hydrocephalus, subdural effusions, and infarcts are among the findings that may be seen.

ACUTE LYMPHOCYTIC MENINGITIS

Acute lymphocytic meningitis is usually a benign, self-limited illness with signs and symptoms similar to but less severe than those of bacterial meningitis. It is usually viral in origin. Enteroviruses (echoviruses, coxsackievirus) and mumps are the most common causes of viral meningitis, but other causes include herpes simplex types I and II, arboviruses, Epstein-Barr virus, and human immunodeficiency virus (HIV). The CSF is clear and demonstrates a lymphocytic pleocytosis, moderately elevated protein, and normal glucose.

As with acute bacterial meningitis, imaging studies are usually normal, although meningeal enhancement and the sequelae of meningitis may be seen.

CHRONIC MENINGITIS

Chronic meningitis is an indolent form of meningitis most commonly caused by hematogenous spread of pulmonary *Mycobacterium tuberculosis*. Less common causes of chronic meningitis include *Cryptococcus neoformans*, *Coccidioides immitis*, *Treponema pallidum*, *Brucella*, and *Candida*.

Chronic meningitis is characterized by a gelatinous exudate within the basal cisterns and sylvian fissures. The exudate contains chronic inflammatory cells and may cause a fibrous arachnoiditis. Sequelae include hydrocephalus, small-vessel occlusion resulting in infarction, and cranial nerve palsies.

Examination of the CSF in chronic meningitis will demonstrate an elevated protein level, a decreased glucose level, and a moderate pleocytosis of monocytes and neutrophils.

Unenhanced CT and MRI may demonstrate a thickened dura, which will appear isodense on CT and isointense on MRI. Contrast-enhanced CT and MRI studies demonstrate enhancement within the basal cisterns and sylvian fissures, which can persist long after treatment.

DIFFERENTIAL DIAGNOSIS OF MENINGITIS

Computed tomography and MRI are helpful in the differential diagnosis of the following entities:

Meningeal Carcinomatosis As in patients with meningitis, noncontrast CT and MRI in patients with meningeal carcinomatosis may be normal or may demonstrate subtle effacement of sulci, high density or signal within the sulci, or hydrocephalus. On contrast-enhanced images, smooth and/or nodular, diffuse leptomeningeal enhancement can be seen.

Sarcoidosis. Central nervous system (CNS) involvement is seen in up to 15 percent of patients with known systemic sarcoidosis. There are two basic patterns of involvement, but chronic basilar meningitis is the most common. Communicating hydrocephalus may develop as a result of the chronic basilar meningitis.

Less commonly, patients with CNS sarcoidosis can present with parenchymal nodules, usually involving basal structures such as the hypothalamus, thalamus, pituitary stalk, and optic chiasm. This is usually associated with extensive arachnoiditis. In addition, infarction can occur secondary to spread of the disease along the Virchow-Robin spaces, resulting in invasion and thrombosis of blood vessels. The nodules may be calcified and usually appear isointense on MRI or hyperdense on CT. They enhance homogeneously and are not usually associated with edema.

Subarachnoid Hemorrhage Following subarachnoid hemorrhage, noncontrast CT may demonstrate hydrocephalus and either effacement of or high density within the cortical sulci and basal cisterns. Noncontrast T1-weighted MRI may demonstrate similar findings. If contrast is inadvertently given to a patient with subarachnoid hemorrhage without a noncontrast study for comparison, subarachnoid blood may be mistaken for enhancement. In addition, if contrast is given to a patient who has had a recent subarachnoid hemorrhage, the leptomeninges may enhance smoothly.

☐ FOCAL LESIONS

PYOGENIC BRAIN ABSCESS

Source of Infection The most common cause of an intracranial abscess is through hematogenous spread from an extracranial source, most commonly the lung, although any transient bacteria may cause intracranial infection. Abscess formation can also occur as a result of retrograde thrombophlebitis from adjacent infection of the paranasal sinuses or mastoid air cells. Children with cyanotic heart disease have a 3 to 11 percent incidence of intracranial abscess. Congenital or acquired breaches in the dura are a less common source of spread of infection. Except in the immunocompromised patient, most intracranial abscesses are solitary lesions.

Most abscesses are caused by pyogenic bacteria; in one-third of cases, more than one organism is responsible. The most frequent organisms isolated from abscesses in adults are aerobic and anaerobic streptococci and staphylococci. In neonates, the most frequent organisms isolated are *Citrobacter*, *Proteus*, *Serratia*, *Pseudomonas*, and *Staphylococcus.* In 20 percent of patients, the source of the infection is not determined.

Evolution Cerebral abscesses develop from focal areas of cerebritis occurring at the corticomedullary junction. Pathologically, early cerebritis lasts from 3 to 5 days and is characterized by vascular congestion, petechial hemorrhage, and edema. If untreated, this eventually results in brain softening and liquefaction necrosis, which characterizes the late stage of cerebritis and lasts from 5 to 14 days. During the early capsular phase, endothelial cells from blood vessels in the cortical gray matter produce fibroblasts that migrate to the area of cerebritis and form the middle wall of the abscess capsule. During the late capsular phase, which lasts from a few weeks to months, more collagen is produced and the abscess wall becomes complete. The inner wall is composed of granulation tissue; the outer wall is composed of glial cells. The abscess capsule is weakest medially because the fibroblasts migrate from the periphery. As the abscess heals, the cavity shrinks.

The area of cerebritis will appear hypointense on T1-weighted images and hyperintense on T2-weighted images, secondary to inflammation and edema. The periphery of the abscess capsule will appear hypointense on T2-weighted images secondary to the presence of debris-laden macrophages. The capsule will enhance with contrast (Fig. 14-1).

Complications Complication of cerebral abscesses include rupture of the abscess cavity, resulting in ventriculitis, meningitis or daughter abscesses, although ventriculitis and meningitis may develop in the presence of an unruptured abscess. Meningitis can occur as a result of direct inflammation of the leptomeninges from an adjacent abscess. Ventriculitis can occur as a complication of meningitis or the placement of a ventricular catheter.

Differential Diagnosis *Glioma* Anaplastic astrocytoma may present as a ring-enhancing lesion with a variable amount of surrounding edema. Classically, the rim enhances uniformly and may be of uniform or irregular thickness. It is not usually thinner medially. Generally, individuals with a primary brain neoplasm will lack the constitutional symptoms associated with abscesses.

Metastasis As with primary brain tumors, metastatic tumors typically have a uniformly enhancing rim and a variable amount of surrounding edema.

Granulomatous Abscess Tuberculomas may present as small iso- or hyperdense homogeneously or ring-enhancing lesions with surrounding edema. True granulomatous abscesses are rare. They are generally hypodense and demonstrate thick ring enhancement, which is difficult to differentiate from a pyogenic abscess.

Infarct Infarcts typically enhance in a gyriform pattern, although ring enhancement can be seen. The clinical picture, location in a vascular distribution, and evolution on follow-up imaging studies should help to differentiate infarct from abscess.

Subacute Hematoma on Computed Tomography Subacute hematomas will demonstrate ring enhancement on contrast CT. As with infarcts and tumors, however, the clinical picture, lack of constitutional symptoms, and evolution on follow-up studies should distinguish hematomas from abscess.

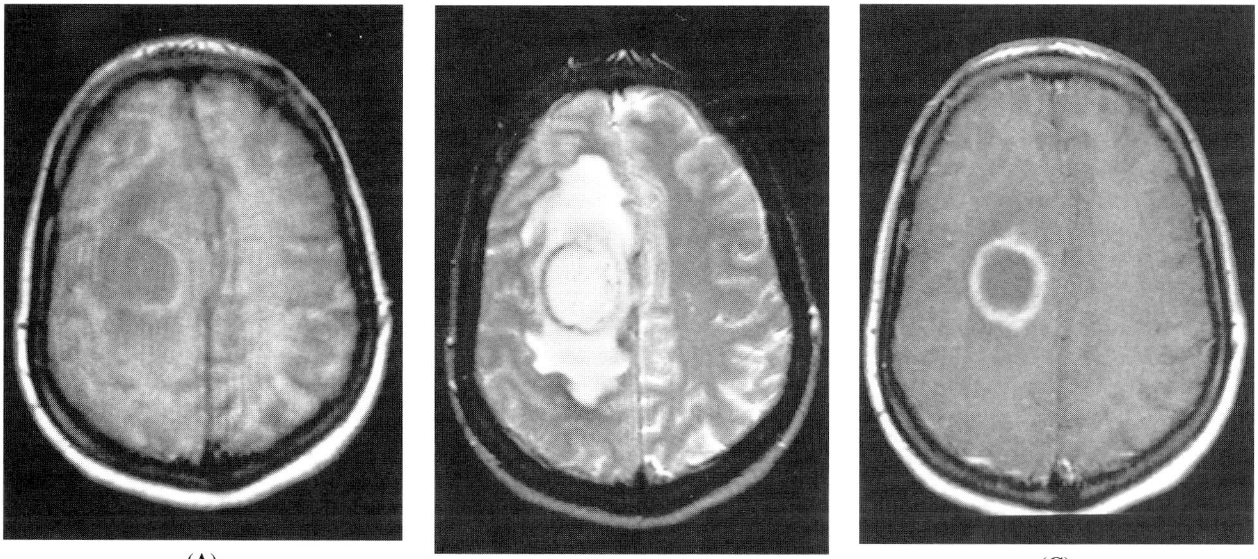

(A) (B) (C)

Figure 14-1 Bacterial abscess caused by *Staphylococcus aureus*. *A*. T1-weighted axial image shows a low-signal-intensity lesion with a peripheral rim of hyperintensity and surrounding edema in the left posterior frontal lobe. *B*. T2-weighted axial image shows a low-signal-intensity rim with central hyperintensity and surrounding hyperintense edema. *C*. Postcontrast T1-weighted axial image shows a relatively smooth, ringlike enhancement with central hypointensity and surrounding edema.

TUBERCULOSIS

Source of Infection Tuberculous meningitis is the result of hematogenous spread of bacilli from a primary lesion in the thorax or genitourinary tract or from direct extension from an intracerebral focus.

Evolution The meningeal exudate, which is frequently seen in the basal cisterns, tends to be thick and adhesive. The basal cisterns and sylvian fissures may be partially or completely obscured by the presence of this purulent exudate and/or inflammatory tissue on unenhanced CT and MRI. Intense enhancement is seen following contrast infusion. Parenchymal nodules (tuberculoma) are also seen with CNS tuberculosis. Definitive diagnosis of tuberculoma may be difficult, since more than 50 percent of patients with intracranial tuberculomas have no evidence of extracranial disease. Generally, tuberculomas are ring-enhancing, although nodular and irregular enhancement has been seen. Old tuberculomas often calcify.

Complications Communicating hydrocephalus may result from obstruction at the level of the basal cisterns. Arteritis involving vessels at the base of the brain or in the sylvian fissures commonly results from surrounding meningeal inflammation. Cerebral infarction may result from arterial and venous involvement.

NOCARDIA

Although controversy still exists as to whether *Nocardia* is a bacterium or a fungus, it is generally considered to be a filamentous bacterium. *Nocardia asteroides* accounts for approximately 90 percent of the roughly 1000 cases diagnosed in the United States each year. The incidence is two to three times higher in men and highest in the fourth through sixth decades. Some 20 percent of patients have no known predisposing factor. In 30 percent, a defect in cellular immunity is suspected. In the remaining 50 percent, a known predisposing factor is present, including immunosuppression, steroid therapy, lymphoma, leukemia, diabetes, collagen-vascular disease, and sarcoid.

The lungs are the most common organ affected (75 percent), followed by the brain (25 to 33 percent) and kidney. The infection is acquired by inhalation of spores and spread hematogenously. Mortality ranges from 20 to 40 percent; the higher mortality is seen in patients with CNS involvement.

Histopathologically, nocardiosis is characterized by multiple or confluent abscesses that may undergo cavitation and necrosis. The organism is visible with Gram's stain or Gomori's methenamine-silver stain. Contrast-enhanced CT and MRI studies demonstrate ring-enhancing lesions similar to pyogenic abscesses or metastases. Indium-111-labeled leukocytes have been used to differentiate nocardial (as well as other) abscesses from metastases.

FUNGUS

Although fungal infections of the CNS are rare, they are increasing in frequency, in part due to an increase in antibiotic use and in part due to the increasing numbers of immunocompromised individuals, particularly patients with acquired immunodeficiency syndrome (AIDS). Fungal pathogens that cause infection in immunocompetent individuals include *Histoplasma*, *Blastomyces*, and *Coccidioides*. Most opportunistic infections in immunocompromised patients are caused by *Aspergillus fumigatus*, *Candida albicans*, *Cryptococcus neoformans*, and *Rhizopus arrhizus*.

Histoplasmosis Histoplasmosis is found worldwide, but infection usually occurs in endemic areas, such as the valleys of the Ohio and Mississippi rivers. It is acquired by inhalation, and although it is usually asymptomatic in immunocompetent hosts, symptomatic individuals exhibit flulike symptoms. Dissemination is rare in healthy individuals but can be seen in immunocompromised patients, infants, and old people. In endemic areas, it is a common opportunistic infection in patients with AIDS. Histoplasmosis of the CNS is seen in individuals with disseminated disease. Various forms of CNS involvement have been described, including meningitis, cerebritis, and ring-enhancing granulomas.

Blastomycosis Blastomycosis is caused by *Blastomyces dermatitidis*. It is a granulomatous disease found in North America, Europe, Africa, and Asia. It is acquired by inhalation and begins as a pulmonary infection. Dissemination occurs from the primary pulmonary focus. Involvement of the CNS is rare; it is reported in up to 10 percent of cases but found in 33 percent at autopsy.

Blastomycosis of the CNS usually presents as a meningitis late in the course of the systemic disease, but it can present with an intracranial mass or spinal epidural granuloma or abscess. Intracranial blastomycosis may be solitary or multiple, isodense or hyperdense on noncontrast CT, and ring-enhancing or homogeneously enhancing with contrast.

Coccidioidomycosis Coccidioidomycosis is caused by *Coccidium immitis*, which is endemic to the southwestern United States and northern Mexico. Patients inhale arthrospores and usually develop a self-limited, asymptomatic pulmonary infection. Dissemination to the CNS is rare, occurring in less than 1 percent of immunocompetent patients. Men and pregnant women have a much higher incidence of dissemination than nonpregnant women. In immunocompromised patients, the disease is either chronically progressive or rapidly fatal.

Basal meningitis is the most common manifestation of dissemination to the CNS, but cerebral abscess formation and caseating granulomas can occur. Hydrocephalus is common secondary to the purulent basal meningitis (Fig. 14-2). Ventriculitis and mycotic aneurysms have also been reported in patients with CNS coccidioidomycosis.

Aspergillosis Aspergillosis can be allergic, toxic, inflammatory, granulomatous, invasive, or disseminated. Infection of the CNS occurs either by direct extension from the nose or paranasal sinuses or by hematogenous dissemination from the lung. Aspergillosis is not common in patients with AIDS, presumably because, unlike immunocompromised patients, they are not neutropenic and neutrophils can destroy *Aspergillus*.

The most common CNS manifestation of aspergillosis is hemorrhagic subcortical infarcts. Less than half of patients with CNS involvement develop meningitis, which is usually focal and adjacent to an area of parenchymal infection. Other manifestations include vasculitis, dural venous sinus thrombosis, granulomas, and abscess formation.

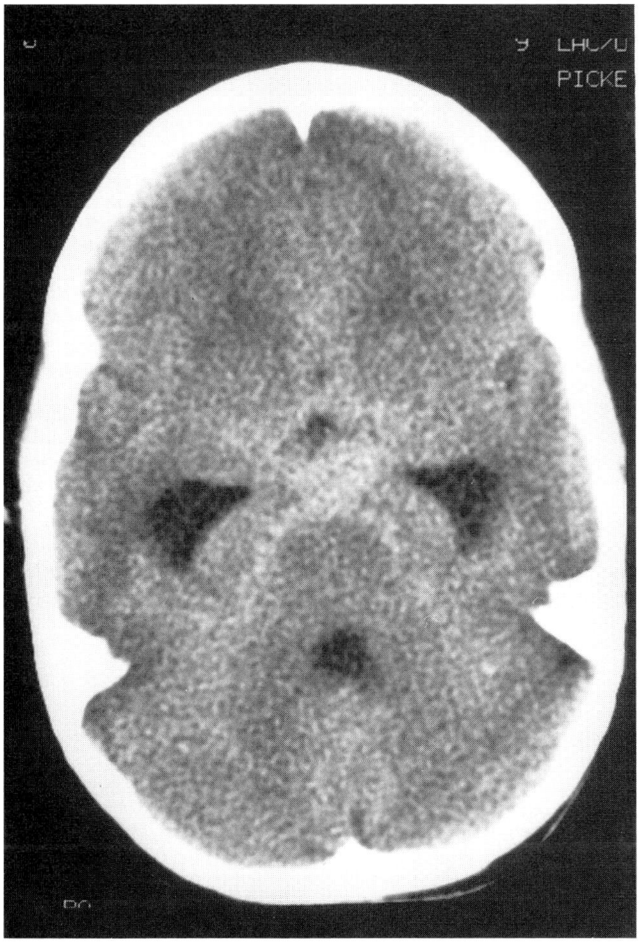

Figure 14-2 Coccidioidomycosis. Axial CT scan shows high-density material in the suprasellar, ambient, and sylvian cisterns as well as in the interhemispheric fissure. Dilatation of both temporal horns is seen, indicating hydrocephalus.

Candidiasis Candidiasis in humans is most often caused by *Candida albicans*. It normally exists in the gastrointestinal tract and mucocutaneous regions. Pregnancy, diabetes, steroid therapy, the use of antibiotics, advanced age, malnutrition, chronic disease, malignancy, immunosuppression, and immune deficiency are all predisposing factors to overgrowth of *Candida* and potential infection. Candidiasis is the most common CNS fungal infection found at autopsy.

Impairment of host defenses leads to hematogenous dissemination from the gastrointestinal tract. The most commonly involved organs are the kidneys, gastrointestinal tract, brain, and respiratory system.

Lesions of the CNS are usually microscopic, although ring-enhancing and homogeneously enhancing lesions have been reported. *Candida* infection can cause ventriculitis, mycotic aneurysms, and focal meningitis; it rarely causes a diffuse meningitis.

Cryptococcosis *Cryptococcosis neoformans* is found worldwide. Clinically, cryptococcosis is the most common CNS fungal infection. As with other nonendemic fungi, it primarily affects immunosuppressed patients, including those with AIDS. It is the most common cause of meningitis-meningoencephalitis in AIDS patients and the third most common CNS pathogen in AIDS (after HIV and *Toxoplasma*); it is seen in 5 percent of patients.

Cryptococcosis produces a usually asymptomatic primary pulmonary infection that reaches the CNS by hematogenous dissemination. Dissemination can occur after resolution of the pulmonary infection. Cryptococcosis of the CNS usually presents as a chronically progressive meningitis but can present as a meningoencephalitis or with an intracranial mass. In immunocompromised patients, the infection spreads along the Virchow-Robin spaces, leading to the formation of gelatinous pseudocysts (cystic lesions filled with yeast cells) in the basal ganglia and thalami.

Radiologic studies may be normal or demonstrate hydrocephalus (the most common abnormal finding), atrophy, infarction, leptomeningeal enhancement, and cryptococcoma formation. The two latter findings are more commonly seen with chronic infection.

Zygomycosis Zygomycosis comprises a group of fungal infections including mucormycosis. *Rhizomucor arrhizus* is the species most frequently responsible for human zygomycosis. It has a worldwide distribution and is common in diabetics.

Rhizomucor arrhizus invades the brain by direct extension from the nose or paranasal sinuses. It spreads to the frontal lobe through the cribriform plate along perivascular and perineural spaces or through the orbital apex into the cavernous sinus. Sequelae of infection include mycotic aneurysm formation, cavernous sinus thrombosis, formation of septic emboli, and occlusion of the internal carotid artery.

Findings on CT include infarcts and abscesses. The abscesses may show ring-enhancement, may enhance homogeneously, or may not enhance.

PARASITIC DISEASES

Toxoplasmosis *Toxoplasma gondii* infection of the CNS is seen in immunosuppressed patients, including patients with AIDS. The classic locations are the basal ganglia and thalami, but toxoplasmosis can occur anywhere at the corticomedullary junction or within the white matter. Typically, well-defined ring-enhancing lesions are seen with surrounding edema and mass effect. Nodular enhancement or lack of enhancement, however, are not uncommon. Rarely, the lesions are hemorrhagic. Unlike the case with intrauterine toxoplasmosis, calcifications are rare following adult infection.

Cysticercosis Cysticercosis is the most common parasitic CNS infection. It results from ingestion of the ova of the pork tapeworm *Taenia solium*. The ova are ingested by humans and hatch in the stomach. From the stomach, they invade the intestinal wall and disseminate throughout the body via the circulatory system. The brain is the second most commonly involved organ (60 to 90 percent) after skeletal muscle. The most common presenting symptoms of CNS involvement are seizures and headache.

Four types of infections may occur: cisternal, parenchymal, ventricular, and mixed. Initially, a parenchymal cyst with a mural nodule (scolex) may be visualized on CT or MRI without surrounding edema or enhancement of the cyst wall (stage 1). When degeneration of the larvae occurs, it incites an intense inflammatory response. It is at this stage that edema develops and there is enhancement of the cyst wall (stage 2). The final stage is represented by calcification of the scolex and cyst—i.e., inactive disease (stage 3). Generally the calcified scolices are better visualized on CT.

In the past, the demonstration of intraventricular cysts was difficult and required CT ventriculography. With MRI, however, intraventricular cysts can be visualized noninvasively. The cysts will appear hypointense to cerebrospinal fluid (CSF) on heavily T2-weighted images and occasionally hyperintense to CSF on proton-density images. Cyst wall and scolex could be identified on T1-weighted images.

Syphilis Syphilis is caused by the spirochete *Treponema pallidum*. Syphilitic involvement of the brain is relatively uncommon today, although it is more common than it was 15 years ago, mainly because of the increased incidence of AIDS. Neurosyphilis may result in a meningitis, a meningovasculitis, or more commonly a parenchymal reaction (gumma). Clinical diagnosis is based on demonstration of the treponemal organism or a positive serum or CSF VDRL/FTA-ABS (Venereal Disease Research Laboratory/fluorescent treponemal antibody-absorption) test.

Meningovasculitis occurs as a result of inflammation in the walls of the subarachnoid vessels and Virchow-Robin spaces, which results in vessel wall thickening, vessel narrowing, and occlusion leading to ischemia and/or infarction. Radiologic imaging will demonstrate ill-defined areas of decreased attenuation (CT) or hyperintensity (T2-weighted MRI). Chronically, patients may develop atrophy. Imaging of patients with syphilitic gumma by CT or MRI will demonstrate a homogeneously enhancing or ring-enhancing mass.

Echinococcosis Hydatid disease or echinococcosis is the larval state of *Echinococcus granulosus*. The definitive host is the dog, and the intermediate hosts are sheep, cattle, and camels. Hydatid disease frequently involves the liver and lungs. Involvement of the CNS is extremely rare. Hydatid cysts of the brain are usually large and may be solitary or multiple. Extradural cysts have been reported. Large intraparenchymal cystic lesions with thin, well-defined margins are seen on unenhanced images (Fig. 14-3). Occasionally, calcification and faint enhancement of the cyst wall may be seen. The lack of intense contrast enhancement and surrounding edema are important features that serve to differentiate this lesion from cerebral abscess.

□ ENCEPHALITIS

Encephalitis is a diffuse inflammation of the brain, usually caused by a virus. The most common viral agent is herpes simplex type I. Other causes of encephalitis include arboviruses, cytomegalovirus (CMV), progressive multifocal leukoencephalopathy, and HIV.

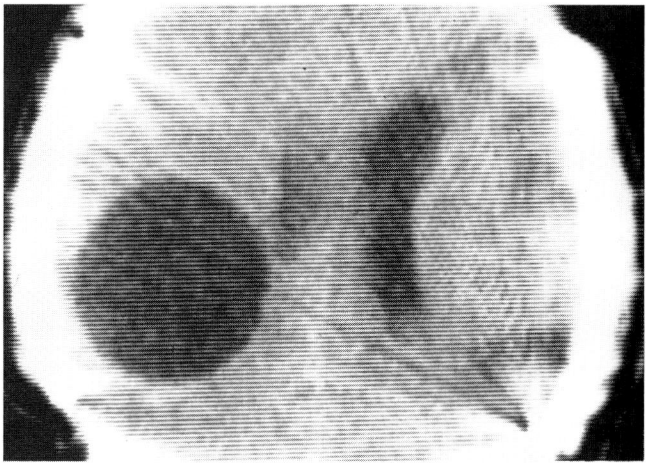

Figure 14-3 *Echinococcus*. Axial CT scan shows a large, low-density mass with smooth margin.

TORCH INFECTIONS

The acronym TORCH stands for toxoplasmosis, rubella, cytomegalovirus, and herpes. All of these infections can be contracted in utero by transplacental transmission during primary or secondary maternal infection or during birth, as the fetus passes through the birth canal. If infection occurs during the first or second trimester, the result will be destructive, causing developmental defects and brain abnormalities. If the infection occurs during or after the third trimester, the result will be a destructive abnormality or no abnormality. TORCH infections may also result in neuronal migration disorders secondary to disruption of migration of the subependymal neuroblast during formation of the neurocortex.

Toxoplasmosis The incidence of congenital toxoplasmosis is approximately 1 per 10,000 births per year. Infection occurs through transplacental transmission. As with all of the TORCH infections, the earlier the fetus is infected, the more severe the anomalies.

The characteristic clinical triad seen in congenital toxoplasmosis encephalitis is hydrocephalus (secondary to aqueductal stenosis), intracranial calcifications (Fig. 14-4), and chorioretinitis, the last being the most common single finding in congenital toxoplasmosis infection. Other neurologic sequelae include atrophy, microcephaly, infarction, hydranencephaly, and neuronal migration disorders such as pachygyria.

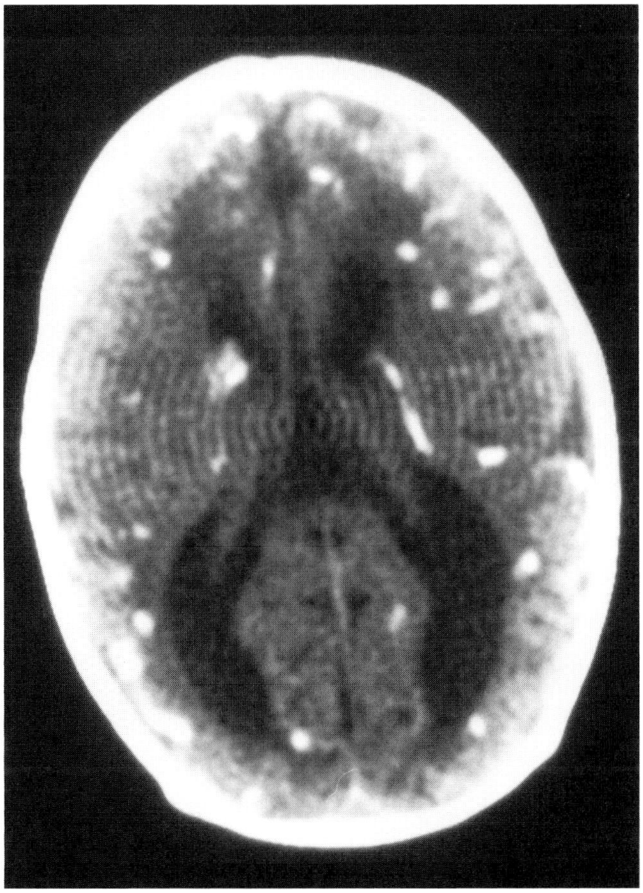

Figure 14-4 Toxoplasmosis. Axial CT scan shows moderate ventriculomegaly with small periventricular and parenchymal calcifications.

Histopathologically, there is an inflammatory infiltrate of the pia-arachnoid. The parasite invades blood vessels, resulting in necrosis of the underlying brain. Calcifications are seen in the basal ganglia, subependymal region, and within areas of brain necrosis.

Rubella Because of immunization and maternal screening programs, congenital rubella infection is now quite rare. The virus is transmitted to the fetus through the placenta during maternal infection. Maternal infection does not necessarily affect the fetus but can result in abortion, stillbirth, or congenital anomalies. The later the fetus is infected, the less severe the damage. Those infected before 12 weeks gestation will have more serious sequelae.

Clinically, rubella can affect multiple organs, including the heart, eyes, and brain. Organs affected tend to be hypoplastic. Infection of the CNS is characterized by a meningoencephalitis. Sequelae include atrophy, hydrocephalus, mental retardation, microcephaly, cataracts, glaucoma, chorioretinitis, and microphthalmia. Deafness is the most common manifestation of late infection.

By inhibiting proliferation of immature, undifferentiated progenitor cells in the germinal matrix, the rubella virus disrupts normal cellular multiplication, resulting in a decreased number of neurons, astroglia, and oligodendroglia. Histopathologically, congenital rubella is characterized by a necrotizing vasculopathy resulting in cytolysis and tissue necrosis.

Although no specific CT or MRI findings have been reported in congenital rubella, calcifications of the cortical and basal ganglia are typically present on CT. In addition, delayed myelination and deep and subcortical white matter lesions may be seen on MRI.

Cytomegalovirus Cytomegalovirus is a DNA (herpes) virus. Humans are the only hosts, and between 50 and 85 percent of women in the United States are seropositive. Also, CMV is the most common cause of congenital CNS infection, which occurs as a result of transplacental transmission during primary or secondary maternal infection.

Gross pathologic findings include porencephaly, encephalomalacia, microcephaly, and hydranencephaly. Histopathologic findings include microglial nodules and intranuclear and intracytoplasmic inclusions.

Since CMV affects multiple organs, patients can present at birth with a wide variety of clinical signs, such as hepatosplenomegaly, jaundice, thrombocytopenia, and chorioretinitis. Central nervous system signs such as seizures, mental retardation, hydrocephalus, and hearing loss are usually seen later. Clinical diagnosis is made by isolating the virus from body fluids, following titers, and identifying the intracytoplasmic inclusions.

Cytomegalovirus causes an encephalitis with radiologic findings and clinical sequelae indistinguishable from toxoplasmosis: hydrocephalus, atrophy, infarction, demyelination, disorders of neuronal migration, gliosis, and calcification, the last usually being paraventricular.

Herpes Simplex Type II Herpes simplex virus type II (HSV-II) is a DNA virus. Although it can occur in all age groups, it is most common in newborns, who usually contract it during their passage through the birth canal of a mother infected with genital herpes. Transplacental and newborn-to-newborn infection are rare but can occur. This virus causes 75 to 90 percent of all neonatal herpes infections. The estimated incidence is 1 per 2000 to 5000 deliveries per year. Mortality has been reported as high as 80 percent. The use of antiviral agents such as vidarabine or acyclovir may improve outcome if they are given early in the course of the infection.

Involvement of the CNS is seen in 30 percent of patients without systemic disease and in two-thirds of patients with systemic disease. Patients with isolated CNS involvement usually present at 2 to 4 weeks of age with lethargy, irritability, and seizures. Patients with systemic disease usually present earlier, between 1 and 2 weeks after birth. They can present with CNS signs, a vascular rash, or respiratory distress.

The infection begins in the white matter and extends to involve the adjacent parenchyma. Computed tomography demonstrates diffuse areas of white matter hypodensity. High density due to petechial hemorrhage, hemorrhagic infarction, gyral calcification, and meningeal contrast enhancement can be seen. Diagnosis is made by isolating the virus from the CSF or skin or by brain biopsy. Histopathologic examination will demonstrate cytolysis and vasculitis. Sequelae of HSV-II infection include multicystic encephalomalacia and diffuse atrophy.

In utero infection can occur but is rare. Transmission occurs via hematogenous spread from the placenta. Affected patients may exhibit microcephaly, microphthalmia, chorioretinitis, hydranencephaly, cerebral and cerebellar necrosis, and intracranial calcification (periventricular, cortical, or white matter) as well as cutaneous and systemic anomalies.

Computed tomography may be more useful in the evaluation of newborns with suspected herpes virus encephalitis, since calcifications are more easily identified on CT and white matter abnormalities may be difficult to identify on T2-weighted MRI because of the lack of myelination.

HERPES SIMPLEX TYPE I

Herpes simplex type I causes a necrotizing encephalitis. It occurs in all age groups but is the more common of the herpes infections to occur in adults. The most common clinical presentation is acute confusion and disorientation, but patients can also present with fever, seizures, headache, and language dysfunction. Initially, CT

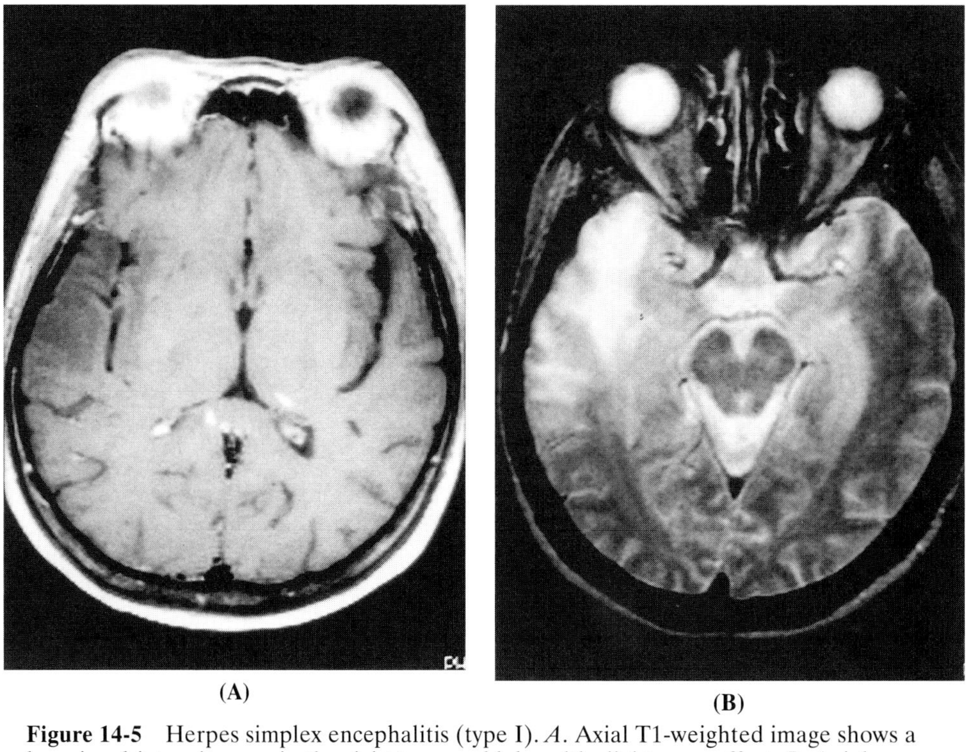

(A) (B)

Figure 14-5 Herpes simplex encephalitis (type I). *A*. Axial T1-weighted image shows a low-signal-intensity area in the right temporal lobe with slight mass effect. *B*. Axial T2-weighted image demonstrates corresponding high-signal-intensity in the right temporal lobe with mild mass effect.

images may appear normal; after a few days, however, CT may demonstrate poorly defined areas of low density in the anterior and medial aspects of the temporal lobe with subtle mass effect. Although the insular cortex and inferior frontal lobes may be involved, the basal ganglia are spared. Magnetic resonance imaging, which is more sensitive than CT, will demonstrate the findings earlier—areas of hypointensity on T1-weighted images which become hyperintense on T2-weighted images (Fig. 14-5). In addition, CT and (less likely) MRI may demonstrate the petechial hemorrhages that are characteristic of herpes encephalitis but are rarely seen. Gyral enhancement is unusual before the second week. Medical therapy (vidarabine or acyclovir) should be started within 5 days of the onset of the illness to be effective. If such an infection is not treated, it will progress rapidly, with spread to the contralateral side and increasing mass effect. This is characteristic of herpes simplex encephalitis type I. A brain biopsy may be necessary for definitive diagnosis. Sequelae include subcortical and periventricular calcification (more common in children), atrophy, and cystic encephalomalacia.

OTHER CAUSES OF ENCEPHALITIS

Listeria *Listeria monocytogenes* is a gram-positive rod. It causes a meningitis or meningoencephalitis more commonly than brain abcess (9 percent). Computed tomography may demonstrate ill-defined areas of low density, gyriform enhancement, meningeal enhancement, and mass effect. Patients can present with isolated brainstem involvement.

Lyme Disease Lyme disease is caused by the tick-borne spirochete *Borrelia burgdorferi*. It was first discovered in Lyme, Connecticut, but it can be found worldwide. The most commonly affected geographic areas are New England, Wisconsin, Minnesota, and the Pacific states. Some 10 to 15 percent of patients with Lyme disease develop CNS complications, generally within weeks to months following the characteristic rash, erythema chronicum migrans. Although CNS manifestations include meningitis, meningoencephalitis, cerebellar ataxia, and myelitis, patients most commonly develop cranial nerve palsies and peripheral neuropathies. Studies by CT and MRI may be normal or may demonstrate deep white matter and subcortical lesions similar in appearance to those of multiple sclerosis or other causes of demyelination. The lesions may or may not enhance. Histopathologically, perivascular infiltrates with demyelinating foci are seen. Diagnosis is made by serologic studies.

Reye's Syndrome The exact etiology of Reye's syndrome is unknown, but it usually occurs following a viral infection such as varicella or influenza A or B. It may also be associated with salicylates or intrinsic metabolic defects. It generally affects children in the first and second decades but can be seen in adults. Generalized symptoms include nausea, vomiting, changes in mental status, and seizures, but the syndrome can progress to unresponsiveness and respiratory arrest. Studies by CT and MRI demonstrate diffuse cerebral edema with or without secondary ventricular compression.

Rickettsia *Rickettsia* is a genus of tick-borne intracellular bacteria that causes Rocky Mountain spotted fever, typhus, Q fever, trench fever, and scrub typhus. The bacteria multiply in endothelial cells, causing a vasculitis that results in thrombosis and infarction. Patients present with generalized symptoms including fever and gastrointestinal disturbance. A rash may develop following onset of the fever. Infection with these organisms produces an encephalitis. Neurologic symptoms include headache, altered mental status, hallucinations, seizures, and sensory and motor deficits.

Acute Disseminated Encephalomyelitis Acute disseminated encephalomyelitis (ADEM), also known as immune-mediated encephalomyelitis, usually results from an immune response to a recent (within 3 weeks) viral infection or vaccination. It can, however, occur spontaneously.

The initial symptoms are generalized and include headache, fever, neck stiffness, and anorexia. Neurologic symptoms, which occur 1 to 3 weeks later, include changes in mental status, seizure, and coma. Patients may die, recover completely, or suffer permanent neurologic and mental deficits, the latter usually occurring in children.

Pathologic changes are the result of vasculitis and demyelination, and the imaging findings reflect the pathologic changes. Magnetic resonance imaging is more sensitive than CT to the subcortical and brainstem foci of demyelination, which are diffuse, bilateral, and asymmetrical. Some of the lesions enhance. Chronic changes include demyelination, parenchymal volume loss, and ventricular dilatation.

A rare hemorrhagic form of the disease exists which is more fulminant and has a high morbidity and mortality. In these patients, the hemorrhages are perivascular and microscopic; they are generally not visible radiologically.

Subacute Sclerosing Panencephalitis Subacute sclerosing panencephalitis (SSPE) is a rare disease, affecting one individual per million per year. It is classified as a slow virus but is usually seen in children and young adults several years after infection with the measles virus. Antibodies to the measles virus are found in the serum and CSF of affected individuals. Histopathologic examination demonstrates atrophy, demyelination, and intranuclear and intracytoplasmic inclusions.

Clinically, patients present with mental and behavioral changes that progress to motor disturbances and seizures. Although the disease is usually slowly progressive, patients generally die within 2 to 6 years.

Initially, CT may be normal or demonstrate diffuse cerebral swelling and/or areas of low density within the subcortical, periventricular white matter and deep gray matter; these do not enhance. Magnetic resonance imaging is more sensitive to the white matter changes. Later, CT and MRI may demonstrate atrophy.

Mumps The mumps vaccine is 75 to 90 percent effective in preventing the disease. Involvement of the CNS is seen in up to 65 percent of patients with mumps. The most common manifestation of CNS involvement is a meningitis with a usually benign outcome. Encephalitis is seen in only 0.2 percent of patients and is fatal in up to 22 percent of cases. Patients may develop seizures as a result of CNS involvement, which is characterized by demyelination and perivascular inflammation. Areas of low density on CT and hyperintensity on T2-weighted MRI are typical but not specific.

Creutzfeldt-Jakob Disease Subacute spongiform encephalitis or Creutzfeldt-Jakob disease is caused by a slow virus. Individuals can be infected through organ transplantation or by the use of contaminated neurosurgical instruments. They usually present in their late fifties with rapidly progressive dementia. Death usually occurs within months. Both CT and MRI demonstrate progressive cerebral and cerebellar atrophy. The white matter appears normal. Diagnosis is made by biopsy. Histopathologic findings include neuronal loss, astrocytic hyperplasia, and cell vacuolation.

☐ AIDS-RELATED INFECTIONS

TOXOPLASMOSIS

Toxoplasmosis of the CNS is among the most common CNS infections in AIDS patients. The classic locations are the basal ganglia and thalami, but toxoplasmosis can occur anywhere at the corticomedullary junction or within the white matter. Typically, well-defined, ring-enhancing lesions are seen, with surrounding edema and mass effect; however, poorly defined areas of low attenuation (CT) or hyperintensity (T2-weighted MRI) are also seen, particularly in patients who are severely immunocompromised. Nodular enhancement, lack of enhancement, and gyral enhancement have also been reported. The differential diagnosis includes other CNS infections and lymphoma. In AIDS patients, it is not uncommon for toxoplasmosis, other infections, and/or lymphoma to occur in the same individual.

PROGRESSIVE MULTIFOCAL LEUKOENCEPHALOPATHY

Progressive multifocal leukoencephalopathy (PML) is caused by a papova (DNA) virus that results in white matter demyelination. Patients who are susceptible include those on immunosuppressive therapy and individuals with tuberculosis, systemic lupus erythematosus, sarcoid, lymphoma, leukemia, and AIDS. Asymmetrical involvement of the parietooccipital lobes in a nonvascular distribution is classic but not invariable. The typical findings are ill-defined areas of homogeneously decreased attenuation in the white matter on CT or high signal intensity on T2-weighted MRI, which have a scalloped peripheral margin, do not enhance, and have no mass effect. Individual cases, however, have been reported with enhancement, mass effect, and atypical and asymmetrical location. At present, no treatment exists and affected patients usually die within 1 year.

CYTOMEGALOVIRUS

Severe infection with CMV has been reported in patients with AIDS. Sites of CMV involvement are usually outside the central nervous system (e.g., the retina). Meningoencephalitis due to CMV is relatively uncommon. The radiologic findings are nonspecific. Unenhanced scans may show ill-defined areas of decreased attenuation (CT) or hyperintensity (T2-weighted MRI) within the white matter. Enhanced scans may also demonstrate periventricular, nodular, or ringlike enhancement.

HUMAN IMMUNODEFICIENCY VIRUS

The HIV virus causes a subacute encephalitis resulting in demyelination. Areas of involvement include the white matter, basal ganglia, cerebellum, and brainstem. Sometimes neither CT nor MRI demonstrates a parenchymal abnormality. However, atrophy, the result of chronic HIV infection, is well demonstrated on both CT and MRI. It can be seen as an isolated abnormality or in conjunction with other AIDS-related abnormalities and will progress over time.

FUNGAL INFECTIONS

Fungal infections occur more commonly in immunocompromised and immune-suppressed patients. The most common fungal infections seen in patients with AIDS are cryptococcosis, coccidioidomycosis, and histoplasmosis, the latter two in endemic areas. In the immunocompetent patient, fungal abscesses evolve more slowly than bacterial abscesses; this is not true for immunocompromised or immune-suppressed patients. There are no specific radiologic features to determine the infecting agent.

SYPHILIS

Syphilis is a risk factor for HIV infection, and neurosyphilis is seen in 1.5 percent of patients with AIDS. Syphilis is more likely to progress to neurosyphilis in patients with

AIDS. Patients can present with a variety of neurologic symptoms, but 42 percent present with ophthalmologic involvement.

☐ QUESTIONS (True or False)

1. *Streptococcus pneumoniae* is the most common cause of bacterial meningitis in adults.
2. Enhancement of the basal cisterns and sylvian fissures can be seen long after treatment for chronic meningitis.
3. Chronic basilar meningitis is the most common type of CNS involvement in sarcoidosis.
4. The lung is the most common extracranial source of an intracranial pyogenic abscess.
5. *Streptococcus* is the organism most frequently isolated from abscesses in neonates.
6. Ventriculitis may occur in the presence of an unruptured abscess.
7. Tuberculomas occur only in patients with pulmonary tuberculosis.
8. The brain is the organ most commonly affected by *Nocardia.*
9. Indium-111-labeled leukocytes have been used to differentiate nocardial abscesses from metastases.
10. Basilar meningitis is the most common manifestation of CNS dissemination in coccidioidomycosis.
11. *Cryptococcosus neoformans* is the most common cause of meningitis in patients with AIDS.
12. Infarction is a sequela of cryptococcal meningitis.
13. Intracranial calcifications are commonly seen following toxoplasmosis infection in adults.
14. Toxoplasmosis is the most common parasitic CNS infection.
15. The organs most commonly affected by cysticercosis are skeletal muscle and brain.
16. Infarction is one of the sequelae of neurosyphilis.
17. Intraparenchymal hydatid cysts are usually large, do not enhance, and lack surrounding edema.
18. Encephalitis is usually caused by a virus, typically herpes simplex type I.
19. TORCH infections can result in disorders of neuronal migration.
20. Hydrocephalus is the most common single finding in congenital toxoplasmosis.
21. Herpes simplex type I causes a necrotizing encephalitis.
22. Patients with *Listeria* encephalitis can present with isolated brainstem involvement.
23. Lyme disease is caused by a tick-borne intracellular bacterium that multiplies in endothelial cells and causes a vasculitis.
24. Studies by CT and MRI in patients with Creutzfeldt-Jakob disease demonstrate rapidly progressive demyelination.
25. *Toxoplasma* is the most common CNS pathogen in patients with AIDS.

☐ ANSWERS

1. T
2. T
3. T
4. T
5. F
6. T
7. F
8. F
9. T
10. T
11. T
12. T
13. F
14. F
15. T
16. T
17. T
18. T
19. T
20. F
21. T
22. T
23. F
24. F
25. T

SUGGESTED READINGS

1. Balakrishnan J et al: Acquired immunodeficiency syndrome: Correlation of radiologic and pathologic findings in the brain. *Radiographics* 10:201–215, 1990.
2. Boesch CH et al: Magnetic resonance imaging of the brain in congenital cytomegalovirus infection. *Pediatr Radiol* 19:91–93, 1989.

3. Buckner CB et al: The changing epidemiology of tuberculosis and other mycobacterial infections in the United States: Implications for the radiologist. *AJR* 196:255–264, 1991.
4. Chang KH et al: Gd-DPTA enhanced MR imaging in intracranial tuberculosis. *Neuroradiology* 32:19–25, 1990.
5. Chang KH et al: GD-DPTA enhanced MR imaging of the brain in patients with meningitis: Comparison with CT. *AJNR* 11:69–76, 1990.
6. Drose JA et al: Infection in utero: US findings in 19 cases. *Radiology* 178:369–374, 1991.
7. Enzman D et al: MR findings in neonatal herpes simplex encephalitis type II. *J Comput Assist Tomogr* 14:453–457, 1990.
8. Haimes AB et al: MR imaging of brain diseases. *AJNR* 10:279–291, 1989.
9. Kesselring J et al: Acute disseminated encephalomyelitis. *Brain* 113:291–302, 1990.
10. Martinez HR et al: MR imaging in neurocysticercosis. *AJNR* 10:1011–1019, 1989.
11. Mathews VP et al: Gd-DPTA-enhanced MR imaging of experimental bacterial meningitis. *AJNR* 9:1045–1050, 1988.
12. Miller DH et al: Magnetic resonance imaging in central nervous system sarcoidosis. *Neurology* 38:378–383, 1988.
13. Osborn A: Infections of the brain and its linings, in *Diagnostic Neuroradiology*. St Louis, Mosby-Year Book, 1994.
14. Ramsey RG, Geremia GK: CNS complications of AIDS: CT and MR findings. *AJR* 151:449–454, 1988.
15. Sherman JL, Stern BJ: Sarcoidosis of the CNS. *AJNR* 11:915–923, 1990.
16. Tassin GB: Cytomegalic inclusion disease. *AJNR* 11:915–923, 1990.
17. Tien RD et al: Intracranial cryptococcosis in immunocompromised patients. *AJNR* 12:283–289, 1991.
18. Tsuchiya K et al: MR imaging vs. CT in subacute sclerosing panencephalitis. *AJNR* 9:943–946, 1988.
19. Weingarten K et al: Subdural and epidural empyemas: MR imaging. *AJNR* 10:81–87, 1989.
20. Whelan MA, Hilal SK: Computed tomography as a guide in the diagnosis and follow-up of brain abscesses. *Radiology* 135:663–671, 1980.
21. Whelan MA, Stern J: Intracranial tuberculoma. *Radiology* 138:75–81, 1980.
22. Whitely RJ: Herpes simplex virus infections of the central nervous system in children. *Semin Neurol* 2:87–96, 1982.
23. Williams AL: Infectious diseases, in Williams AL, Haughton VM (eds): Cranial computed tomography: A comprehensive text. St Louis, Mosby-Year Book, 1985, pp 269–315.
24. Zee CS et al: MR imaging of neurocysticercosis. *J Comput Assist Tomogr* 12;927–934, 1988.
25. Zee CS et al: MR imaging of cerebral toxoplasmosis: Correlation of computed tomography and pathology. *J Comput Assist Tomogr* 9:797–799, 1985.
26. Zee CS et al: Unusual neuroradiological feature of intracranial cysticcercosis. *Radiology* 137:397–407, 1980.
27. Zimmerman RD, Weingarten K: Neuroimaging of cerebral abscesses. *Neuroimaging Clin North Am* 1:1–16, 1991.
28. Zimmerman RA et al: Evolution of cerebral abscess: Correlation of clinical features with computed tomography. *Neurology* 27:14–19, 1977.
29. Zimmerman RD et al: CT in the early diagnosis of herpes simplex encephalitis. *AJNR* 134:61–66, 1980.

CHAPTER 15

Head Trauma

Fong Y. Tsai

Trauma is the third leading cause of death in the United States and the leading cause of death among young adults and teenagers. There has been a continuous increase in acute trauma, not just from automobile accidents and falls but also from assaults, child abuse, and other violent behavior. Head trauma ranks highest of all types of fatal injuries. It may be the result of a blunt blow or a penetrating injury. Often, head trauma, results in prolonged disability, creating societal and family burdens as well. The evaluation of these patients has become an important part of neuroradiologic practice.

The neuroimaging signs of head trauma may fall into one of three major categories:

1. Calvarial and basal skull fractures
2. Intracranial extraaxial hematoma
3. Intracerebral injury

☐ CALVARIAL AND BASAL SKULL FRACTURES

Skull radiography has been a major diagnostic examination for head trauma for many decades, even after the introduction of computed tomography (CT). Not until recently have data supported the limited value of skull radiographs in the evaluation of head trauma. Although skull radiographs have continued to be used for the evaluation of depressed or basal skull fractures and their extension, there has recently been a change in the management of depressed fractures. Computed tomography has largely replaced skull radiographs for the evaluation of head trauma. However, skull radiographs may be the preferable diagnostic modality for restless patients and those who cannot tolerate excessive motion. During the skull radiography procedure, overextension of the neck should be avoided until the cervical spine is known to be free of injury.

Depressed skull fractures with overlying scalp lacerations often occur in adults, but this association is not as frequent in children. Depressed fractures may lacerate the dura and the cerebral cortex, inducing a hematoma. Depressed bone fragments should be removed carefully en bloc to avoid additional injury although not all need to be elevated. In fact, Braakman (see "Suggested Readings") has recommended that there be no elevation attempt if the fracture overlies a dural sinus. The rationale for elevation of a depressed fracture is to prevent further brain injury and seizure. However, Jennet and coworkers have found that the incidence of seizure is not increased without elevation versus surgical elevation of the depression.

Fractures of the anterior cranial fossa usually involve the facial and frontal bones. They may extend to the orbital surface of the frontal bone and cause lacerations of the dura as well as disruptions of the optic foramen. Leakage of cerebrospinal fluid (CSF) and pneumocephalus can occur from a frontal skull fracture when it extends to the sphenoid, ethmoid, and frontal sinuses. A fracture of the middle cranial fossa may involve the petrous bones, either as a transverse or longitudinal fracture. Transverse fractures have a higher incidence of seventh- and eighth-cranial-nerve injury and a lesser incidence of CSF otorrhea; the relative incidence of the complications is reversed with longitudinal fractures. Longitudinal fractures occur more frequently than transverse fractures in a ratio of 5:1. Fractures of the posterior cranial fossa may extend to the petrous bones. There is also a risk of injury to the cerebellum and brainstem.

Complications of basal skull fractures include infections and cranial nerve palsies. Pneumocephalus is commonly found with basal skull fractures, but it often resolves spontaneously. If there is persistent pneumocephalus and/or CSF leakage, a CT with intrathecal contrast may be necessary to identify the site of the dural injury for surgical repair.

Computed tomography can delineate the extent of a fracture and any complications. High-resolution CT can clearly demonstrate the basal foramina, complicated middle ear structures, and the optic foramen. Computed tomography is more suitable in evaluating a depressed fracture in acute trauma and is also very useful in identifying the inner table of the frontal sinus. Complications of calvarial and basilar fractures can be divided into five categories:

1. *Frontal bone*: sinus involvement leading to infection, CSF rhinorrhea
2. *Skull base*: sphenoid sinus, pituitary injury, CSF rhinorrhea, cerebral artery injury, carotid cavernous fistula
3. *Petrous bone*: seventh- and eighth-cranial-nerve palsies, CSF otorrhea, ossicular disruption
4. *Midline*: dural sinus injury
5. Leptomeningeal cyst or growing fracture

Although skull radiographs are occasionally used for evaluating skull fractures, CT is now the primary tool for the evaluation of head trauma. Emergent CT is the first imaging modality used to evaluate acute head trauma after a neurologic examination. Prompt CT diagnosis is crucial to determine treatment. Trauma patients are often restless and uncooperative, and they may also have organ injuries. New spiral CT techniques enable us to perform the examinations with greater speed. The scout view may be used in screening for skull fractures and evaluating the upper cervical spine. The routine CT examination should be performed with both brain and bone windows. A depressed skull fracture may mimic an extraaxial hematoma, and a small hematoma may be overlooked without the proper window setting. After reviewing the examination, if there is a question, the subdural (wide) window setting may be adjusted to evaluate a small epidural hematoma (EDH) or subdural hematoma (SDH). Additional thin sections with high-resolution bone algorithm techniques for specific areas such as the petrous bone or skull base are deferred for later evaluation.

The following are the main indications for emergent CT:

1. Loss of consciousness for more than 5 min
2. Persistent neurologic deficit
3. Bleeding diathesis or on anticoagulation
4. Glasgow Coma Scale score less than 10
5. All penetrating wounds

MECHANISMS OF HEAD INJURY

A head injury may be caused by closed head trauma or by a penetrating wound. The primary mechanisms of acute brain tissue injury are coup or contrecoup injuries. However, a severe closed head trauma or gunshot wound may produce additional remote brain tissue injury due to a shifting or gliding mechanism.

☐ INTRACRANIAL EXTRAAXIAL HEMORRHAGE

Normal dura consists of two layers, the outer periosteal dura and the inner meningeal dura. The two layers are split to form the dural sinuses, falx, tentorium, and interhemispheric fissures. The periosteal dura is at the outer wall of the major dural sinuses, adjacent to the calvarium, and the meningeal dura is at the lateral wall. The characteristic appearance of extraaxial bleeding is directly related to the anatomy of dura, arachnoid, and pia mater, which provide the coverage of the brain and the periosteum of the skull. Based upon the location of the hemorrhage, it may be categorized into four types:

1. Epidural hematoma
2. Subdural hematoma
3. Subarachnoid hemorrhage
4. Intraventricular hemorrhage

EPIDURAL HEMATOMA

An EDH lies beneath the calvarium, external to the periosteal dura. It rarely extends beyond a suture margin due to the firm attachment of the periosteal dura to the suture margin. An EDH most frequently occurs over the convexity from a lacerated meningeal or periosteal artery at the fractured bone edges. It is associated with an underlying skull fracture in 22 to 90 percent of cases. Approximately 2 percent of all hospitalized head injury patients have an EDH. Although this occurs in only 1 percent of all cases, it may reach up to 15 percent of all fatal head traumas. An EDH may also occur secondary to venous bleeding from a dural sinus injury. An arterial EDH may further disrupt the dura by expanding in size. The classic "lucid" interval, which is a period of mild symptoms, is related to an EDH. A venous EDH rarely increases in size, as an arterial bleed can. Posterior fossa and midline EDHs are often the result of venous bleeding due to a dural sinus injury.

An EDH is almost always the result of a coup injury at the site of impact. Conversely, a SDH is often the result of a contrecoup injury away from the impact site. Unlike EDHs, SDHs are frequently associated with underlying brain injury. An EDH may extend beyond the boundary of the tentorium and may cross the tentorium (from the posterior fossa) and extend into the supratentorial region. An extension in the reverse direction may also occur. Extension of a SDH is limited by the tentorium. An EDH may cross the midline by displacing the interhemispheric fissure and falx away from the inner table while a SDH will follow the subdural space beneath the meningeal dura and enter the interhemispheric fissure. An EDH occurs unilaterally most frequently and occurs bilaterally less than 5 percent of the time.

Because of the firm sutural attachment of the dura, an EDH may have a more abrupt margin and a biconvex appearance on CT or magnetic resonance imaging (MRI), and the inner margin may be flat (Fig. 15-1). The typical EDH appears as a homogenous, high-density, biconvex lesion on CT, but it is possible for it to appear as a heterogenous density due to mixing of clotted and unclotted blood. There is no definite advantage to MRI over CT in the evaluation of an EDH, although MRI may show medial displacement of the dura with a hypointense line. An EDH appears isointense on T1- and hyperintense on T2-weighted MRI. With active bleeding, an EDH may appear mixed (with both hypo- and hyperintensity). As an EDH evolves into a subacute or chronic hematoma, CT will demonstrate decreasing density (isointensity or low density) and MRI will show hyperintensity on T1- and T2-weighted images.

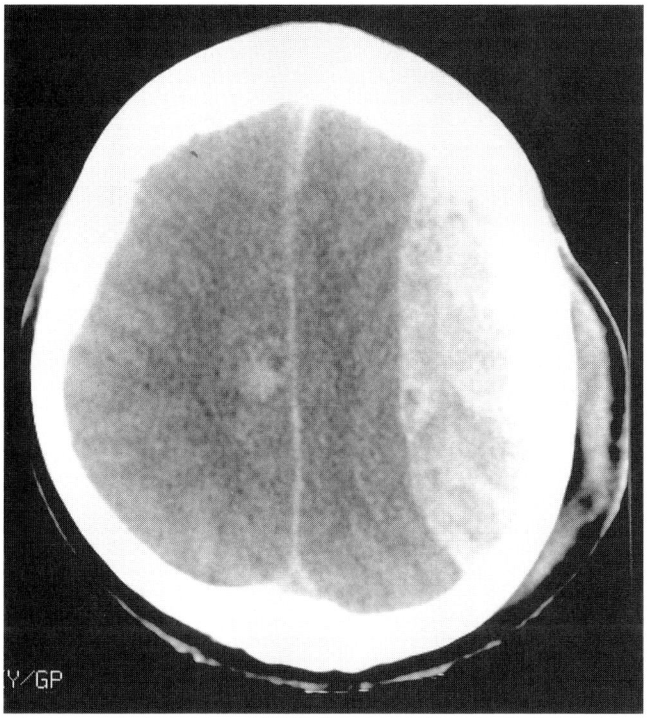

Figure 15-1 Epidural hematoma. Computed tomography shows a mixed high-density left temporal epidural hematoma (EDH) with shearing injury hemorrhage at the corpus callosum.

SUBDURAL HEMATOMA

A SDH is one that occurs in the subdural space between the meningeal dura and arachnoid mater. A SDH may occur from the rupture of bridging cortical veins, the bending of vessels from deceleration, or by direct injury to pial veins, great veins, or pacchionian granulations. Lacerations of the cortex or contusions frequently occur in patients suffering from a SDH. In those patients, the SDH alone may not be the major part of the mass effect; an associated intracerebral injury may also contribute to it. The prognosis may be worse than the size of the SDH would indicate. The incidence of SDHs ranges from 10 to 20 percent of all head trauma, but it may reach 30 percent of all fatal traumas.

Due to the confined subdural space, a SDH tends to extend along the meningeal dura and the underlying arachnoid, forming a crescent-shaped hematoma with a long tail (unlike an EDH, which has an abrupt end). The high-density crescent-shaped SDH may blend in with the dense calvarium if a wide window setting is not used. A typical acute SDH appears as a homogenous, high-density, crescent-shaped hematoma following along the convexity of the cerebral hemisphere. An atypical CT appearance of an acute SDH may occur because of several different circumstances:

1. Anemia resulting in a lower-density blood collection
2. Hyperacute blood that is still in liquid form and not yet clotted
3. Rebleeding with a mixing of preexisting chronic blood and fresh blood
4. Mixing of blood with CSF

An acute EDH or SDH is removed by a craniotomy. The mortality rate of EDHs ranges from 5 to 10 percent, but the mortality rate of SDHs may reach 50 percent or even higher. A small EDH or SDH may not require surgical intervention if there is no significant brainstem compression. A SDH may evolve from high density into an isodense lesion in the subacute phase; rebleeding into a chronic SDH may produce an isodense or mixed-density hematoma.

A SDH is usually a crescent-shaped density on CT, but occasionally an acute SDH may have a spindle form, like an EDH; however, a SDH always has a long tail. If a SDH is located in the interhemispheric fissure, it may be confused with a subarachnoid hemorrhage (SAH), but a SDH is always a thick, sausage-shaped density, in contrast to the thin, linear, density typical of SAH. A SDH may extend from the convexity to the interhemispheric fissure and the tentorial edge. As a rule, a SDH often produces a midline shift with parenchymal contusions, but it can be bilateral, in which case there will be no significant midline shift.

About 15 percent of all SDHs may be bilateral, but they occur more frequently with head trauma related to child abuse.

SUBACUTE AND CHRONIC SUBDURAL HEMATOMA

The organization of a SDH is accomplished by fibroblasts and phagocytes, with a proliferation of blood vessels starting from the inner surface of the dura. During evolution, the organizing SDH is vulnerable to rebleeding. If there is no rebleeding, a SDH will become chronic. The old hematoma may become a black-brown fluid and have a low-density appearance on CT. With longer survival, the residuum of the blood clot becomes a thin membrane, which is firmly attached to the dura.

In the evolution of an acute SDH, the inner surface of the hematoma starts to decrease in density about 3 or 4 days after the injury. If the CT examination is done during this time, it may have an irregular isodense inner margin and a high-density outer margin. This may lead to an underestimation of the size of the SDH. Upon complete spontaneous resolution of a SDH, a small residual membrane may be attached to the dura, and this may calcify.

Although an isodense SDH may be difficult to identify, displacement of the cortex or buckling of the white matter may provide evidence of an isodense SDH. Contrast-enhanced CT may further confirm the diagnosis by enhancing a displaced membrane, cortical vein, or cortex. The hematoma, itself may enhance as well.

After an acute SDH evolves, it may become organized and/or calcified, or it may spontaneously resolve. Some SDHs may increase in size if untreated. Rebleeding from the outer membrane of a chronic SDH may occur without any significant trauma. During evolution or rebleeding, the inner margin of the SDH is usually not as smooth as it is in the acute phase. It may have several layers, representing different stages of hemorrhage and/or fluid-fluid levels. A chronic or subacute SDH may appear spindle-shaped due to retraction of the clot. A chronic SDH typically appears as an area of low density on CT.

SUBDURAL HYGROMA

The mechanism of a traumatic acute subdural hygroma does not differ from that of a SDH, but a hygroma is the result of a posttraumatic leak of the arachnoid membrane. The ruptured membrane acts as a one-way valve to prevent backflow and resorption of the CSF from the subdural space. On CT, a subdural hygroma cannot be distinguished from a chronic SDH because they have the same uniform low density, but they *can* be differentiated by MRI characteristics. A chronic SDH will demonstrate a higher signal intensity than the CSF signal intensity of a subdural hygroma.

Magnetic resonance imaging has less importance in the evaluation of an acute SDH than in that of a subacute or chronic SDH. Computed tomography is able to identify most acute SDHs. However, MRI can distinguish cortical hemorrhage from SDH or EDH more easily than CT. In the acute stage, MRI shows the signal characteristic of iso- or hypointensity on T1-weighted images and hypointense blood on T2-weighted images. In the early subacute stage, MRI shows high-signal intensity on T1-weighted images and low-signal intensity on T2-weighted images (intracellular methemoglobin) (Fig. 15-2). In the late subacute and early chronic stages, the SDH appears as high signal (from extracellular methemoglobin) on all pulse sequences. In the chronic stage, the blood signal may be variable and may appear as hypo- or isointense or hyperintense on T1-weighted images. This differs from a chronic parenchymal hemorrhage in that the signal change is due to dilution of methemoglobin.

SUBARACHNOID HEMORRHAGE

Subarachnoid hemorrhage is very common in patients with head trauma. Subarachnoid blood stems primarily from laceration of the pial vessels or a small superficial cortical injury with blood leakage into the subarachnoid

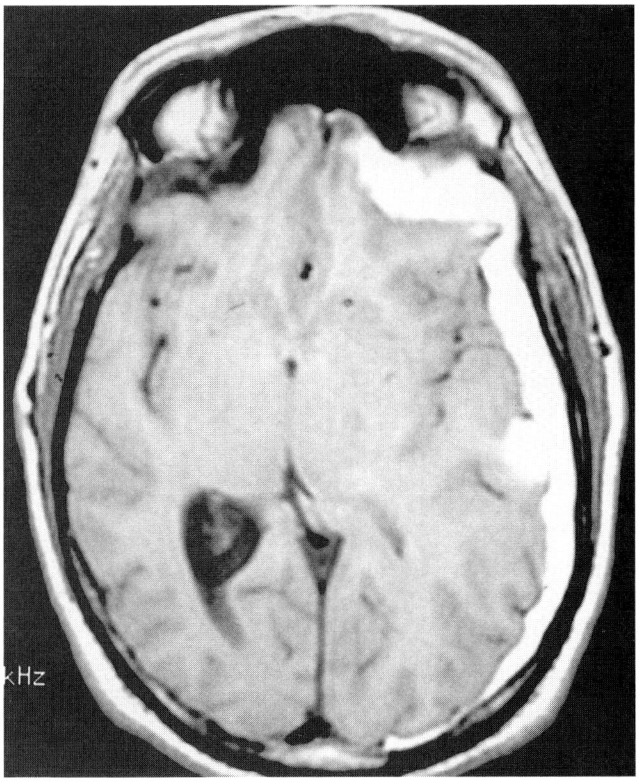

Figure 15-2 Subdural hematoma. On MRI, a T1-weighted spin-echo image shows a high-intensity subdural hematoma (SDH) in the left cranial fossa extending from the frontal to the occipital regions. A cortical hemorrhagic contusion is also seen at the left temporal cortex.

space. A traumatic SAH usually localizes in the interpeduncular fossa or sylvian fissures; however, it may spread diffusely throughout the entire subarachnoid space. A traumatic SAH may be an isolated finding in head trauma, associated with an intracerebral contusion or extracerebral hemorrhage, such as an intraventricular hemorrhage.

INTRAVENTRICULAR HEMORRHAGE

A traumatic intraventricular hemorrhage (IVH) is quite commonly seen on CT after head trauma. Computed tomography may detect a very small volume of intraventricular blood. Bleeding in an IVH may stem from subependymal vein injury, involving ventricular portions of the corpus callosum or fornices of the choroid plexus. An IVH may accompany intracerebral or extracerebral hemorrhages. An IVH is more frequently seen as a ventricular extension of an intracerebral hematoma.

A small amount of intraventricular blood may not be life-threatening, but it may induce acute hydrocephalus, cerebral swelling, or a severe increase of intracranial pressure, requiring an emergent ventriculostomy. The sequelae of a traumatic IVH and/or a SAH may also include posttraumatic hydrocephalus due to the blockage of CSF absorption. For the evaluation of an acute SAH or IVH, CT is superior to MRI.

INTRACEREBRAL INJURY

The intracerebral injury primarily relates to the line of impact: coup contusions are situated beneath the impact, contrecoup contusions are in the contralateral hemisphere. Contusions along the line of force (other than these two) are intermediary coup contusions. The posterior fossa tends to be exempt from this kind of injury.

There are two additional contusions that are not directly related to coup and contrecoup contusions:

1. Momentary shifting contusions occurring at the cerebellar tonsils due to downward shifting into the foramen magnum.
2. Gliding or stretching contusions, in which the sudden gliding produces overstretching. Gliding contusions occur more often in white matter and the cortex of both frontal and paramedial central convolutions.

According to pathologic findings, the term *contusion* applies to all types of intracerebral injury produced by the force of impact to the head. Morphologically, three major types of contusion can be differentiated:

1. Contusion hemorrhage
2. Contusion necrosis
3. Contusion tear

CONTUSION HEMORRHAGE AND HEMATOMA

Hemorrhagic cortical contusions represent about half of all intracerebral injuries. A hemorrhagic contusion usually occurs in the part of the brain adjacent to firm structures, such as the orbital roof, anterior temporal fossa, and sphenoid ridge. A contusion hemorrhage is a small hemorrhage initially but can potentially develop into a space-occupying lesion. As a rule, however, few enlarge to form a hematoma. Traumatic intracerebral hemorrhage is the result of leakage of blood from injured brain parenchyma. The bleeding may stop secondary to vascular spasm or thrombosis. Rebleeding may occur and form a delayed hematoma, resulting in Bollinger's late traumatic apoplexy. Delayed hematomas may occur as quickly as a few hours after the initial injury, but most occur between 2 and 5 days afterward. It has been reported that severely contused areas or areas being compressed by overlying hematomas can undergo delayed cortical hematoma formation. Delayed hematomas are often associated with the worst prognosis. Hemorrhage that is less than 12 h old cannot be differentiated on MRI from other edematous lesions. Computed tomography is the primary tool for the evaluation of acute hematoma in head trauma (Fig. 15-3). After the acute phase, the hematoma starts to decrease in density on the outside. It may then become isodense at the subacute stage and have low density at the chronic stage. Contrast-enhanced CT may show a ringlike enhancement along the peripheral margin of the hematoma. Hyperacute hematoma that is less than 1 day old may appear as isointense on T1-weighted images and hyperintensity on T2-weighted images due to intracellular oxyhemoglobin. Once intracellular hemoglobin turns into deoxyhemoglobin, blood signals may appear with slight hypointensity on T1-weighted images and hypointensity on T2-weighted images during the acute stage within a 3-day window. The blood may become intracellular methemoglobin after 3 days, with hyperintense signals on T1-weighted images and hypointense on T2-weighted images. Once the hemorrhage lasts more than 1 week, methemoglobin will leak from the intracellular to the extracellular space and appear hyperintense on all sequences. As the blood evolves progressively from hemichromatosis to hemosiderosis, the chronic hematoma will appear hypointense, since the surroundings are isointense, at the center on T1-weighted images, hypointense at the rim, and hyperintense at the center on T2-weighted images.

CONTUSION NECROSIS AND CONTUSION TEAR

These two types of contusions are the result of shearing forces. Contusion necrosis typically occurs at the crest of convolutions. It is usually associated with a few small hemorrhages (or even without hemorrhage at all).

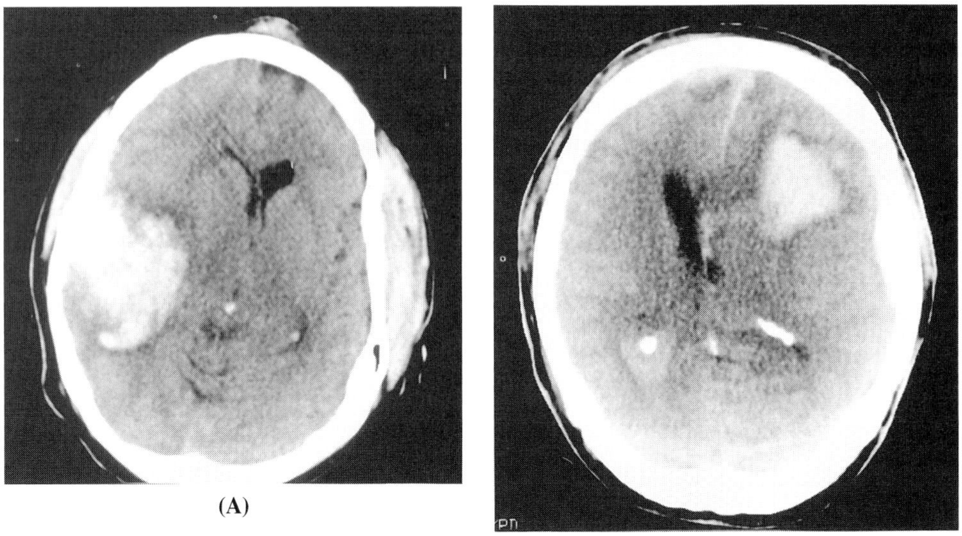

(A)

(B)

Figure 15-3 Intracranial hematoma. *A*. Computed tomography shows a huge hematoma of the right temporal lobe with brain herniation (subfalcial) as a contrecoup contusion from an impact at the left temporal area. *B*. Computed tomography shows a left frontal lobe hematoma dissecting into the left frontal horn and right trigone. A small right frontal hemorrhagic contusion also presents just under the inner table.

Conversely, contusion tears occur deep within the parenchyma, as in the corpus callosum, the septum pellucidum, the pyramids of the brainstem, or deep white matter. Strich observed swelling of white matter in patients with severe brain injury. This finding is known as a shearing axonal injury of the white matter. Shearing injuries are the result of severe head trauma with disruption of the nerve fibers at the juncture between gray and white matter. This is a typical example of a contusion tear as described by Lindenberg. Computed tomography usually shows hemorrhage at the corticomedullary junction and deep parenchymal small areas of petechial hemorrhages or a diffused swelling pattern with effacement of the sulci and small ventricles. If the patient has severe clinical symptoms and the CT demonstrates hemorrhage at the corpus callosum with small ventricles, shearing injury should be suspected.

The value of CT in head trauma has been well established. It will identify significant intracranial hematomas in severe head trauma without any difficulty. Frequently, patients with severe head trauma are identified as having diffuse brain injury even if no significant or obvious hemorrhage is seen on the CT. However, a comatose patient's condition may be due to diffuse cerebral swelling or edema secondary to trauma. Cerebral swelling may be due to increasing blood volume and hyperemia or due to the slowing of capillary circulation and increased water content. Cerebral swelling may also be secondary to loss of autoregulation of blood flow. The patient may recover completely without residual morphologic damage. Cerebral swelling or edema can be diffuse or focal and may produce effacement of sulci or cisterns as well as compression of cerebral ventricles. Cerebral injuries on CT, based upon the density difference, may be divided into the following: hematoma, hemorrhagic contusion, isodense contusion, edematous contusion, and edema. Computed tomography can confidently identify the high density of hemorrhage and the low density of edema. However, isodense traumatic contusions, when petechial hemorrhage mixes with edema fluid, may not be so easily identified on CT. Magnetic resonance imaging is superior in identifying the contusions with subtle signal intensity change in gray and white matter. Thus, MRI is the imaging modality of choice in evaluating diffuse brain injuries such as a shearing injury or diffuse swelling. However, it may not be suitable for the evaluation of head trauma in the acute stage due to the patient's unstable condition or because of the patient's excessive restlessness. It is better to perform MRI during the subacute stage, several days after the initial trauma.

A shearing injury usually shows a small area of abnormal density in the white matter and spares the cortical gyrus. This is in contrast to a cortical contusion. The MRI manifestations of a shearing injury depend upon the presence of hemorrhage and the age of the contusion. As usual, the T1-weighted spin-echo MRI is often normal, but the T2-weighted images will show multiple foci of hyperintensity at the corticomedullary junction of white matter or deep parenchyma, especially at the corpus callosum. The hyperintense lesions may dissolve as the lesion evolves. However, MRI may show hypointense areas in the white matter on T2-weighted spin-echo or gradient-echo sequences if there is hemorrhage. The gradient-echo sequence is more sensitive in identifying small hemorrhagic foci than the regular spin-echo sequence. The signal changes will depend upon the blood degradation.

BRAINSTEM INJURY

Brainstem injury often accompanies fatal head injuries. The mortality and morbidity associated with brainstem injury are very high. Brainstem injuries may occur at the time of the original trauma, with direct impact from the clivus or tentorium, or from shearing forces. A secondary injury may be the result of mechanical stresses secondary to tentorial herniation, with hypoxic injury or Duret hemorrhage. Duret hemorrhage may be due to the laceration of perforating arteries or venous congestion from dural sinus compression. Computed tomography may not identify brainstem injuries if there is no significant hemorrhage or density change, but secondary signs may be seen with obliteration of mesencephalic and/or ambient cisterns secondary to swelling or edema. Magnetic resonance imaging may identify small or isodense brainstem injuries that are not seen on CT.

☐ PENETRATING INJURIES

Penetrating injuries may be the result of knife or gunshot wounds. The incidence of gunshot injuries has increased. The damage to the brain from a bullet depends upon the caliber and velocity. Once the bullet penetrates the skull, it passes through the meninges and enters the brain. If the bullet has lost much of its energy, it may proceed slowly and either stop in the brain, deflect to the other side, or follow tangentially along the skull. If the bullet has great velocity, it may result in a massive path of necrosis and produce an exit wound. A shotgun injury usually produces a large entrance wound with multiple pellet channels. This differs greatly from the injury caused by a single bullet.

Skull radiographs may provide valuable information for a gunshot wound to the head. However, the smaller bone fragments may not show up on a skull radiograph and may require the use of CT. A CT scan can also provide a three-dimensional evaluation of the path of the bullet, the bone fragments, and the extent of brain injury, not only from the bullet but also from the shock waves of impact.

☐ THE ROLE OF MAGNETIC RESONANCE IMAGING IN HEAD TRAUMA

Although MRI is superior to CT in the evaluation of intracranial hemorrhage, CT is more obtainable and more tolerant of the patient's motion. Despite the fact that the fast spin-echo technique of MRI can decrease imaging time, it is not suitable for acute hemorrhage and requires additional technique such as the gradient-echo pulse sequence. Computed tomography is superior to MRI in evaluating skull fracture, bone fragments, and a bullet. Magnetic resonance imaging is the preferred modality in the evaluation of subacute or chronic head injuries and secondary sequelae such as diffuse cerebral swelling, ischemia, and vascular injuries. It is superior to CT in the evaluation of isodense intracranial injuries, shearing injury (Fig. 15-4) and posterior fossa trauma. However, CT should remain the primary imaging modality for the evaluation of acute head trauma.

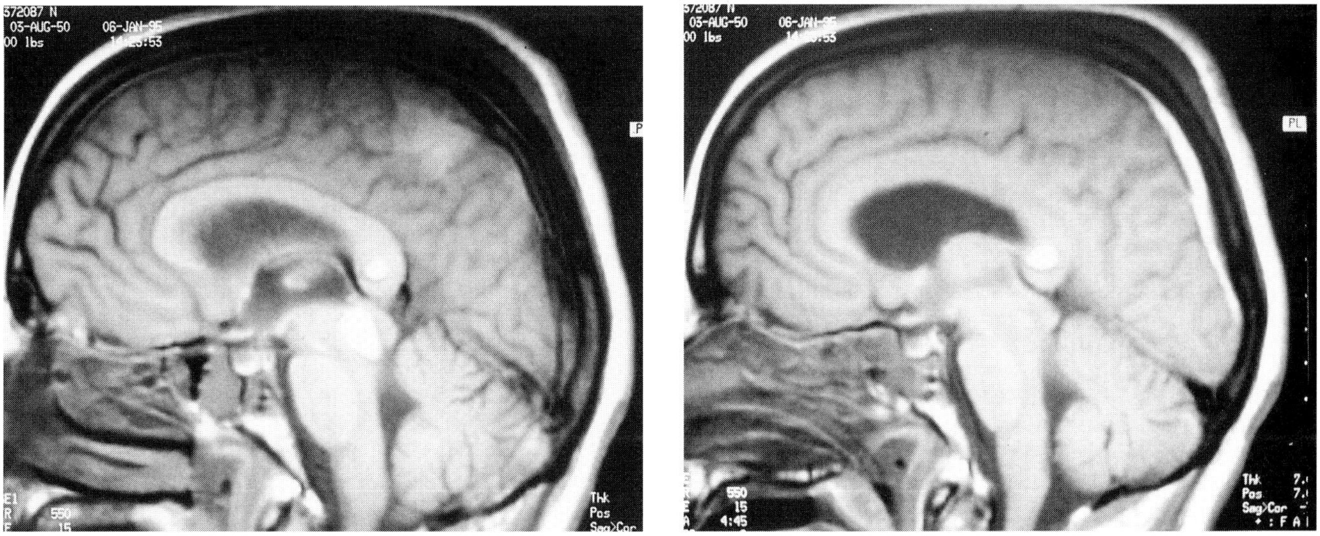

(A) (B)

Figure 15-4 *A* and *B*. Saggital T1-weighted MRI shows a high-signal intensity subacute SDH in the parieto-occipital region and small areas of high-signal intensity in the splenium of corpus callosum and midbrain, consistent with hematomas due to shearing injury.

SUGGESTED READINGS

1. Adams JH et al: Diffuse axonal injury due to non-missile head injury in humans: An analysis of 45 cases. *Ann Neurol* 12:557–563, 1982.
2. Annegers JF, Kurland LT: The epidemiology of central nervous system, in Odom GL (ed): *Central Nervous System Trauma Research, Status Report*. Washington DC, National Institutes of Health, 1979, pp. 1–8.
3. Baker CC et al: Epidemiology of trauma deaths. *Am J Surg* 140:144–150, 1980.
4. Baykaner K et al: Observation of 95 patients with extradural hematomas and review of the literature. *Surg Neurol* 30:339–341, 1988.
5. Becker DP et al: The outcome from severe head injury with early diagnosis and intensive management. *J Neurosurg* 47:491, 1977.
6. Braakman R: Depressed skull fracture: Data, treatment and follow-up in 225 consecutive cases. *J Neurol Neurosurg Psychiatry* 35:395, 1972.
7. Bradley WG: MR appearance of hemorrhage in the brain. *Radiology* 189:15–26, 1993.
8. Braun J et al: Acute subdural hematoma mimicking epidural hematoma on CT. *AJNR* 8:171–173, 1987.
9. Caplan LR, Zervas NT: Survival with permanent midbrain dysfunction after surgical treatment of traumatic subdural hematoma: The clinical picture of a Duret hemorrhage. *Ann Neurol* 1:587–589, 1977.
10. Carey ME et al: A bacteriological study of craniocerebral missile wounds from Vietnam. *J Neurosurg* 34:145, 1971.
11. Chakeres DW, Bryan RN: Acute subarachnoid hemorrhage: In vitro comparison of magnetic resonance and computed tomography. *AJNR* 7:223–228, 1986.
12. Clifton GL: Traumatic lesions, in Rosenberg RN, Grossman RG (eds): *The Clinical Neurosciences*. New York, Churchill Livingstone, 1983, pp 1269–1311.
13. Clifton GL et al: Neurological course and correlated computerized tomography findings after severe closed head injury. *J Neurosurg* 52:611, 1980.
14. Clifton GL et al: Neuropathology of early and late deaths after head injury. *Neurosurgery* 8:309, 1981.
15. Cooper PR et al: Traumatically induced brain stem hemorrhage and the computerized tomographic scan: Clinical, pathological, and experimental observations. *Neurosurgery* 4:115–124, 1979.
16. Cordobes F et al: Intraventricular hemorrhage in severe head injury. *J Neurosurg* 58:217–222, 1983.
17. Cordobes F et al: Post traumatic diffuse axonal brain injury: Analysis of 78 patients studied with computed tomography. *Acta Neurochir* 81:27–35, 1986.
18. Crockhard HA: Early intracranial pressure studies in gunshot wounds of the brain. *J Trauma* 15:339, 1975.
19. Davis KR et al: Computed tomography in head trauma. *Semin Roentgenol* 12:53–62, 1977.
20. Dawson SL et al: The contrecoup phenomenon: Reappraisal of a classic problem. *Hum Pathol* 11:155–166, 1980.
21. Freytag E: Autopsy findings in head injuries from firearms. *Arch Pathol* 76:215, 1963.
22. Friede RL, Roessman U: The pathogenesis of secondary mid-brain hemorrhages. *Neurology* 16:1210–1216, 1966.
23. Garniak A et al: Skull x-rays in head trauma: Are they still necessary? *Eur J Radiol* 6:89–91, 1986.
24. Gentry LR et al: MR imaging of head trauma: Review of the distribution and radiopathologic features of traumatic lesions. *AJR* 150:663–672, 1988.
25. Gentry LR et al: MR imaging of head trauma: Review of the distribution and radiopathologic features of traumatic lesions. *AJR* 150:663–672, 1988.
26. George B et al: Frequency of primary brainstem lesions after head injuries: A CT analysis from 186 cases of severe head trauma. *Acta Neurochir (Wein)* 59:35–43, 1981.
27. Goldstein M: Traumatic brain injury: A silent epidemic. *Ann Neurol* 27:327, 1990.
28. Greenberg J et al: The "hyperacute" extra-axial intracranial hematoma: Computed tomographic findings and clinical significance. *Neurosurgery* 17:48–56, 1985.
29. Gugliamini P et al: Post traumatic leptomeningeal cyst in infancy. *Neurosurgery* 9:11–14, 1981.
30. Han JS et al: Head trauma evaluated by magnetic resonance and computed tomography: A comparison. *Radiology* 150:71–77, 1984.
31. Hesselink JR et al: MR imaging of brain contusions: A comparative study with CT. *AJR* 150:1133–1142, 1988.
32. Holbourn AHS: Mechanics of head injuries. *Lancet* 2:438–441, 1943.
33. Jennet B et al: Epilepsy after non-missile depressed skull fracture. *J Neurosurg* 41:208, 1974.
34. Kaufman HH et al: Isodense acute subdural hematoma. *J Comput Assist Tomogr* 4:557–559, 1980.
35. Kaufman HH et al: Delayed and recurrent intracranial hematomas related to disseminated intravascular clotting and fibrinolysis in head injury. *Neurosurgery* 7:445, 1980.
36. Kelly AB, Zimmerman RA: Head trauma: Comparison of MR and CT—Experience in 100 patients. *AJNR* 9:699–708, 1988.
37. Kim KS et al: Computed tomography in the isodense subdural hematoma. *Radiology* 128:71–74, 1978.
38. Lende RA, Erickson TC: Growing skull fractures of childhood. *J Neurosurg* 18:479–489, 1961.
39. Lindenberg R: Pathology of craniocerebral injuries, in Newton TH, Potts DG (eds): *Radiology of the Skull and Brain: Anatomy and Pathology*. St Louis, Mosby, 1977, pp 3049–3087.
40. Masters SJ: Evaluation of head trauma: Efficacy of skull films *AJR* 135:539–547, 1980.
41. Mittl RL et al: Prevalence of MR evidence of diffuse axonal injury in patients with mild head injury and normal head CT findings. *AJNR* 15:1583–1598, 1994.
42. Nanassis K et al: Delayed post-traumatic intracerebral bleeding. *Neurosurg Rev* 12:243–251, 1989.
43. Pozzati E et al: Extradural hematomas of the posterior cranial fossa: Observations on a series of 32 consecutive cases treated after the introduction of computed tomographic scanning. *Surg Neurol* 32:300–303, 1989.
44. Reed D et al: Acute subdural hematomas: Atypical CT findings. *AJNR* 7:417–421, 1986.
45. Shenkin HA: Acute subdural hematoma: Review of 39 consecutive cases with a high incidence of cortical rupture. *J Neurosurg* 57:254–257, 1982.
46. Sklar EML et al: Magnetic resonance applications in cerebral injury. *Radiol Clin North Am* 30:353–366, 1992.
47. Snow RB et al: Comparison of magnetic resonance imaging and computed tomography in the evaluation of head injury. *Neurosurgery* 18:45–52, 1986.

48. St John JN, Dila C: Traumatic subdural hygroma in adults. *Neurosurgery* 9:621–626, 1981.
49. Stone JL et al: Traumatic subdural hygroma. *Neurosurgery* 8:542–550, 1981.
50. Strich SJ: Shearing of nerve fibers as a cause of brain damage due to head injury: A pathological study of twenty cases. *Lancet* 1:2443–2448, 1961.
51. Tsai FY et al: *Neuroradiology in Head Trauma*. Baltimore, MD, University Park Press, 1983, pp 3049–3087.
52. Tsai FY et al: Diagnostic and prognostic implications of computerized tomography of head trauma. *J Comput Assist Tomogr* 2:323–331, 1978.
53. Tsai FY et al: The contrast enhanced CT scan in the diagnosis of isodense subdural hematoma. *J Neurosurg* 50:64–69, 1979.
54. Tsai FY et al: Computed tomography in child abuse head trauma. *J Comput Assist Tomogr* 4:277–286, 1980.
55. Tsai FY et al: Computed tomography of posterior fossa trauma. *J Comput Assist Tomogr* 4:291–305, 1980.
56. Tsai FY et al: CT of brainstem injury. *AJNR* 1:23–29, 1980.
57. Zimmerman RA et al: Computed tomography of shearing injuries of the cerebral white matter. *Radiology* 127:393–396, 1978.
58. Zuccarello M et al: Traumatic primary brainstem hemorrhage: A clinical and experimental study. *Acta Neurochir (Wein)* 67:103–113, 1983.
59. Zuccarello M et al: Epidural hematomas of the posterior cranial fossa. *Neurosurgery* 8:434–437, 1981.
60. Zulch KJ: Delayed post-traumatic apoplexy. *Neurosurg Rev* 12:252–253, 1989.

☐ QUESTIONS (True or False)

1. Skull radiography is the diagnostic exam of choice for the evaluation of head trauma.
2. Seventh- and eighth-cranial-nerve palsies are commonly associated with transverse fractures of the petrous bone.
3. Pneumocephalus and infection are common complications of basal skull fractures.
4. An epidural hematoma (EDH) lies external to the periosteal dura and frequently extends beyond the suture margin.
5. Epidural hematomas are typically crescent-shaped.
6. An EDH is almost always the result of a coup injury at the site of impact in cases of head trauma.
7. Subdural hematomas (SDH) occur from the rupture of bridging cortical veins.
8. Lacerations of the cortex or contusion frequently occur in patients with an SDH.
9. A chronic SDH appears as low density on CT.
10. Subarachnoid blood is primarily from a small laceration of the meningeal artery.
11. Subarachnoid hemorrhages (SAHs) are often associated with interventricular hemorrhage.
12. Traumatic SAHs usually localize in the interpeduncular fossa or subarachnoid space.
13. Computed tomography is not sensitive for small volumes of intraventricular blood.
14. Intraventricular hemorrhage (IVH) may induce hydrocephalus, cerebral swelling, or severe increases in intracranial pressure.
15. Magnetic resonance imaging is superior to CT for the evaluation of acute SAH or IVH.
16. Shearing injuries are the result of disruption of the nerve fibers at the junction of the gray and white matter.
17. CT findings of shearing injuries show subcortical petechial hemorrhages of a diffuse swelling pattern.
18. Gradient-echo sequences are less sensitive than spin-echo techniques in identifying small hemorrhagic foci.
19. Magnetic resonance imaging is superior to CT in the evaluation of intracranial subacute hemorrhage.
20. Magnetic resonance imaging is superior to CT in evaluating skull fractures, bone fragments, and a bullet injury.
21. Magnetic resonance imaging is superior to CT in the evaluation of subacute and chronic head injuries.

☐ ANSWERS

1. F
2. T
3. T
4. F
5. F
6. T
7. T
8. T
9. T
10. F
11. T
12. T
13. F
14. T
15. F
16. T
17. F
18. F
19. T
20. F
21. T

CHAPTER 16

Intracranial Hemorrhage

William G. Bradley

The diagnosis of hemorrhage in the brain by either computed tomography (CT) or magnetic resonance imaging (MRI) is generally critical to patient management. The initial presentation is usually abrupt and may well be life-threatening. The management of a patient presenting with stroke generally begins with a CT to exclude or confirm the presence of hemorrhage. The correct CT or MRI diagnosis of an intracranial hematoma may lead to a lifesaving craniotomy and evacuation. The correct exclusion of hemorrhage may clear the way for anticoagulation.

The role of the radiologist in the management of intracranial hemorrhage is to diagnose its presence, suggest its cause, and estimate when and exactly where it occurred. The presence of associated findings—for instance, the flow voids of an arteriovenous malformation (AVM) (Fig. 16-1) or an aneurysm, the mass effect and enhancement of a tumor, or the multiplicity of metastases (Fig. 16-2)—may suggest the cause. The location may point to the cause, hypertensive bleeds being more central in the basal ganglia while amyloid angiopathy (Fig. 16-3) occurs more peripherally in elderly patients. The associated findings of cortical and deep white matter infarcts may suggest the presence of vasculitis, cocaine abuse, or a coagulopathy (e.g., lupus).

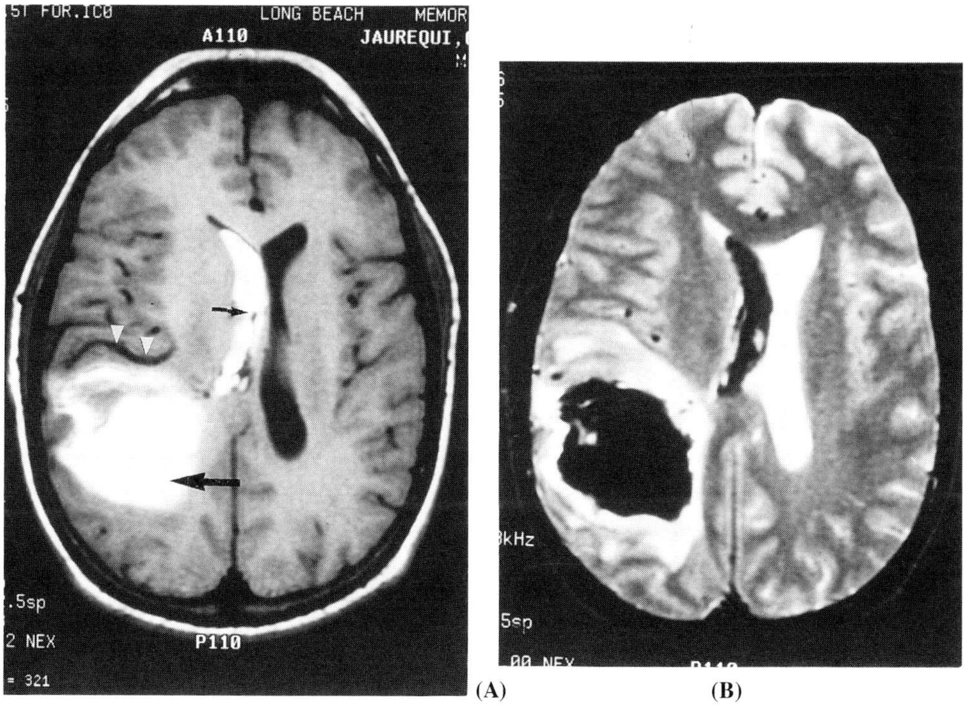

(A) (B)

Figure 16-1 Early subacute hematoma. Thirty-year-old man with known arteriovenous malformation and 4-day history of obtundation. *A*. On MRI, T1-weighted axial image demonstrates hyperintensity in hematomas within right parietal lobe (*large arrow*) and right lateral ventricle (*small arrow*). Note also flow voids of dilated arterial feeders of the arteriovenous malformation (*arrowheads*) [spin echo 500/20] (SE). *B*. T2-weighted axial image demonstrates central hypointensity within both right parietal and right lateral ventricular hematomas. The combination of high signal on the T1-weighted image and low signal on the T2-weighted image is indicative of intracellular methemoglobin.

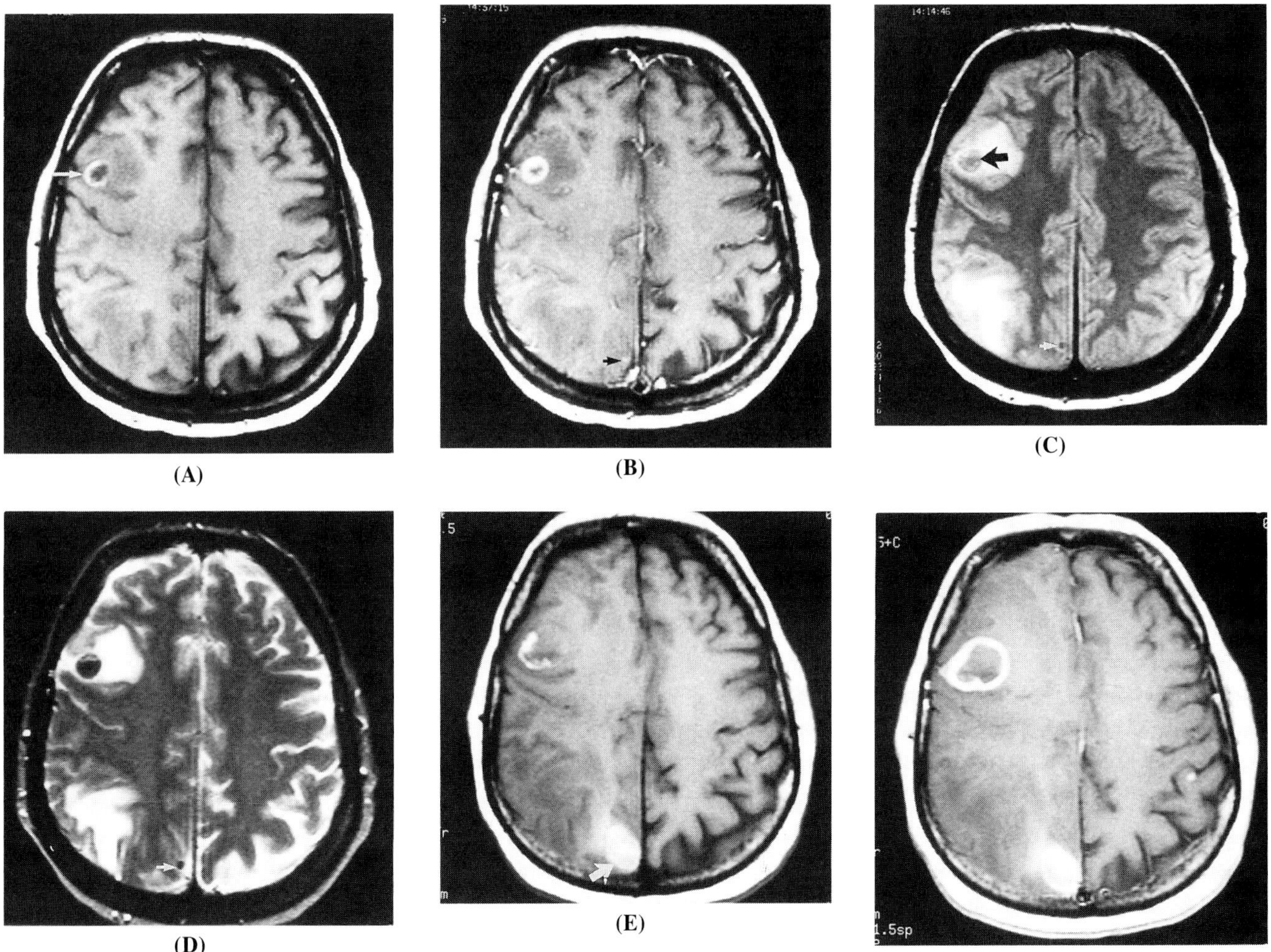

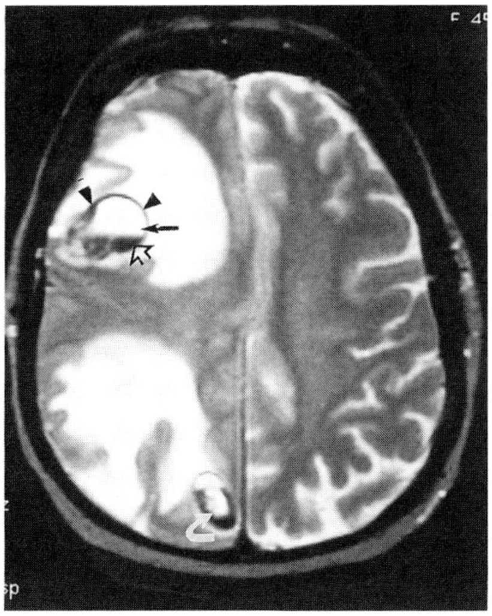

Figure 16-2 Forty-six-year-old woman with hemorrhagic metastatic melanoma. *A*. On MRI, unenhanced T1-weighted axial section demonstrates hyperintensity (*small arrow*) consistent with methemoglobin (SE 500/15). *B*. Enhanced axial section demonstrates larger area of hyperintensity than noted in *A*, indicating tumoral enhancement. Note also punctate focus of enhancement just anterior to the torcula (*small arrow*), suggestive of possible additional lesion (SE 500/15 with gadolinium). *C*. Proton-density-weighted image demonstrates edema around right frontal lesion (*large arrow*), which has now become hypointense, suggesting T2 shortening from hemorrhage. A second, larger area of edema is noted in the right parietal lobe. The punctate focus of enhancement noted in *B* anterior to the superior sagittal sinus now appears hypointense (*small arrow*) (SE 3000/22). *D*. T2-weighted axial image demonstrates marked hypointensity and a fluid level in the right frontal lesion. The combination of findings on the unenhanced T1- and T2-weighted images indicates that the marked hypointensity is due to intracellular deoxyhemoglobin centrally with intracellular methemoglobin peripherally. The slightly more intense nondependent portion represents lysed red cells. Note the marked hypointensity of the punctate right parafalcine lesion (*arrow*) without any evidence of surrounding edema. This is characteristic of hemorrhagic pial metastases (SE 3000/90). *E*. Four months later, the follow-up unenhanced study demonstrates increasing size of all lesions, particularly the posterior right parafalcine lesion (*arrow*). The hyperintensity of the right frontal and parafalcine regions is indicative of methemoglobin on this nonenhanced image (SE 500/20). *F*. Gadolinium-enhanced follow-up image through the same level as *E* demonstrates irregular rim enhancement, particularly of the right frontal lesion, indicative of tumor. No definite enhancement is noted in the right parafalcine lesion posteriorly due to the high background signal of the methemoglobin (SE 500/20 with gadolinium). A new left parietal lesion is also noted (*small arrow*). *G*. T2-weighted image demonstrates fluid levels in both hemorrhagic lesions. The hyperintensity noted in the nondependent position represents serosanguineous fluid (*small arrow*). The marked hypointensity noted in the dependent position (*open arrow*) represents a combination of intracellular deoxyhemoglobin centrally and methemoglobin peripherally. The central hyperintensity in the posterior right parafalcine lesion (*curved arrow*), which remains hyperintense on both T1- and T2-weighted images, represents extracellular methemoglobin. Note also the well-defined hemosiderin rim (*arrowheads*) of the right frontal lesion, which has broken through its lateral margin by recurrent tumor growth (as evidenced by the area of enhancement in *F*) (SE 3000/90).

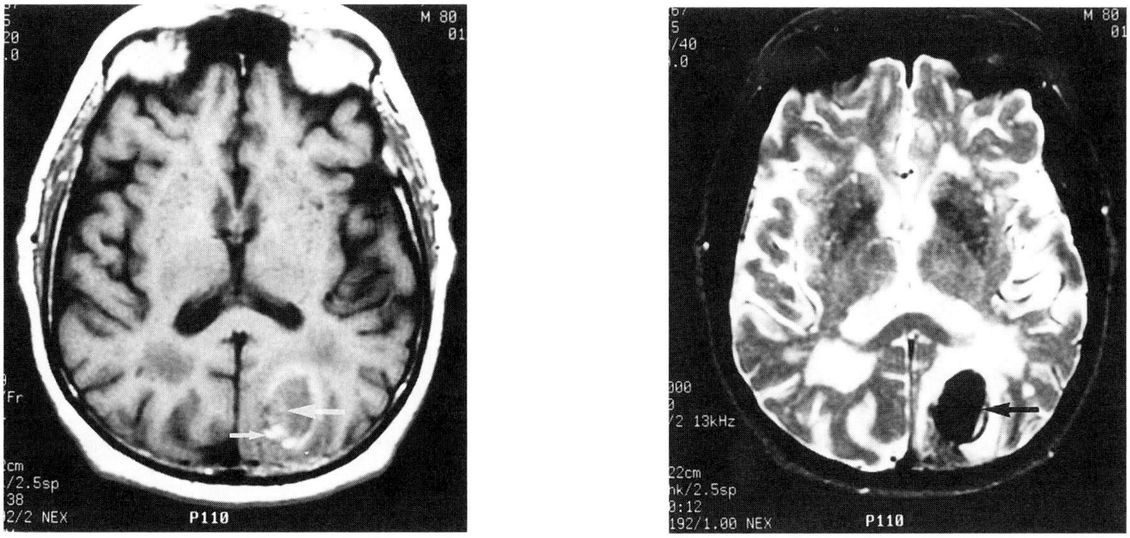

(A) (B)

Figure 16-3 Acute hematoma in an 80-year-old man with 3-day history of "memory loss." *A*. On MRI, T1-weighted axial section demonstrates central isointensity to brain (*large arrow*) with peripheral rim of hyperintensity (*small arrow*) (SE 500/20). *B*. T2-weighted axial image through the same level as *A* demonstrates marked hypointensity (*large arrow*) on this 1.5-T image (SE 3000/90). The combination of findings indicates that the hematoma has a markedly shortened T2 with a small peripheral component of shortened T1. The 3-day history and the presence of persistent mass effect and edema indicates that most of this hemorrhage is in the intracellular deoxyhemoglobin form with early oxidation to methemoglobin at the periphery.

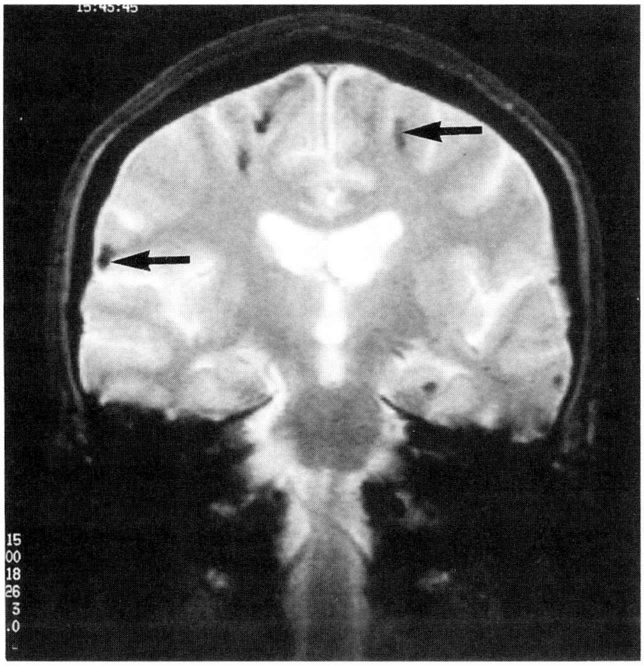

Figure 16-4 Shearing injury. On MRI, low-flip-angle gradient-echo image demonstrates multiple areas of low signal intensity (*arrows*) consistent with magnetically susceptible hemorrhage in this patient, following head trauma in a motor vehicle accident. Shearing injury (diffuse axonal injury) classically involves the gray/white junction, as shown here.

The history (as always) plays a key role in narrowing the differential diagnosis. Known head trauma should prompt a search for coup and contrecoup hematomas as well as associated shearing injury (Fig. 16-4) and subarachnoid, intraventricular, and extraaxial hemorrhage. Knowledge of a coexisting blood dyscrasia or the use of anticoagulants may suggest the cause of hemorrhage following trivial trauma.

The evaluation of intracranial hemorrhage is most often attempted by CT in the acute setting and by MRI in the elective setting. The MRI appearance of most lesions in the brain has a direct correlate in CT. Most lesions, being edematous, appear dark on both unenhanced CT scans and T1-weighted MRI images, i.e., those acquired with a short repetition time (TR) (approximately 500 ms) and a short echo time (TE) (approximately 20 ms) in which T1 contrast predominates. Such lesions also appear bright on T2-weighted MRI images, i.e., those acquired with a long TR (approximately 3000 ms) and a long TE (approximately 80 ms) in which T2 contrast predominates. Hemorrhage, on the other hand, may be bright or dark on T1- or T2-weighted images, depending on the *age* of the hematoma and the integrity of the red cell membrane (1-7). The combination of appearance on T1- and T2-weighted images defines five stages of hemorrhage that can be distinguished by MRI (Table 16-1).

On CT, acute intracranial hemorrhage is usually hyperdense, reflecting a protein effect (Fig. 16-5). Depending on the compartment involved, this lasts for several days, and then the hemorrhage fades to isodensity and, eventually, hypodensity. On MRI, hemorrhage (Table 16-1) evolves in a changing pattern of variable signal

Table 16-1
EVOLUTION OF PARENCHYMAL HEMATOMAS ON MRI

Stage	Time	Compartment	Hemoglobin	T1WI	Intensity on T2WI
Hyperacute	<24 h	Intracellular	Oxyhemoglobin	–	↑
Acute	1–3 days	Intracellular	Deoxyhemoglobin	↓	↓
Subacute					
Early	3+ days	Intracellular	Methemoglobin	↑↑	↓↓
Late	7+ days	Extracellular	Methemoglobin	↑↑	↑↑
Chronic					
Center	14+ days	Extracellular	Hemichromes	–	↑
Rim		Intracellular	Hemosiderin	↓	↓↓

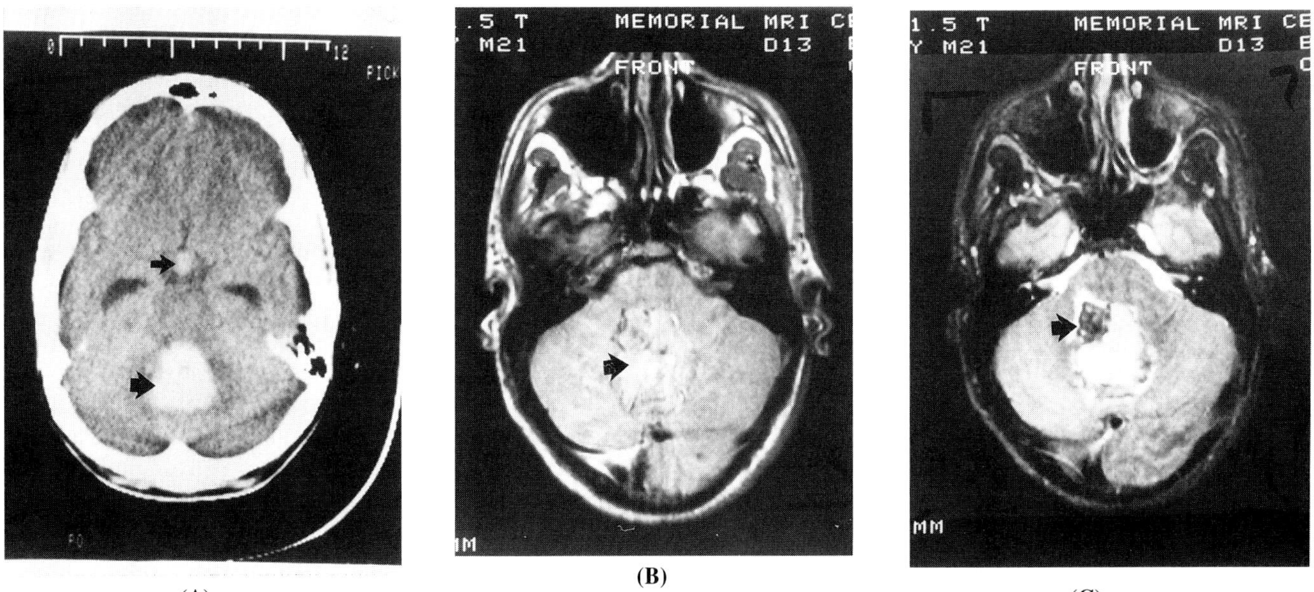

(A) (B) (C)

Figure 16-5 Acute intraventricular hemorrhage in a 21-year-old man 16 h postictus. *A*. Computed tomography demonstrates blood in the anterior recesses of the third ventricle (*small arrow*) and in a massively enlarged fourth ventricle (*large arrow*). *B*. On MRI, proton-density-weighted image demonstrates enlarged fourth ventricle with signal intensity only slightly greater than that expected from CSF (*arrow*). *C*. T2-weighted image demonstrates focal area of low signal intensity (*arrow*), representing retracted clot containing deoxyhemoglobin.

intensity, which depends on the specific form of hemoglobin present (i.e., oxyhemoglobin, deoxyhemoglobin, or methemoglobin) (Fig. 16-6), on whether the red cells are intact or lysed, on the type of MRI signal (that is, routine spin echo, fast spin echo, or gradient echo), and on the degree of T1- or T2-weighting (7).

The appearance of hemorrhage also depends on the specific intracranial compartment involved—subarachnoid, intraventricular, subdural, epidural, intratumoral, or intraparenchymal. Different zones may also be defined from the inner core to the outer rim of parenchymal hematomas. Because there are unpaired electrons in the heme iron of deoxyhemoglobin and methemoglobin, some basic concepts of paramagnetism must be understood to fully appreciate the different T1 and T2 characteristics. Paramagnetic phenomena such as the "electron-proton dipole-dipole interaction" and "magnetic susceptibility effects" both enter into a discussion of the MRI appearance of hemorrhage.

□ PARAMAGNETISM IN HEMORRHAGE

There are two primary mechanisms for T1 and T2 shortening in hemorrhage: "bound-water effects" and "paramagnetic effects" (7, 11). Free, "bulk-phase" water—such as cerebrospinal fluid (CSF)—has very high natural motional frequencies (or, alternatively, very short molecular correlation times). Because these natural motional frequencies are much higher than the Larmor frequencies used in MRI, T1 relaxation is inefficient and the T1 relaxation time of CSF is longer than that of any other substance in the body (approximately 2700 ms) (11).

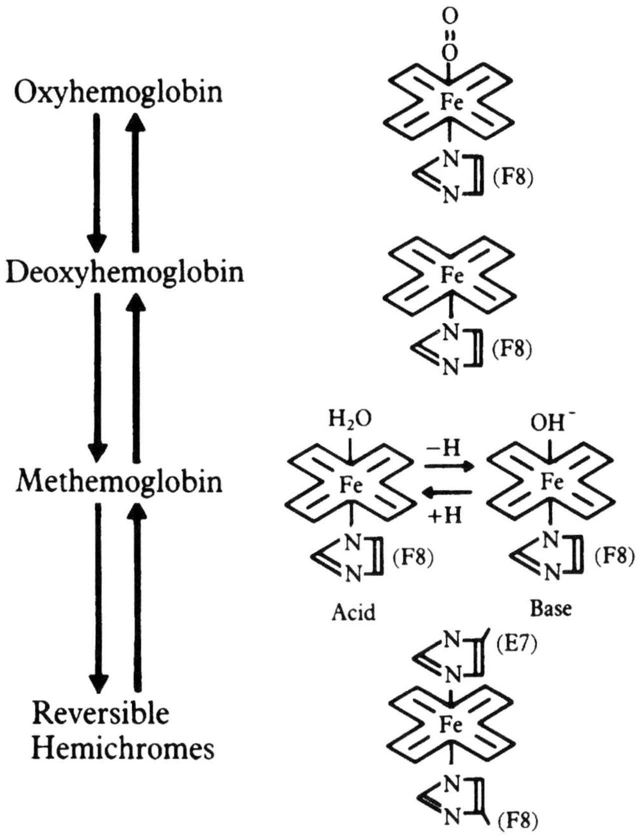

Figure 16-6 Oxidative denaturation of hemoglobin. In the circulating form, hemoglobin goes from the oxy state (as it leaves the pulmonary circulation) to the deoxy state (as it leaves the capillary circulation). Although there is a higher concentration of deoxyhemoglobin in venous blood (30 percent) compared to arterial blood (5 percent), oxyhemoglobin is the predominant form throughout the circulation. The heme iron in both oxy- and deoxyhemoglobin is in the ferrous (Fe^{2+}) state. The heme iron in the oxy form is diamagnetic (i.e., it has no unpaired electrons) and therefore exhibits no paramagnetism. There are four unpaired electrons on the heme iron in deoxyhemoglobin, which is, therefore, paramagnetic. When the hemoglobin is removed from the high-oxygen environment of the circulation, the heme iron undergoes oxidative denaturation to the ferric (Fe^{3+}) state, forming methemoglobin. The combination of five unpaired electrons on the heme iron and a water molecule at the sixth coordination site (in the acid form, which predominates at physiologic pH) results in T1 shortening. Continued oxidative denaturation forms low-spin (diamagnetic) ferric hemichromes where the sixth coordination site is occupied by a second histidine group from the now denatured globin chain. [Reproduced with permission from Bradley WG: Hemorrhage and vascular abnormalities, in Bradley WG, Bydder GM (eds): *MRI Atlas of the Brain*. London, Dunitz, 1990, pp 201–264.]

When protein is added to pure water, the polar water molecules are attracted or "bound" to the charged side groups of the protein, forming a hydration layer. Water in this hydration layer environment has longer molecular correlation times and shorter T1 relaxation times than pure CSF (i.e., approximately 400 to 1000 ms, depending on protein concentration). Thus the T1 of nonparamagnetic, proteinaceous oxyhemoglobin is much less than that of CSF and approaches that of brain parenchyma (11).

Considerably greater T1-shortening is possible due to the dipole-dipole interaction resulting from paramagnetic substances such as gadolinium or methemoglobin in aqueous solution. Such paramagnetic substances (12) (defined by the presence of unpaired electrons) may shorten the T1 of aqueous solutions into the range of several hundred milliseconds, which is considerably shorter than that possible with diamagnetic species (i.e., those *not* having unpaired electrons).

A similar statement can be made for T2 shortening. Proteinaceous solutions of sufficient concentration can bind sufficient water to cause observable T2 shortening compared to brain. Such "solutions" are really more like mucinous gels (11) and contribute to the T2 shortening observed at high hematocrit as water is resorbed from a hematoma (7). Substantially greater T2 shortening is observed from the magnetic susceptibility effects resulting from compartmentalization of paramagnetic deoxy- or methemoglobin inside intact red cells (7). In general, the greater the number of unpaired electrons, the greater the paramagnetic effect (13).

The interaction between the dipole of the unpaired electrons and that of a hydrogen nucleus falls off as the sixth power of the distance between them. Hydrogen nuclei must be able to approach the paramagnetic center within a distance of 3Å (12), or there will be negligible T1 shortening. In methemoglobin, the water molecules can closely approach the heme iron; but in deoxyhemoglobin, they cannot because of the configuration of the protein. Therefore, methemoglobin demonstrates paramagnetic T1 shortening but deoxyhemoglobin does not.

Paramagnetic substances also become more strongly magnetized than diamagnetic substances when placed in a magnetic field. Exactly *how* magnetized a substance becomes is quantified by the "magnetic susceptibility" coefficient, which is the ratio of the induced to the applied magnetic field. Paramagnetic substances such as hemosiderin have high magnetic susceptibilities and become more magnetized than diamagnetic substances when placed in an external magnetic field. This leads to focal "hot spots," which create local regions of magnetic nonuniformity. These, in turn, lead to rapid dephasing of spins and signal loss on T2*-weighted *gradient-echo* images (13–17). As water protons diffuse through these magnetically nonuniform regions, they lose phase coherence in proportion to the interecho time. This dephasing decreases the signal intensity on T2-weighted *spin-echo* images as well (1, 6, 18). Because the induced field (and thus the induced nonuniformity) is proportional to the strength of the applied magnetic field (through the magnetic susceptibility coefficient), both T2*- and T2-shortening are greater at higher fields (1, 5, 14). To the extent that dephasing results from diffusion through the field gradients (19) resulting from these nonuniformities, T2 decreases as the square of the field strength (1) at constant bandwidth. As the receiver bandwidth is decreased on low and midfield systems, however, the sensitivity to susceptibility effects is increased somewhat, partially reflecting the longer TEs required to accommodate the longer echo sampling times. As the time available for diffusion decreases (e.g., with the short echo spacing of hybrid RARE techniques such as *fast spin echo* or *turbo spin echo*), the sensitivity to this magnetic susceptibility decreases (20, 21), although some workers maintain that this decrease is not significant (22). To summarize, the sensitivity to the magnetic susceptibility effects of hemorrhage increases as one progresses from fast spin echo to routine spin echo to gradient echo, from T1- to T2- (or T2*)-weighting, from short to long interecho times or echo spacing, and from lower to higher field strengths.

Dephasing can also result from the diffusion of water molecules across red cell membranes when the magnetic susceptibility inside the red cell differs from that outside (Fig. 16-2). For example, when paramagnetic deoxyhemoglobin or methemoglobin is present within intact red blood cells in an acute or early subacute hematoma, the induced magnetic field inside the red cell is much greater than that outside in the nonparamagnetic plasma. Water molecules diffusing across the red cell membrane thus experience a magnetic field gradient that results in dephasing and T2 shortening (Fig. 16-2) (19).

Clot retraction also causes T2 shortening (23–26). Since this effect does not depend on field strength, it contributes more to the observed T2 shortening at lower fields than at higher fields. Patients with hemorrhagic diatheses or those on anticoagulants, therefore, may not demonstrate the expected T2 shortening following acute hemorrhage, particularly when imaged at lower field strengths.

☐ OXIDATION OF HEMOGLOBIN

The MRI appearance of hemorrhage, which is variable, depends on the structure of hemoglobin and its various oxidation products (27) (Fig. 16-6). In the circulation, hemoglobin alternates between the oxy and deoxy forms. As the blood passes through the high-oxygen environment of the lungs, molecular oxygen (O_2) is bound, forming oxyhemoglobin. When the blood then passes through the lower-oxygen environment of the capillaries, the O_2 is given off, forming deoxyhemoglobin. To bind oxygen reversibly, the iron in the hemoglobin (the "heme iron") must be maintained in the reduced, ferrous (Fe^{2+}) state. When the red cell is removed from the high-oxygen environment of the circulation, deoxyhemoglobin undergoes denaturation to methemoglobin and the heme iron becomes oxidized to the ferric (Fe^{3+}) form.

Changes in the conformation of the hemoglobin molecule result from changes in the oxidation state of the heme iron. The heme iron is normally held in a nonpolar crevice in the deoxyhemoglobin. It is held by a covalent bond to a histidine attached at the F8 position of the globin chain and by four hydrophobic van der Waals forces to nonpolar groups on the globin molecule. The sixth coordination site of the heme iron is occupied by molecular oxygen in oxyhemoglobin and is vacant in deoxyhemoglobin (Fig. 16-6). In methemoglobin, the sixth coordination site is occupied by either a water molecule or a hydroxyl ion, depending on whether the methemoglobin is in the acid or base form, respectively (6). At physiologic pH, the acid form predominates. With continued oxidative denaturation, methemoglobin is converted to derivatives known as hemichromes (27). The iron in these compounds remains in the ferric state. An alteration of the tertiary structure of the globin molecule occurs, such that the sixth coordination site of the heme iron becomes occupied by a ligand from within the globin molecule (the distal histidine at E7).

Following red cell lysis, the hemoglobin is broken down into the heme iron and the globin molecule. The iron is initially stored as ferritin, which is water-soluble ferric hydroxide–phosphate micelles attached to the iron storage protein, apoferritin (28, 29). With localized iron overload (12) and depletion of apoferritin, hemosiderin is formed, which represents water-insoluble clumps of ferritin particles (28).

While the oxidation state of the heme iron has everything to do with its function, it has nothing at all to do with its appearance on MRI. The MRI appearance depends on whether there are unpaired electrons or not (i.e., on whether or not the species is paramagnetic).

The magnetic properties of hemoglobin were initially described almost 150 years ago by Faraday (30) and subsequently by Pauling and Coryell (31). Basically, oxyhemoglobin and the hemichromes are diamagnetic (i.e., they have no unpaired electrons) and deoxy- and methemoglobin are paramagnetic. Deoxyhemoglobin has four unpaired electrons and methemoglobin has five. Since seven unpaired electrons is the maximum possible (e.g., gadolinium), deoxy- and methemoglobin are, indeed, quite paramagnetic.

Paramagnetism per se does not ensure T1 shortening in aqueous solution; the paramagnetic centers must also be accessible to surrounding water protons. Quantitation of T1 shortening requires consideration of the magnitude of the magnetic moment of the paramagnetic dipole (that is, the number of unpaired electrons), the electron spin relaxation time, the concentration of paramagnetic dipoles, the average distance from surrounding water protons, and the relative motions of the protons and the paramagnetic centers (6, 12). Theories of proton relaxation by paramagnetic solutes are based on translational diffusion and the distance of closest approach of the proton and paramagnetic ions, which determines an "outer sphere of influence" (32). It has also been shown that there can be a contribution to the relaxation from exchange between the solvent and water ligands in the first coordination sphere of the paramagnetic ion, that is, "inner-sphere effects" (32).

Although deoxyhemoglobin is paramagnetic, it does not cause T1 shortening. Because the electron spin relaxation time of deoxyhemoglobin is very short and water molecules are unable to approach the heme iron within a distance of 3Å, the T1 of an aqueous solution of deoxyhemoglobin is not short (33). In fact, the T1 of an acute hematoma is prolonged (compared to brain) due to the higher water content (34). The frequencies corresponding to the electron spin relaxation time of methemoglobin, on the other hand, are much closer to the Larmor frequencies used in MRI. Also water molecules are better able to approach the paramagnetic center in methemoglobin than in deoxyhemoglobin (32). Thus, methemoglobin causes significant T1 shortening in aqueous solutions, while deoxyhemoglobin does not.

☐ EVOLVING PARENCHYMAL HEMATOMA

In order to properly stage hemorrhage by MRI, both T1- and T2-weighted images must be acquired. Five stages of an evolving hematoma can be described (7): hyperacute (intracellular oxyhemoglobin, first few hours), acute (intracellular deoxyhemoglobin, 1 to 3 days), early subacute (intracellular methemoglobin, about 3 to 7 days), late subacute (extracellular methemoglobin, more than 7 days), and chronic (older than 2 weeks) (Table 16-1).

During the first few hours (hyperacute phase), the hematoma consists of a mixture of oxy- and deoxyhemoglobin (Fig. 16-7), initially as a liquid suspension of intact red cells and, as thrombosis progresses and plasma is resorbed, an increasingly solid conglomerate of intact red cells (1, 24–26). Over the next few days (acute phase), the hematoma consists primarily of deoxyhemoglobin within intact red cells (1) (Fig. 16-3). The term *hyperacute* was first adopted (35) to describe the stage preceding deoxyhemoglobin, which was defined as "acute" by Gomori (1). Both hyperacute and acute hematomas on MRI appear dense on CT and are labeled "acute."

During the subacute period, which begins after several days, deoxyhemoglobin undergoes oxidative denaturation, forming methemoglobin (6). Early in this phase (Fig. 16-8), the red cells are intact. Later in this phase (after approximately 1 week), red cell lysis occurs (Fig. 16-9).

In parenchymal hematomas, modified macrophages (microglia or "gitter cells") move in from the periphery by the end of the second week and remove the iron from the extracellular methemoglobin (7). This marks the beginning of the chronic phase, when the heme iron is deposited at the periphery as a rim of hemosiderin and ferritin (26) within macrophages (Fig. 16-10). The center of the hematoma is eventually left with non-iron-containing, nonparamagnetic heme pigments, such as hematoidin (36).

A note of caution: although it is useful to describe the evolution of a hematoma in these well-defined stages, in fact the several stages may coexist (8). For example, at the time hemosiderin and ferritin are first deposited at the periphery of a hematoma (indicating the beginning of the chronic stage), free methemoglobin is present in the outer core (late subacute stage) and intracellular deoxyhemoglobin or even oxyhemoglobin may still be found in the inner core from the acute and hyperacute stages, respectively. By convention, the hematoma is described in terms of the most mature form of hemoglobin present (7).

HYPERACUTE PHASE

In the first few hours on short-TR–short-TE T1-weighted images, hyperacute hematomas (mainly oxyhemoglobin) are iso- to hypointense to brain due to their longer T1 times, reflecting their higher water content (24–26). The T2 relaxation time reflects both the fluid-solid character of the fresh hematoma (Fig. 16-11) (23–26) and the relative amounts of oxyhemoglobin and deoxyhemoglobin. Ninety-five percent of arterial blood is oxyhemoglobin (28), which is diamagnetic and does not cause T2 shortening. Because most nontraumatic bleeds are arterial (such as that resulting from aneurysmal rupture, and/or the rupture of microaneurysms in hypertension), there may be no significant T2 shortening in the center of the hematoma initially (Fig. 16-7). Close inspection usually reveals an irregular border (Fig. 16-7) of low intensity surrounding the isointense bulk of the hematoma. This is believed to represent deoxyhemoglobin, produced within a few minutes by deoxygenation of the red cells at the periphery of the hematoma by the adjacent, actively metabolizing brain. The minimum concentration of deoxyhemoglobin that produces visible T2 shortening throughout the rest of the hematoma depends on the field strength (1), the bandwidth, and the imaging technique, gradient echoes being more sensitive than spin echoes (13, 17), which are more sensitive still than fast spin-echo techniques. It should be stressed, however, that during the first few hours, the diagnosis of hemorrhage is more easily made by CT than by MRI.

ACUTE PHASE

After the initial 24 h, deoxyhemoglobin is normally found within clotted, intact red cells (1, 17). As noted above, although deoxyhemoglobin is magnetically susceptible, it does not cause T1 shortening. T2 shortening results from the dephasing due to diffusion of water molecules in and out of the red cell (Fig. 16-3). Since the magnetic susceptibility effects increase with field strength, the low-intensity appearance of an acute hematoma on T2-weighted images may be more obvious at higher fields (1). Low flip angle, short TR, T2*-weighted, gradient echo images are also more sensitive to susceptibility effects than T2-weighted spin-echo images (13-17) (Fig. 16-4). Since high-field and gradient-echo techniques increase the sensitivity to

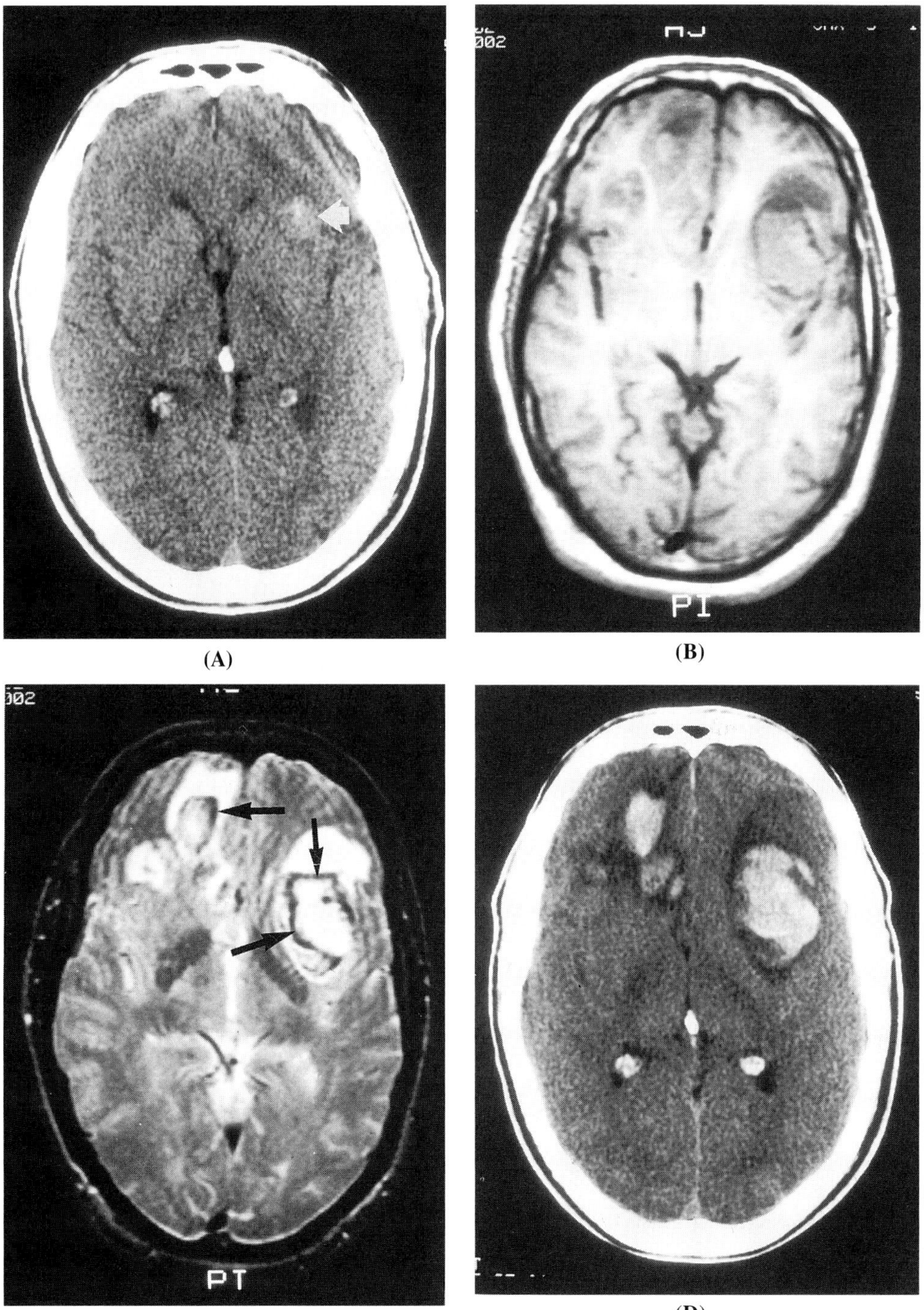

(A) (B) (C) (D)

Figure 16-7 Hyperacute posttraumatic parenchymal hematoma. *A*. Initial CT following motor vehicle accident demonstrates hyperdensity in left frontal lobe (*arrow*) consistent with parenchymal hematoma. *B* and *C*. On MRI, a study performed a few minutes later demonstrates apparent "blooming" of the parenchymal hematomas in both frontal lobes. This hyperacute hemorrhage (oxyhemoglobin) is slightly hypointense brain on the T1-weighted image *B*. and somewhat hyperintense brain on the T2-weighted image *C*., with surrounding very hyperintense vasogenic edema. Note also the low-intensity "borders" on the T2-weighted image (*arrows*), felt to represent early deoxyhemoglobin formation at the point of contact between the hematoma and the still metabolizing brain. *D*. Given the apparent discrepancy in the appearance of the initial CT study in *A* with the MRI study obtained a few minutes later in *B* and *C*, a repeat CT was performed a few minutes later, demonstrating hyperdense hematomas comparable to those seen on the MRI study. The hyperdensity on CT represents a protein density effect. (Courtesy of Robert Lukin, MD, University of Cincinnati.)

magnetic susceptibility effects through different mechanisms, they are additive (13) and produce marked signal loss when applied together.

During both the hyperacute and acute phases, progressive concentration of red cells by thrombosis also causes T2 shortening (23, 25, 37, 38). This reflects both clot retraction and increasing hematocrit. Formation of the fibrin clot (from polymerization of fibrinogen) and clot retraction (by platelets) both shorten T2 (23). Such effects can be seen in plasma clots alone without any magnetically susceptible species (23). Prior to clot retraction, therefore, T2 shortening may be minimal (24, 25).

The T2 shortening resulting from increasing hematocrit increases with increasing field strength, like the magnetic susceptibility effects. The mechanism reflects increasing protein concentration and binding of water protons (11, 39, 40). T2 shortens progressively as the hematocrit approaches 100 percent (23). Dehydration of red blood cells is also known to occur during the acute phase and can cause a selective decrease in T2 (41–45).

It should be stressed that it may not be possible to distinguish among the various mechanisms that lead to T2 shortening in acute hemorrhage. Specifically, the signal loss noted in about 24 h on long-TR–long-TE T2-weighted images may be due to deoxygenation, hemoconcentration,

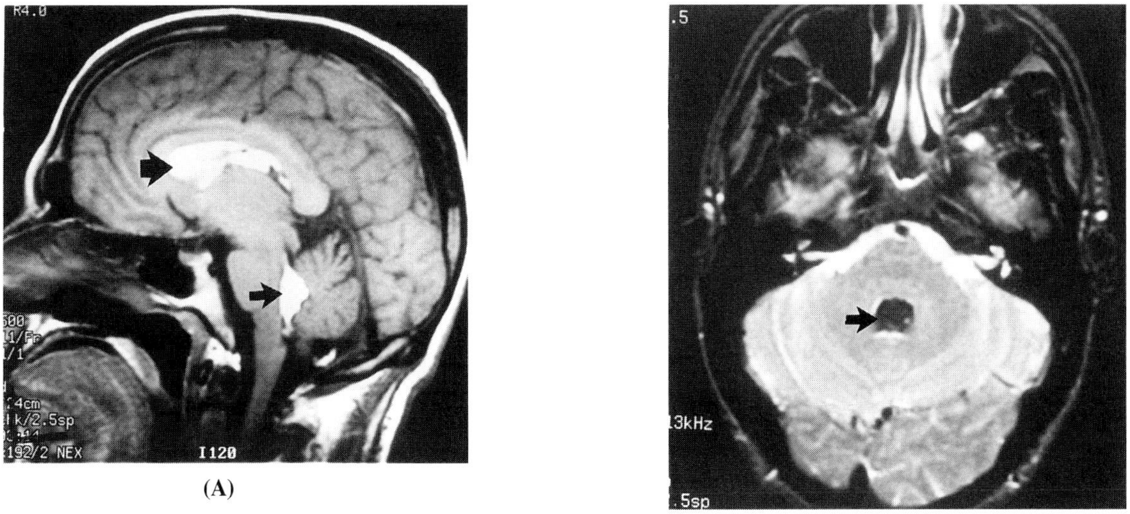

(A) (B)

Figure 16-8 Early subacute intraventricular hemorrhage. *A*. On MRI, sagittal T1-weighted image demonstrates high signal intensity in the third and fourth ventricles (*arrows*). On a T1-weighted image, it can only be stated that this is methemoglobin, without further subdividing it into early or late subacute hemorrhage. *B*. On the T2-weighted image, the hemorrhage in the fourth ventricle turns dark (*arrow*), indicating the presence of early subacute hemorrhage (intracellular methemoglobin).

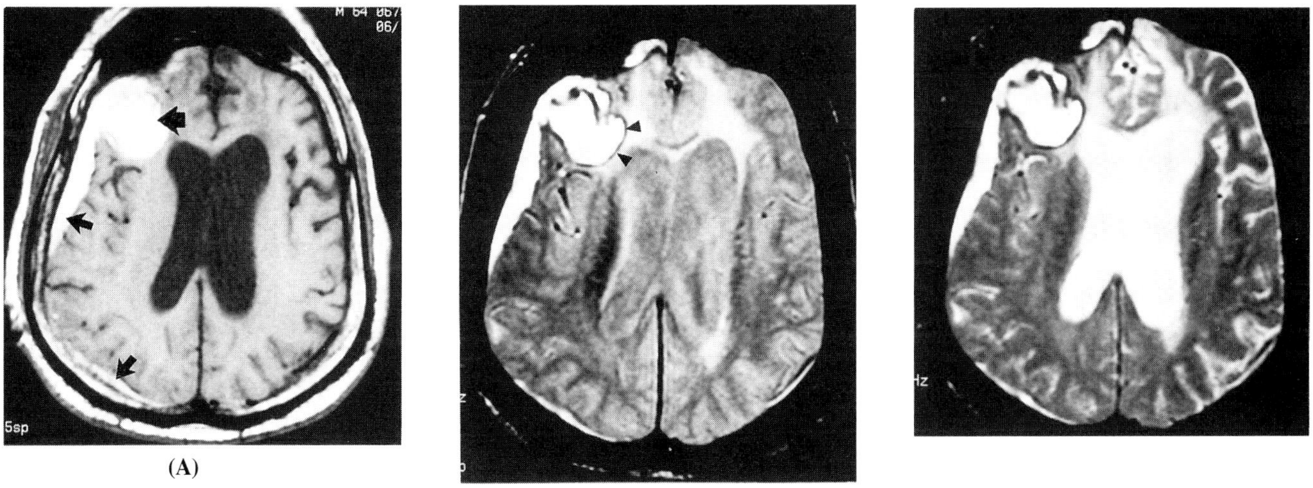

(A) (B) (C)

Figure 16-9 Late subacute hemorrhage 3 weeks following head trauma to a 64-year-old man. *A*. On MRI, a T1-weighted axial image demonstrates high-intensity subdural hematomas of the right convexity (*small arrows*) as well as a right subfrontal parenchymal hematoma (*large arrow*). The ventricles are dilated due to associated communicating hydrocephalus from subarachnoid hemorrhage. *B*. Proton-density-weighted axial image demonstrates persistent hyperintensity of the subdural and parenchymal hematomas relative to lower-intensity CSF. A hemosiderin rim (*arrowheads*) is now becoming visible around the parenchymal hematoma (SE 3000/20). *C*. T2-weighted axial image demonstrates persistent hyperintensity of the subdural and parenchymal hematomas, which are now isointense with hyperintense CSF. The combination of high signal intensity on the T1-weighted image with persistent high signal intensity on the T2-weighted image is indicative of extracellular methemoglobin. The hemosiderin rim surrounding the parenchymal hematoma is more apparent with additional T2-weighting, indicating the beginning of the chronic stage.

red blood cell dehydration, and/or clot retraction. Further, the relative influence of these factors on T2 shortening depends on the operating field strength (23).

EARLY SUBACUTE PHASE

The subacute phase is defined by the oxidation of deoxyhemoglobin to methemoglobin (6). In the early subacute phase, the red cells are still intact (46). With the formation of methemoglobin, T1 is markedly shortened due to a dipole-dipole interaction, resulting in increased intensity on T1-weighted images (6, 46) (Figs. 16-1 and 16-8). For parenchymal hematomas, the formation of methemoglobin begins peripherally (Fig. 16-3) due to "intrinsic tissue factors" (47). In addition, oxygen is needed for the oxidation of the heme iron, and the oxygen level is higher in the normal

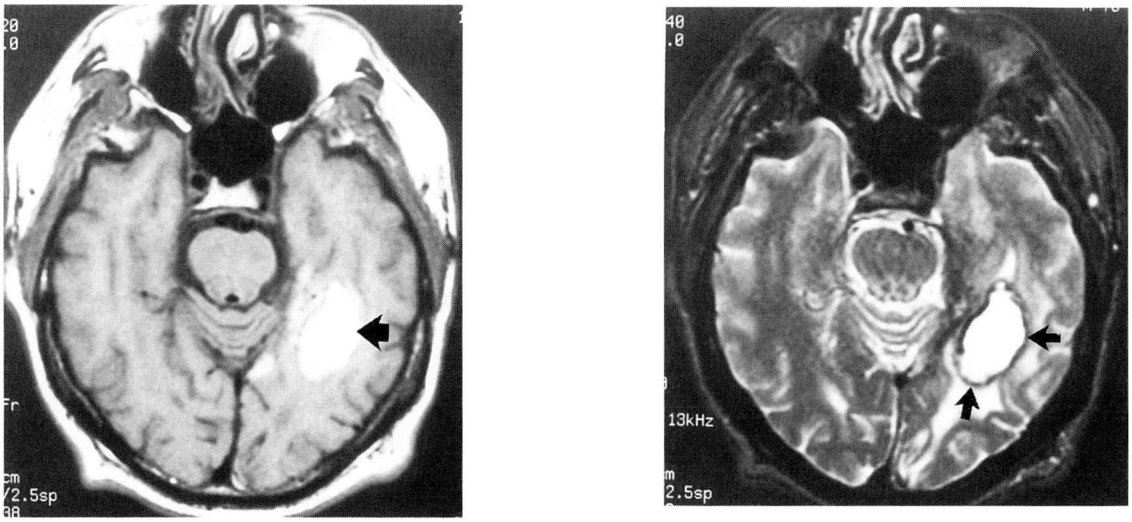

(A) (B)

Figure 16-10 Chronic hematoma. *A*. On MRI, a T1-weighted image demonstrates methemoglobin in the left posterior temporal hematoma (*arrow*). *B*. T2-weighted image demonstrates surrounding rim of ferritin- and hemosiderin-laden macrophages appearing dark (*arrows*). The central high signal intensity is due to the persistent presence of extracellular methemoglobin.

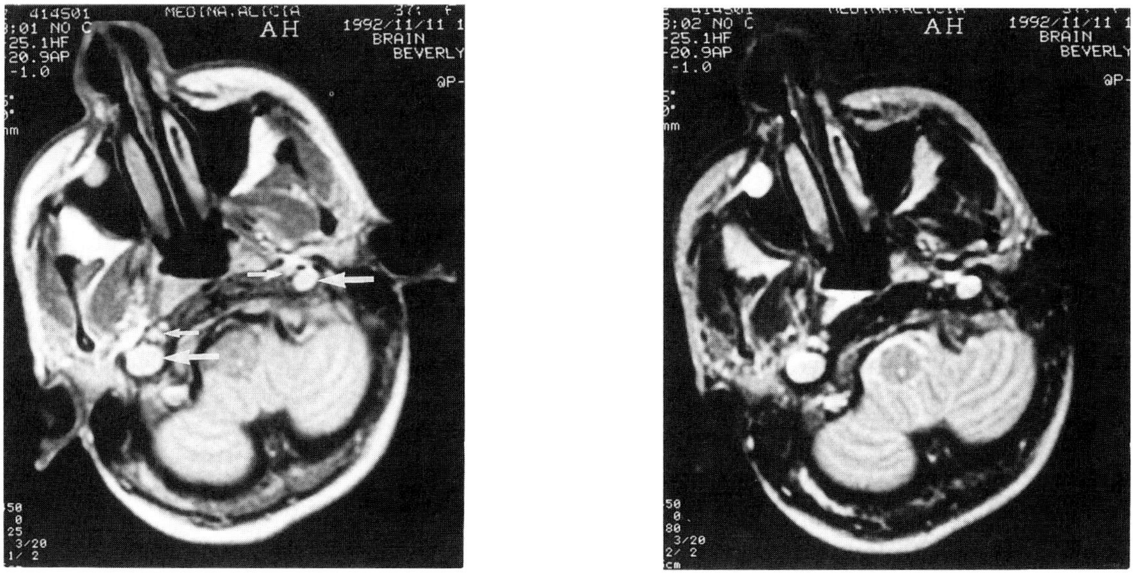

(A) (B)

Figure 16-11 Hyperacute hemorrhage (stagnant oxyhemoglobin) in a 35-year-old heroin addict who had a cardiopulmonary arrest immediately prior to the acquisition of these images. *A*. On MRI, the proton-density-weighted image demonstrates high intravascular signal due to complete absence of motion in the jugular veins (*large arrow*) and carotid arteries (*small arrows*) (SE 3000/25). *B*. T2-weighted axial section through the same level as *A* demonstrates intravascular hyperintensity due to long T2 of unclotted intracellular oxyhemoglobin (SE 3000/80). (The patient was subsequently resuscitated.)

surrounding brain than in the center of the hematoma. Later, the center becomes oxidized to methemoglobin as well. Interestingly, the pattern of methemoglobin formation is exactly the opposite for partially thrombosed intracranial aneurysms, as the oxygen tension is higher in the central lumen than at the periphery (46).

In the early subacute phase, the red cells are still intact. Since methemoglobin is magnetically susceptible, the middle of the red cell becomes more magnetized than the plasma on the outside. Thus the magnetic nonuniformity that causes T2 shortening with intracellular deoxyhemoglobin persists with intracellular methemoglobin.

T1-weighted images are better suited to distinguish acute hemorrhage (long T1) from subacute hemorrhage (short T1). Since methemoglobin has five unpaired electrons (compared to four for deoxyhemoglobin), the T2 of the hematoma should be additionally shortened in the transition from the acute to early subacute phase, although this may be difficult to document.

It should be mentioned that other substances besides methemoglobin can have a short T1. Fat also appears bright on T1-weighted images and, like early subacute hemorrhage, fades on T2-weighted conventional spin-echo images (although not nearly to the same degree as hemorrhage). High protein content (e.g., in a craniopharyngioma) may simulate subacute hemorrhage. Enhancement with gadolinium leads to T1 shortening, which can appear like methemoglobin. The distinction of methemoglobin from these other causes of T1 shortening is usually accomplished on the basis of the lesion morphology or the finding of other stages of hemorrhage in the vicinity.

LATE SUBACUTE PHASE

Late subacute hemorrhage is bright on *both* T1- and T2-weighted images. By the late subacute phase, red cell lysis has occurred. On T1-weighted images, both early and late subacute hemorrhage appears bright, since water molecules can pass freely across the red cell membrane. As lysis occurs, the T2 shortening that had resulted from compartmentalization of methemoglobin is lost (Fig. 16-9). In addition, the high water content of the lysed red cells leads to increases in both T2 and proton density (compared to brain) (48). Obviously, T2-weighted images are necessary to accurately distinguish early (short-T2) from late (long-T2) subacute hemorrhage (7).

CHRONIC PHASE

In the chronic phase, paramagnetic hemosiderin and ferritin (having high magnetic susceptibilities) are found within macrophages in a dark rim surrounding the hematoma on T2-weighted images (Figs. 16-9 and 16-10) (29). In order for ferritin and hemosiderin to be formed, red cells containing methemoglobin must first lyse (29). Thus, initially, there is always a bright ring of free methemoglobin just inside the darker hemosiderin ring on T2-weighted images. Eventually the hematoma is reduced to a hemosiderin-lined slit (Fig. 16-12). Like deoxyhemoglobin, intracellular paramagnetic hemosiderin causes preferential T2 shortening (1).

☐ SUBDURAL AND EPIDURAL HEMATOMAS

Like parenchymal hemorrhage, subdural hematomas (SDHs) have five stages of evolution and thus five different appearances on MRI (7, 49, 50). Since the dura is so well vascularized, however, the oxygen tension remains high and the temporal progression from one stage to the next is slower in the extraaxial compartment than in the brain itself (49). The first four stages are the same as for a parenchymal hematoma, with the same T1 and T2 characteristics. The chronic stage is characterized by continued oxidative denaturation of methemoglobin, forming nonparamagnetic hemichromes (27). The T1 of such compounds is greater than that of paramagnetic methemoglobin; thus the intensity of chronic subdural hematomas is less than that of subacute subdural hematomas, particularly on T1-weighted images. Chronic SDHs (Fig. 16-13) are less intense than subacute subdurals (Fig. 16-9) but more intense than CSF due to their higher protein content (39, 49, 50). In the extraaxial compartments during the chronic phase, there is no hemosiderin rim per se because there are no tissue macrophages to surround the

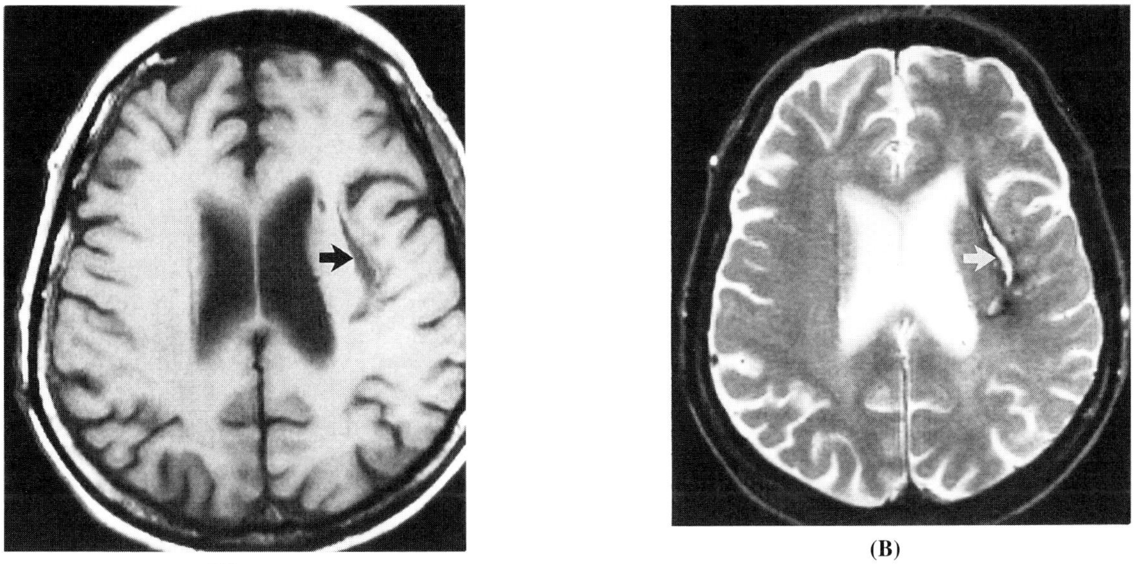

(A) (B)

Figure 16-12 Chronic hematoma in a 61-year-old woman who had a documented hemorrhage 9 months previously and now presented with seizures. *A*. On MRI, T1-weighted image demonstrates slitlike encephalomalacia in the high external capsule (*arrow*) (SE 500/20). *B*. T2-weighted axial image demonstrates hemosiderin-lined slit (*arrow*) from chronic hemorrhage (SE 3000/90).

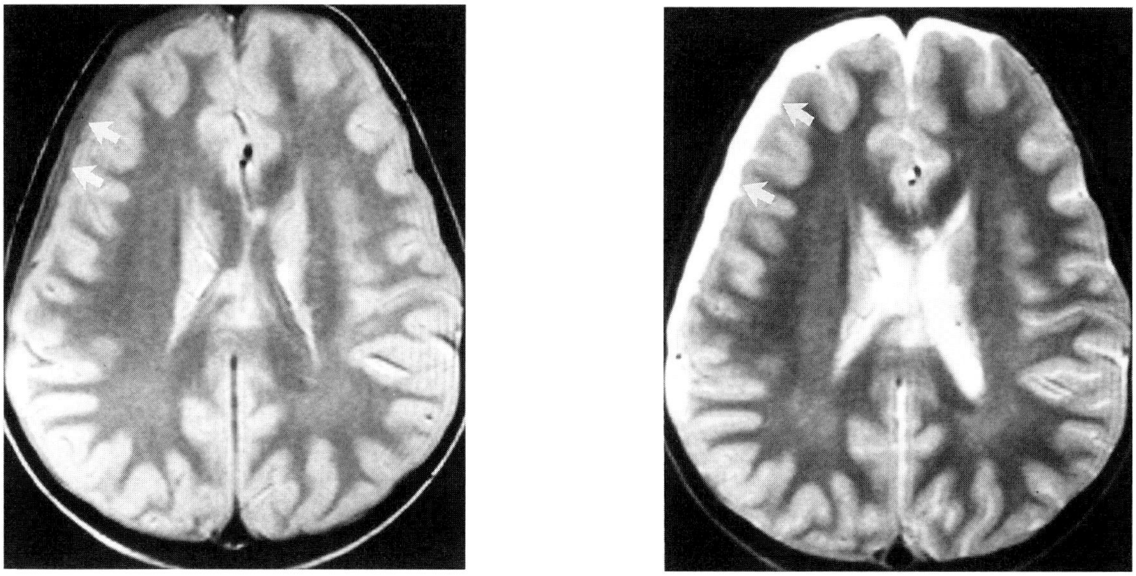

(A) (B)

Figure 16-13 Chronic subdural hematoma in a 5-year-old boy 6 months following head trauma. *A*. On MRI, a so-called proton-density-weighted image demonstrates subdural hematoma of the right convexity (*large arrows*) with slightly higher intensity than the CSF in the lateral ventricles (*small arrows*) (SE 3000/22). The slightly higher signal intensity of the proteinaceous chronic subdural hematoma actually represents T1 shortening from hydration-layer water. *B*. T2-weighted image demonstrates a similar high signal intensity in the subdural collection (*arrows*) and the CSF. On such images, the effects of subtle T1 shortening due to elevated protein concentration are not apparent (SE 3000/90). (Reproduced with permission from Bradley WG: Hemorrhage and brain iron, in Stark DD, Bradley WG (eds): *Magnetic Resonance Imaging*, 2d ed. St Louis, Mosby Year-Book, 1992, p 753.)

hematoma. In the case of recurrent bleeding into a subdural hematoma, however, there may be hemosiderin staining of the membrane that forms along the inner border of the subdural collection. Like the hemosiderin surrounding a parenchymal hematoma, this will also turn dark on T2-weighted images.

In our experience, most elderly patients present in the subacute phase several weeks after the veins bridging the subdural space have been torn by minor trauma. Subdural hematomas are often bilateral and may be of different ages. When recurrent bleeding occurs in a subdural hematoma, the separate events may be distinguishable by the different signal intensities on MRI.

Epidural hematomas (EDHs) evolve in a manner similar to SDHs. They are distinguished from the latter on the basis of classic morphology (i.e., bilenticular EDH versus medially concave SDH) and by the low intensity of the fibrous dura mater (7) between the hematoma and the brain. Like an acute SDH, an acute EDH has deoxyhemoglobin within intact red blood cells, resulting in T2 shortening and low intensity on T2-weighted images, particularly at high field. On the basis of intensity characteristics alone, therefore, it may be difficult to separate the low-intensity dura from the low-intensity hematoma during this phase. In cases of atypical morphology (i.e., bilenticular SDH), it may be difficult to accurately distinguish a subdural from an epidural collection. In the late subacute phase of an epidural hematoma, methemoglobin has been formed and the red cells have lysed, providing excellent contrast between the high-intensity EDH and the low-intensity dura. Unfortunately, during the late subacute stage of a SDH with recurrent bleeding, the hemosiderin-stained membrane can simulate the dura, potentially leading to the mistaken diagnosis of EDH in morphologically atypical cases.

☐ SUBARACHNOID AND INTRAVENTRICULAR HEMORRHAGE

Subarachnoid and intraventricular hemorrhage differs from intraparenchymal, subdural, or epidural hemorrhage in that it is admixed with CSF. Like the extraaxial hematomas, however, subarachnoid and intraventricular hemorrhage have high ambient oxygen levels and thus "age" more slowly than parenchymal hematomas (Fig. 16-10).

Immediately after subarachnoid hemorrhage, there is a small decrease in T1 (6, 51–53), reflecting the increase in hydration-layer water (44) due to the higher protein content of the bloody CSF. This leads to subtle signal increase in the CSF on T1- and proton-density-weighted images ("dirty CSF") (Fig. 16-14) (51–53), which is much more obvious on FLAIR images (Fig. 16-15). As has been shown in vitro (6), significant quantities of methemoglobin are not formed until several days after the hemorrhage. Several days to a week postictus, signal intensity increases in the subarachnoid space due to methemoglobin formation (Fig. 16-16). In cases of milder subarachnoid hemorrhage, the red cells may be resorbed by the time significant methemoglobin formation would have

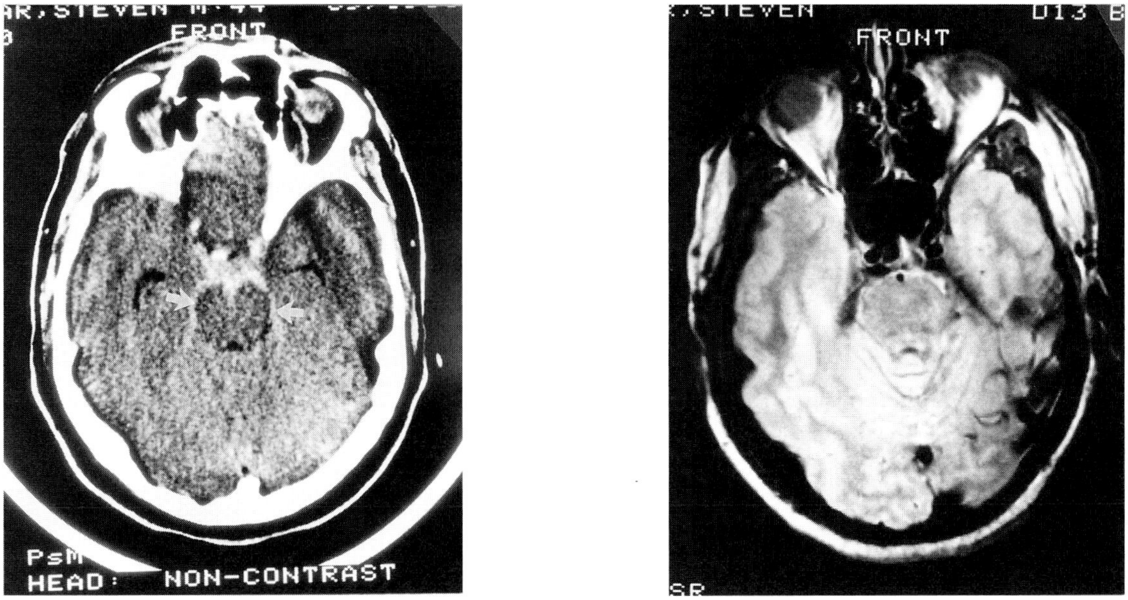

(A) (B)

Figure 16-14 Acute subarachnoid hemorrhage. *A.* On this unenhanced CT study, high density is noted in the interpeduncular and perimesencephalic cisterns (*arrows*), indicative of subarachnoid hemorrhage. *B.* On MRI, subtle high signal intensity is noted in a similar location on the proton-density-weighted image. Since CSF is normally isointense to hypointense to brain on a proton-density-weighted conventional spin-echo image, the high signal noted here anterior to the pontine isthmus is subtly suggestive of subarachnoid hemorrhage. This reflects the protein content of the serum with subsequent mild reduction in T1 of the CSF. This appearance has been called "dirty CSF."

occurred; therefore, the anticipated short-T1 appearance will not be seen. For these reasons, CT is still advocated for the early diagnosis of subarachnoid hemorrhage (6, 7).

A short-T2 appearance may be observed in subarachnoid or intraventricular (Fig. 16-1) hemorrhage when massive bleeding has occurred. When a fluid-fluid level is present, the short-T2 component is dependent, reflecting intact red cells. When short T2 is seen throughout, a subarachnoid or intraventricular *thrombus* may be present. In chronic, repeated subarachnoid hemorrhage, hemosiderin may be seen staining the leptomeninges, leading to a short-T2 appearance known as "superficial siderosis" (54) (Fig. 16-17).

☐ INTRATUMORAL HEMORRHAGE

Hemorrhage is common in the higher-grade gliomas and certain highly vascular metastases, such as melanoma (Fig. 16-2), choriocarcinoma, and carcinoma of the lung, kidney, thyroid, and breast. (Melanoma can also appear bright without hemorrhage due to the paramagnetic free radical on the melanin.)

The diagnosis of a neoplastic source of hemorrhage may be difficult in the subacute setting. Since methemoglobin is already hyperintense, it may be difficult to appreciate marginal gadolinium enhancement against an already intense background. In such cases, CT with and without contrast may be useful, as the subacute hemorrhage is usually hypodense on CT. (Similarly, during the acute phase of a neoplastic hemorrhage, the hyperdensity on CT may make marginal enhancement difficult to appreciate; simultaneously, the background deoxyhemoglobin on a T1-weighted MRI is hypointense, facilitating the detection of marginal enhancement with gadolinium.)

Early pial metastases are notoriously difficult to detect without gadolinium due to the lack of associated vasogenic edema and T2 prolongation (55). Should these metastases be hemorrhagic (Fig. 16-2), they may actually be hypointense on T2-weighted images due to intracellular deoxyhemoglobin and methemoglobin.

When a hematoma results from a primary or metastatic tumor (or other source), fluid-fluid levels may be seen (Fig. 16-2*G*). The dependent portion is often hypointense on T2-weighted images due to the presence of intact red cells containing deoxyhemoglobin or methemoglobin. The nondependent fluid is more intense than CSF on proton-density- and T2-weighted images but not as intense as methemoglobin on T1-weighted images. These signal characteristics are indicative of mild T1 shortening due to the proteinaceous serosanguinous serum (39).

When followed sequentially, intratumoral hemorrhage may appear to evolve more slowly than parenchymal hematomas, reflecting the much lower ambient oxygen levels (56). Delayed evolution of hematomas is, therefore, seen both in the setting of low O_2 (not enough to oxidize the heme iron from ferrous deoxyhemoglobin to ferric methemoglobin) and high O_2 (which keeps the methemoglobin reductase systems powered to drive methemoglobin back to deoxyhemoglobin). The optimal O_2 tension for hemoglobin oxidation is approximately 20 mmHg (57).

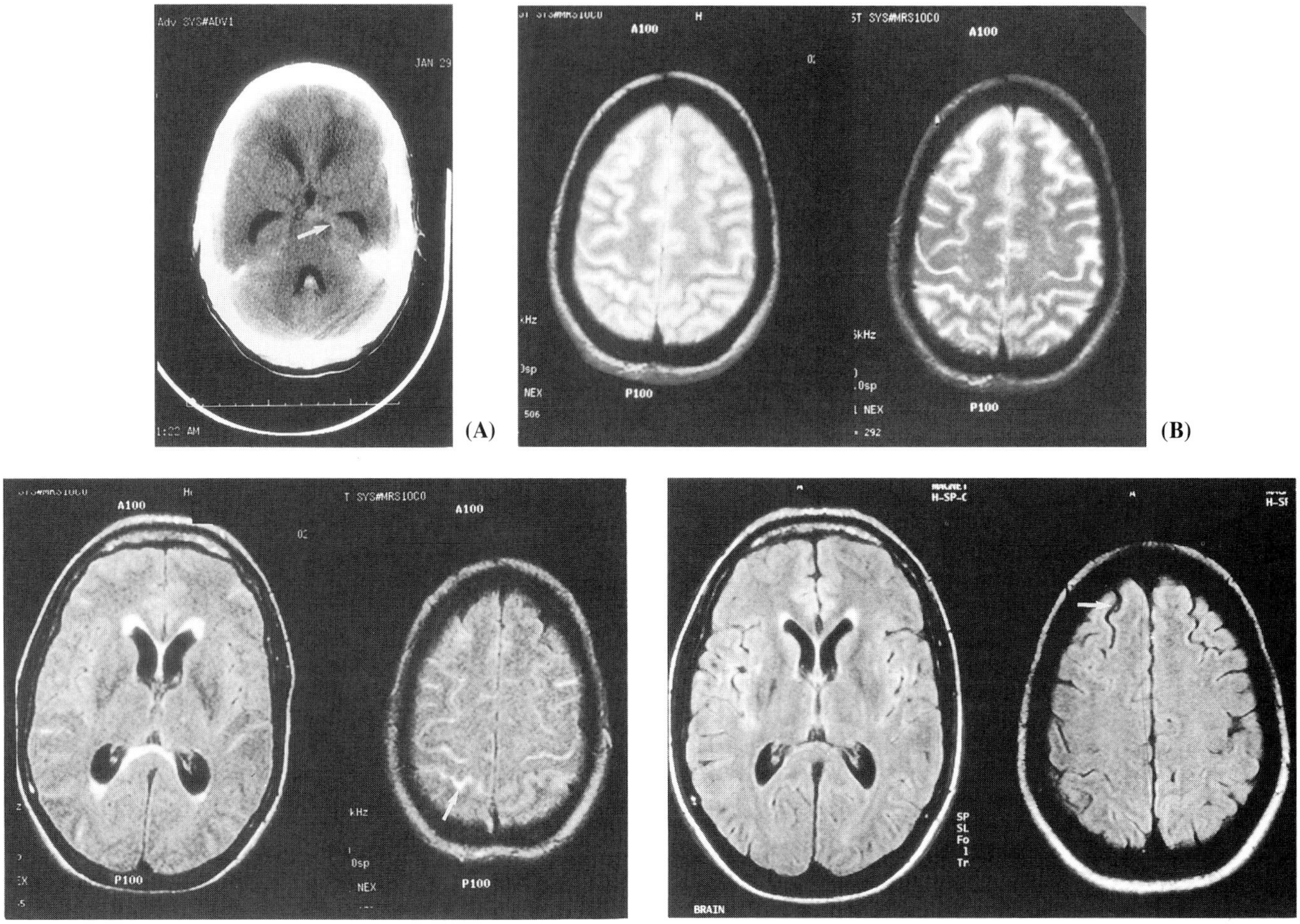

(A) (B) (C) (D)

Figure 16-15 Acute subarachnoid hemorrhage using turbo FLAIR (fluid attenuated inversion recovery) technique. *A*. Computed tomography demonstrates hyperdensity (*arrow*), indicative of subarachnoid hemorrhage. *B*. On MRI, proton-density and T2-weighted images show no apparent abnormality in the intensity of the CSF. *C*. Turbo FLAIR demonstrates low-intensity CSF within the lateral ventricles but high-intensity CSF in the cortical sulci (arrow), suggestive of subarachnoid hemorrhage. *D*. Two weeks later, the patient was scanned using the same turbo FLAIR technique, demonstrating the anticipated low-signal-intensity CSF within the cortical sulci (*arrows*) following clearing of the subarachnoid hemorrhage. (Courtesy of Michael Brant-Zawadzki, MD, Newport Beach, CA.)

When tumors bleed in the brain, macrophages move in to surround the hemorrhage, just as in the nonneoplastic situation. Hemosiderin/ferritin rims are seen in the chronic setting. With renewed tumor growth, the hemosiderin rim may become disrupted (46) (Fig. 16-2*G*). While this is a useful sign of neoplastic hemorrhage, it is less than 100 percent specific, as rebleeding from any cause (e.g., hypertension, AVM) can produce disruption of an earlier hemosiderin rim.

☐ PITUITARY HEMORRHAGE

Pituitary hemorrhage (Fig. 16-18) may be seen in the setting of an adenoma or a previously normal gland either spontaneously (Simmonds's syndrome) or during pregnancy (Sheehan's syndrome). Prior to the use of MRI, pituitary hemorrhage was presumed to cause acute panhypopituitarism ("pituitary apoplexy"). In the MRI era, pituitary hemorrhage is often diagnosed in asymptomatic individuals—most often in the setting of bromocriptine therapy for microadenoma. At most, these patients may have a mild headache, presumably due to the associated mild subarachnoid hemorrhage.

☐ SUMMARY

Although MRI *can* detect a hyperacute hematoma (on the basis of an irregular low-intensity border on T2-weighted images) and although it *can* detect acute subarachnoid hemorrhage (using FLAIR), CT remains more convincing in these circumstances. After 12 to 24 h, MRI becomes more sensitive than CT in the detection of hemorrhage. It is also more specific than CT as to the timing of the hemorrhage. As it evolves, hemorrhage passes through five well-defined and easily identified stages on MRI. Knowledge of these stages may be useful to approximately date a single hemorrhagic event or to suggest that multiple hemorrhagic events have occurred at different times. As stressed throughout this chapter, it is important to acquire *both* T1- and T2-weighted images to adequately characterize and stage hemorrhage.

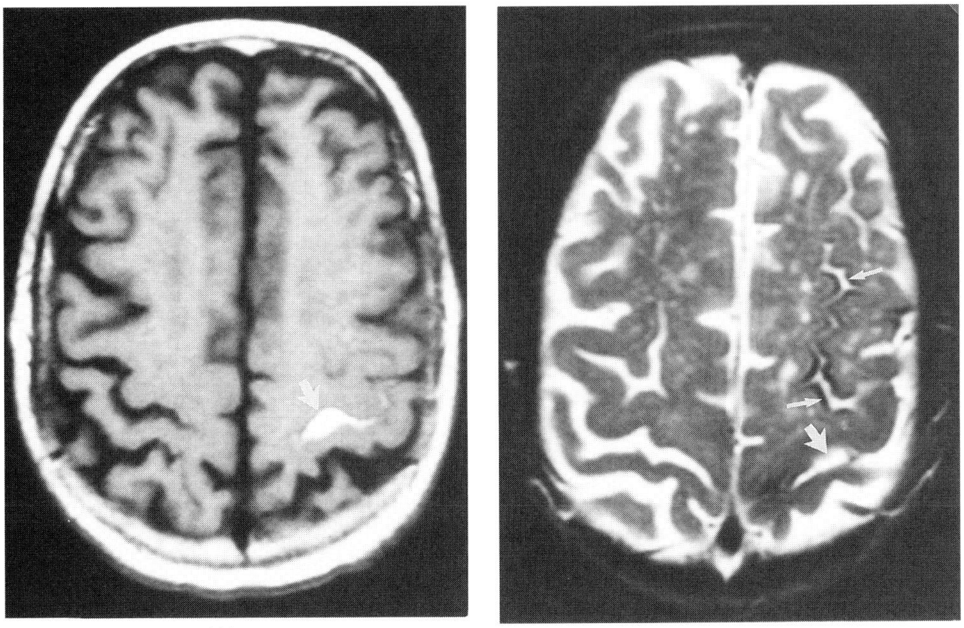

(A) (B)

Figure 16-16 Subacute, subarachnoid hemorrhage. *A*. On MRI, high signal intensity (*arrow*) is noted within the left central sulcus, consistent with methemoglobin. *B*. T2-weighted image demonstrates persistent high signal intensity (indistinguishable from CSF) in the left central sulcus (*arrow*). Low signal intensity is also noted in the sulci more anteriorly, indicative of early hemosiderin staining of the leptomeninges (*small arrows*) on this T2-weighted image.

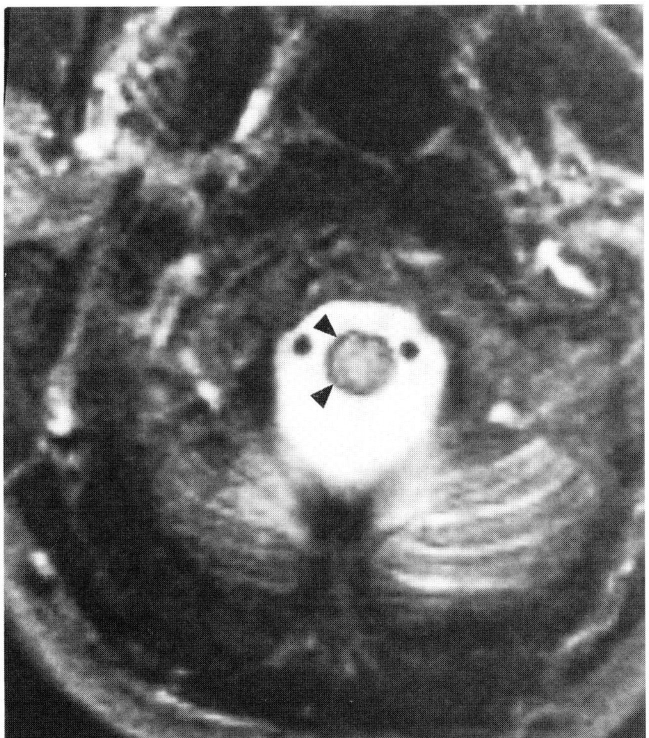

Figure 16-17 Superficial siderosis due to recurrent bleeding from multiple cavernous angiomas in a 62-year-old Hispanic man with a 1-week history of altered mental status. On MRI, T2-weighted axial section through the upper cervical cord demonstrates linear hypointensity surrounding cord (*arrowheads*) secondary to superficial siderosis.

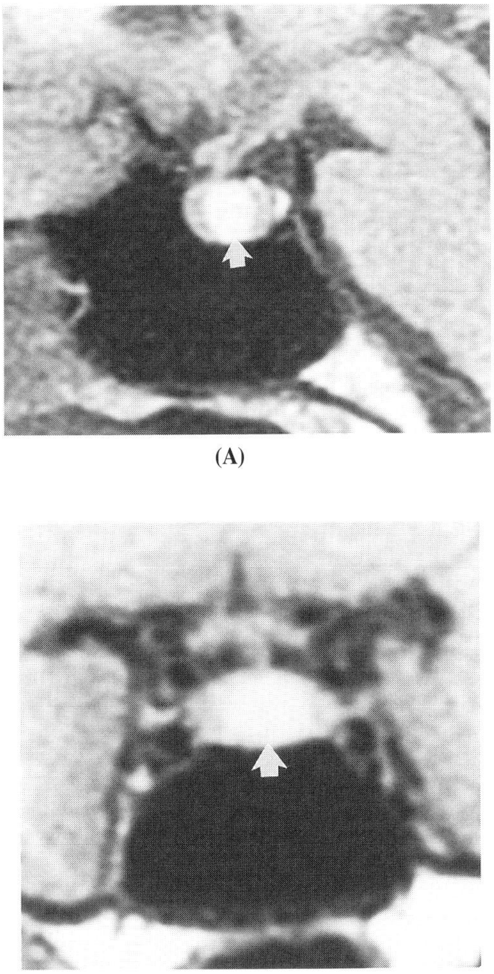

(A)

(B)

Figure 16-18 Pituitary hemorrhage. On MRI, high signal intensity is noted within this enlarged pituitary gland (*arrow*) following initiation of bromocriptine treatment for a microadenoma. Although the patient had a mild headache (the cause for the examination), there was no evidence of "pituitary apoplexy." *A*. Sagittal SE (450/15). *B*. Coronal SE (450/15).

SELECTED READINGS

1. Gomori JM et al: Intracranial hematomas: Imaging by high field MR. *Radiology* 157:87–92, 1985.
2. DeLaPaz RL et al: NMR imaging of intracranial hemorrhage. *J Comput Assist Tomogr* 8:599–607, 1983.
3. Sipponen JT et al: Nuclear magnetic resonance (NMR) imaging of intracerebral hemorrhage in the acute and resolving phases. *J Comput Assist Tomogr* 7:954–959, 1983.
4. Hayman LA et al: Pathophysiology of acute intracerebral and subarachnoid hemorrhage: Applications to MR imaging. *AJNR* 10:457–481, 1989.
5. Brooks RA et al: MR imaging of cerebral hematomas at different field strengths: Theory and applications. *J Comput Assist Tomogr* 13:194–206, 1989.
6. Bradley WG, Schmidt PC: Effect of methemoglobin formation on the MR appearance of subarachnoid appearance. *Radiology* 1156:99–103, 1985.
7. Bradley WG: Hemorrhage and brain iron, in Stark DD, Bradley WG (eds): *Magnetic Resonance Imaging*, 2d ed. St Louis, Mosby-Year Book, 1992, pp 201–264.
8. Zyed AM et al: MR imaging of intracerebral blood: Diversity in the temporal pattern at 0.5 and 1.0 T. *AJNR* 12:469–474, 1991.
9. Zimmerman RD et al: Acute intracranial hemorrhage: Intensity changes on sequential MR scans at 0.5 T. *AJNR* 9:47–57, 1988.
10. Zimmerman RD, Deck MDF: Intracranial hematomas: Imaging by high field MR. *Radiology* 159:565, 1986.
11. Fullerton GD: Physiologic basis of magnetic relaxation, in Stark DD, Bradley WG (eds): *Magnetic Resonance Imaging*, 2d ed. St Louis, Mosby-Year Book, 1992, pp 88–108.
12. Bloembergen N et al: Relaxation effects in nuclear magnetic resonance absorption. *Phys Rev* 73:679–712, 1948.
13. Atlas SW et al: Intracranial hemorrhage: Gradient-echo MR imaging at 1.5 T: Comparison with spin-echo and clinical applications. *Radiology* 168:803–807, 1988.
14. Mills TC et al: Partial flip angle MR imaging. *Radiology* 162:531–539, 1987.
15. Hardy PA et al: Cause of signal loss in MR images of old hemorrhagic lesions. *Radiology* 174:549–555, 1990.
16. Edelman RR et al: MR of hemorrhage: A new approach. *AJNR* 7:751–756, 1986.
17. Seidenwurm D et al: Intracranial hemorrhagic lesions: Evaluation with spin-echo and gradient-refocused MR imaging at 0.5 and 1.5 T. *Radiology* 172:189–194, 1989.
18. Wesbey GE et al: Translational molecular self-diffusion in magnetic resonance imaging: Effects and applications, in James TL, Margulis AR (eds): *Biomedical Magnetic Resonance*. San Francisco, University of California Press, 1984, pp 63–76.
19. Packer KJ: The effects of diffusion through locally inhomogeneous magnetic fields on transverse nuclear spin relaxation in heterogeneous systems: Proton transverse relaxation in striated muscle tissue. *J Magn Reson* 9:438–443, 1973.
20. Feinberg DA, Oshio K: GRASE (gradient- and spin-echo) MR imaging: A new fast clinical imaging technique. *Radiology* 181:597, 1991.
21. Norbash AM et al: Intracerebral lesion contrast with spin-echo and fast spin-echo pulse sequences. *Radiology* 185:661, 1992.
22. Jones KM et al: Brain hemorrhage: Evaluation with fast spin-echo and conventional dual spin-echo images. *Radiology* 182:53–58, 1992.
23. Clark RA et al: Acute hematomas: Effects of deoxyhemoglobin, hematocrit, and fibrin-clot formation and retraction on T2 shortening. *Radiology* 174:201–206, 1990.
24. Hayman LA et al: MR imaging of hyperacute intracranial hemorrhage in the cat. *AJNR* 10:681–686, 1989.
25. Hayman LA et al: T2 effect of hemoglobin concentration: Assessment with in vitro MR spectroscopy. *Radiology* 168:489–491, 1988.
26. Hayman AL et al: Effect of clot formation and retraction on spin-echo MR images of blood: An in vitro study. *AJNR* 10:1155–1158, 1989.
27. Wintrobe MM et al: *Clinical Hematology* Philadelphia, Lea & Febiger, 1981, pp 88–102.
28. Rapoport SI: *Introduction to Hematology*. New York, Harper & Row, 1971, p 31.
29. Thulborn KR et al: Role of ferritin and hemosiderin in the MR appearance of cerebral hemorrhage: A histopathologic biochemical study in rats. *AJNR* 11:291–297, 1990.
30. Pauling L, Coryell C: The magnetic properties and structure of hemoglobin, oxyhemoglobin, and carbonmonoxyhemoglobin. *Proc Natl Acad Sci USA* 22:210–216, 1936.
31. Pauling L, Coryell C: The magnetic properties and structure of the hemochromogen and related substances. *Prod Natl Acad Sci USA* 22:159–163, 1936.
32. Koenig SH et al: Interactions of solvent with the heme region of methemoglobin and fluoromethemoglobin. *Biophys J* 34:397–408, 1981.
33. Singer JR, Crooks LE: Some magnetic studies of normal and leukemic blood. *J Clin Eng* 3:357–363, 1978.
34. Zimmerman RD et al: Acute intracranial hemorrhage: Intensity changes on sequential MR scans at 0.5 T. *AJNR* 9:47–57, 1988.
35. Bradley WG: Hemorrhage and brain iron, in Stark DD, Bradley WG (eds): *Magnetic Resonance Imaging*. St Louis, Mosby-Year Book, 1988, pp 721–769.
36. Whisnant JP et al: Experimental intracerebral hematoma. *Arch Neurol* 9:586–592, 1963.
37. Bydder GM et al: Clinical use of rapid T2-weighted partial saturation sequences in MR imaging. *J Comput Assist Tomogr* 11:17–34, 1987.
38. Rapoport S et al: Venous clots: Evaluation with MR imaging. *Radiology* 162:527–530, 1987.
39. Fullerton GD et al: Frequency dependence of magnetic resonance spin lattice relaxation of protons in biological materials. *Radiology* 151:135–138, 1984.
40. Fullerton GD et al: The influence of macromolecular polymerization on spin lattice relaxation of aqueous solutions. *Magn Reson Imaging* 5:353–370, 1987.
41. Alanen A, Kormano M: Correlation of the echogenicity and structure of clotted blood. *J Ultrasound Med* 4:421–425, 1985.
42. Chin HY et al: Temporal changes in red blood cell hydration: Application to MRI of hemorrhage. *Neuroradiology* 33(suppl):79–81, 1991.
43. Enzmann DR et al: Natural history of experimental intracerebral hemorrhage: Sonography, computed tomography and neuropathology. *AJNR* 2:517–526, 1981.

44. Fabry ME, Eisenstadt M: Water exchange across red cell membranes: II. Measurement by nuclear magnetic resonance T1, T2, and T12 hybrid relaxation: The effects of osmolarity, cell volume and medium. *J Membr Biol* 42:375–398, 1978.
45. Taber KH et al: Change in red blood cell relaxation with hydration: Application to MR imaging of hemorrhage. *J Mag Res Imaging* 2:203–208, 1992.
46. Gomori JM, Grossman RI: Head and neck hemorrhage, in Kressel HY (ed): *Magnetic Resonance Annual*. New York, Raven Press, 1987, pp 71–112.
47. Taber KH et al: Temporal changes in the oxidation state in vitro blood. *Invest Radiol* 25:240–244, 1990.
48. Hackney DB et al: Subacute intracranial hemorrhage: Contribution of spin density to appearance on spin echo images. *Radiology* 165:199, 1987.
49. Fobben ES et al: MR characteristics of subdural hematomas and hygromas at 1.5 T. *AJNR* 10:687, 1989.
50. Ebisu T et al: Nonacute subdural hematoma: Fundamental interpretation of MR images based on biochemical and in vitro MR analysis. *Radiology* 171:449, 1990.
51. Chakeres DW, Bryan RN: Acute subarachnoid hemorrhage: In vitro comparison of magnetic resonance and computed tomography. *AJNR* 7:223–228, 1987.
52. Yoon HC et al: MR of acute subarachnoid hemorrhage. *AJNR* 9:405–408, 1988.
53. Satoh S, Kadoya S: Magnetic resonance imaging of subarachnoid hemorrhage. *Neuroradiology* 30:361, 1988.
54. Gomori J et al: High field MR imaging of superficial siderosis of the central nervous system. *J Comput Assist Tomogr* 9:972–975, 1985.
55. Paako E et al: Meningeal Gd-DTPA enhancement in patients with malignancies. *JCAT* 14:542, 1990.
56. Destian S et al: MR imaging of hemorrhagic intracranial neoplasms. *AJR* 152:137–144, 1989.
57. Kelly WM, Johnson BA: Understanding intracranial hemorrhage: A practical approach. *MRI Decisions* 7:9–22, 1993.

CHAPTER 17

Intracranial Aneurysms

William O. Bank
Wayne J. Olan
Edwin R. Hudson
Michael Lefkowitz

Radiological evaluation of intracranial aneurysms has evolved continually since the first angiographic demonstration of an aneurysm by Egaz Moniz in 1927. While selective cerebral angiography maintains an important role in pretreatment planning and has become the "surgical approach" of the endovascular therapist in those aneurysms that can be occluded with coils or other devices, the "gold standard" role of angiography in diagnosing and characterizing these lesions has been slipping recently, as three-dimensional computed tomography (CT) and magnetic resonance imaging (MRI) techniques evolve. Holographic images based on these latter modalities allow the neurosurgeon, in the operating room, to look at a single three-dimensional hologram on which he can see the data previously portrayed on multiple films with multiple images.

After a short historical divergence, we will review the anatomic, pathologic and clinical aspects of intracranial aneurysms and then attempt to place into perspective the strengths and weaknesses of the available imaging modalities.

☐ HISTORICAL BACKGROUND

History depends upon a means of recording. To the neuroradiologist, the history of aneurysms begins with the classic article by Egaz Moniz in 1933: "Aneurysme intracranien de la carotide interne droite rendu visible par l'angiographie cerebrale" (Aneurysm of the right internal carotid demonstrated by cerebral angiography; see "Suggested Readings"). His subsequent monograph *L'Angiographie Cerebrale* is a classic that adds perspective to the progress we have made in the past six decades.

In fact, the first anatomic description of an intracranial aneurysm dates back to the time of the American Revolution, when Biumi described an intracavernous aneurysm of the internal carotid artery. The first antemortem diagnosis of an intracranial aneurysm is attributed to Hutchinson, who described a 40-year-old woman, first seen by him in 1861, with a third-nerve palsy and headache. The presence of a bruit led him to diagnose an aneurysm. His diagnosis was confirmed 11 years later, when the patient died of an unrelated illness and postmortem examination disclosed an egg-shaped aneurysm of the cavernous internal carotid artery (ICA). Skeptical interventional neuroradiologists favor the diagnosis of a chronic carotid-cavernous fistula.

Progress in diagnostic capabilities led to improvements in the modes of treatment available. Magnuss reported successful treatment of an ICA aneurysm by ICA ligation in 1927. Dott successfully treated a 53-year-old man with a subarachnoid hemorrhage from an ICA bifurcation aneurysm in 1931 by packing it with muscle. Dandy, using a vascular clip developed by his mentor Harvey Cushing, successfully obliterated a posterior communicating aneurysm in a 43-year-old man with oculomotor palsy. The greatest improvement in neurosurgical results, however, occurred with the advent of the operating microscope in the seventies.

☐ ANATOMIC AND PATHOLOGICAL CONSIDERATIONS

Like many pathologic processes, most aneurysms are classified by their morphology as saccular or fusiform, with an element of pathogenesis involved in naming the third and fourth categories: dissecting aneurysms and traumatic pseudoaneurysms. While pathologic features are specific and differentiate between these types, these features can be masked by specimen handling in the operating room or necropsy suite. While the clinical presentation of each type can vary from asymptomatic to intracranial hemorrhage with coma or death, it is usually possible to differentiate between them.

☐ SACCULAR ANEURYSMS

DEVELOPMENTAL/DEGENERATIVE ANEURYSMS

- Intracranial developmental/degenerative aneurysms are true aneurysms.
- Deficient, collagenized tunica muscularis protrudes through a focal defect in the internal elastic membrane to produce a circumscribed outpouching, usually at an arterial bifurcation.
- The muscularis and elastic laminae terminate at the aneurysm neck or "face," and the sac or dome of the aneurysm consists of intima, adventitia, and occasionally thrombus.
- When they appear to arise from the lateral wall of an artery like the basilar trunk, skeptics (like the authors) remember the presence of small arteries that may provide the necessary bifurcation to preserve a cohesive theory of origin.
- Most saccular aneurysms appear to have a degenerative origin.
- Atherosclerotic changes are commonly present in adjacent arteries.
- Abnormal mural shear-stress probably accounts for their initiation and growth and contributes to the development of intra-aneurysmal thrombosis and rupture.

ONCOTIC ANEURYSM

- Infiltration of the arterial wall by neoplasm, either primary or metastatic, is an even rarer cause of intracranial aneurysm, the oncotic aneurysm.
- It has been reported in patients with meningioma, pituitary adenoma, glioma, and metastatic atrial myxoma and choriocarcinoma.
- Irradiation of the brain has also been implicated in the induction of aneurysm formation.

MYCOTIC ANEURYSM

- Infection, either local or "metastatic," weakens the arterial wall and accounts for 2.5 to 4.5 percent of intracranial aneurysms.
- *Streptococcus viridans* is the most common bacterial cause.
- *Aspergillus* is the most common fungal cause.
- Most mycotic aneurysms are due to infective emboli that lodge in branch arteries; thus they are typically found on peripheral branches of the middle cerebral artery.
- Although saccular in appearance, these are usually pseudoaneurysms and are associated with a high incidence of intraparenchymal hemorrhage and with high mortality.
- The incidence of mycotic aneurysms declined with the introduction of antibiotics but has increased again with the arrival of immune deficiencies.
- Mycotic aneurysms are frequently associated with bacterial endocarditis.

FLOW-RELATED ANEURYSM

- The high-flow states encountered in patients with arteriovenous malformations (AVM) and arteriovenous fistulas (AVF) contribute to the development of aneurysms.
- The association of AVM/AVF and aneurysms has been given a prevalence varying from 3 to 23 percent.
- Aneurysms occurring in a vascular territory remote to the AVM/AVF probably reflect a shared predisposition to vascular problems.
- Truly flow-related aneurysms are encountered on a feeding pedicle, the so-called pedicle aneurysms (Fig. 17-1); within the nidus of the malformation itself, there are intranidal or nidal aneurysms.
- These aneurysms tend to be thin-walled and prone to rupture with changes in the arterial pressure.
- They presumably account for a major cause of intracranial hemorrhage in patients with AVM/AVF.
- Aneurysms are demonstrated in close to 60 percent of all cases in which superselective angiography is performed; 42 percent of these are nidal.

☐ FUSIFORM ANEURYSMS

Fusiform aneurysms are comparable to the atherosclerotic aneurysms of the abdominal aorta in which weakening of the media results in elongation and widening of the artery. They typically occur in older patients and involve the supraclinoid ICA and the vertebrobasilar system. More recently, fusiform aneurysms of middle cerebral branches have been reported. These aneurysms present the neurosurgeon with the problem of reimplantation of the artery distal to the segment involved in the aneurysm, since it supplies normal brain.

While subarachnoid and intracerebral hemorrhage are uncommon in fusiform aneurysms, either can occur. More commonly, these patients present with cranial neuropathies, brainstem infarction, and/or hydrocephalus.

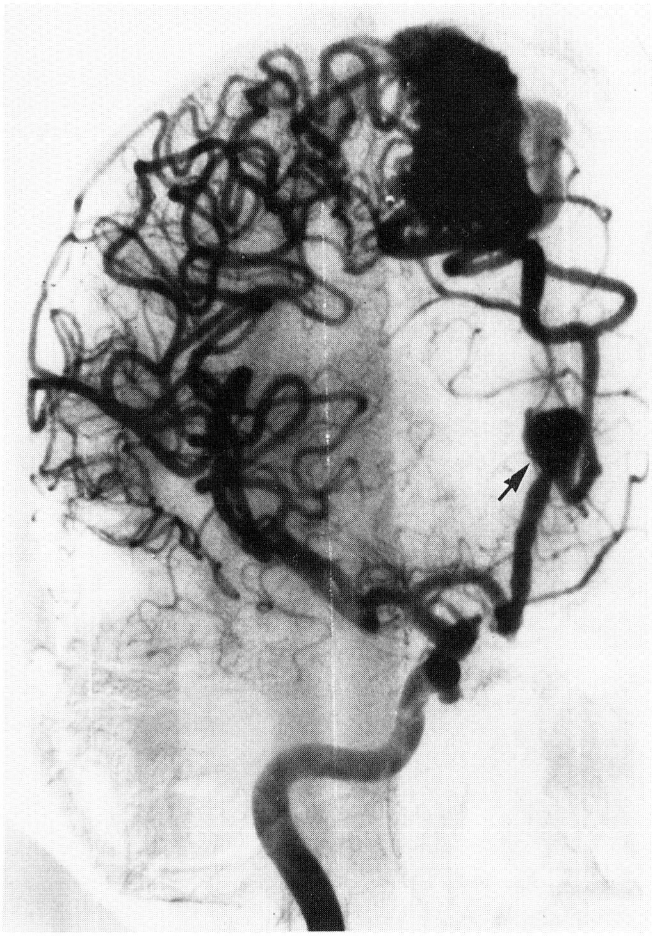

Figure 17-1 Flow-related aneurysms. A right internal carotid injection shows an AVM supplied by the right anterior cerebral artery as well as the right middle cerebral artery. An associated aneurysm is seen along the dilated, slightly irregular feeding artery (pericallosal artery) (*arrow*).

☐ DISSECTING ANEURYSMS

A small tear in the intima or intima and internal elastic membrane can result in the dissection of blood within the arterial wall. When this intramural hematoma extends into the subadventitial plane, the resultant focal widening of the artery is referred to as a dissecting aneurysm. These are usually seen in the cervical ICA or vertebral artery but can extend intracranially, especially in the vertebrobasilar system, and have been reported as isolated intracranial lesions.

Patients with a history of cervical trauma and/or fibromuscular dysplasia seem to be more prone to developing arterial dissections, but this problem can occur with no evidence of predisposing condition or antecedent trauma.

☐ TRAUMATIC PSEUDOANEURYSMS

Direct trauma to the arterial wall can produce a complete laceration of an artery that results in a paravascular hematoma. Lysis of clot centrally with cavitation and communication to the arterial lumen results in the production of an apparent saccular aneurysm. The absence of any component of arterial wall at the periphery of this lesion makes it a traumatic pseudoaneurysm. Traumatic pseudoaneurysms account for less than 1 percent of aneurysms.

While usually associated with penetrating injury and involving the cervical carotid or vertebral arteries, these pseudoaneurysms can occur intracranially. Foreign bodies that penetrate the cranial vault can occur through foramina or fissures. Arterial laceration can be related to surgical misadventure, can occur against a fracture fragment, or may be caused by impaction of the artery against an edge of the falx or tentorium.

EPIDEMIOLOGY AND ASSOCIATED CONDITIONS

- Intracranial aneurysms are relatively common, occurring in 1 to 8 percent of autopsy and angiographic series. (It must be remembered that aneurysms can be difficult to identify at autopsy in uninjected specimens.)
- There is a female predominance of 3:2.
- Other risk factors include systemic hypertension and increasing age.
- Most saccular aneurysms are found in the middle-aged and elderly populations. They are uncommon in children and rare in infants (Fig. 17-2).
- When present in the pediatric population, aneurysms tend to be large and are found more commonly in the posterior fossa.
- Relatives of a patient who has experienced rupture of an aneurysm have an incidence of intracranial aneurysm slightly greater than that of the population at large.
- A rare autosomal dominant form of familial intracranial aneurysm exists. Ronkainen and coworkers have reported a 10 percent incidence of aneurysms in 21 Finnish families screened by MR angiography, and Leblanc and colleagues found aneurysms in 29 percent of siblings when both a mother and one other child had an aneurysm.
- Patients with coarctation of the aorta, fibromuscular dysplasia (Fig. 17-3), connective tissue disorders (Ehlers-Danlos syndrome, Marfan's syndrome, systemic lupus erythematosus), and phakomatoses such as neurofibromatosis and tuberous sclerosis have a reported increased incidence of saccular aneurysms.
- Adult polycystic kidney disease is associated with intracranial aneurysms in 15 percent of cases.
- Anomalies of the circle of Willis, such as trigeminal artery, are associated with an increased incidence of aneurysm (Fig. 17-4).

☐ GIANT ANEURYSM

- Approximately 5 percent of intracranial aneurysms are greater than 2.5 cm in diameter and are classified as giant aneurysms.

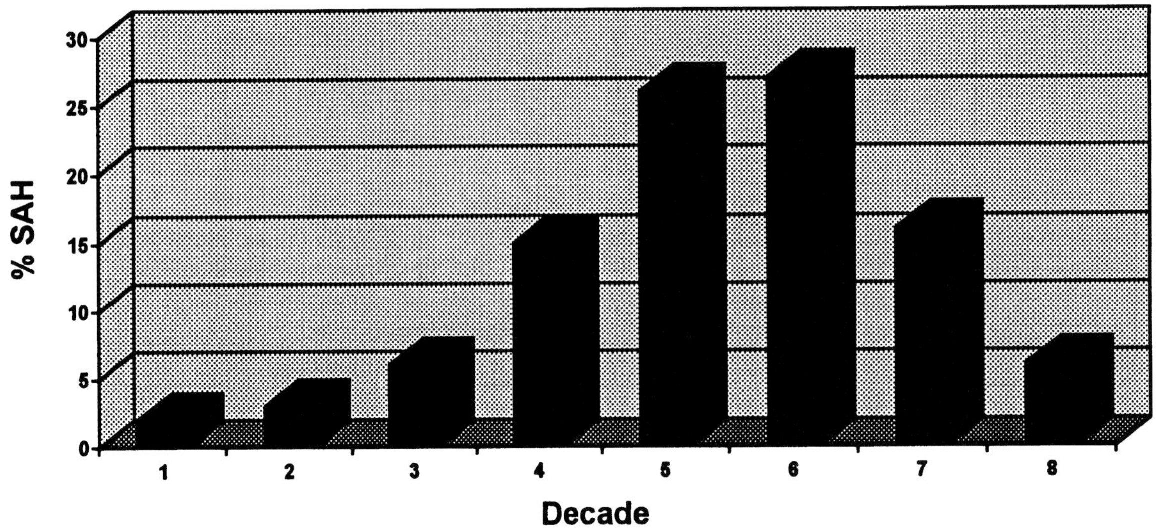

Figure 17-2 Age distribution for aneurysmal subarachnoid hemorrhage.

- Although only 10 percent of aneurysms arise in the posterior fossa, one-half to two-thirds of giant aneurysms are found in this location. Table 17-1 lists the locations of giant aneurysms in the large series reported by Drake.
- Some 60 percent of giant aneurysms contain thrombus, making size as represented on CT and MRI more reliable than that seen on angiography (Fig. 17-5).

Table 17-1
LOCALIZATION OF 173 GIANT INTRACRANIAL ANEURYSMS

Aneurysm Location	Percentage (N°)		
Supratentorial	**39(67)**		
Internal carotid artery		28(48)	
Cavernous segment			5 (9)
Para-ophthalmic segment			14(24)
@ posterior communicating artery			4 (7)
@ bifurcation			5 (8)
Anterior communicating artery		2 (4)	
Middle cerebral artery		9(15)	
Incisural	**42(73)**		
Posterior cerebral artery		8(13)	
Basilar apex		24(42)	
Superior cerebellar artery		10(18)	
Infratentorial	**19(33)**		
Basilar trunk		8(13)	
Vertebrobasilar junction		7(12)	
Vertebral artery		4 (8)	

* Data from Drake CG: Giant intracranial aneurysms: Experience with surgical treatment in 174 patients. *Clin Neurosurg* 26:12–95, 1979.

- Most giant aneurysms are saccular, although a subset of fusiform giant aneurysms has been identified; these are referred to as serpentine aneurysms.

CLINICAL CONSIDERATIONS

Asymptomatic aneurysms can be discovered on CT scans or MRI studies done for other reasons. Careful evaluation of angiograms done for carotid vascular disease also discloses unsuspected intracranial aneurysms that may mandate modification of treatment for carotid stenosis.

Some patients with aneurysms become symptomatic secondary to mass effect on adjacent structures. Hydrocephalus can occur if the cerebral aqueduct is compressed by a basilar apex aneurysm. Aneurysms arising from the ICA within the cavernous sinus (3 percent of

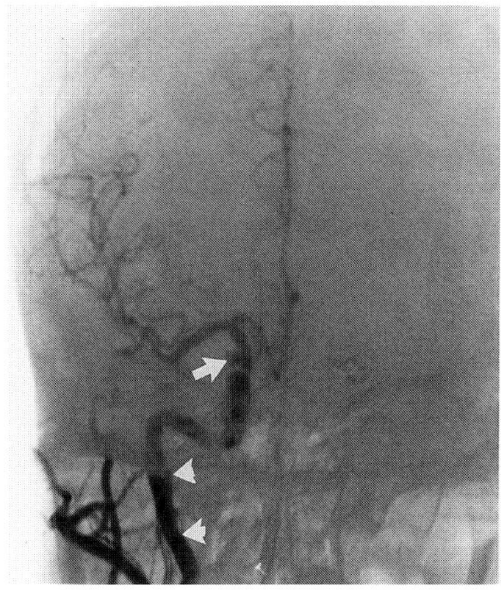

Figure 17-3 Fibromuscular dysplasia associated with intracranial aneurysm. An AP angiogram shows an aneurysm at the junction of internal carotid artery and posterior communicating artery (*arrow*). The cervical portion of the internal carotid artery shows "string of beads" appearance of fibromuscular dysplasia (*arrowheads*).

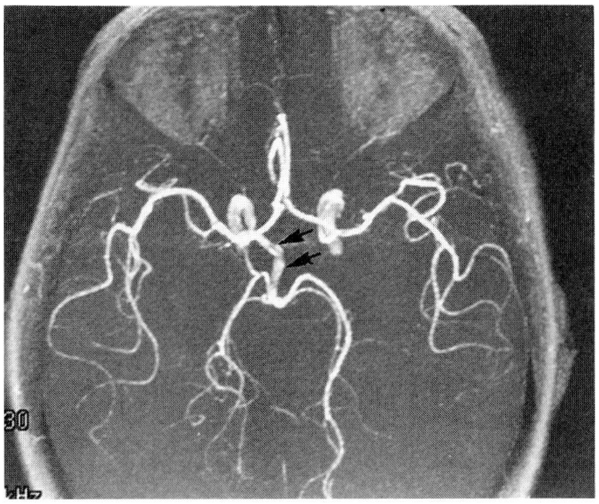

(A)

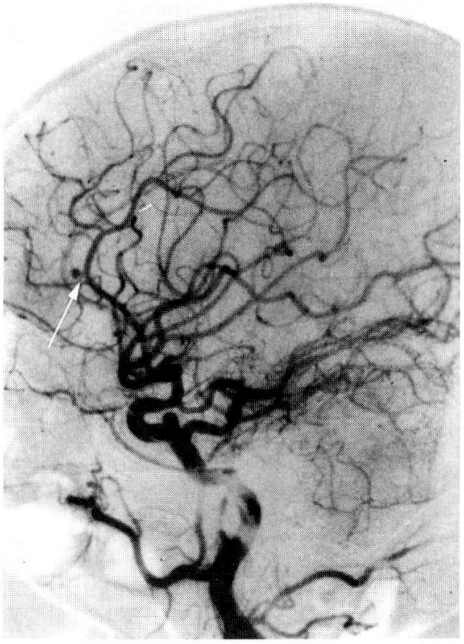

(B)

Figure 17-4 Aneurysms associated with the trigeminal artery. *A*. Magnetic resonance angiogram demonstrates the presence of a trigeminal artery on the right side (*arrows*) as well as a posterior communicating artery on the right side. The left posterior communicating artery is not present. An aneurysm is seen at the left middle cerebral bifurcation. *B*. Conventional aneurysm (right common carotid injection, lateral view) shows the presence of the trigeminal artery as well as the posterior communicating artery. A small pericallosal artery aneurysm is seen (*arrow*).

intracranial aneurysms) may rupture into that sinus, causing sudden onset of a carotid-cavernous fistula with proptosis, chemosis, and an audible bruit. Growth of unruptured cavernous carotid aneurysms can produce cranial nerve deficits, most commonly a partial oculomotor palsy. Oculomotor nerve palsy, classically without pupil sparing, is associated with posterior communicating artery aneurysms, aneurysms of the bifurcation of the ICA, bifurcation and basilar apex aneurysms.

Usually, however, patients with intracranial aneurysms present with rupture of that aneurysm and associated subarachnoid hemorrhage (SAH). The classic symptom is the sudden onset of severe, disabling headache. If symptoms do not progress to focal neurologic deficit, obtundation, or coma, the patient will at least stop whatever he or she is doing. Neck ache and neck stiffness follow.

The patient with an intracranial aneurysm has an annual risk of rupture estimated to be 2 percent per year. This can be a devastating event and is associated with mortality as high as 45 percent. After an initial SAH, the risk of a second hemorrhage is about 7 percent per week for the next 6 weeks. Patient outcome is related to clinical status at presentation, usually assessed using the grading scale devised by Hunt and Hess or one of several related variants (Table 17-2).

The mean size of aneurysms at time of rupture is 21 mm, suggesting a likelihood that hemorrhage is related to aneurysmal size. Indeed, aneurysms less than 10 mm in diameter appear less prone to rupture, but there is no minimum size for rupture, and in view of the associated grave mortality, aneurysms of any size must be considered at risk for rupture. Interestingly, giant aneurysms

Table 17-2
GRADING SCALES FOR CLINICAL STATUS OF PATIENTS AFTER SUBARACHNOID HEMORRHAGE

Hunt and Hess[a]

Grade	Symptoms on Presentation
I	Asymptomatic or mild headache and neck stiffness
II	Moderate to severe headache and neck stiffness Neurologic deficit limited to cranial nerve palsy
III	Somnolence, confusion, or focal neurologic deficit
IV	Stupor, moderate to severe hemiparesis, decerebrate reactions
V	Profound coma, decerebrate rigidity, moribund

WFNS (World Federation of Neurological Surgeons)[b]

Grade	Glasgow Coma Scale	Motor Deficit
I	15	Absent
II	13–14	Absent
III	13–14	Present
IV	7–12	Present or absent
V	3–6	Present or absent

[a]Hunt WE, Hess RM: Surgical risk as related to time of intervention in the repair of intracranial aneurysms. *J Neurosurg* 28:14–20, 1968.
[b]Drake CG: Report of World Federation of Neurological Surgeons Committee on a Universal Subarachnoid Haemorrhage Grading Scale. *J Neurosurg* 68:985–986, 1988.

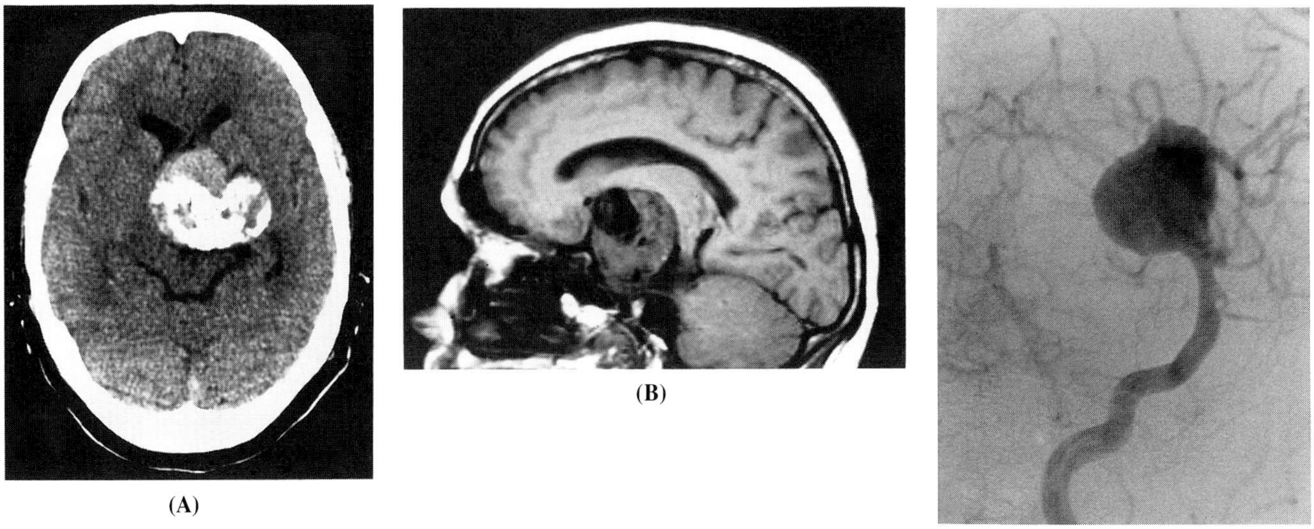

(A) (B) (C)

Figure 17-5 Giant aneurysm. *A*. An axial CT shows a giant aneurysm in the suprasellar region. The aneurysm has a small patent lumen with a large portion containing thrombus. *B*. Sagittal T1-weighted MRI shows the giant aneurysm with a small patent lumen and a large thrombus. *C*. Cerebral angiogram demonstrates the patent aneurysmal lumen, which appears to arise from the supraclinoid portion of the internal carotid artery. The internal carotid bifurcation is seen through the aneurysm.

are considered less likely to be associated with SAH, although they still presented with SAH in 36 percent of patients in Drake's series.

Certain aneurysms are associated with less common forms of intracranial hemorrhage: aneurysms located at the anterior communicating artery and basilar apex are associated with intraventricular hemorrhage; middle cerebral aneurysms produce intraparenchymal hemorrhages; aneurysms of the middle and distal anterior cerebral artery may hemorrhage into the subdural space. Data from the Cooperative Study on the Timing of Aneurysm Surgery show the incidence of intraventricular, intraparenchymal, and subdural hemorrhage on the initial CT scan to be 20, 19, and 1 percent respectively.

LOCATION

Most intracranial aneurysms occur in close proximity to the circle of Willis, as indicated in Table 17-3. The incidence at any given site varies among the different series and between studies done on symptomatic patients and autopsy studies. A good rule of thumb places one-third each at the anterior and posterior communicating arteries, 20 percent at the middle cerebral artery (MCA) bifurcation or trifurcation, and 10 percent in the posterior fossa. About half of the posterior fossa aneurysms occur at the basilar apex.

Most aneurysms arise at an asymmetrical bifurcation, along the outer wall of dominant vascular curves. They are not infrequently associated with such anatomic variants as hypoplasia of one segment of the circle of Willis, vascular fenestrations, persistent embryonic caroticovertebral connections (hypoglossal, trigeminal), duplication of the vertebral or middle cerebral artery, and azygous anterior cerebral artery. Some 20 to 45 percent of patients with aneurysms will harbor multiple aneurysms; when they are bilateral, symmetrical, so-called mirror image aneurysms are not unusual. The development of aneurysms on previously normal anterior communicating arteries after unilateral carotid artery occlusion emphasizes the relationship of aneurysm formation and altered shear-stress relationships.

Ongoing research into the origin, growth, and rupture of aneurysms has become quite sophisticated, using mathematical models, computer flow simulations, viscoelastic replicas in systems with mechanical pumps to

Table 17-3
LOCALIZATION OF INTRACRANIAL ANEURYSMS BASED ON ANGIOGRAPHIC AND AUTOPSY DATA

	Percentage	
Location	Angiographic Data[a]	Autopsy Data[b]
Internal carotid artery	30	50
Middle cerebral artery	22	15
Anterior cerebral artery	39	26
Vertebrobasilar artery	7	7
Other	2	2
Total number of aneurysms	3521	83

[a]Data from Kessel NF et al: The international cooperative study on the timing of aneurysm surgery. *J Neurosurg* 73:18–47, 1990.
[b]Data from Hounpian EM, Pool JL: A systematic analysis of intracranial aneurysms from the autopsy file of Presbyterian Hospital. *J Neuropathol Exp Neurol* 17:409–423, 1958.

produce controllable pulsatile flow, and surgically produced animal models.

☐ EVALUATION BY COMPUTED TOMOGRAPHY

UNENHANCED COMPUTED TOMOGRAPHY

- An enhanced CT scan is the examination of choice for the initial imaging evaluation of a patient with symptoms suggesting SAH.
- It should be performed without delay, especially if the patient is awake and oriented; this may change.
- The sensitivity of CT scanning to the disclosure of subarachnoid blood approaches that of lumbar puncture.
- In addition to making the diagnosis of SAH, the pattern of hemorrhage on CT can help to determine which aneurysm bled in patients with multiple aneurysms.
- Hemorrhage that preferentially fills the sylvian fissure, especially when associated with an intraparenchymal hematoma, suggests rupture of MCA aneurysms on that side.
- Hemorrhage concentrated within the anterior interhemispheric fissure suggests rupture of an anterior communicating artery aneurysm, especially when associated with intraventricular extension of hemorrhage.
- Inundation of the ventricular system with fresh blood, with ballooning of the third ventricle, is frequently seen in posterior fossa aneurysms.

Caution must be exercised in evaluating intraventricular blood, since small amounts of blood may reflux from the subarachnoid space into the fourth ventricle, passing through the third ventricle to layer in the occipital horn of one or both lateral ventricles. The finding of a small amount of blood in this location is less ominous than intraventricular blood associated with focal ventricular ballooning or an intraparenchymal tract or hematoma. A small amount of blood layered in one occipital horn cannot be relied upon for lateralizing the source of bleeding, since it is definitely related to the position of the patient's head prior to scanning.

In evaluating a CT scan that exhibits extensive subarachnoid blood, it is important to play with the window and level controls in search of the aneurysm within the clot. Focal distortion of adjacent anatomic structures, calcification within the wall of the aneurysm, and intraluminal thrombus can reveal the location of the aneurysm. Approximately 5 percent of aneurysms in the Cooperative Study on the Timing of Aneurysm Surgery were evident on unenhanced CT scans.

CONTRAST-ENHANCED COMPUTED TOMOGRAPHY AND CT ANGIOGRAPHY

In the age of the spiral or helical fast scanner, contrast-enhanced CT plays an important role in patients with SAH. While Heiserman and Bird report a case in which an enhanced CT located the aneurysm in a patient in critical clinical status, "allowing emergency craniotomy without preoperative angiography . . . ," they neglected to cite the clinical outcome. The neurosurgeon in that case

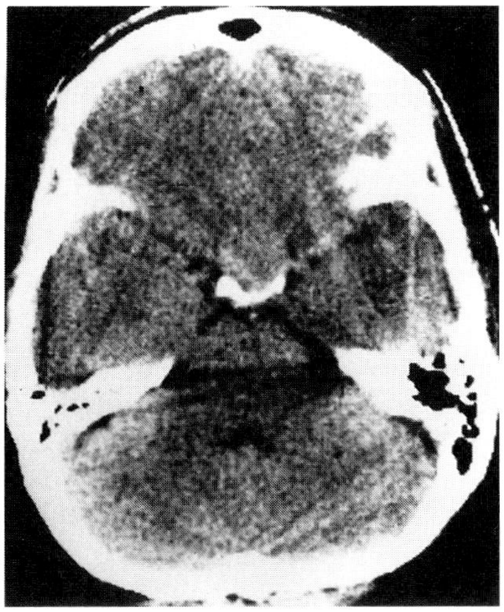
(A)

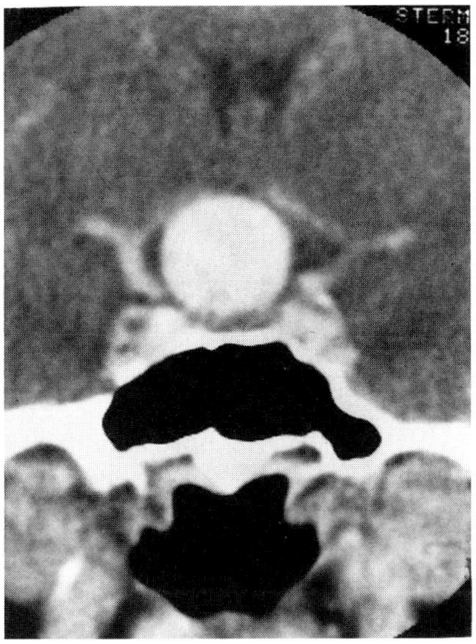
(B)

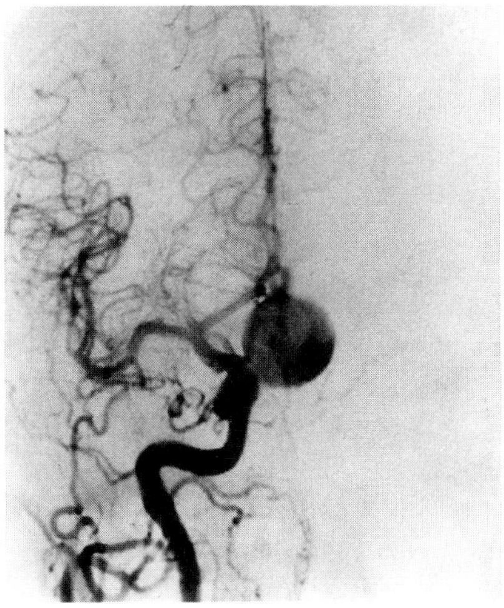
(C)

Figure 17-6 A large aneurysm in the suprasellar region, simulating a suprasellar neoplasm. *A*. Axial noncontrast CT scan shows a high-density mass in the suprasellar cistern. *B*. Coronal contrast-enhanced CT scan shows a large enhancing mass in the suprasellar cistern. *C*. A right common carotid angiogram shows a large aneurysm arising from the supraclinoid portion of the right internal carotid artery at the posterior communicating artery, situated in the suprasellar region.

operated without information that could have proved very important.

Conventional CT images obtained after contrast enhancement may, indeed, demonstrate an aneurysm (Fig. 17-6). They may also miss aneurysms less than 5 mm in diameter or those near the skull base in regions of beam-hardening artifact. By bolus injecting 75–100 mL of nonionic contrast agent at 2.5 ml/sec and obtaining a 1-mm helical scan through the circle of Willis (40–50 mm) after an 18-s delay, you will have the advantage of immediately available contrast-enhanced images plus the data to process for three-dimensional CT angiography (3D CTA) (Fig. 17-7). The 3D CTA can be processed during angiography and be available to the neurosurgeon by the time of surgery, even if surgery is done immediately after angiography.

Imaging by 3D CTA allows the creation of unusual oblique projections, not readily obtainable by conventional angiography, that add to the neurosurgeon's knowledge of the aneurysm to be confronted. Additionally, the data can be used to create a hologram that provides the neurosurgeon with a single, stereoscopically three-dimensional, life-sized image of the aneurysm. (Unfortunately it is not feasible to reproduce these images in a book. They can be viewed in displays at the American Society of Neuroradiology (ASNR) and Radiological Society of North America (RSNA). To imagine them, think of stacking 70 translucent axial slices, one on top of the other, and then looking at the stack from any side.) This image can be created in the projection from which the surgeon will approach the aneurysm, making it possible to check the size of the clips that are to be used in that particular case on the image without wasting time during the actual procedure. An extra advantage to the holograms lies in the as yet unexplained fact that beam-hardening and metallic-spray artifacts are attenuated and tend to disappear from the image.

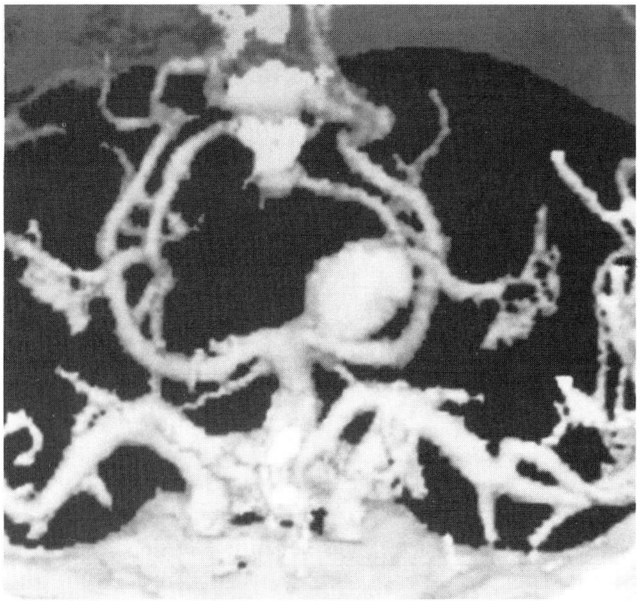

Figure 17-7 A posterior cerebral artery aneurysm demonstrated by CT angiography.

☐ EVALUATION BY MAGNETIC RESONANCE

MAGNETIC RESONANCE IMAGING

The advent of MRI brought clinicians a more complete evaluation of patients with unruptured intracranial aneurysms than had been available with CT and angiography. With MRI, we can see anatomic displacements secondary to mass effect more clearly, evaluate the extent of intraluminal thrombus, see clot adjacent to an aneurysm, have an approximation of the age of that clot, and identify old blood breakdown products that signify a previous hemorrhage.

The MRI appearance of flowing blood is complex, depending on its velocity, direction, and turbulence as well as the specific imaging sequences chosen. Unlike CT, in which the only way to vary the image is to vary the window and level setting, the MRI signal intensity of hemorrhage and blood breakdown products depends upon the age of the thrombus and the imaging parameters. The appearance of aneurysms on routine MRI is therefore quite variable, depending on the imaging sequence chosen, the state of turbulence, direction and velocity of flow within the aneurysm, and the presence or absence of thrombus.

Completely thrombosed aneurysms are encountered occasionally, but in most cases a central flow void is present within the lumen of the aneurysm. In many cases, this flow void is continuous with the flow void of the parent artery and indicates a high-flow jet through the neck of the aneurysm. The stenosis that produces the jet may be real, produced by the neck of the aneurysm or thrombus, or it may be caused by the disordered flow in the parent artery that helped produce the aneurysm.

Slow flow within an aneurysm can result in even-echo rephasing, an additional clue to the presence of an aneurysm. Proper choice of flip angle on gradient-echo pulse sequences can produce flow-related enhancement, making flowing blood in the lumen appear bright. The presence of significant hemorrhage adjacent to the aneurysm limits the usefulness of these sequences, however, since both flowing blood and blood breakdown products can be hyperintense. Gated cine techniques have been used to create loops that demonstrate the pulsatility and changes in signal intensity occurring within an aneurysm during the cardiac cycle.

Thrombus within the lumen of an aneurysm can produce a typical onionskin appearance. Unlike hematomas, in which the subacute blood breakdown product methemoglobin is first seen peripherally, the lamina nearest the lumen of the aneurysm contain methemoglobin that is hyperintense on both T1- and T2-weighted images. The more peripheral lamina contain the more chronic blood breakdown products, such as hemosiderin, and are strikingly hypointense on T2-weighted images.

Like all other imaging modalities, MRI has definite limitations. Air within a pneumonized anterior clinoid process can mimic a flow void in an aneurysm of the paraclinoid segment of the ICA. Calcifications within the wall of an aneurysm are more accurately identified on CT and plain films.

Although MRI techniques can identify and help characterize aneurysms and some authors identified hyperintensity on T2-weighted images in patients with acute SAH (mid- and low-field imaging systems), it is a general rule that MRI exhibits limited sensitivity to the presence of acute SAH. Since it can be identified on CT scans, it is unlikely that the poor visualization of subarachnoid blood on MRI is related to rapid dilution and clearance from the subarachnoid space. Artifacts related to cerebrospinal fluid (CSF) pulsation may provide a better explanation. The complementary roles of CT and MRI in acute SAH must not be forgotten.

MAGNETIC RESONANCE ANGIOGRAPHY

Magnetic resonance angiography (MRA) is really an evolving group of techniques that permit noninvasive visualization of arteries and/or veins. Each approach to MRA capitalizes upon the differences between flowing blood and adjacent stationary tissue. Clinically useful methods currently in use can be divided into two categories: time-of-flight (TOF) and phase-contrast (PC) acquisitions. Sequential slice acquisitions and volume acquisitions, called "two-dimensional" and "three-dimensional" respectively, are possible with both TOF and PC acquisitions. The source images obtained in either way can be postprocessed retrospectively to create composite images in any desired orientation, most commonly using the maximum intensity projection (MIP) algorithm.

As in the case of 3D CTA, the source images can be used to create holograms that provide true stereoscopic 3D images, as opposed to 2D projections of a 3D data set. In fact, superimposition of separate life-sized or same-scale holograms from CT bone window data and MRI data creates a single 3D image that can be examined and understood as the examiners merely move their heads from side to side or up and down.

The TOF sequences rely on flow-related enhancement to provide contrast between flowing blood and adjacent tissues. Intracranially, TOF volume acquisitions can accurately depict the arteries of the circle of Willis and significant portions of the anterior, middle, and posterior cerebral arteries. Medium-sized aneurysms are usually well seen as areas of abnormal signal intensity adjacent to the parent artery. Segmentation of source data can be performed to isolate regions of interest and minimize vessel overlap.

Since current MRA sequences are limited to a 512 × 512 matrices at best, resolution of MRA falls short of conventional angiography: this can limit sensitivity in the detection of small aneurysms. Insensitivity to slow flow and intravoxel dephasing from disordered flow limit the sensitivity of TOF volume acquisitions in large or lobulated aneurysms with irregular and/or slow flow. Signal loss from intravoxel dephasing can be minimized by reducing voxel size and echo time (TE) while other parameters are held constant. Because large aneurysms are usually well seen by MRI techniques, MRA and MRI complement each other in the evaluation of moderate and large aneurysms. Clinical comparison of TOF volume acquisitions with arterial digital subtraction angiography has shown that this technique can demonstrate aneurysms as small as 3 to 4 mm in diameter. Some small aneurysms are apparent only on the source images; this can be related to artifacts associated with the MIP post-processing algorithms. For this reason, close attention must be paid to the interpretation of both projection and source images, with an awareness that the pulse sequences employed for TOF MRA produce heavily T1-weighted source images, so the high signal intensity of a subacute thrombus may stimulate flow on MIP images. Multiple overlapping thin-slab acquisition (MOTSA) is a hybrid MRA technique that combines advantages of both 2D and volume MRA. Using this technique, intracranial aneurysms as small as 2.8 mm in diameter were detected.

Phase-contrast (PC) techniques rely on differences in phase shift between moving blood and the stationary tissue in a magnetic field gradient. These techniques involve subtraction of two acquisitions that are subjected to bipolar gradient pulses and are characterized by marked background suppression. Because multiple acquisitions are required to visualized motion in different directions, 3D PC acquisitions require more time than corresponding TOF acquisitions. Comparison of TOF and PC techniques suggests that PC acquisitions may better depict large aneurysms (greater than 15 mm), while TOF sequences visualize intraluminal clot not seen on PC MRA because of the inherent background suppression of stationary tissue.

In screening of patients at increased risk for aneurysms, such as patients with adult polycystic kidney disease and relatives of patients with ruptured aneurysms, MRA has a dominant role. In the quest for small aneurysms, careful choice of technique is as important to MRA as it is to conventional angiography. If holograms cannot be made from the data, multiple segmentations of the source images should be made and multiple projections of each segmentation should be inspected to minimize vessel overlap. Alternative projection algorithms may also improve discrimination of aneurysms and vascular loops. Routine MR images, source images, and the projection images must be carefully inspected to avoid missing aneurysms that may be all too easily seen retrospectively. Considering the 1 percent incidence of intracranial aneurysms in the general population, it is not surprising that careful inspection of intracranial MRI and MRA obtained for other indications occasionally reveals an unsuspected aneurysm.

☐ CEREBRAL ANGIOGRAPHY

TECHNICAL CONSIDERATIONS

Cerebral angiography remains the gold standard in the quest for intracranial aneurysms. The early evolution of the technical aspects of cerebral angiography are well documented in Newton and Potts and in Osborn. Since the publication of these books, improvements in the resolution of digital subtraction angiography (DSA) systems has all but replaced cut-film angiography. Selective arterial DSA can be performed with smaller (less traumatic) catheters, more projections, less contrast agent, and less time than cut-film angiograms. Each of these factors reduces the incidence of complications. (In our own experience, supervising the performance of cerebral angiograms by residents and fellows, more than 70 percent of diagnostic angiograms can be performed using one 4-French catheter, one guide wire, and 50 mL of nonionic contrast agent; only during the treatment of large AVMs do we exceed 100 mL. Review of fluoroscopy time and total contrast agent used provides an accurate indicator of a given resident's progress.)

Another advantage to the use of DSA techniques lies in the hardware and software now available. Since the early 1980s, 1024 × 1024 resolution has been available. Modern DSA suites provide biplane imaging, stereoscopic biplane imaging, and rotational subtraction angiograms with multiple oblique projections during a single contrast injection. A brief presentation on the possibilities of viewing sequentially paired images from a rotational angiogram rapidly led to the development of true stereoscopic rotational angiograms that provide unprecedented visualization of aneurysms. Software has also been created that allows placement of cursors on several different projections of an aneurysm from a single rotational angiogram, and the computer will then determine the best obliquity to identify the neck or face of the aneurysm. This is as important to the neurosurgeon as it is to the interventional neuroradiologist.

Intracranial aneurysms are frequently multiple. In evaluating a patient suspected of having an intracranial aneurysm or when an aneurysm is coincidentally discovered during evaluation of cervical carotid disease, a complete angiogram must be obtained. Although this approach was traditionally described as panangiography or four-vessel angiography, it is more important to think in terms of the locations that must be well seen. The angiogram must thoroughly evaluate the cavernous and supraclinoid ICAs without superimposition of external carotid branches. (In aneurysm patients, selective catheterization beyond mild to moderate bifurcation stenoses improves sensitivity with little additional risk if small catheters are used with careful technique and runoff is good.)

Supratentorially, one must clearly visualize the origins of each ophthalmic artery, each posterior communicating artery, each anterior choroidal artery, the anterior communicating artery, and the major trunks of each MCA. Infratentorially it is necessary to see both vertebral arteries from C1 to the vertebrobasilar junction, the origins of each (there may be more than two!) posterior inferior cerebellar arteries (PICA), each anterior inferior cerebellar artery (AICA), each superior cerebellar artery (SCA), and the precommunicant (P1) segment of each posterior cerebral artery (PCA). Additionally, the main trunk of the basilar artery must be opacified well enough to exclude the possibility of fenestration, since aneurysms may arise on one limb and not be visible if that limb is not opacified.

A routine angiogram for aneurysm would consist of a minimum of three projections in each internal carotid artery (frontal, lateral, and transorbital oblique) and three projections in the dominant vertebral artery (lateral, Townes, and exaggerated Waters or transfacial), provided that reflux opacifies the contralateral vertebral artery to provide good visualization of the opposite PICA. Hypoplasia of the preconfluent segment of one vertebral artery demands selective injections in both.

When an aneurysm is identified, careful evaluation of the images must be performed to confirm that all necessary information has been obtained for the neurosurgeon. Not only must the neck or face of the aneurysm be identified, but care must be taken to delineate adjacent arteries that may be displaced or incorporated in the aneurysmal wall. Nor should the venous phase of the angiogram be neglected, especially in the angiographic frontal and lateral projections: neurosurgeons need information about the venous drainage of the brain, especially if the aneurysm might be approached by a skull base approach and one of the sinuses might be ligated.

CAROTID OCCLUSION TESTING

Certain giant aneurysm involving the cavernous ICA, proximal MCA, and basilar artery are amenable to trapping and placement of a bypass graft to the distal circulation. Although small-caliber grafts from arteries such as the superficial temporal artery have frequently failed to provide enough blood flow, large-caliber sphenous vein grafts from the cervical internal or external carotid artery to the intracranial circulation (MCA, ICA, PCA, and SCA) can completely vascularize most territories. In these cases, it is important to know your neurosurgeon's intentions and preferences, since carotid occlusion testing may provide information that aids in determining the exact placement of the graft.

ANGIOGRAPHY AFTER RECENT SUBARACHNOID HEMORRHAGE

Although many neurosurgeons, especially those who use modified skull base approaches, can visualize and clip more than one aneurysm through the same craniotomy, when patients with multiple aneurysms present with SAH, it is important to try to identify the aneurysm that has ruptured. The respective roles of MRI and CT have been discussed. In angiography, identification of contrast extravasation is an uncommon but definitive observation associated with high mortality. The largest or most irregular aneurysm is a more likely source of bleeding, and focal vasospasm and/or mass effect are also useful indicators. The probability of aneurysmal rupture is also related to location in the following progression: anterior communicating artery, PICA, basilar apex, posterior communicating artery, ACA, and PCA.

SUBARACHNOID HEMORRHAGE AND NORMAL ANGIOGRAMS

Approximately 10 percent of patients who present with SAH will exhibit normal cerebral angiograms in the acute phase. In these patients it is important to complete the study by injecting both external carotid arteries and, if they are normal, by imaging the cervical region while injecting the vertebral arteries. This is done to exclude AVM/AVF. In some cases that appeared normal (especially late at night), an aneurysm has proved to have been present and visible but was not seen on that initial examination. In about one-fourth of the cases of initially normal angiograms, no aneurysmal opacification occurred on the initial angiogram, but subsequent follow-up angiography has documented its existence. In some cases, nonaneurysmal SAH may be responsible for hemorrhage seen in the basilar cisterns on CT.

INTRAOPERATIVE, POSTOPERATIVE, AND INTERVENTIONAL NEUROANGIOGRAPHY

With modern microsurgical and neuroanesthetic techniques, nearly all intracranial aneurysms can be obliterated with preservation of the parent vessel. Most vascular neurosurgeons request either intraoperative or postoperative angiography to verify obliteration of the aneurysm and preservation of the parent vessel. If surgery is to occur within 24 h, a sheath should be left in the groin to serve as an arterial pressure monitoring line and provide access in the operating room.

Angiography plays an important role in the evaluation of patients with cerebral vasospasm associated with SAH, whether it precedes or follows surgery. When vasospasm is detected, angioplasty is frequently the treatment of choice. Finally, progress continues in the field of interventional neuroradiology, and many aneurysms that can be clipped can also be occluded by endovascular techniques that obviate the need for craniotomy.

□ SUMMARY

Evolution in the neuroradiologic evaluation and in neurosurgical and neuroradiologic treatment of intracranial aneurysms has altered attitudes concerning this condition. After confirmation of SAH with emergent CT, meticulous panangiography remains the procedure of choice to exclude aneurysmal rupture. It can also serve as an avenue for treatment, serving as an adjunct to or instead of traditional neurosurgical clipping. Both CTA and MRA play a role in delineating the 3D anatomy of aneurysms, and MRI provides information about the presence of intraluminal thrombus, mass effect, and any focal ischemic change. In addition, MRA plays an important role in the screening evaluation of otherwise asymptomatic patients with a strong family history or other suspicion of aneurysm. The importance of each of these modalities will change continually as technology evolves.

SUGGESTED READINGS

1. Atlas SW et al: Partially thrombosed giant intracranial aneurysms: Correlation of MR and pathologic findings. *Radiology* 162:111–114, 1987.
2. Bank WO et al: Traumatic aneurysm of the basilar artery. *AJR* 130:975–977, 1978.
3. Barami K, Ko K: Ruptured mycotic aneurysm presenting as an intraparenchymal hemorrhage and nonadjacent acute subdural hematoma: Case report and review of the literature. *Surg Neurol* 4:290–293, 1994.
4. Barrow DL, Prats AR: Infectious intracranial aneurysms: Comparison of groups with and without endocarditis. *Neurosurgery* 27:562–572, 1990.
5. Biondi A, Scialfa G, Scotti G: Intracranial aneurysms: MR imaging. *Neuroradiology* 30:214–218, 1988.

6. Biumi F: Observationes anatomicae, scholiis illustratae: Observatio V. In Sandifoert E (ed): *Thesaurus Dissertationum*. Vol 3. Milan, Lichtmans, 1778.
7. Blatter DD et al: Cerebral MR angiography with multiple overlapping thin slab acquisition: Part II. Early clinical experience. *Radiology* 193:379–389, 1992.
8. Branch CL et al: Left atrial myxoma with cerebral emboli. *Neurosurgery* 16:675–680, 1985.
9. Chakeres DW, Bryan RN: Acute subarachnoid hemorrhage: In vitro comparison of magnetic resonance and computed tomography. *AJNR* 7:223–228, 1986.
10. Chong BW et al: Blood flow dynamics in the vertebrobasilar system: Correlation of a transparent elastic model and MR angiography. *AJNR* 15:733–745, 1994.
11. Dandy WE: Intracranial aneurysm of the internal carotid artery: Cured by operation. *Ann Surg* 107:654–659, 1938.
12. Drake CG: Giant intracranial aneurysms: Experience with surgical treatment in 174 patients. *Clin Neurosurg* 26:12–95, 1979.
13. Drake CG: Report of World Federation of Neurological Surgeons Committee on a Universal Subarachnoid Haemorrhage Grading Scale. *J Neurosurg* 68:985–986, 1988.
14. Gonzalez CF et al: Intracranial aneurysms: Flow analysis of their origin and progression. *AJNR* 13:181–188, 1992.
15. Heiserman JE, Bird CR: Cerebral aneurysms, in intracranial vascular lesions. *Neuroimaging Clin North Am* 4:799–822, 1994.
16. Holmes B, Harbaugh RE: Traumatic intracranial aneurysms: A contemporary review. *J Trauma* 35:855–860, 1993.
17. Hutchinson J: Aneurysm of the internal carotid within the skull diagnosed eleven year before the patient's death: Spontaneous cure. *Trans Clin Soc Lond* 8:127–131, 1875.
18. Inagawa T: Multiple intracranial aneurysms in elderly patients. *Acta Neurochir (Wien)* 106:119–126, 1990.
19. Juvela S, Porras M, Heiskanen O: Neurosurgical forum: Natural history of unruptured aneurysms. *J Neurosurg* 80:773–774, 1994.
20. Hounpian EM, Pool JL: A systematic analysis of intracranial aneurysms from the autopsy file of Presbyterian Hospital. *J Neuropathol Exp Neurol* 17:409–423, 1958.
21. Kahn MT et al: Serpentine aneurysms of the posterior circulation: Report of two cases. *Br J Neurosurg* 4:217–223, 1990.
22. Kessel NF et al: The international cooperative study on the timing of aneurysm surgery. *J Neurosurg* 73:18–47, 1990.
23. Kurino M et al: Mycotic aneurysm accompanied by aspergillotic granuloma: A case report. *Surg Neurol* 42:160–164, 1994.
24. Leblanc R et al: Angiographic screening and elective surgery of familial cerebral aneurysms: A decision analysis. *Neurosurgery* 35:9–19, 1994.
25. Ljunggren B et al: Aneurysmal subarachnoid hemorrhage: Total annual outcome in a 1.46 million population. *Surg Neurol* 22:435–438, 1984.
26. Matsummura M et al: Unruptured intracranial aneurysms in polycystic kidney disease. *Acta Neurochir* 79:94–99, 1986.
27. Meyer FB et al: Cerebral aneurysms in childhood and adolescence. *J Neurosurg* 70:420–425, 1989.
28. Moniz E: Aneurysme intracranien de la carotide interne droite rendu visible par l'arteriographie. *Rev Otoneuroophthalmol* 11:746–748, 1933.
29. Nadel L et al: Intracranial vascular abnormalities: Value of MR phase imaging to distinguish thrombus from flowing blood. *AJNR* 11:1133–1140, 1990.
30. Newton TH, Potts DG (eds): Angiography, in *Radiology of the Skull and Brain*. Vol 4. St Louis, Mosby, 1974.
31. Osborn AG: *Handbook of Neuroradiology*. St Louis, Mosby-Year Book, 1991.
32. Osborn AH: *Introduction to Cerebral Angiography*. New York, Harper & Row, 1980.
33. Penta HJ et al: Feeding artery pedicle aneurysms: Association with parenchymal hemorrhage and arteriovenous malformation in the brain. *J Neurosurg* 80:631–634, 1994.
34. Rinkel GJE et al: Non-aneurysmal perimesencephalic subarachnoid hemorrhage: CT and MR patterns that differ from aneurysmal rupture. *AJNR* 12:829–834, 1991.
35. Ronkainen A et al: A ten percent prevalence of asymptomatic familial intracranial aneurysms: Preliminary report of 110 magnetic resonance angiography studies in members of 21 Finnish familial intracranial aneurysm families. *Neurosurgery* 35:208–213, 1994.
36. Rosenorn J et al: The risk of rebleeding from ruptured intracranial aneurysms. *J Neurosurg* 67:329–332, 1987.
37. Rosenorn J et al: Unruptured intracranial aneurysms: An assessment of the annual risk of rupture based on epidemiological and clinical data. *Br J Neurosurg* 2:369–377, 1988.
38. Seigle JM et al: Multiple oncotic intracranial aneurysms and cardiac metastasis from choriocarcinoma: Case report and review of the literature. *Neurosurgery* 20:39–42, 1987.
39. Shuaib A et al: Subarachnoid hemorrhage and normal angiography: Should the angiogram be reviewed by a second neuroradiologist? *Can J Neurol Sci* 15:413–416, 1988.
40. Stehbens WE: Etiology of intracranial berry aneurysms. *J Neurosurg* 70:823–831, 1989.
41. Strother CM et al: Aneurysm hemodynamics: An experimental study. *AJNR* 13:1089–1095, 1992.
42. Turjman P et al: Aneurysms related to cerebral arteriovenous malformations: Superselective angiographic assessment in 58 patients. *AJNR* 15:1601–1605, 1994.
43. van Alphen HA, Gao YZ: Multiple cerebral de novo aneurysms. *Clin Neurol Neurosurg* 93:13–18, 1991.
44. Wiebers DO et al: The significance of unruptured intracranial aneurysms. *J Neurosurg* 66:23–29, 1987.
45. Wilson FM et al: Multiple cerebral aneurysms: A reappraisal. *Neuroradiology* 31:232–236, 1989.
46. Zimmerman RD et al: Acute intracranial hemorrhage: Intensity changes on sequential MR scans at 0.5%. *AJNR* 9:47–57, 1988.

☐ QUESTIONS (True or False)

1. Saccular aneurysms include the following:
- **a.** Developmental/degenerative aneurysms
- **b.** Oncotic aneurysms
- **c.** Mycotic aneurysms
- **d.** Flow-related aneurysms
- **e.** Dissecting aneurysms

2. Regarding flow-related aneurysms:
- **a.** The high-flow states encountered in patients with arteriovenous malformation contribute to the development of aneurysms.
- **b.** Aneurysms are not associated with AV fistulas.
- **c.** True flow-related aneurysms are encountered on a feeding pedicle.

d. Aneurysms associated with AVM are a major cause of intracranial hemorrhage.
e. Superselective angiography demonstrates a much higher incidence of aneurysm associated with AVM as compared to conventional angiography.

3. Increased incidence of saccular aneurysm is reported in the following conditions:
a. Fibromuscular dysplasia
b. Marfan's syndrome
c. Sarcoidosis
d. Coarctation of the aorta
e. Ehlers-Danlos syndrome

4. Regarding giant aneurysm:
a. Approximately 25 percent of intracranial aneurysms are giant aneurysms.
b. They are aneurysms greater than 2.5 cm in diameter.
c. One-half to two-thirds of giant aneurysms are found in the posterior fossa.
d. For showing aneurysm size, CT and MR are more reliable than angiography.
e. It can be saccular or fusiform.

5. Regarding location of intracranial aneurysms:
a. Approximately 30 percent are at the anterior communicating artery.
b. Approximately 30 percent are at the posterior communicating artery.
c. Approximately 20 percent are at the middle cerebral artery bifurcation.
d. Approximately 15 percent are at the basilar tip.
e. Some 20 percent of patients with aneurysm may have multiple aneurysms.

☐ ANSWERS

1. a. T
b. T
c. T
d. T
e. F

2. a. T
b. F
c. T
d. T
e. T

3. a. T
b. T
c. F
d. T
e. T

4. a. F
b. T
c. T
d. T
e. T

5. a. T
b. T
c. T
d. F
e. T

CHAPTER

18

Intracranial Vascular Malformation

Mark Mehringer

Vascular malformations of the brain are most simply divided into four categories, according to their histopathology. These are arteriovenous malformations, capillary telangiectasias, cavernous angiomas, and venous malformations. Combinations of these types may occur.

Arteriovenous malformations (AVMs) are subdivided into parenchymal (*pial*) and dural types. Parenchymal AVMs exist when there is a primitive, congenital communication between arteries and veins without an intervening capillary bed. This abnormal tangle of connecting vessels is referred to as the nidus. Because the nidus offers less resistance to blood flow than a normal capillary bed, a shunt or sump effect exists, with resultant increased flow through the AVM vessels. The feeding and draining vessels are typically enlarged. The presence of a nidus and arteriovenous shunting are hallmarks of a parenchymal AVM.

☐ ARTERIOVENOUS MALFORMATIONS

PARENCHYMAL

Incidence

- Arteriovenous malformations are the commonest and most important congenital vascular anomaly.
- Their estimated incidence is 0.15 percent in the general population and 3 percent in patients with cerebral hemorrhage.
- They are almost always solitary, but a small number (2 percent) may be multiple.
- When they are multiple, they may be associated with one of two syndromes, Rendu-Osler-Weber or Wyburn-Masson syndrome.
- Rendu-Osler-Weber syndrome consists of multiple capillary telangiectasias of skin and mucosa plus brain and pulmonary arteriovenous malformations.
- Wyburn-Mason syndrome consists of cutaneous nevi plus retinal and cerebral arteriovenous malformations along the optic pathway.

Age and Gender

- The incidence of AVMs is equal between males and females.
- These lesions are congenital and at least 25 percent of patients have symptoms in childhood; however, AVMs most often present in adulthood between 20 and 40 years of age. By age 50, most AVMs have become manifest.

Location

- Approximately 80 to 90 percent of parenchymal AVMs are supratentorial.
- They may occur anywhere in the brain, but a classic appearance is one in which the malformation has a wedge shape, with its base near the brain surface and its apex toward the ventricular wall.
- Malformations may also be either entirely superficial or deep.

Pathology Grossly, an AVM is a tangle of tortuous dilated arteries and veins with an interposed nidus. There is no capillary bed and brain parenchyma is not present within the nidus. Brain around the AVM may be atrophic and gliotic and there may be evidence of prior hemorrhage. Mass effect is notably absent unless there has been recent hemorrhage or there is a large aneurysm or varix. The walls of the dilated feeding arteries and draining veins may show vasculopathic changes with focal stenoses or occlusion. Aneurysms on feeding arteries, within the nidus or in the circle of Willis are seen in 10 percent of cases.

Imaging ***Plain Films*** Plain skull radiographs may show intracranial calcifications and enlarged vascular grooves and foramina, but the amount of information imparted does not warrant their routine use.

Cerebral Angiography

- Cerebral angiography remains the definitive study for displaying the gross morphology and hemodynamics of an AVM. This display, in turn, allows optimum therapeutic planning.
- The location of the nidus, the origin and number of feeding arteries, the presence of aneurysms, and the size, location and configuration of draining veins are all important information provided by the arteriogram (Fig. 18-1*A* and *B*).
- The use of microcatheters for subselective arteriography may allow even better anatomic detail and is an entree to endovascular therapy.
- A pitfall for angiography is the thrombosed arteriovenous malformation. Thrombosis occurs when an AVM has bled and hematoma compresses the malformation or when vasculopathic changes result in stenoses or occlusion of feeding arteries. Angiography may be normal in a thrombosed AVM. Arteriovenous shunting may be absent or reduced and, in fact, flow may be stagnant.

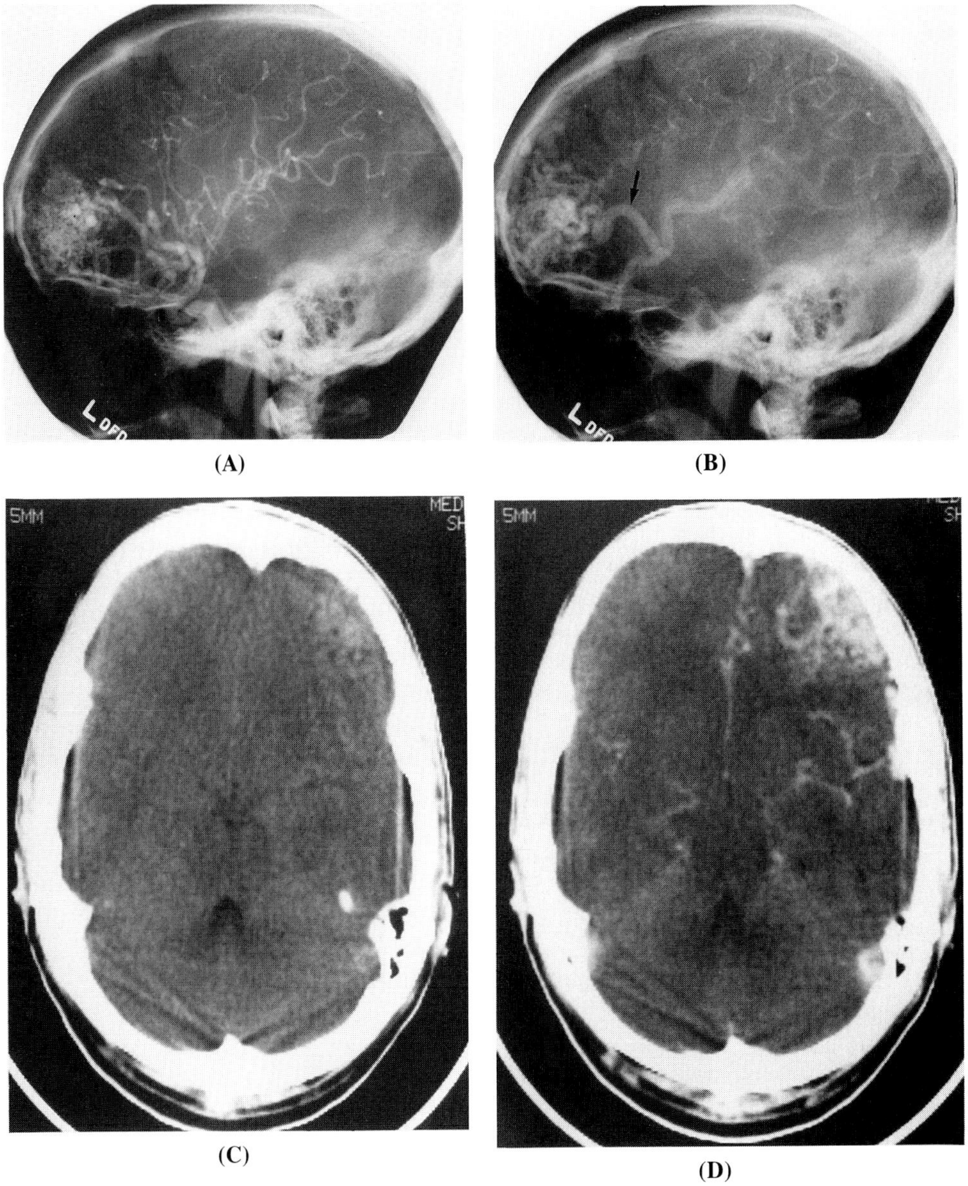

Figure 18-1 *A*. Arterial phase of the cerebral arteriogram. The enlarged anterior, middle cerebral artery feeders and nidus are evident. *B*. The late arterial phase of the cerebral arteriogram shows an enlarged, early draining vein coming out of the nidus (*arrow*). *C*. A noncontrast CT scan shows subtle increased density in the left frontal lobe. There is no mass effect and no edema corresponding to an arteriovenous malformation. *D*. A contrast enhanced CT shows an area of curvilinear enhancement, consistent with nidus of arteriovenous malformation. Dilated feeding arteries and draining veins are also seen.

Computed Tomography

- Arteriovenous malformations may be indiscernible on non-contrast-enhanced computed tomography (CT). The pool of circulating blood in the nidus and feeding and draining vessels is usually slightly hyperintense to brain parenchyma and may be detectable if the vascular structures are large enough.
- They are easily detectable on a contrast-enhanced scan as curvilinear, serpiginous areas of enhancement. Typically, there is little or no mass effect.
- The noncontrast scan is useful for identifying calcifications and is especially useful for showing acute hemorrhage.
- Both enhanced and nonenhanced scans are usually appropriate (Fig. 18-1*C* and *D*, Fig. 18-2*A* and *B*).

Magnetic Resonance Imaging

- Magnetic resonance imaging (MRI) offers many advantages for imaging AVMs. The appearance of an AVM on MRI is variable and will depend upon the scanning parameters employed as well as characteristics of the malformation, such as the rate and direction of flow and the presence of new or old hemorrhage.
- The presence of flow void within enlarged feeding arteries and draining veins and within the nidus are characteristic of AVMs. On T1- and T2-weighted images, flow voids have a dark signal. The latter are more sensitive to flow than the former.
- On gradient-echo images, flow has bright signal. This may be useful for differentiating dark signal on T1- and T2-weighted images due to rapidly flowing blood from dark signal due to calcification or hemosiderin, because flow has bright signal on gradient-echo sequences, but calcification and hemosiderin will remain dark.
- Magnetic resonance imaging has several advantages over CT in evaluating AVMs. In addition to identifying acute and chronic hemorrhage, MRI is superior to CT scanning for the ease with which it can supply images in multiple planes. This, in turn, leads to better anatomic localization of the nidus and sizing of the nidus.
- Location referable to surrounding anatomic structures and the size of the AVM are important criteria for determining therapeutic options.
- Flow void within the nidus, feeding arteries, and draining veins may be absent if there is decreased flow due to compressed by hematoma, thrombosis, or vasospasm.

DURAL ARTERIOVENOUS FISTULA

Dural arteriovenous (AV) fistulas are a distinct subgroup of vascular malformations that have traditionally been grouped with AVMs, probably because they are often high-flow lesions with arteriovenous shunting. Their pathophysiology and clinical course, however, differ from those of parenchymal AVMs and some controversy surrounds their description.

Incidence

- Dural AV fistulas make up 10 to 15 percent of intracranial vascular malformations, and one-third of posterior fossa AVMs are dural.

Age and Gender

- Most dural AV fistulas are clinically manifest between 40 and 60 years of age.
- Women are affected more often than men, especially in cases of dural malformations involving the cavernous sinus.

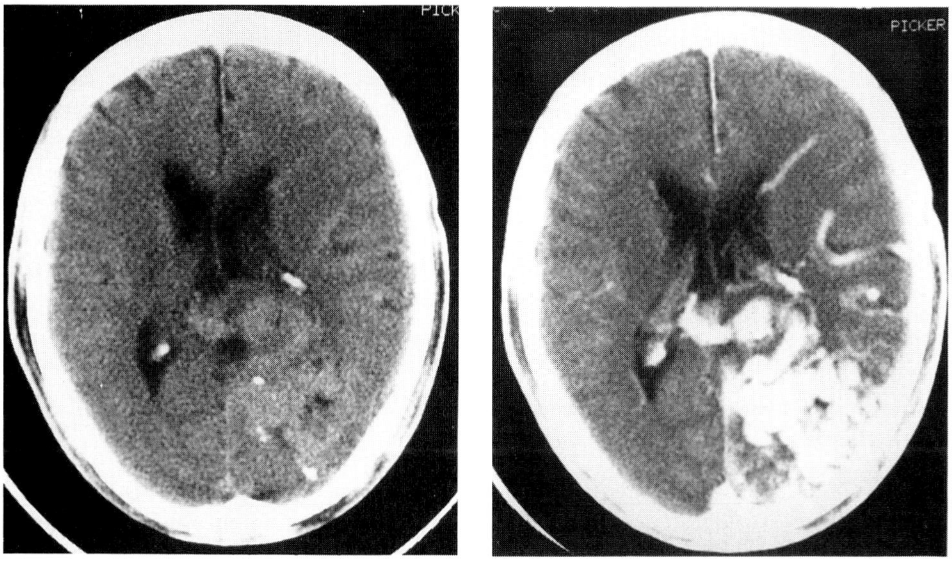

(A) (B)

Figure 18-2 *A*. A noncontrast CT scan of an arteriovenous malformation in the splenium of the corpus callosum and left occipital lobe. Nonclotted blood in the malformation is of slightly higher density than gray matter and there is calcification. In this instance there is also mass effect. *B*. A contrast-enhanced CT scan shows serpentine and punctate enhancement in the enlarged arteries, veins, and nidus.

Location
- Dural AV malformations can be associated with any dural sinus but most frequently involve the transverse, sigmoid, and cavernous sinuses.

Pathology A dural malformation exists when there is an arterial connection from a meningeal artery to a dural sinus. Although this can be a single point fistula, more often numerous small microfistulas exist. There may be numerous small, dilated feeding arteries, but there is no nidus, as would be seen in a parenchymal AVM. There is some controversy regarding the pathophysiology of dural AV malformations. In most cases, these lesions probably arise as a response to sinus thrombosis. Exactly how this happens is uncertain, but it may represent an attempt at recanalization of the sinus run amok. In addition to the fistula, the dural sinus may have vasculopathic changes. Vasculopathic changes in the involved dural sinus may be residua of preceding thrombosis or a response to increased or turbulent flow. These changes include focal stenoses or occlusion of the sinus. Compromise of the sinus lumen in the face of an arterial fistula raises intracranial venous pressure and may increase symptomatology due to venous infarct, hemorrhage, or communicating hydrocephalus.

Imaging ***Plain Films*** Plain films may show enlarged meningeal artery grooves or foraminas, but—as with pial malformations—the amount of information provided does not warrant their routine use.

Cerebral Angiography
- Cerebral angiography is of more value than any other study for demonstrating and defining a dural arteriovenous malformation (Fig. 18-3*D*).
- Salient features that should be looked for include the number and site of arterial feeders and characteristics of the venous drainage, such as which sinus is involved, vasculopathic changes in the sinus, and the exact drainage pattern of the sinus itself.
- The best arteriograms will be obtained by selectively catheterizing the meningeal feeders, and this should be done when possible. As with parenchymal AV malformations, arteriography may be an entree to endovascular treatment.

Computed Tomography Because feeding meningeal arteries may be difficult to separate from the adjacent bone of the skull, CT may be normal in cases of dural AVM. Enlarged draining veins are more likely to be identified than enlarged arteries (Fig. 18-3*A* and *B*). Complications such as hemorrhage, infarction, or hydrocephalus may be appreciated.

Magnetic Resonance Imaging
- Magnetic resonance imaging is more useful than CT, but less useful than angiography in the evaluation of dural AVMs (Fig. 18-3*C*).
- Magnetic resonance imaging is less useful for studying dural AV malformations than pial malformations. The identification of enlarged cortical veins without any AVM nidus suggests a dural AVM.
- Complications such as infarction, sinus thrombosis, and hydrocephalus are well displayed by MRI.

CAVERNOUS ANGIOMAS

Incidence Because cavernous angiomas are usually occult to angiography, they were formerly thought to be uncommon. Cross-sectional imaging, particularly MRI, has detected many more of these lesions. It is now apparent that they are among the commonest types of malformation. There is a tendency for multiplicity in up to 50 percent of cases, and there is also a familial predisposition.

Age and Gender
- Cavernous angiomas can present at any age but usually do so between 20 and 40 years.
- They may be discovered incidentally on scans or present with seizures or various neurologic symptoms, particularly if they are associated with hemorrhage.
- There is no predilection as to gender.

Location
- Cavernous angiomas can occur anywhere in the central nervous system and may even be extradural.
- They are most common in a supratentorial location in the frontal and temporal lobes, less common in the posterior fossa, and even less common in the spinal cord.

Pathology Cavernous angiomas are composed of a spherical cluster of endothelium-lined sinusoidal spaces with stagnant blood, blood clot, and blood degradation products within. Hemosiderin may stain the surrounding brain, and calcification is common. Overlap with other vascular malformations, particularly capillary telangiectasias, may occur. An important pathologic differentiating point is the lack of any neural tissue within the malformation, in distinction to other types of malformation, in which brain tissue is interspersed in the malformation.

Plain Films Although there may be calcification within some cavernous angiomas, no other finding that could be seen on plain films is expected. Routine use of plain films is not warranted.

Cerebral Angiography Cavernous angiomas are slow-flowing vascular malformations without enlarged feeding arteries, draining veins, or AV shunting. Occasionally a faint stain may be seen within the sinusoidal spaces of the angioma. However, these lesions

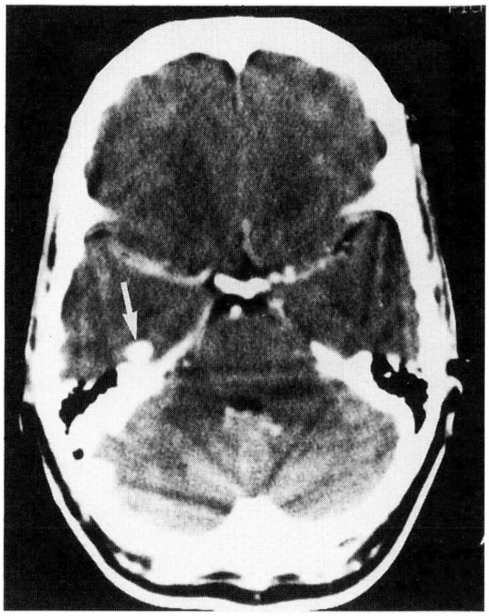

(A)

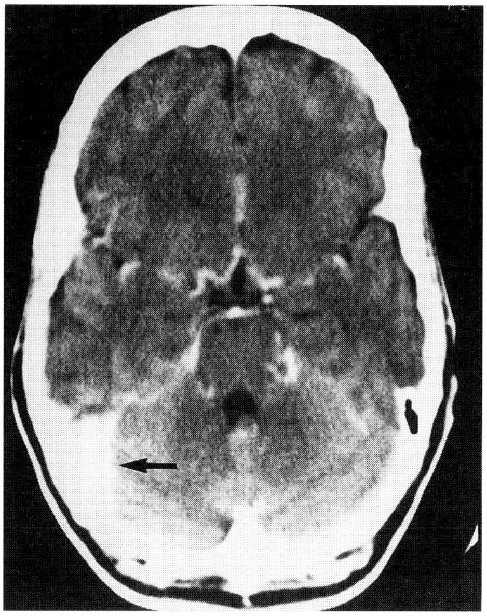

(B)

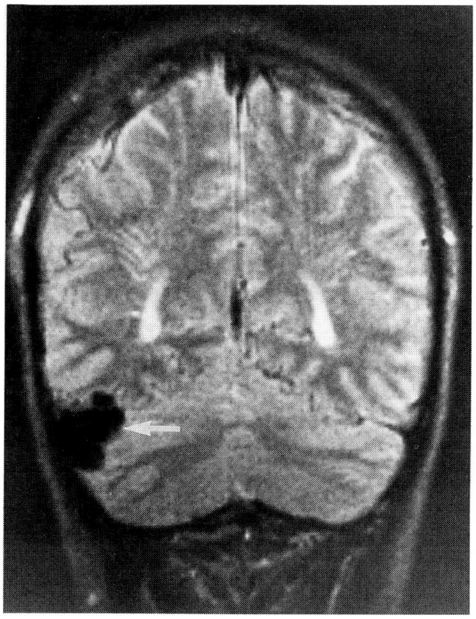

(C)

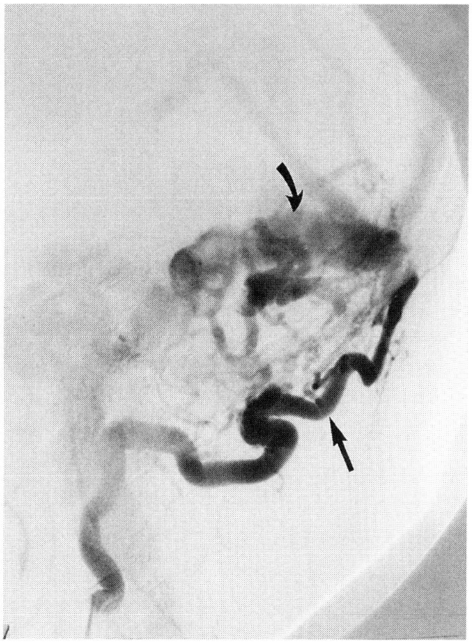

(D)

Figure 18-3 *A*. A contrast-enhanced CT scan shows a small ovoid area of enhancement (*arrow*) anterior to the right petrous temporal bone. This rather subtle finding corresponds to an enlarged venous collateral in a dural arteriovenous malformation. *B*. An additional enhanced CT slice shows increased enhancement and fullness of the right transverse sinus (*arrow*). *C*. A coronal T2-weighted MRI shows dark flow void in the enlarged right transverse sinus (*arrow*) *D*. A lateral view of the arterial phase of a selective right occipital arteriogram shows rapid shunting from the markedly enlarged occipital artery (*arrow*) into the right transverse sinus (*curved arrow*), confirming the dural AV fistula.

are usually occult to angiography; hence they are often referred to as "occult malformations." A previously high-flow arteriovenous malformation may also become occult on an arteriogram if it has thrombosed and a capillary telangiectasia may be occult. It is important to remember that vascular malformations may be mixed. There is an association of venous angiomas with cavernous angiomas, and the presence of a typical venous angioma on an arteriogram does not mean that there is not also a cavernous angioma present (Fig. 18-4*B*).

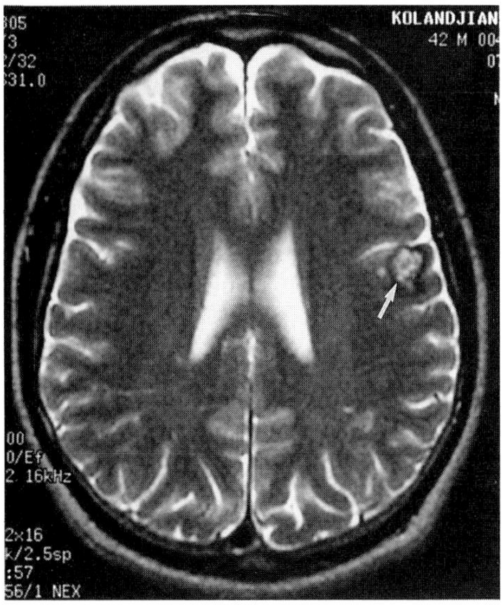

(A)

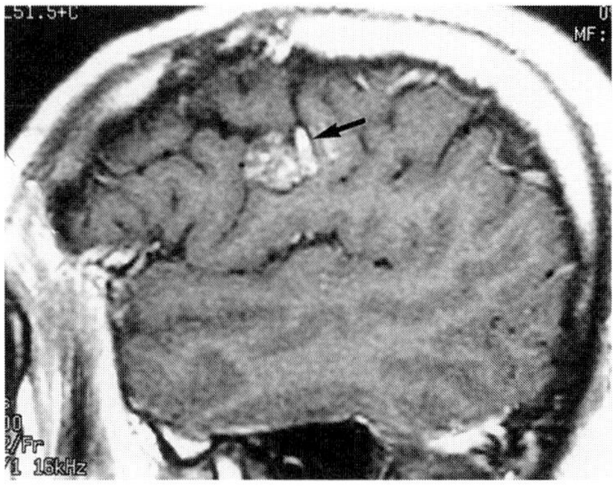

(B)

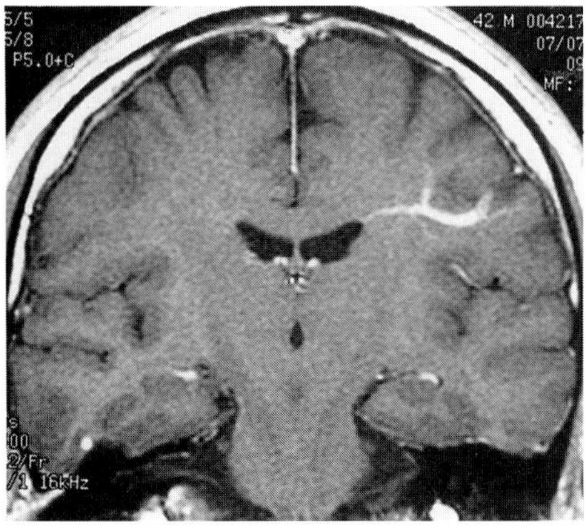

(C)

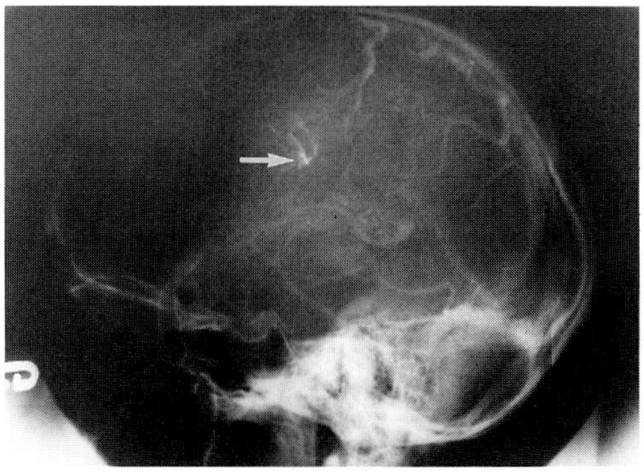

(D)

Figure 18-4 *A*. An axial T2-weighted MRI shows a left frontal lobe lesion with a peripheral dark rim and bright speckled or "popcorn" appearance internally (*arrow*). This is compatible with a cavernous angioma. *B*. A sagittal postcontrast enhanced T1-weighted MRI shows the cavernous angioma anteriorly and a more tubular enhancing structure behind it (*arrow*), suggesting an associated venous angioma and cavernous angioma. *C*. A coronal T1-weighted postcontrast MRI section at a level just posterior to the cavernous angioma shows typical enhancement in a slowly flowing transcortical venous angioma. *D*. Lateral view of the venous phase of a left carotid arteriogram shows the venous angioma end-on (*arrow*). The cavernous angioma, as expected, was not shown. The arterial phase was normal.

Computed Tomography

- On CT, cavernous angiomas are at least isodense to brain and are usually hyperdense. Calcification is often present and may be intense.
- It seems intuitively true that contrast enhancement would be present in a vascular malformation, but in fact enhancement is variable, from none to intense.
- There is no mass effect or edema and there are no enlarged vessels. These lesions can be confused with a low-grade tumor, granuloma, or hematoma on CT.

Magnetic Resonance Imaging

- Magnetic resonance imaging is the definitive study for cavernous angiomas, far surpassing other techniques where the malformation is occult or findings are nonspecific.
- The angioma is a round, well-circumscribed area that has mixed signal due to the presence of various blood products. It has been described as "popcornlike" in appearance. There is a circumferential ring of hemosiderin that is dark and has a blooming effect on T2-weighted images and particularly on gradient-echo images (Fig. 18-4*A*). The hemosiderin is present because of prior hemorrhage or seepage of blood from the angioma.
- Because of their increased sensitivity to susceptibility effect, gradient-echo sequences are most useful for detecting multiple and small cavernous angiomas.
- Contrast enhancement is usually present (Fig. 18-4*B*). The differentiation of a cavernous angioma from a hemorrhagic tumor may be a challenge, but the evolution of hemorrhage in a tumor contrasts with the static appearance of the angioma. A complete hemosiderin ring and lack of mass effect and edema favor a cavernous angioma. With time, the hematoma will resorb and collapse; an angioma will not collapse and in fact may grow slowly.
- If the angioma has an acute bleed, it is more difficult to differentiate from a hemorrhagic tumor; with time, however, it will evolve to the typical appearance of an angioma.

CAPILLARY TELANGIECTASIAS

Incidence The exact incidence of capillary telangiectasias is unknown because they are usually asymptomatic lesions, detected incidentally by imaging, and cannot be definitively differentiated from cavernous angiomas by imaging. They may, in fact, be found in association with cavernous angiomas. Although they may occur in association with Osler-Weber-Rendu syndrome, they usually do not.

Age and Gender

- Capillary telangiectasias are usually discovered incidentally at autopsy or on imaging in middle-aged and elderly patients.
- There is no sexual predilection.

Location

- Capillary telangiectasias show a propensity for the pons but may occur elsewhere in the brain and spinal cord.
- Lesions may be multiple.

Pathology Capillary telangiectasias are usually small lesions of several centimeters in diameter or less. They are composed of a collection of dilated capillary spaces with interspersed normal brain tissue. There may be gliosis and hemorrhage surrounding the lesion, but a clinically manifest hemorrhagic event is unusual. If there is a history of hemorrhage, the possibility of an associated cavernous angioma or arteriovenous malformation should be considered.

Imaging ***Plain Films*** Plain films have no role in the evaluation of capillary telangiectasias.

Angiography Capillary telangiectasias are usually occult on cerebral arteriograms. They may have a faint blush or stain, which is more likely to be seen if a prolonged injection is performed. This author does not recommend prolonged contrast injections in the brain. Patients with Osler-Weber-Rendu disease may have capillary telangiectasis of the brain, but if they have a vascular malformation of the brain, they are more likely to have an AVM than a capillary telangiectasia.

Computed Tomography A faint blush may be seen on contrast-enhanced scans, but the lesions are usually occult.

Magnetic Resonance Imaging

- These lesions usually show contrast enhancement on T1-weighted images and are manifest as a small nodular area of bright signal in the pons after contrast administration.
- They may be isointense on T1- and T2-weighted images.
- They seldom bleed and therefore usually do not have blood products associated with them. They can be associated with other vascular malformations; if they have a bleed, they may be indistinguishable from a cavernous angioma.
- The bottom line is that these are usually asymptomatic incidental findings.

VENOUS ANGIOMAS

Incidence

- Venous angiomas are probably developmental venous anomalies rather than true vascular malformations.
- They are the commonest vascular malformation of the brain at autopsy and have been reported to occur in as many as 26 percent of the population. They are usually solitary.

Age and Gender

- Venous angiomas are usually an incidental finding on a CT or MRI.
- They may present at any age but are usually asymptomatic.
- There is no sexual predilection.

Location

- The typical location of these lesions is in the deep white matter of the cerebrum and cerebellum.
- The most common location is adjacent to the frontal horn of the lateral ventricle.

Pathology Venous angiomas are composed of an aggregate of radially oriented dilated medullary veins that drain into an enlarged transcortical vein, which, in turn, connects to a deep vein, cortical vein, or dural sinus. Although hemorrhage is reported with these lesions, it is uncommon, and the presence of hemorrhage raises the suspicion of an associated cavernous angioma (Fig. 18-4*B*). Venous angioma in the cerebellum may bleed more often than cerebral lesions. Normal brain surrounds the angioma and is interspersed between the dilated medullary veins. Since these are more likely vascular anomalies than malformations, they may be the only venous drainage for the adjacent normal brain; therefore it would seldom be appropriate to remove them.

Imaging ***Plain Films*** Plain films have no role in evaluating venous angiomas.

Cerebral Angiography

- Venous angiomas have a characteristic angiographic appearance. The dilated medullary veins and single draining vein create a "medusa head," "star on a stick," or "spoke wheel" appearance (Fig. 18-4*D*).
- Arteries are normal, neither enlarged nor increased in number. There should be no shunting or early appearance of the malformation, which should appear and persist in the venous phase only.

- Early venous filling has been reported but is atypical.

Computed Tomography

- On nonenhanced scans, venous angiomas are usually occult.
- After contrast enhancement, the radial tangle of converging medullary veins will be displayed as an aggregate of linear or punctate dense structures, depending upon their orientation within the CT slice.
- The draining vein likewise will be tubular, ovoid, or round, depending upon its orientation. It will drain into a cortical vein, subependymal vein, or dural sinus.
- There is no mass effect or edema and rarely any hemorrhage.

Magnetic Resonance Imaging

- Magnetic resonance imaging shows the same morphologic appearance—"medusa head" lesion—as seen on a CT scan.
- Flow within the draining transcerebral vein is usually fast enough to have a flow void on non-contrast-enhanced sequences but may be slow enough for flow-related enhancement.
- After contrast administration, the draining vein and tributaries are usually enhanced (Fig. 18-4*C*).

☐ QUESTIONS (TRUE OR FALSE)

1. What is the single best technique to detect cavernous angiomas?
   - **a.** Angiography
   - **b.** Radionuclide imaging
   - **c.** MRI with gradient-echo technique
   - **d.** MRI with spin-echo technique
   - **e.** Contrast-enhanced CT

2. Capillary telangiectasias are
   - **a.** Easily differentiated from cavernous angiomas
   - **b.** A significant cause of brainstem hemorrhage
   - **c.** Best demonstrated by angiography
   - **d.** Usually an incidental finding
   - **e.** Notable for their mass effect

3. Venous angiomas are
   - **a.** Usually multiple
   - **b.** Best removed surgically
   - **c.** Associated with AV shunting by arteriography
   - **d.** Often a cause of hemorrhage
   - **e.** None of the above

4. Dural AV fistulas may
   - **a.** Be difficult to appreciate on MRI and CT scans
   - **b.** Be best imaged by angiography
   - **c.** Cause symptoms related to intracranial venous hypertension
   - **d.** Be a response to a thrombosed dural sinus
   - **e.** All of the above

5. Arteriovenous malformations
   - **a.** Have a nidus
   - **b.** Typically have enlarged feeding arteries and draining veins with AV shunting
   - **c.** May have associated aneurysms
   - **d.** May hemorrhage
   - **e.** All of the above

6. Occult malformations
   - **a.** Are "occult" to angiography
   - **b.** Are best imaged by MRI
   - **c.** May be a cause of hemorrhage
   - **d.** Include cavernous angiomas, capillary telangiectasias, and thrombosed AVMs
   - **e.** All of the above

7. Symptoms from vascular malformations
   - **a.** May be due to hemorrhage
   - **b.** May be due to vascular "steal" or shunting of blood away from normal brain
   - **c.** May be due to intracranial venous hypertension
   - **d.** Are least likely to be due to mass effect
   - **e.** All of the above

☐ ANSWERS

1. **a.** F
   b. F
   c. T
   d. F
   e. F

2. **a.** F
   b. F
   c. F
   d. T
   e. F

3. **a.** F
   b. F
   c. F
   d. F
   e. T

4. **a.** T
   b. T
   c. T
   d. T
   e. T

5. **a.** T
b. T
c. T
d. T
e. T

6. **a.** T
b. T
c. T
d. T
e. T

7. **a.** T
b. T
c. T
d. T
e. T

SUGGESTED READINGS

1. Atlas SW: Intracranial vascular malformations and aneurysms, in *Magnetic Resonance Imaging of the Brain and Spine.* New York, Raven Press, 1991.
2. Barkovich AJ: Anomalies of cerebral vasculature, in *Pediatric Neuroimaging*, 2d ed. New York, Raven Press, 1995.
3. Berenstein A, Lasjaunias P: *Surgical Neuroangiography*, vol 4. Berlin, Springer-Verlag, 1992.
4. Grossman RI, Yousem DM: Vascular diseases of the brain, in *Neuroradiology: The Requisites.* St. Louis, Mosby, 1994.
5. Osborn AG. Intracranial vascular malformations, in *Diagnostic Neuroradiology.* St. Louis, Mosby, 1994.

CHAPTER

19

Cerebral Infarction and Ischemic Disease

Ay-Ming Wang
Tereasa M. Simonson
William T. C. Yuh

☐ PATHOLOGY

The terms *cerebral infarct*, *cerebral softening*, and *encephalomalacia* are used to denote an area of brain tissue necrosis localized to a particular arterial territory and secondary to occlusion of the feeding arterial tree. Arterial occlusion of sufficient duration can produce ischemic cerebral necrosis, in which the pathologic features undergo a series of identical sequential changes regardless of the distribution of the affected arterial territory. Two main types of infarctions are generally recognized: anemic infarcts, in which the lesions of ischemic necrosis remain relatively unaltered, and hemorrhagic infarcts, which tend to involve the cortical ribbon and the basal ganglia selectively. Obstruction of an artery by thrombus or embolus is the usual cause of ischemia, but failure of the circulation and hypotension from cardiac decompensation or shock can also produce infarction if severe and sufficiently prolonged. More than any other organ, the brain depends from minute to minute on an adequate supply of oxygenated blood. Unconsciousness occurs within 10 seconds of the beginning of asystole in the patient with a complete atrioventricular block, if the patient is upright. In animal experiments, the complete cessation of blood flow for longer than 3 min produces irreversible brain damage.

GENERAL PATHOLOGIC FEATURES

Anemic Infarction *Initial Phase (First 48 H)* During the first 6 h, no visible alteration is observed, although the neural tissue is already irreversibly damaged. From 8 to 48 h, the damaged zone becomes pale and the demarcation between the white and gray matter becomes indistinct. Edematous swelling is apparent and a certain degree of vascular congestion, which is more marked in the cortex, can be seen. Microscopically, 6 h after the event, the neurons within the infarcted vascular territory demonstrate of ischemic changes such as retraction of the cell body, cytoplasmic eosinophilia, disappearance of Nissl bodies, pyknosis, and nuclear hyperchromasia. The glial cells also undergo comparable changes. The capillary blood vessels show endothelial swelling accompanied by exudation of edematous fluid and extravasation of red blood cells. Between 24 and 48 h there is evidence of phagocytic activity with an exudation of neutrophil leukocytes.

From 3 to 10 Days The phagocytic process increases while the edematous reaction remains. The softened tissue becomes more friable and the boundaries of the infarcted territory become better defined.

After 10 Days Liquefaction begins, and after the third week, the cavitation becomes more evident. The area of necrosis is then replaced by yellowish gray tissue causing depression of the cortical surface.

After a Few Months A cystic cavity is organized in the softened area. This cavity has ragged outlines, is intersected by vascular connective tissue strands, and is covered on its outer border by a thin meningeal membrane that is visible on the cortical surface. During the phase of cicatrization, the residual cystic cavity becomes surrounded by a glial proliferation that is at first protoplasmic, then fibrillary, while a few foamy compound granular corpuscles remain along the numerous vascular connective tissue strands that run across the cavity.

Hemorrhagic Infarction Hemorrhagic infarction has frankly hemorrhagic features consisting of petechial zones that are sometimes confluent and are situated in the cortex. These hemorrhagic areas may involve the entire zone of infarction but tend most often to predominate along boundary zones supplied by meningeal arterial anastomoses or, in the case of middle cerebral infarcts, in the basal ganglia. The anemic infarction may have microscopic hemorrhagic extravasations, but it is regarded as distinct from hemorrhagic infarction.

PATHOPHYSIOLOGY AND ETIOLOGY

Hemodynamic Factors *Anastomotic Collateral Pathways* In the course of arterial occlusion, the degree of ischemic infarction is related to the anastomotic collateral circulation by arteries at the base of the brain (circle of Willis, ophthalmic artery) and by superficial corticomeningeal anastomoses. When cerebral arterial occlusion occurs, if there is an effective and adequate anastomotic substitution network of blood supply, no infarction will be seen. However, if there is no anatomically effective anastomotic blood supply network, massive infarction of the corresponding cerebral territory can be seen. The anastomotic arrangement of the vascular tree varies from case to case, a fact that is related to the variable anastomotic collateral circulation.

Site of Occlusion Proximal occlusion of a large vessel such as the internal carotid artery may produce an infarct limited to the distal arterial territory or the junction of two vascular territories (watershed or boundary zone infarct), because collateral circulation is in general adequate in the proximal arterial territory, in this case from the posterior communicating and ophthalmic arteries. However, if there is an insufficient collateral network due to anatomically absent or occluded collaterals as a result of thrombus extension, the infarct will be massive and involve the entire arterial territory. In distal arterial occlusion—i.e., involving an end-artery such as the middle cerebral artery—the only possibility of collateral circulation will depend on the presence of a superficial pial anastomotic network that is often precarious. As a result, the infarct proximal to this superficial anastomotic network will usually be extensive.

Type of Occlusion In general, thrombosis leading to gradual arterial occlusion will permit the adaptation of an anastomotic substitution network of blood supply. The resulting infarct is then usually pale and of relatively limited extent. By contrast, emboli produce complete and sudden occlusion, and if collateral circulation is inadequate, they result in extensive infarct. In addition, the frequency of cortical hemorrhages in the marginal territories is due to reperfusion through blood vessels that were initially damaged by sudden ischemia. Migration or secondary fragmentation of the embolus is the cause of hemorrhages observed in the proximal part of the ischemic territory in the course of sudden reentry of arterial blood pressure (reperfusion injury).

Etiologic Factors *Atherosclerosis* Atherosclerosis is the chief etiologic factor in the production of cerebral infarction. In the brain, atherosclerosis affects mainly large blood vessels, carotid arteries in their cervical course, and the basilar artery. It predominates at sites of bifurcation, at sites of arterial curvature, and where the arteries are fixed. The internal carotid and basilar arteries are the most heavily involved, both at their origins and at their terminations. The arteries of the convexity are less severely and less often affected than the vessels of the base. A gradual increase in plaque size and local changes—intraluminal hemorrhage, calcification, and mural thrombosis—lead to increasing arterial stenosis. It is generally believed that arterial stenosis involving at least 75 percent of the original lumen of the artery is necessary to cause a significant decrease in blood flow. The course of the arterial stenosis produced by arteriosclerosis is variable. Mural thrombosis can fragment and give rise to arterial emboli. Thrombosis may cause the complete occlusion of the arterial lumen and, as a result, a new event, stagnation thrombus, may develop in the first sizable collateral branch.

Cardiac Emboli Cardiac emboli are a frequent cause of complete cerebral arterial occlusion, whether they originate from an atrial thrombus in mitral stenosis or atrial fibrillation, from a mural thrombus in the course of myocardial infarction or endocarditis, or from a cardiac prosthesis.

Other Causes Arteritis is a rare cause of cerebral infarction. Collagen diseases, especially polyarteritis nodosa, may affect several small superficial arterioles and the deep intracerebral small vessels, causing small-vessel infarct. In children, otitis media and rhinopharyngitis can occasionally result in internal carotid artery occlusion, causing cerebral infarction. Herpes zoster occasionally causes infarction of the basal ganglia. Traumatic neck injury can cause carotid or vertebral artery dissection, resulting in brain infarction. Intravascular thrombosis from vascular malformation can also cause cerebral infarction. Vascular spasm due to subarachnoid hemorrhage, head trauma, or migraine can cause cerebral infarction. Embolism from coagulopathy, fat, or air is a rare cause of infarction. Basal arterial vascular occlusive disease and fibromuscular dysplasia are also rare causes of cerebral infarction.

Cerebral infarction can be caused by hypoperfusion due to intracranial hypertension from closed head injury or pseudotumor cerebri; decreased cardiac output from myocardial infarction, arrhythmias, tamponade, cardiac surgery, and congestive heart failure; and shock and decreased circulatory volume. Hypoperfusion usually results in watershed infarction. Hypoxia/anoxia (such as carbon monoxide poisoning) has a predilection for infarction of the basal ganglia.

Venous sinus occlusive disease can cause venous infarcts. Venous thrombosis or stenosis usually causes interstitial brain edema and may result in cerebral hemorrhage.

Other Cerebrovascular Lesions of Ischemic Nature Cerebral infarcts due to atherosclerosis or emboli account for the most frequent manifestations of ischemic cerebrovascular pathology. However, other pathophysiologic mechanisms may cause cerebrovascular lesions.

LACUNAE These are small lesions consisting of foci of cerebral necrosis with irregular borders. They eventually form cystic cavities that are surrounded by a zone of reactive gliosis. They are most often pale but are sometimes orange-yellow because of the presence of old hemorrhages. Their size usually ranges from 2 to 10 mm, rarely exceeding 15 mm. The lenticular nuclei, pons, thalamus, internal capsule, and caudate nuclei are the most frequent sites in decreasing order of frequency. Lacunae are usually multiple and are characteristically found in older populations suffering from long-standing hypertension. They are the result of thrombotic occlusion of small intraparenchymal arterioles in which the walls have developed hyalinosis and sclerosis due to elevated blood pressure.

GRANULAR ATROPHY OF THE CEREBRAL CORTEX This is seen in certain forms of arteriopathic dementia and is characterized by the presence of small punched-out foci of cavitated cicatricial softening, situated entirely in the cortex and accompanied by focal glial scars and zones of cortical ribbon thinning. The lesions are bilateral and are often distributed along the crests of the gyri, at the junction of the middle and anterior cerebral artery territories, and at the junction of the middle and posterior cerebral artery territories. These watershed lesions are indicative of previous total circulatory ischemia related either to bilateral internal carotid artery thrombosis or to cardiac insufficiency. Thromboangiitis obliterans and hypertension have been reported to narrow small cortical arteries, also causing granular atrophy in rare cases.

BINSWANGER'S SUBCORTICAL ENCEPHALOPATHY This is characterized by diffuse lesions in the cerebral white matter and is seen in certain forms of arteriopathic dementia. The changes consist of diffuse demyelination of the white matter, which spares the U fibers and affects mainly the parietooccipital regions. In addition to the demyelinating process, numerous juxtaposed microscopic foci of lacunar disintegration associated with astrocytic gliosis are seen. This form of subacute leukoencephalopathy of atherosclerotic origin is apparently due to selective involvement of the deep arterial branches that supply the cerebral white matter.

☐ CLINICAL FINDINGS

Stroke is the third leading cause of death in the United States, following myocardial infarction and cancer, and is the leading cause of disability. There are 500,000 new strokes each year; 85 percent of these are ischemic and 15 percent are hemorrhagic. At the present time, the economic costs of stroke in terms of health care expenditures and lost productivity are estimated at approximately $15 billion per year in the United States. Thus, stroke appears to be the third most costly disease affecting adults.

Stroke presents clinically as a sudden loss of cerebral function usually manifest by hemiparesis and/or aphasia. There are five clinical classifications for cerebral ischemia (Table 19-1).

The original definition of a transient ischemic attack (TIA) was a period of neurologic deficit of less than 20 min without apparent permanent neurologic deficit. This definition has been changed to an ischemic event with temporary loss of focal neurologic function lasting for less than 24 h without apparent permanent neurologic deficit. On the basis of this definition, most TIAs are believed to represent small strokes.

The acronym RIND (reversible ischemic neurologic deficit) was introduced to cover an individual with neurologic deficits lasting more than 24 h but less than 3 weeks. It is an unnecessary term and is not commonly used. The term *stroke in evolution* is used to describe a changing neurologic state as compared to disease onset. The evolution and resolution of neurologic deficits resulting from strokes generally take months to complete.

INCIDENCE

The incidence of stroke in men is approximately 30 percent higher than it is in women, but the incidence increases sharply with age regardless of sex. In patients over age 55, the incidence of stroke doubles for each decade of life, remaining higher in men than in women up to the ninth decade, when the pattern is reversed.

RISK FACTORS

There are many risk factors for thromboembolic stroke (Table 19-2). Hypertension is probably the most important risk factor for stroke and diabetes mellitus is the second. The association of hypertension and diabetes mellitus is particularly pernicious.

Table 19-1
CLINICAL CLASSIFICATION OF CEREBRAL ISCHEMIA

Subclinical ischemia and infarction without symptoms
Transient ischemic attack (TIA)
Reversible ischemic neurologic deficit (RIND)
Stroke in evolution (progression)
Complete stroke

Table 19-2
RISK FACTORS FOR THROMBOEMBOLIC STROKE

Hypertension
Older age (>65 years)
Diabetes mellitus
Other metabolic abnormalities
  Hypothyroidism
  Hyperlipidemia
  Hyperuricemia
Obesity
Smoking
Alcohol abuse
Heart disease
Hypercoagulable state
  Primary
    Protein C deficiency
    Protein S deficiency
    Antithrombin III deficiency
  Secondary
    Antiphospholipid-positive arteritis
    Lupus anticoagulant use
    Homocystinuria
Platelet hyperaggregability

CLINICAL FEATURES

The symptoms and signs of stroke have traditionally been described in terms of the involved cerebral artery. Stroke occurs in the internal carotid artery/middle cerebral artery territory approximately two times more often than in the vertebrobasilar artery territory. Embolic strokes characteristically have an acute onset of neurologic deficit that reaches its peak almost at once. Thrombotic strokes may have the same abrupt onset, but many are comparatively slower and evolve over a period of several minutes, hours, or days, in a series of steps rather than smoothly.

Internal Carotid Artery Transient monocular blindness (amaurosis fugax) occurs as an intermittent symptom before the onset of stroke in approximately 25 percent of cases of symptomatic carotid occlusion. The clinical manifestations of internal carotid artery occlusion are variable. Occlusion is frequently silent, owing to the efficacy of the collateral circulation; however, in other instances it may cause a massive infarction involving the anterior two-thirds or all of the cerebral hemisphere, including the basal ganglia, and can lead to death in a few days. Most often the infarct involves all or some part of the middle cerebral artery territory; but when the anterior communicating artery is very small, the ipsilateral anterior cerebral artery territory is affected as well. If the two anterior cerebral arteries arise from a common origin on one side, infarction may involve the territories of both. When the posterior cerebral artery receives its main blood supply from the internal carotid artery instead of the basilar artery, its territory is included in the infarction. Not infrequently, the territory of the anterior choroidal artery is also affected.

Symptomatic occlusion of the internal carotid artery usually produces a picture resembling that of middle cerebral artery occlusion: contralateral hemiplegia, hemihypesthesia, and aphasia (with involvement of the dominant hemisphere). When the anterior cerebral artery territory is occluded, there will be the additional symptoms of stupor or semicoma. If one internal carotid artery has been occluded previously, occlusion of the other may cause bilateral cerebral infarction. The clinical effect in this case will include coma with quadriplegia and continuous horizontal metronomic conjugate eye movements. Other signs of carotid artery occlusion include pulseless arms, faintness on arising from the horizontal position or recurrent loss of consciousness when walking, headache and neck pain, unilateral or bilateral transient blindness or dimness of vision with exercise, premature cataracts, retinal atrophy and pigmentation, atrophy of the iris, leukomas, peripapillary arteriovenous anastomoses in the retinas, optic atrophy, claudication of jaw muscles, perforation of the nasal septum, saddle nose deformity, facial atrophy (unilateral or bilateral), indolent infections of the face, abnormal facial pigmentation, and loss of hair.

Middle Cerebral Artery Strokes in the middle cerebral artery territory are the most common. The middle cerebral artery supplies the lateral part of the cerebral hemisphere through its cortical branches. The areas of the frontal lobe include area 4, the contraversive centers for lateral gaze, and the motor speech area (of Broca) in the dominant hemisphere. The areas of the parietal lobe include the sensory cortex (area 5) and the angular and supramarginal gyri. The areas of the temporal lobe include most of the lateral surface of the temporal lobe and the insula. The penetrating branches of the middle cerebral artery supply the putamen, part of the head and body of the caudate nucleus, outer globus pallidus, posterior limb of the internal capsule, and corona radiata. The middle cerebral artery may be occluded in its stem, blocking the flow in the deep penetrating cortical branches as well as the superficial ones, or its major branches may be occluded individually.

Most internal carotid artery occlusions are thrombotic, whereas most middle cerebral artery occlusions are embolic. The classic clinical picture of total occlusion of the middle cerebral artery consists of contralateral hemiplegia, hemianesthesia, and homonymous hemianopia. In addition, there is aphasia with left hemispheric stroke and amorphosynthesis with right hemispheric stroke.

Anterior Cerebral Artery Through its cortical branches, the anterior cerebral artery supplies the anterior three-fourths of the medial surface of the cerebral hemisphere, including the medial-orbital surface of the frontal lobe, frontal pole, a strip of the lateral surface of the cerebral hemisphere along the superior border, and the anterior four-fifths of the corpus callosum. The deep branches of anterior cerebral artery, which arise near the circle of Willis, run chiefly to the anterior limb of the caudate nucleus.

The clinical picture of stroke in the territory of the anterior cerebral artery depends on the location and size of the infarct. Occlusion of the stem of the anterior cerebral artery proximal to its connection with the anterior communicating artery is usually well tolerated because adequate collateral circulation is provided from the opposite side. Maximal disturbance occurs when both anterior cerebral arteries arise from the occluded stem; in this case, the medial parts of both cerebral hemispheres will be infarcted. This results in paraplegia, incontinence, and abulic and aphasic symptoms. Complete infarction due to occlusion of one anterior cerebral artery distal to the anterior communicating artery is rare (0.6 percent of all infarcts) and results in sensorimotor deficits of the opposite foot and leg and a lesser degree of paresis of the arm, with sparing of the face.

Anterior Choroidal Artery The anterior choroidal artery usually arises from the distal internal carotid artery above the origin of the posterior communicating artery. It typically supplies part of the posterior limb and genu of the internal capsule, medial globus pallidus, optic tract, temporal lobe uncus, amygdaloid nucleus, and choroid plexus of the lateral ventricle. Isolated spontaneous occlusion of the anterior choroidal artery is extremely rare. The anterior choroidal artery occlusion syndrome consists of contralateral hemiplegia, hemihypesthesia, and homonymous hemianopia.

Vertebrobasilar Arteries ***Posterior Cerebral Artery*** In approximately 70 percent of the normal population, both posterior cerebral arteries arise from the basilar artery, and only thin posterior communicating arteries join this system to the internal carotid arteries. In 20 to 25 percent of cases, one posterior cerebral artery arises from the basilar artery and the other from the internal carotid artery. In the remainder, both posterior cerebral arteries arise from the internal carotid arteries. In the most common situation, the posterior cerebral artery supplies the posterior one-third of the convexity and most of the inferior temporal lobe. It also supplies the occipital lobe and posterior limb of the internal capsule. Infarcts of the hemispheric posterior cerebral artery are second in frequency to infarcts of the middle cerebral artery. Three categories of syndromes related to occlusion of the posterior cerebral artery are commonly observed: anterior and proximal syndromes (involving interpeduncular and perforating thalamic branches), cortical syndromes (inferior temporal and medial occipital), and bilateral cortical syndrome.

Anterior and proximal syndromes include the following:

Thalamic syndromes are manifest by severe sensory loss, both deep and cutaneous, of the opposite side of the body, accompanied by a transitory hemiparesis related to occlusion of the thalamogeniculate branches.

Central midbrain syndromes are manifest by oculomotor palsy with contralateral hemiplegia, paralysis of vertical gaze, stupor or coma, and movement disorders, most often ataxic tremor due to occlusion of paramedian branches on one or both sides.

Anteromedial-inferior thalamic syndrome cause deep sensory loss and hemiataxia or tremor due to occlusion of the thalamoperforate branches.

Cortical syndromes are caused by occlusion of hemispheric branches to the temporal and occipital lobes giving rise to a homonymous hemianopia.

The bilateral cortical syndrome may occur as a result of occlusion of the upper basilar artery when the posterior communicating arteries are extremely small. This lesion may result in bilateral homonymous hemianopia, sometimes accompanied by unformed visual hallucinations.

Vertebral Artery The vertebral arteries are the main arteries of the medulla. Each artery supplies the lower three-fourths of the pyramid, medial leminiscus, all or nearly all the retroolivary region (the lateral medullary region), restiform body, and posteroinferior part of the cerebellar hemispheres. The relative size of the vertebral arteries varies markedly; in approximately 10 percent of cases, one vertebral artery is so small that the other is essentially the only artery of supply to the brainstem. If one vertebral artery is extremely small and the other vertebral artery is occluded without collaterals through the circle of Willis, an infarction equivalent to occlusion of the basilar artery or of both vertebral arteries will occur. When there are two good-sized arteries, occlusion on one side may occur without any recognizable signs or symptoms.

If the subclavian artery is blocked proximal to the origin of the vertebral artery, exercise of the arm on that side may draw blood from the vertebrobasilar system into the arm, sometimes resulting in the symptoms of basilar insufficiency called the subclavian steal syndrome.

The posteroinferior cerebellar artery is usually a branch of the vertebral artery, but it can have a common origin with the anteroinferior cerebellar artery from the basilar artery. The posteroinferior cerebellar artery supplies the entire posteroinferior cerebellum, tonsil, and ipsilateral inferior cerebellar vermis. This artery also often supplies the posterolateral medulla. Sometimes a posteroinferior cerebellar artery infarct produces a classic Wallenberg syndrome, although vertebral artery occlusion is a more common cause of this syndrome. The Wallenberg (lateral medullary) syndrome is manifest by the features of ipsilateral Horner's syndrome, ataxia, facial pain, numbness, impaired sensation, dysphagia, hoarseness, diminished gag reflex, diminished taste, nystagmus, diplopia, and oscillopsia as well as hiccups. Contralateral symptoms include numbness and decreased pain and temperature sensation in the trunk and limbs (spinothalamic tract).

Basilar Artery Territory The branches of the basilar artery may be conveniently grouped as follows: (1) paramedian, seven to ten in number, supplying a wedge of the pons on either side of the midline; (2) short circumferentials, five to seven in number, supplying the lateral two-thirds of the pons and the middle and superior cerebellar peduncles; (3) long circumferential, two on each side (superior and anterior inferior cerebellar arteries), running laterally around the pons to reach cerebellar hemispheres; and (4) several paramedian branches at the bifurcation of the basilar artery into the posterior cerebral arteries supplying the medial subthalamic zone. Occlusion of these branches may produce the following syndromes: (1) medial midpontine syndrome—occlusion of the paramedian branch of the midbasilar artery occlusion, (2) lateral midpontine syndrome—occlusion of the short circumferential artery, (3) medial superior pontine syndrome—occlusion of the paramedian branches of the upper basilar artery, and (4) lateral superior pontine syndrome—occlusion of the superior cerebellar artery. When only the distal basilar artery is occluded, symptoms occur due to lesions in the thalami, posterior limb of internal capsule, mesencephalon, pons, and posterior temporal and occipital lobes. Occlusion of the main trunk of the basilar artery results in the locked-in syndrome, a condition characterized by loss of all voluntary except vertical eye movements with maintained consciousness.

STROKES IN CHILDREN

Cerebral infarcts in children are extremely rare. Common causes are congenital heart disease with cerebral thromboembolism (most common), dissection (traumatic, spontaneous), infection, drug abuse, blood dyscrasias, and clotting disorders. Uncommon causes are fibromuscular dysplasia, Marfan's syndrome, collagen vascular disease, moyamoya disease, neurofibromatosis type 1, and vasculitis.

☐ RADIOLOGIC FINDINGS

COMPUTED TOMOGRAPHY

For the evaluation of occlusive cerebrovascular disease, the noncontrast CT scan of the head can delineate the regions or territories supplied by major cerebral arteries and detect intracranial hemorrhage, brain edema, mass effect, hydrocephalus, blood clots in the cerebral vessels, and calcifications. In addition, the contrast-enhanced CT scan of the head can depict the normal and occluded vessels as well as abnormal enhancement of the areas of the injured brain with breakdown of the blood-brain barrier. The key role of CT in the evaluation of occlusive cerebrovascular disease is to exclude the presence of intracranial hemorrhage.

Ischemic Infarction The CT findings of stroke are related to the time between ischemic or symptom onset and scanning. Ischemic infarction can be divided into four stages: hyperacute (to 24 h), acute (24 h to 7 days), subacute (8 to 21 days), and chronic (more than 21 days).

Hyperacute Stage The major roles of CT in this stage are to exclude, first, the presence of hemorrhage (noncontrast CT study) and, second, the disease entities such as brain tumors that could clinically mimic stroke (contrast CT study). With the improved spatial and contrast resolution of today's state-of-the-art CT scanners, the detection of infarcted brain tissue has improved markedly. However, the sensitivity of CT for early detection of ischemic infarction remains limited and only about half of all strokes are visualized within the first 48 h. The detectable noncontrast CT changes associated with hyperacute stroke are as follows: subtle mass effect with effacement of the surface sulci in cerebral cortical infarction and ventricular compression in deep cerebral infarction, loss of distinction between gray and white matter density due to the slightly decreased cerebral gray matter density from the cytotoxic brain edema, and visualization of a hyperdense cerebral artery. The larger the area of cytotoxic brain edema in the infarction, the more likely the ischemic infarction will be seen on a high-quality CT study between 6 and 12 h after the ictus.

The gray matter hypodensity reflects the presence of cytotoxic brain edema, which usually begins immediately after the onset of cerebral hypoperfusion. Cytotoxic brain edema is caused by a redistribution of sodium and water from the extracellular to the intracellular compartment, with minimal change in the overall water content of the brain. It is not associated with changes in the blood-brain barrier and is reversible if perfusion is restored. Because the blood-brain barrier is intact in cytotoxic brain edema, there is usually no pathologic enhancement on the contrast-enhanced CT study in the hyperacute stage of stroke. Visualization of pathologic enhancement requires at least 24 h after the ictus for blood-brain barrier damage to be sufficient to allow leakage of contrast material on the contrast-enhanced CT study.

Increased density in a cerebral artery, most commonly in the horizontal (M1) segment of the middle cerebral artery and also commonly in the basilar artery, can be seen in the superacute stage of stroke on the noncontrast CT study. It represents an intraluminal thrombus or embolus (see Figure 19-1).

The use of intravenously administered iodinated contrast agents in hyperacute or acute stroke is controversial. Some studies claim that contrast-enhanced CT is of

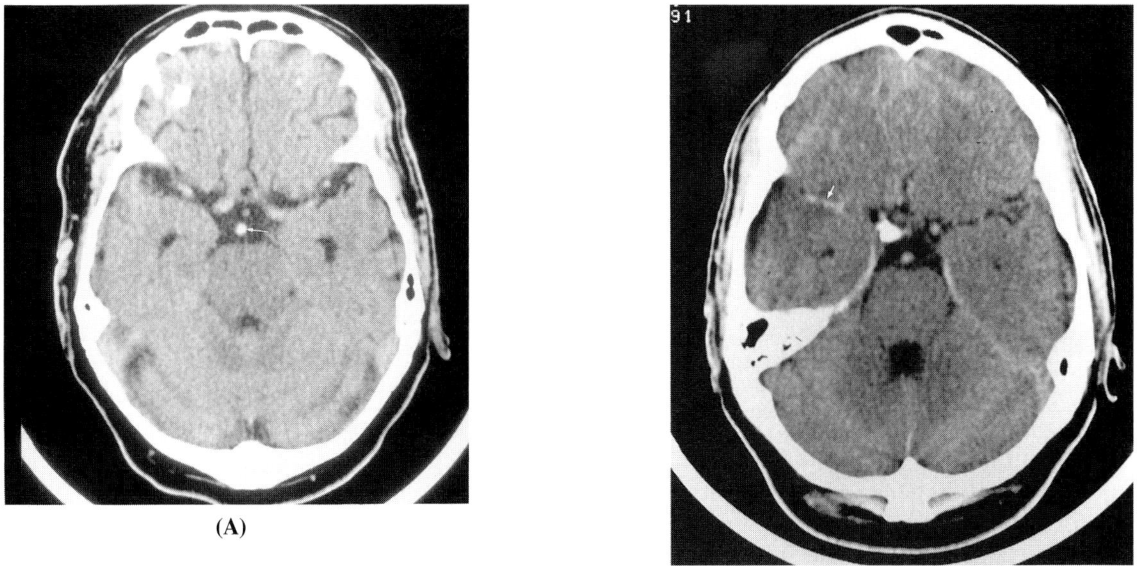

(A)

(B)

Figure 19-1 Noncontrast head CT. The hyperdense cerebral artery sign (thrombus or embolus) seen in hyperacute and acute stages of infarct: (*A*) at the tip of the basilar artery (*white arrow*), (*B*) At the right proximal middle cerebral artery (*white arrow*). Follow-up studies of these cases show infarctions in the arterial distributions.

great value in the diagnosis and characterization of infarcts, whereas other reports suggest that the prognosis is poorer for stroke patients receiving intravenously administered iodinated contrast material because of the neurotoxicity of such agents. Contrast material may cause ischemic but not yet infarcted brain tissue to undergo irreversible damage. It has been concluded that there are few indications for a contrast-enhanced CT in a suspected case acute infarction. If contrast material is given in the hyperacute or acute stages, the CT may show enhancement of the normal cortical gray matter and normal vessels but no enhancement in the zone of infarction or occluded vessels.

Acute Stage During the first week of the stroke, the CT hypodensity involving infarcted cerebral gray and white matter in a vascular distribution gradually becomes more sharply delineated. Cerebrocortical infarcts are typically triangular or wedge-shaped in configuration, and deep cerebral infarcts are usually round or oval. Brain edema and mass effect usually reach their maximum during the third to fifth days.

Subacute Stage On the contrast-enhanced CT study of the head, enhancement within the infarction usually appears during the second week after the ictus. The pattern of enhancement involving the cortex may be gyroform. Ring enhancement is seen in deep gray matter. Homogeneous enhancement can also be seen. The patterns of enhancement are nonspecific and reflect the underlying pathophysiologic mechanism, including disruption of the blood-brain barrier, enhanced capillary filling of the affected gyri (luxury perfusion), reactive hyperemia, and neovascularity.

Brain edema and mass effect decrease during the subacute stage and are usually resolved completely by 2 to 3 weeks. The attenuation values of the infarcted brain increase briefly as the brain edema subsides. Some infarcts show normal density (fogging effect) on noncontrast and contrast-enhanced CT during the subacute stage and then revert to hypodensity. Fogging can occur in all or part of an infarct and represents the phase of phagocytization of necrotic brain after the resolution of edema. Areas affected by fogging may enhance intensely. At this time, ischemic infarcts may develop secondary hemorrhagic transformation, which is often associated with embolic infarcts. Due to the lack of autoregulation in the capillary beds of embolic infarcts, exposure to systemic arterial pressure after fragmentation and lysis of the clot produces hemorrhagic transformation following reestablishment of normal antegrade flow. These reperfusion hemorrhages are usually petechiae and clinically silent. They are difficult to see on the noncontrast CT study but are visualized easily by MRI.

Chronic Stage The areas of infarction are replaced by a well-defined and sharply marginated focal zone of cystic encephalomalacia and gliosis involving both cerebral gray and white matter. On noncontrast CT of the head, the cystic encephalomalacia is isodense to cerebrospinal fluid (CSF), whereas the gliotic rim is slightly hyperdense. Dilatation of the ipsilateral ventricle and sulci and retraction of the midline structure toward the infarcted brain are often seen.

The degree of contrast enhancement begins to decrease at the third week after ictus and is unusual after the second month. A ribbon of preserved cortex may be seen overlying a zone of infarction because the outer layer of cerebral cortex is more resistant to ischemic infarction than the deep structures.

A large chronic infarct affecting the motor cortex or internal capsule can cause atrophy of the ipsilateral cerebral peduncle, pons, and contralateral cerebellum. The mechanism of this atrophy is antegrade degeneration of axons and myelin sheath after injury to the proximal portion of the axon or the cortical neuronal cell body (Wallerian degeneration) as well as functional disuse or crossed cerebellar diaschisis. This appears as crossed cerebellar atrophy, which can be demonstrated on CT but is better seen on MRI. Calcification may also occasionally be seen in the old infarct.

Hemorrhagic Infarction Hemorrhagic infarction occurs within 24 h of the ischemic event, whereas hemorrhagic transformation usually is delayed 7 to 10 days and is due to reperfusion. Hemorrhagic infarction is most common in embolic stroke and in large infarcts. Acute hemorrhagic infarction may appear as small, slightly hyperdense bands within a larger hypodense infarct. These hemorrhages are most commonly seen in the cerebral cortex or at the margin of the infarct, but they can also be seen centrally in the deep cerebral gray matter. The hemorrhages can become confluent, resulting in more striking hyperdensity. Such predominant hyperdensity combined with extension into the cerebral white matter can mimic a nontraumatic primary intracerebral hematoma, which tends to be more homogeneous in density, round or oval in shape, and more sharply defined than the hemorrhagic infarct. Noncontrast CT can define an acute cerebral hemorrhage as a hyperdense lesion, but it cannot differentiate a subacute (isodense) or chronic (hypodense) cerebral hemorrhage from the nonhemorrhagic infarction.

Hemorrhagic transformation may be due to embolic migration and collateral supply distal to the arterial thrombotic occlusion. It appears as petechial hemorrhage and may be underdiagnosed by CT; MRI has been reported to be more sensitive than CT in differentiating the subacute and chronic nonhemorrhagic infarction from the hemorrhagic infarction. Also, MRI can better identify hemorrhagic transformation because it can detect the presence of methemoglobin and hemosiderin by their characteristic signal-intensity changes on T1- and T2-weighted images. Contrast CT may also demonstrate rim enhancement along the hemorrhage margin.

MAGNETIC RESONANCE IMAGING

The typical MRI findings in ischemic disease are summarized in Table 19-3.

Infarction (Complete Ischemia) ***Superacute and Acute Stages*** The MRI findings in acute cerebral ischemia are summarized in Table 19-4.

VASCULAR ABNORMALITIES Absence of the flow-void phenomenon is most obvious in the larger blood vessels, such as internal carotid and basilar arteries. Arterial enhancement is more apparent in smaller distal branches of the cerebral arteries, especially in the tributaries of the middle cerebral artery, due to slow flow (Figure 19-2*A*). The presence of arterial enhancement tends to be more prominent than the absence of the flow-void phenomenon. Both are more sensitive than the dense-artery sign demonstrated on CT. Vascular abnormalities are more frequently seen in patients with cortical infarcts. The early demonstration of arterial enhancement seems to represent slow flow rather than a blood clot and probably indicates inadequacy of collateral flow. Thus, it can reliably predict the severity of the brain tissue ischemia.

MASS EFFECT Mass effect is often seen in acute infarct, but it may be subtle in the first few hours and usually becomes maximal at 24 h. Mass effect is more apparent in cortical infarcts than in subcortical infarcts and is probably related to cytotoxic edema.

PARENCHYMAL SIGNAL CHANGES Vasogenic edema develops after blood-brain barrier breakdown occurs and is associated with the shift of intravascular water and leakage of protein into the interstitium. This results in increased signal intensity on T2-weighted images owing to the macromolecular binding of free water. Signal intensity changes (hyperintensity) on T2-weighted images are not reliably present until 8 h after the onset of symptoms and become maximal at 24 h.

PARENCHYMAL ENHANCEMENT Parenchymal enhancement is usually not seen during the first week in patients with complete stroke. This is probably due to the significant interruption of blood and contrast agent delivery to the ischemic zone.

MENINGEAL ENHANCEMENT This occurs in one-third of the acute cortical infarcts. Peak incidence is within the first 3 days after ictus. It is best seen with large, supratentorial cortical cerebral infarcts. It usually resolves after 1 week. Possible explanations for meningeal enhancement are as follows: reactive hyperemia related to arterial collaterals, venous engorgement, local vasodilation, and irritation of meninges by adjacent infarcted tissue.

Subacute Stage The subacute stage is characterized by the neoproliferation of blood vessels to reestablish flow to the ischemic tissue. There are two types of proliferation: (1) marginal proliferation, which is the reestablishment of blood circulation to the injured brain tissue by the ingrowth of neovascularity at the margins of the ischemic zone, and (2) transmedullary proliferation, which is the reestablishment of blood circulation to the injured brain tissue by the ingrowth of neovascularity at the pial surface from the subarachnoid space.

Table 19-3
TYPICAL MRI FINDINGS IN THREE ISCHEMIC STROKE MODELS

	Vascular						
	Flow Void	AE	Mass Effect (Positive or Negative)	Signal Change[a]	PE	Size of Lesion Demonstrated by Gadolinium and T2-Weighted Image	Comments
Complete ischemia							
Acute (< 7 days)							
Cortical	+	+ +	+ + +	+ + +	−		
Noncortical	−	−	±	+ +	−	$T_2 > Gd$	Usually severe symptoms Usually infarction
Subacute (7 days to 3 months)							
Cortical	±	−	+	+ +	+ + +	$T_2 > Gd$	
Noncortical	−	−	±	+ +	+		AE usually disappears after day 7, whereas PE starts
Chronic (> 3 months)							
Cortical	±	−	+b	+	−		
Noncortical	−	−	+b	+	−	T2 > Gd	Usually infarction
Incomplete ischemia							
Acute	−	−	+	±	+ + +		
Subacute or chronic	−	−	−	±	−	GdσT2	Usually minimal symptoms
Watershed ischemia							
Acute	−	−	+ +	+ +	+ +	GdσT2	Usually severe symptoms with infarction
Subacute or chronic	−	−	+	+ +	−	T2 > Gd	

[a]Changes usually after 8 h.
[b]Negative mass effect.
Abbreviations: AE = arterial enhancement; PE = parenchymal enhancement; Gd = gadolinium.
Source: From Yuh WTC, Crain MR: Magnetic resonance imaging of acute cerebral ischemia. *Neuroimaging Clin North Am* 2:428, 1992, with permission.

VASCULAR ABNORMALITIES Absence of normal flow void in major cerebral vessels persists. Arterial enhancement disappears. The rate of disappearance of arterial enhancement varies with the rate of revascularization. This enhancement will disappear as the faster blood flow is established often by 1 week.

MASS EFFECT Mass effect may be evident during the first 2 weeks. After 1 month, negative mass effect may be seen as a result of parenchymal loss.

PARENCHYMAL SIGNAL CHANGES Abnormal hyperintensity on T2-weighted images persists.

PARENCHYMAL ENHANCEMENT As revascularization occurs and arterial enhancement fades, parenchymal enhancement starts to progress in both intensity and thickness (Figure 19-2*B*).

Chronic Stage VASCULAR ABNORMALITIES Absence of normal flow void in major cerebral vessels persists. Arterial enhancement resolves.

MASS EFFECT Negative mass effect due to brain tissue loss in infarction predominates. Ex vacuo dilatation of ipsilateral ventricular system and CSF sulci is observed.

PARENCHYMAL SIGNAL CHANGES Hyperintensity persists on T2-weighted images and on fluid-attenuated inversion recovery (FLAIR) images.

PARENCHYMAL ENHANCEMENT A progressively thick gyriform parenchymal enhancement occurs in the involved brain tissue from a few weeks to several months after the ictus. It eventually fades and disappears in the chronic stage as an intact blood-brain barrier is reestablished and the reparative process ceases.

Table 19-4
MRI FINDINGS IN ACUTE CEREBRAL ISCHEMIA

Mechanism	MRI Findings	Possible Causes	Estimated Time[a]
Flow kinetics	Absent flow	Slow flow; occlusion	Early
	Arterial enhancement	Accentuation of flow derangement	Early
Biophysiologic	T1 morphologic change	Cytotoxic edema (free water)	2–4 h
	T2 signal change	BBB[b] breakdown; vasogenic edema; macromolecular binding	8 h
	T1 signal change	BBB breakdown; vasogenic edema; macromolecular binding	16–24 h
Combination	Delayed parenchymal enhancement[d]	Impaired delivery of significant contrast agent	$>$24 h[c]
	Early exaggerated enhancement[e]	Intact delivery of contrast agent; BBB leakage; focal hyperemia	2–4 h[e]

[a]Time at which findings generally could first be detected by available MR examinations; this does not necessarily imply the exact time of onset.
[b]BBB = blood-brain barrier.
[c]Usually not detected before 5 to 7 days.
[d]Typical findings in completed cortical infarctions.
[e]Found in cases with transient or partial occlusions and in watershed infarctions.
Source: From Yuh WTC et al: MR imaging of cerebral ischemia: Findings in the first 24 hours. *AJNR* 12:621–629, 1991, with permission.

Incomplete Ischemia (Reversible or Minimal Neurologic Deficits) This condition is related either to a partially intact blood supply or transient interruption of blood supply by an arterial occlusion, embolic phenomenon, or iatrogenic insult with development of sufficient collateral circulation. The distinctive MRI findings are early or intense parenchymal contrast enhancement and limited parenchymal T2-signal abnormalities.

Superacute and Acute Stages VASCULAR ABNORMALITIES Arterial enhancement is absent (in most cases) or it may resolve in 24 to 48 h. Absence of flow void may be seen in large cerebral vessels.

MASS EFFECT Brain swelling producing mass effect can be seen in the first few hours after the ictus and persists up to 24 h but usually improves and disappears in several days.

PARENCHYMAL SIGNAL CHANGES Parenchymal signal changes are absent or minimal on T2-weighted images.

PARENCHYMAL CONTRAST ENHANCEMENT Early (a few hours) or intense parenchymal contrast enhancement on T1-weighted images is seen in the gray and white matter as well as subcortical gray matter in the entire vascular distribution distally. Parenchymal enhancement tends to approximate or exceed the signal T2 abnormalities. This is the key to differentiating complete from incomplete ischemia on MRI.

MENINGEAL ENHANCEMENT Meningeal enhancement may occasionally be seen.

PATIENT PROGNOSIS AND MRI FINDINGS On MRI, arterial enhancement, parenchymal enhancement, and signal abnormalities may have predictive values for stroke outcome. Parenchymal enhancement is inversely related to the presence of arterial enhancement, whereas the extent of parenchymal signal abnormalities is directly related to the presence of arterial enhancement. The presence of early arterial enhancement with associated extensive signal abnormalities suggests severe acute infarct, whereas the presence of early parenchymal enhancement without severe signal abnormalities or arterial enhancement is typical in incomplete ischemia and suggests a less severe insult. An exception is early resolution of arterial enhancement, which may indicate a favorable outcome. Early parenchymal enhancement limited to the watershed zone may indicate a more severe outcome.

Watershed Infarction Ischemic brain tissue injury at the very distal end of the vascular distribution, due to intact but inadequate perfusion between two adjacent major vessels, is called watershed infarction. It is caused by local hypotension owing to systemic hypotension or a proximal vascular stenosis/occlusion with intact but inadequate antegrade or collateral blood flow. No ischemic changes are observed in the vascular territory proximal to the watershed zone.

The following findings have been reported in watershed infarction.

Vascular Abnormalities Arterial enhancement is absent. Flow void is absent in a distal branch vessel feeding one or both adjacent vascular territories.

Mass Effect There is brain swelling in acute stage, then loss of brain parenchyma during the subacute or chronic stage.

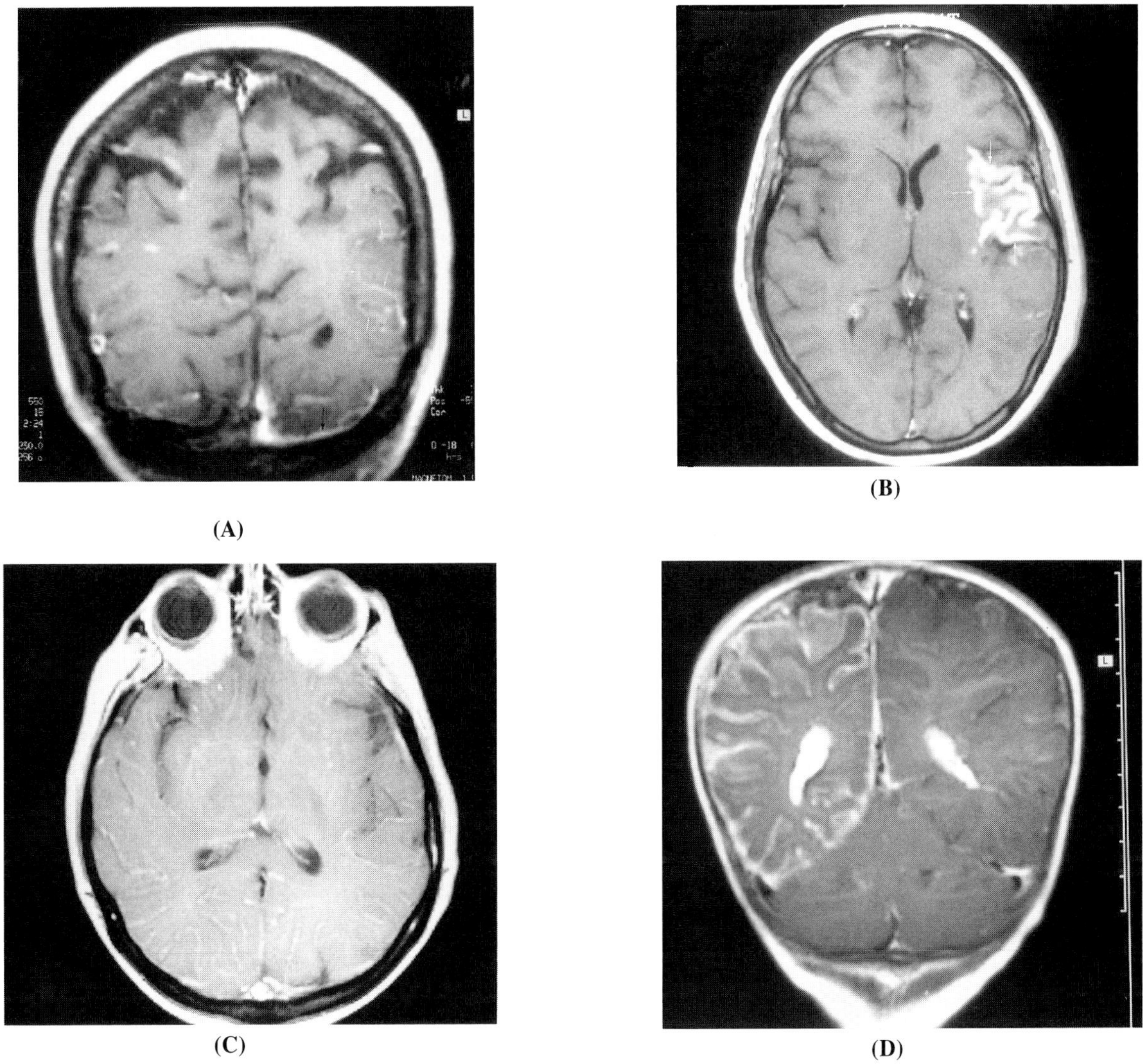

Figure 19-2 Contrast-enhanced T1-weighted MRI. *A*. Intraarterial enhancement in the distal left middle cerebral artery at the left parietal lobe, complete ischemia; dural enhancement (*arrow*) is also seen. *B*. Early gyrus enhancement (*white arrow*), incomplete ischemia of the left insular cortex and left frontoparietal operculum. *C*. Diffuse pial-leptomeningeal enhancement of vasculitis in a patient with Sjögren's syndrome. *D*. Diffuse enhancement of the enlarged cortical veins in the right parietal lobe associated with cortical atrophy in a patient of Sturge-Weber disease.

Parenchymal Signal Changes on T2-Weighted Images Abnormal hyperintensity localized at the watershed zone is maximal at 2 to 3 days and persists into the chronic stages.

Parenchymal Enhancement There is early, intense parenchymal enhancement that approximates the intensity and extent of parenchymal signal changes. It represents the equivalent of incomplete ischemia with early parenchymal enhancement but absence of arterial enhancement on contrast-enhanced T1-weighted images while retaining the typical severe signal parenchymal abnormalities and mass effect of complete infarction on noncontrast MRI.

Hemorrhagic Infarction Hemorrhage almost never occurs as the primary manifestation of arterial occlusion. It occurs as hemorrhagic transformation of initially ischemic lesions. It typically occurs when an occluded vessel recanalizes and ischemic areas are reperfused following embolus fragmentation and lysis. Most hemorrhagic infarction is demonstrated 24 to 48 h following the ischemic event. The incidence of hemorrhagic infarction is higher in patients with embolic as compared with thrombotic arterial occlusion. Hemorrhagic infarction has a predilection for two particular areas, i.e., the basal ganglia and cerebral cortex. The incidence of hemorrhagic infarction demonstrated by MRI is higher than that demonstrated by CT, because subacute and chronic hemorrhage is better appreciated on the MRI study. The MRI findings of intracranial hemorrhage vary according to the age of the hemorrhage, state of oxidation of the hemoglobin, paramagnetic properties, magnetic field strength, and pulse sequence.

Hyperacute Clots Oxyhemoglobin is initially present in hyperacute clots (a few minutes to a few hours). It has ferrous iron with no unpaired electrons and is therefore diamagnetic. It does not affect the T1 or T2 relaxation time. Hyperacute clots appear isointense on T1-weighted and T2-weighted images. Hyperintense edema may surround the hemorrhage on T2-weighted images.

Acute Clots and Deoxyhemoglobin After a few hours of hemorrhage, hemoglobin desaturates from oxyhemoglobin to deoxyhemoglobin. By 24 to 72 h after clot formation begins, most intracerebral hematomas contain deoxygenated intracellular hemoglobin. Deoxyhemoglobin has ferrous iron with four unpaired electrons and is therefore strongly paramagnetic. However, it is shielded from interaction with water molecules by a hydrophobic cleft in the globin protein and therefore does not affect T1 relaxation. However, intracellular deoxyhemoglobin does appear moderately hypointense on proton-density [balanced, long repetition time (TR), short echo time (TE)] images and profoundly hypointense on T2-weighted images as well as on gradient-refocused sequences at high field strength (may be isointense at low field strength).

Subacute Clots and Methemoglobin The early subacute stage of intracerebral hemorrhage begins a few days after the initial ictus. Oxidative denaturation of hemoglobin progresses and deoxyhemoglobin gradually converts to intracellular methemoglobin. It starts from the periphery of the hematoma and then progresses centrally, because the center of the hematoma is extremely hypoxic. Methemoglobin is ferric iron, which has five unpaired electrons and is strongly paramagnetic. In its conversion to methemoglobin, the globin protein undergoes structural changes and the ferric iron is no longer contained in a hydrophobic cleft. It appears hyperintense on T1-weighted images, first in the periphery of the hematoma and then progressing to its center. Because the methemoglobin is contained within intact red blood cells, it appears as hypointense on T2-weighted and gradient-refocused sequences.

In the late subacute stage (around 1 week after the ictus), further hemoglobin oxidation and cell lysis begin at the periphery of the hematoma. Methemoglobin is released in the extracellular space, creating a more homogeneous environment. Surrounding brain edema subsides and mass effect gradually diminishes. It appears hyperintense on both T1- and T2-weighted images.

Chronic Clots and Iron Storage In the early chronic stage, the resolving clot contains a relatively uniform pool of dilute extracellular methemoglobin surrounded by a vascularized wall that contains activated macrophages. It appears homogeneously hyperintense on both T1- and T2-weighted images and has a pronounced low-signal rim on T2-weighted images. The macrophages contain two iron-storage substances: ferritin and hemosiderin. Edema and mass effect disappear.

In adults, macrophages laden with iron storage products remain around the margins of old clots for years. Hemosiderin is ferric iron but water insoluble and does not affect T1-weighted images; therefore it appears isointense. It is very hypointense on T2-weighted and gradient-refocused images. In infants, all of the hemosiderin may be removed.

Wallerian Degeneration Wallerian degeneration is antegrade degeneration of an axon and its myelin sheath after injury to the proximal portion of the axon or the neuronal cell body. It is a common neuropathologic finding in the corticospinal tracts after cerebral infarction. On MRI, findings are related to three stages (time interval after the ictus): (1) In the first 10 weeks, there are usually no signal abnormalities. Occasionally, hypointensity is seen in corticospinal tracts on T2-weighted images due to intact myelin lipid structures while relative water content has diminished. (2) At 10 weeks to 12 months after the ictus, there is increased extracellular water content, producing hypointensity on T1-weighted and hyperintensity on T2-weighted images in the ipsilateral brainstem. Contrast enhancement may be present. Initially, the ipsilateral midbrain may be enlarged slightly. (3) One year after the ictus, Wallerian degeneration is characterized by volume loss and gliosis. On MRI, ipsilateral brainstem atrophy is seen, with or without signal alterations (hypointense on T1-weighted and hyperintense on T2-weighted images). Only during the end stage of Wallerian degeneration will the brain CT be positive, demonstrating ipsilateral midbrain atrophy.

MAGNETIC RESONANCE ANGIOGRAPHY

Flowing blood itself provides an intrinsic contrast for MRI study. There is no need for the intravenous administration of contrast agents. Clinical brain MRI is performed using spin-echo pulse sequences in which flowing blood appears dark (signal-flow void). In gradient refocused echo-pulse sequences and phase contrast imaging, the flowing blood can appear much brighter than stationary tissues and can be used to generate magnetic resonance angiography (MRA). Such angiography generally employs one of two MR techniques: time of flight (TOF) or phase contrast (PC), and then displays the result in multiple projections using a maximum-intensity-projection (MIP) algorithm. Time-of-flight MRA is the most widely used MRA technique and relies on the inflow of fully magnetized blood into the imaging plane. This flow-related enhancement is frequently encountered in flow-compensated gradient-echo MR images obtained perpendicular to the axis of the blood vessel. The TOF information can be obtained as a series of two-dimensional (2D) images or as a three-dimensional (3D) volume data set. The sequential 2D TOF MRA is usually used for the study of carotid bifurcation or venous anatomy, whereas 3D TOF MRA is used for the study of intracranial arterial vessels and/or carotid bifurcation. The TOF MRA technique has the advantage of providing high contrast between vessels and soft tissue. This is due to strong flow-related enhancement, which is maintained even in the setting of relatively slow flow.

However, minor motion by the patient during a 2D TOF MRA scan can cause a severe "stair-step" misregistration artifact. This misregistration artifact may not be apparent in a 3D TOF MRA data acquisition. Because TOF MRA gives T1 weighting to surrounding tissue, extracellular methemoglobin and fat may have hyperintense signal mimicking blood flow. Careful evaluation of the spin-echo images can be helpful to separate flowing blood from these artifacts.

The main disadvantages of using 3D volume TOF MRA is the potential saturation of slowly moving spins in areas far downstream within the volume or distal to severe stenosis. Thin, overlapping, stacked 3D volume TOF MRA and magnetization transfer (reduction of background signal from stationary tissue without affecting the flow enhancement from blood) have been used to improve this limitation. Although the direction of the blood flow cannot be detected by TOF MRA, application of an appropriately positioned saturation pulse can eliminate the observed inflow from one large intracranial vessel such as the internal carotid artery and allows the extent of collateral flow (from the circle of Willis) to the territory of severely stenotic or occluded internal carotid artery to be evaluated.

Usually, the 3D TOF MRA protocol is as follows: a 28- to 60-slice (slice thickness = 0.7–1.0 mm) 3D volume is obtained in the axial plane through the region of interest with a field of view of 16 to 20 cm, TR of 40 ms, TE of 5 to 9 ms, and flip angle of 15 to 20°.

Three-dimensional TOF MRA can reliably identify and confirm distal internal carotid, distal vertebral, and basilar artery occlusion. It works well as an adjunct to brain MRI. Two- or three-dimensional TOF MRA also is very valuable to demonstrate stenosis or occlusion of the carotid bifurcation, and apparent degree of carotid bifurcation stenosis correlates well with digital subtraction angiography (DSA). Although with more severe stenosis (greater than or equal to 70 percent) TOF MRA tends to overestimate stenosis due to complex flow patterns, the degree of error is considered to be acceptable. Time-of-flight MRA is particularly useful in old patients, very sick patients, and children to evaluate large-vessel occlusive disease noninvasively.

Phase-contrast (PC) MRA generates MR vascular images by detecting changes in the phase transverse magnetization as the blood moves along a magnetic field gradient. It therefore relies on alteration in spin phase for image contrast. Three-dimensional PC MRA is obtained with flow encoding and displayed as a maximum intensity projection (MIP) in multiple views. Two-dimensional PC MRA is used for localizer and for flow direction and velocity of intracranial and extracranial vasculature. Cardiac-gated (cine) 2D PC MRA is used to study the aortic arch.

Phase-contrast MRA requires a significantly longer time to acquire the data compared with TOF MRA and this is one of its disadvantages.

ANGIOGRAPHY

Intraarterial contrast cerebral angiography is still the most precise and definitive radiologic study for the evaluation of intracranial and cervicocranial vasculature. It provides high-quality anatomic detail of the intracranial and extracranial blood vessels as well as hemodynamic evaluation of their circulations. However, it is an invasive study and carries a higher complication rate (four times higher) in patients with occlusive vascular disease than in patients with nonischemic brain disease. Most of these neurologic complications are transient, but permanent neurologic deficits occur in 0.15 to 0.6 percent and the mortality rate is 0.1 to 0.5 percent.

With a combination of modern digital equipment and 1024 × 1024 matrix, the resolution of DSA approaches that of a standard cut-film cerebral angiogram. The benefits of lower concentration and amounts of contrast material required for DSA as well as immediate imaging display have made DSA widely accepted for the evaluation of cerebral vascular disease.

Extracranial Cervicocranial Angiography *Atherosclerosis* DETERMINE DEGREE OF CAROTID STENOSIS Cerebral ischemic disease may be caused by either a hemodynamic effect or emboli from atherosclerotic plaques usually located at the extracranial carotid artery bifurcation. Since recent studies from the North American Symptomatic Carotid Endarterectomy Trial (NASCET) and the European Carotid Surgery Trial demonstrated definite benefit from carotid endarterectomy only in symptomatic patients with narrowing of the internal carotid artery lumen diameter greater than 70 percent, accurate determination of maximum stenosis is extremely important. At least two angiographic projections are required to measure the maximum stenosis and to profile the plaque adequately.

Stenosis of the internal carotid artery origin is the most common and can be divided into three categories: complete occlusion, clinically significant stenosis, and hemodynamically insignificant stenosis. Percentage of stenosis is calculated by determining the ratio between the stenosis and normal distal internal carotid artery and multiplying by 100. Sometimes the cervical internal carotid artery stenosis is so severe as to appear occluded on the short image acquisition with rapid contrast injection, but a thin trickle of delayed antegrade flow can be found on the prolonged image acquisition with slow contrast injection. This pseudoocclusion or "string" sign can be treated with carotid endarterectomy, but it can be missed by duplex sonography as well as MRA.

IDENTIFY TANDEM LESIONS Such lesions may be identified in the carotid siphon or intracranial circulation. A tandem lesion is a distal stenosis in patients with high-grade stenosis of the cervical internal carotid artery. The incidence is approximately 2 percent. It is commonly seen in the carotid siphon and is occasionally seen in the horizontal segment of the middle cerebral artery.

EVALUATE EXISTING AND POTENTIAL COLLATERAL CIRCULATION In the evaluation of cerebral infarction and ischemic disease, the demonstration of collateral circulation is very important and helps to predict the clinical outcome. It also helps the surgeon decide whether a shunt across the carotid bifurcation for endarterectomy will be necessary. There are three major collateral circulations: the circle of Willis, extracranial to intracranial, and intracranial pial as well as leptomeningeal collaterals.

1. Circle of Willis (most important collaterals). The following vessels make up the circle of Willis: two internal carotid arteries, horizontal (A1) segments of both anterior cerebral arteries, anterior communicating artery, two posterior communicating arteries (anterior circulation), horizontal (P1) segments of both posterior cerebral arteries, and basilar artery (posterior circulation). The circle of Willis is complete in 20 to 25 percent of the population. Normal variants (incomplete circle of Willis) include hypoplasia of one or both posterior communicating arteries (34 percent), hypoplastic or absent A1 segment, and hypoplastic or absent P1 segment with a fetal origin of the posterior cerebral artery from the internal carotid artery.
2. Extracranial to intracranial collaterals (important). There are potential collaterals to the internal carotid artery via the middle meningeal artery to ethmoidal branches of the ophthalmic artery, artery of the foramen rotundum to the inferolateral trunk of the internal carotid artery, and accessory meningeal artery to the inferolateral trunk. Other collaterals include the occipital artery to the vertebral artery, ascending pharyngeal artery to the vertebral artery, ascending pharyngeal artery to the internal carotid artery, facial artery to the internal carotid artery, posterior auricular artery to the internal carotid artery, and extracranial-intracranial surgical bypass.
3. Intracranial pial or leptomeningeal collaterals may develop, but they are often inadequate to prevent neurologic deficit.

ASSESS FOR POSSIBLE PLAQUE ULCERATION AND INTRAVASCULAR THROMBI Identification of plaque ulcerations is important in lesions without significant stenosis. However, significant inaccuracies in the cerebral angiographic diagnosis of ulceration in the carotid origin have been reported in the literature. Ulcers may not be visualized unless they are imaged tangentially. The valley between two adjacent atheromatous plaques in the arterial wall may mimic an ulcer. These ulcer mimics generally have a broader margin toward the arterial lumen, with a narrow deeper portion toward the arterial wall. True plaque ulcerations generally are larger in their deeper intramural portion and have undercutting margins in relation to the edges of the orifice into the arterial lumen.

Fibromuscular Dysplasia Fibromuscular dysplasia (FMD) predominantly affects middle-aged and older women. It occurs in the mid- and upper cervical segments of the internal carotid artery and may extend into the petrous portion. It may be focal or extend over several centimeters along the vessel. Fibromuscular dysplasia may also occur in the upper cervical segment of the vertebral arteries. Bilateral involvement is present in about 75 percent of cases. It is usually an incidental finding but occasionally may result in severe stenosis, giving rise to ischemic cerebral symptoms. The dissecting aneurysm is another complication. It produces a characteristic "string of beads" appearance in the affected vessel. In most cases, the luminal stenosis is less than 40 percent; however, occasionally, higher-grade stenosis may occur producing significant hemodynamic cerebral ischemia.

Dissecting Aneurysm This condition is usually identified in the mid- and upper cervical segments of the internal carotid arteries or in the infraforaminal segment of the vertebral arteries. It may develop as a result of penetrating or blunt injury to the neck, spontaneously, or from rapid forced or spontaneous vigorous head and neck rotation, flexion, or extension. It may be seen spontaneously in association with fibromuscular disease, cystic medial necrosis, or atherosclerotic disease with subintimal ulceration, or it may be idiopathic. It may be iatrogenic from catheter angiography. It may also occur as a result of chiropractic neck adjustments. It usually represents a dissecting hematoma within the wall of the internal carotid artery or vertebral artery. Dissection may produce a string sign, appearing as a tapered narrowing of the vessel proximally and distally. Occasionally, there is complete occlusion of the involved arterial lumen. In most instances, associated cerebral infarctions are the result of embolization from a site on the dissection to the brain. The emboli usually form at the site of the initial arterial injury that caused the dissection. The intramural clot of the dissection usually resolves completely by 6 to 8 weeks, and follow-up cerebral angiography may demonstrate a normal appearing vessel.

On MRI, spin-echo sequences can identify subintimal hematomas as well as the stenotic or occluded true lumen. An increase in the external diameter of the artery and narrowing of the true lumen can be demonstrated on both MRI and TOF MRA. However, subacute intramural hematomas may be a potential pitfall in the diagnosis of arterial dissection by the TOF MRA technique because the bright methemoglobin and bright flowing blood will both be displayed in the maximum-intensity projection. Dissections are easily identified on spin-echo MRI as a bright ring around the flow void in the axial plane or parallel bright lines on either side of the flow void in the sagittal and coronal planes. Magnectic resonance angiography can assist in showing the extent of dissection. Both MRI and TOF MRA are valuable non-invasive studies for use in the diagnosis and follow-up of carotid or vertebral artery dissection (Figure 19-3).

Takayasu's Arteritis This condition is rare and affects mainly young women. The proximal portions of the brachiocephalic arteries along with other large arteries arising from the aorta distally are predominantly involved. The stenosis may have a smooth luminal contour, and the narrowings are caused by a round-cell infiltration.

Intracranial Cerebral Angiography Intraarterial contrast digital subraction cerebral angiography is often not performed during the hyperacute stage of stroke unless thrombolytic therapy is being entertained or other causes of cerebral infarction besides atherosclerotic vascular disease are being considered. The angiographic findings of acute cerebral infarction are as follows: arterial occlusion (with or without meniscus), slow antegrade flow with delayed arterial emptying, collateral and retrograde filling, bare (nonperfused) areas, vascular blush

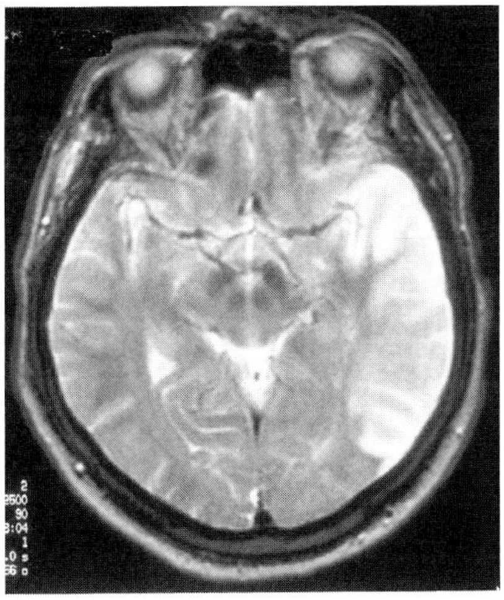

(A)

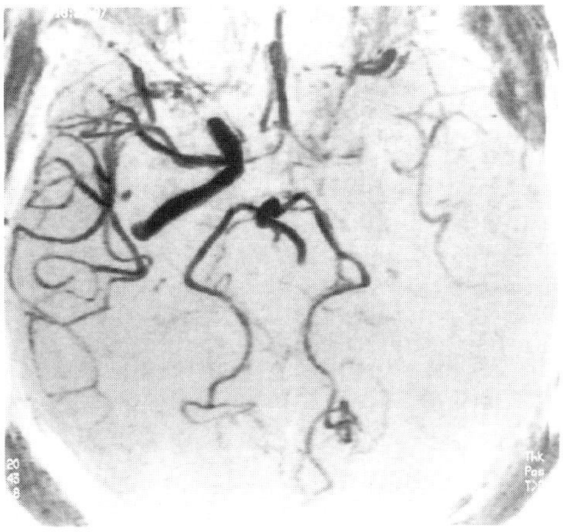

(B)

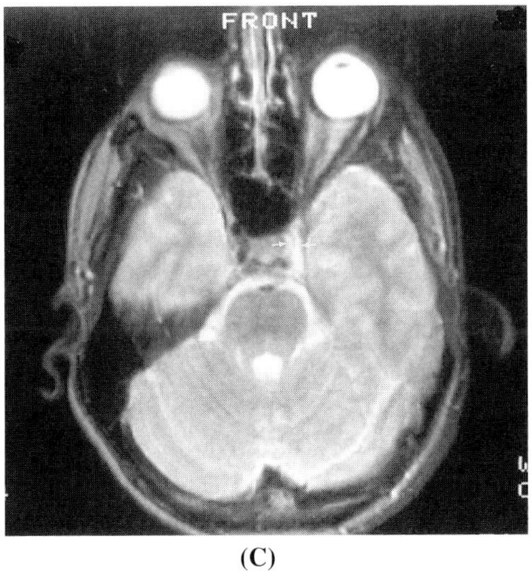

(C)

Figure 19-3 Internal carotid artery dissection. *A*. Axial T2-weighted image through the circle of Willis shows abnormal increased signal intensity in the left frontoparietal operculum and temporal lobe. There is a flow signal void in the major vessels of the circle of Willis. *B*. Three-dimensional time-of-flight MRA shows occlusion of the left internal carotid artery with inadequate collaterals through the circle of Willis and occlusion of the distal branches and decreased flow in the proximal portion of the left middle cerebral artery. *C*. Another patient with complete occlusion of the left internal carotid artery (lack of flow signal void in the cavernous segment of the left internal carotid artery) on T2-weighted image (*white arrow*) but no signal alteration of the parenchyma; adequate collaterals were demonstrated on a three-dimensional time-of-flight MRA (not included).

(luxury perfusion), arteriovenous shunting with early venous drainage, and sometimes variable mass effect. The intracranial occlusive arterial diseases are summarized as follows.

Atherosclerosis In the evaluation of atherosclerotic vascular diseases, adequate intracranial arterial contrast DSA should be included along with extracranial cervicocranial arterial contrast DSA. A very small percentage of patients with significant extracranial carotid bifurcation disease may also have significant incranial arterial stenosis, particularly diabetic and hypertensive patients. The intracranial atherosclerotic vascular diseases usually involve the siphon of the internal carotid artery, middle cerebral artery, and basilar artery.

Embolic Disease Brain emboli arise from atherosclerotic ulcers in the extracranial cervical vessels or from the heart in association with atrial fibrillation, recent myocardial infarction, prolapsed mitral valve, bacterial endocarditis, paradoxical venous emboli through cardiac septal defects and atrial myxoma, as well as from extracranial dissection of the carotid and vertebral arteries. It may occasionally be seen iatrogenically from catheter cerebral arteriography. It is the most frequent cause of infarcts of the middle cerebral artery territory. Larger emboli may persist for 3 to 5 days before fragmentation and lysis, whereas small emboli may lyse within minutes to several hours. An embolic clot rarely becomes fixed and organized, causing a permanent vascular occlusion. Cerebral angiographic findings may be variable depending on when the arteriogram is performed.

Arteritis Primary cerebral arteritis is the disease process principally within the blood vessels, whereas secondary arteritis results from conditions that primarily affect the meninges of the brain such as pyogenic, tuberculous, and fungal meningitis as well as leptomeningeal sarcoidosis. Primary CNS arteritis may be a reflection of a systemic collagen vascular or autoimmune disease or related to a granulomatous arteritis affecting cerebral arteries. Both primary and secondary cerebral arteritis usually involves the large arteries at the base of the brain or smaller arteries over the convexities. Cerebral arteriole involvement can be found in some of the primary arteridites; however, cerebral angiography often fails to demonstrate these abnormalities. Parenchymal changes will be evident on brain MRI studies if the disease is severe enough to be demonstrated by DSA. If the MRI shows no abnormalities, the cerebral angiogram is unlikely to demonstrate signs of vasculitis. Occasionally, postradiation treatment and sickle-cell disease can also produce intracranial occlusive arterial vascular disease. The cerebral angiographic findings are nonspecific and show multiple relatively longer segments of smooth concentric tapered narrowings along the course of the large- and medium-sized cerebral arteries. Arteritis usually involves bilateral cerebral arteries; occasionally, however, it is unilateral, particularly several weeks after a herpes zoster ophthalmicus infection.

Moyamoya Disease Moyamoya disease is a rare progressive cerebrovascular occlusive disease of unknown etiology. It may produce cerebral ischemia (more often in children) and intracranial hemorrhages (more often in adults) which can be demonstrated on CT and MRI studies. *Moyamoya* is a Japanese word meaning "puff of smoke." The name reflects the vascular blush resulting from the dilatation of the penetrating arteries to the basal ganglia and thalamus due to progressive bilateral stenosis or occlusion of the supraclinoid portion of the internal carotid arteries extending to the proximal portions of both interior and middle cerebral arteries. Transdural, leptomeningeal, and parenchymal collateral vessels are necessary to supply the ischemic brain. Although most commonly seen in Japan, it can be found worldwide.

A similar appearance can be seen in patients with sickle-cell occlusive vascular disease as well as in older individuals with slowly progressive atherosclerotic occlusive vascular disease involving these vessels.

Cerebral angiography is needed to confirm the diagnosis. The cerebral angiographic findings are as follows: (1) Bilateral occlusion or stenosis of the supraclinoid portions of the internal carotid artery extending to the proximal portions of the anterior and middle cerebral arteries. (2) Penetrating arteries arising from the distal internal carotid artery, anterior choroidal artery, and posterior communicating artery become markedly dilated, particularly their intraparenchymal small branches. (3) Intraparenchymal anastomoses between the dilated arterioles and capillaries in the territory that would have been supplied by the occluded segments of the proximal portions of the middle and anterior cerebral arteries. (4) Retrograde flow will develop through the penetrating arteries distal to the occluded segment, reestablishing antegrade flow in the distal middle and anterior cerebral arteries.

☐ CEREBRAL VENOUS AND DURAL SINUS OCCLUSIVE DISEASE

A large number of disease processes can cause cerebral venous and/or dural sinus thrombosis, which can be divided into three groups: (1) local disease such as infection, trauma, neoplasm, and arterial infarction as well as subarachnoid hemorrhage; (2) systemic conditions such as pregnancy, puerperium, collagen vascular disease, migratory thrombophlebitis, inflammatory bowel disease, cardiac disease, Behçet's disease, and hematologic disorders; and (3) idiopathic conditions. Direct involvement of a dural sinus, venous stasis, hypercoagulable states, and increased blood viscosity resulting from polycythemia or dehydration are the common causes of cerebral venous and dural sinus thrombosis.

Table 5
COMPARISON OF CT AND MRI IN EVALUATING CEREBRAL INFARCTION

CT LIMITATIONS:	Difficult to detect: Cerebral ischemia without infarct Superacute ischemic infarct Posterior fossa infarct Petechial reperfusion hemorrhage
CT ADVANTAGE:	Superacute hemorrhage
MRI LIMITATIONS:	Superacute hemorrhage

For the patient's safety, MRI should not be performed under the following conditions:	Internal cardiac pacemakers
	Cochlear implants
	Cerebral aneurysm clips
	Certain types of
	  Prosthetic heart valves
	  Neurostimulators
	  Bone-growth stimulators
	  Implantable drug infusion pumps

MRI ADVANTAGES:	Superacute and early acute infarct Absence of bone artifact Multiplanar ability High sensitivity to tissue water changes Direct visualization of cerebral vessels (flow-signal void) (MRA)

The clinical findings are dependent on the location and extent of the thrombosis, rate and degree of propagation into the cerebral veins and dural sinuses, and presence of collateral venous drainage as well as the degree of recanalization. It is a serious, potentially lethal problem that may present a confusing, nonspecific clinical picture. Strokelike symptoms with a slow onset, especially in a clinical setting with known predisposition to venous thrombosis, suggest the diagnosis.

COMPUTED TOMOGRAPHY

The role of CT in the evaluation of cerebral venous and dural sinus thrombosis is to detect complications such as hemorrhage (particularly the white matter), infarctions, brain edema, and hydrocephalus, and to visualize the thrombosed veins. On noncontrast CT of the head, the thrombosed veins and dural sinuses can be visualized directly as foci of significantly increased density ("cord" sign) for the first week after the thrombosis has formed. The positive cord sign has been reported in fewer than 20 percent of cases of cerebral venous/dural sinus thrombosis. Unfortunately, this sign is of limited usefulness because state-of-the-art CT scanners can visualize routinely the intrinsic mild hyperdensity (relative to cerebral gray matter) of unclotted intraluminal blood in the cerebral veins and dural sinuses. On contrast-enhanced CT of the brain, there is enhancement of the surrounding collateral venous channels and normal enhancement of the dura with a hypodense central portion relative to its enhanced peripheral portion producing the "empty delta" sign, which is best seen in patients with superior sagittal sinus thrombosis. The empty delta sign was reported as a pathognomonic sign for superior sagittal sinus thrombosis; however, the incidence of this sign is variable from 25 to 70 percent. Spiral CT angiography with the intravenous administration of contrast material can reliably demonstrate the occluded dural sinus and can be used as a follow-up study for monitoring the progress of treatment.

MAGNETIC RESONANCE IMAGING

In cerebral venous occlusion and dural sinus thrombosis, MRI findings vary with clot age and presence of collaterals (Fig. 19-4*A*, *B*). The findings are as follows:

Detection of Thrombus

Superacute thrombi: Flow-signal void is absent, and the clots appear isointense on T1- and T2-weighted images.

Acute thrombi: Clots appear hyperintense on T1-weighted and hypointense on T2-weighted images.

Subacute thrombi: Clots appear hyperintense on T1- and T2-weighted images.

Chronic thrombi: Normal signal void is absent in the clotted sinus with collateral venous drainage (presence of signal void) around the clotted sinus.

Brain Parenchymal Changes ***No MRI Signal Abnormalities*** Brain swelling with sulcal effacement without signal abnormalities on T2-weighted images may represent

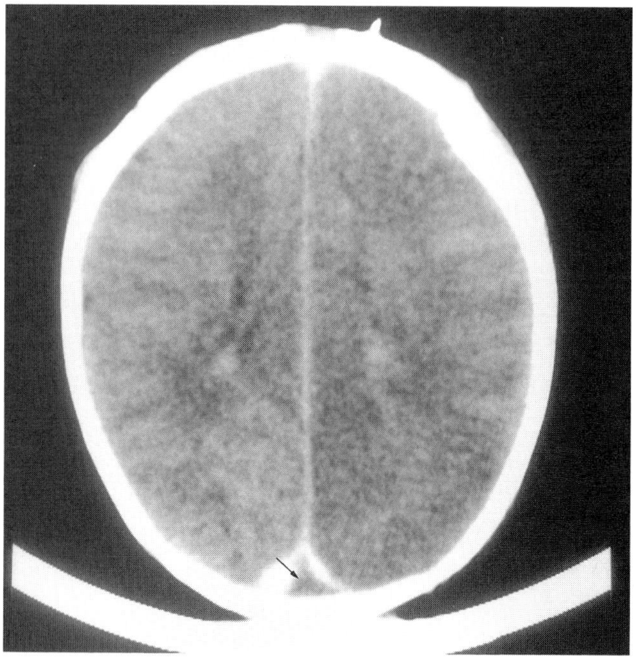

(A)

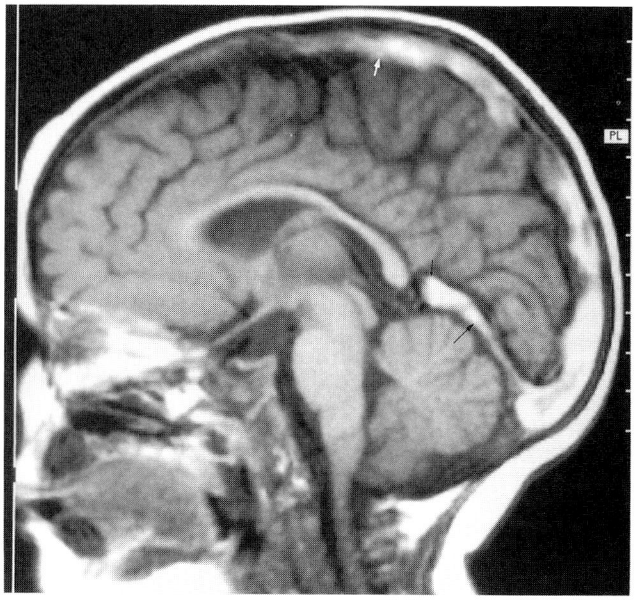

(B)

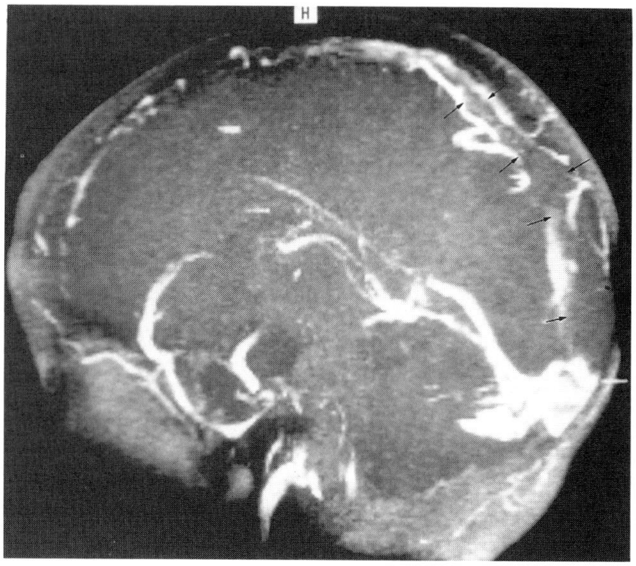

(C)

Figure 19-4 Cerebral venous and dural sinus thrombosis in three different patients. *A*. Head CT with contrast shows thrombosis with presence of a negative delta sign in the superior sagittal sinus (*arrow*) with severe edema of the left parieto-occipital region, which is not in an arterial territory. *B*. T1-weighted midsagittal image shows thrombotic clots in the superior sagittal sinus (*white arrow*) and the straight sinus (*arrow*). *C*. Two-dimensional sequential time-of-flight MRA shows occlusion of the superior sagittal sinus (*arrows*).

the earliest and/or mildest degree of venous occlusion. In this case, the compliant venous bed has dilated without significant elevation of venous pressure. There is no significant increase or shift in interstitial fluid from the vascular bed toward the ventricle and therefore there is no accompanying signal abnormality on T2-weighted images. This distention of the venous bed without associated interstitial edema may result in persistent brain swelling without abnormal signal on T2-weighted images for months or years.

Magnetic Resonance Signal Abnormalities without Hematoma Brain swelling with signal abnormalities on T2-weighted images with interstitial brain edema but no hematoma is the next stage of venous occlusive disease. The abnormal signal on T2-weighted images is usually periventricular, basal ganglia, and thalamic in location, and it is always less extensive than the overall area of mass effect. Bithalamic edema suggests deep venous thrombosis. Hydrocephalus develops due to the combination of the alteration of the fluid exchange between the blood and tissue compartments of the brain with the production of edema and mass effect. This results in compromising the third ventricle as well as obstruction of the foramen of Monro. The increased shift of interstitial bulk fluid from the vascular bed toward the lateral ventricles occurs because of impaired venous drainage, decreased CSF absorption caused by elevated dural sinus pressure, and increased CSF production caused by increased pulsation of the choroid plexus.

Magnetic Resonance Signal Abnormalities with Hematoma The cortical sulcal effacement and abnormal signal on T2-weighted images likely represent reversible venous congestion and pressure-driven interstitial edema and should not be considered as venous infarctions. When patients are treated for the underlying venous-occlusive process by successful thrombolytic treatment or sinojugular venous graft, the sulcal effacement, abnormal signal on T2-weighted images, and hydrocephalus as well as clinical symptoms may rapidly resolve. All of these parenchymal findings suggest that the pathophysiology of cerebral venous and dural sinus occlusive disease is different from that of cerebral arterial occlusive vascular disease. The evolution of MRI brain parenchymal changes through five stages is correlated with dural sinus pressure in Table 19-6.

Contrast Enhancement Patterns on T1-Weighted Images These enhancement patterns include absence of arterial enhancement; negative delta sign presents in the clotted sinus, whereas normal dural sinus enhances homogeneously; absence of abnormal parenchymal enhancement; and presence of cortical vein enhancement as collaterals.

VENOUS MAGNETIC RESONANCE ANGIOGRAPHY

Both 2D sequential TOF or 3D phase-contrast venous MRA are reliable to demonstrate the occluded cerebral veins and clotted dural sinus (Figure 19-4*C*). They are noninvasive studies and are particularly useful in screening cerebral venous and dural sinus thrombosis in children and gravely ill patients and in the planning and follow-up of interventional endovascular thrombolytic treatment for cerebral venous and dural sinus occlusive vascular disease.

CEREBRAL ANGIOGRAPHY AND DURAL SINUS VENOGRAPHY

The venous phase of arterial contrast cerebral angiography is a precise diagnostic study for cerebral venous and dural sinus thrombosis. However, it is an invasive study, and now MRA has been widely used to replace conventional cerebral angiography as a screening study for this disease. A catheter can be placed on the dural sinus to measure dural sinus pressure and deliver a thrombolytic agent (urokinase) to the blood clot with great success.

□ NEW DEVELOPMENTS IN THE MRI EVALUATION OF ISCHEMIA

MAGNETIC RESONANCE SPECTROSCOPY

Spin-echo images show no abnormalities in the first minutes and hours after a stroke despite the profound and sometimes irreversible biochemical changes that are occurring. Proton (^{1}H) MR spectroscopy can be used to evaluate the acid-base balance (i.e., presence of lactate in ischemic tissue). Spectral changes caused by ischemia are detectable within minutes after the ischemic event due to altered cellular metabolism. Phosphorus 31 (^{31}P) spectroscopy can evaluate the decrease in cellular energy subtrates and the increase in their breakdown products. Although intense research interest centers around spectroscopy, its clinical application has been limited because of long acquisition times.

DIFFUSION MAGNETIC RESONANCE IMAGING

Diffusion imaging can also detect hyperacute changes due to ischemia before morphologic abnormalities develop on conventional spin-echo MRI. Diffusion maps of the brain can be calculated and display regions of slower water proton diffusion due to restriction of water in the intracellular compartment in cytotoxic edema. This decrease in the calculated apparent diffusion coefficient

Table 19-6
VENOUS SINUS OCCLUSIVE DISEASE

Stage	MRI Findings	Dural Sinus Pressure
1	None	< 20 mmHg
2	Brain edema without T2 signal abnormalities	20–25 mmHg
3	Mild to moderate edema with T2 signal abnormalities	30–40 mmHg
4	Severe brain edema with T2 signal abnormalities with or without hemorrhage	40–50 mmHg
5	Massive edema with T2 signal abnormalities with or without hemorrhage	> 50 mmHg (assume)

(ADC) appears bright on the ADC map. The ADC increases to appear dark in the vasogenic edema stage, probably because of the increase in extracellular bulk water, which is freely diffusable.

PERFUSION MAGNETIC RESONANCE IMAGING

Perfusion mapping can be done using fast MRI techniques, such as echo-planar, to acquire rapid sequential images tracking a tight intravenously administered bolus of contrast material through the brain. The contrast material causes T2 shortening or loss of signal, which can be graphed over time. These data can then be used to calculate relative cerebral blood flow, blood volume, and mean transit time through the tissue. These calculations can then be displayed as gray-scale maps.

These new experimental techniques may serve to increase our understanding of the pathophysiology of ischemia. Whether these techniques will prove practical in acute stroke evaluation remains to be seen. Acute stroke evaluation strategies of the future need to be extremely rapid, reliable, and convenient in order to facilitate therapeutic intervention before irreversible, irreparable damage is done.

SUGGESTED READINGS

1. Adams RD, Victor M: *Principles of Neurology*, New York, McGraw-Hill, 1981.
2. Atlas SW: *Magnetic Resonance Imaging of the Brain and Spine*. New York, Raven Press, 1991.
3. Baker LL et al: Recent advances in MR imaging: Spectroscopy of cerebral ischemia. *AJR* 156:1133–1143, 1990.
4. Bryan RN et al: Diagnosis of acute cerebral infarction: Comparison of CT and MR imaging. *AJNR* 12:611–620, 1991.
5. Crain MR et al: Cerebral ischemia: Evaluation with contrast-enhanced MR imaging. *AJNR* 12:631–639, 1991.
6. Crockard HA et al: Acute cerebral ischaemia: Concurrent changes in cerebral blood flow, energy metabolites, pH, and lactate measured with hydrogen clearance and 31P and 1H nuclear magnetic resonance spectroscopy: II. Changes during ischaemia. *J Cereb Blood Flow Metab* 7:394–402, 1987.
7. Duijn JH et al: Human brain infarction: Proton MR spectroscopy. *Radiology* 183:711–718, 1992.
8. Edelman RR et al: Cerebral blood flow: Assessment with dynamic contrast-enhanced T2*-weighted MR imaging at 1.5 T. *Radiology* 176:211–220, 1990.
9. Elster AD, Moody DM: Early cerebral infarction: Gadopentetate dimeglumine enhancement. *Radiology* 177:626–632, 1990.
10. Escourolle R, Poirier J: *Manual of Basic Neuropathology*, Philadelphia, Saunders, 1978.
11. Goldberg HI: Angiography of extracranial and intracranial occlusive cerebrovascular disease. *Neuroimaging Clin North Am* 2:487–507, 1992.
12. Harris KG et al: Diagnosing intracranial vasculitis: The roles of MR and angiography. *AJNR* 15:317–330, 1994.
13. Hayman LA et al: Mechanisms of MR signal alteration by acute intracerebral blood: Old concepts and new theories. *AJNR* 12:899–907, 1991.
14. Heiserman JE: The role of magnetic resonance and angiography in the evaluation of cerebrovascular ischemic disease. *Neuroimaging Clin North Am* 2:753–767, 1992.
15. Johnson BA, Fram EK: Cerebral venous occlusive disease: Pathophysiology, clinical manifestations, and imaging. *Neuroimaging Clin North Am* 168:199–202, 1992.
16. Levy D et al: Carotid and vertebral artery dissections: Three-dimensional time-of-flight MR angiography and MR imaging versus conventional angiography. *Radiology* 190:97–103, 1994.
17. Moseley ME et al: Diffusion-weighted MR imaging of acute stroke: Correlation with T2-weighted and magnetic susceptibility-enhanced MR imaging in cats. *AJNR* 11:423–429, 1989.
18. Mueller DP et al: Arterial enhancement in acute ischemia: Clinical and angiographic correlation. *AJNR* 14:661–668, 1993.
19. Osborn AG: CT of acute cerebral infarction. *Imaging Decisions* 1:3–14, 1994.
20. Osborn AG: *Diagnostic Neuroradiology*. St Louis, Mosby-Year Book, 1994.
21. Rumbaugh CL et al: *Cerebrovascular Disease: Imaging and Interventional Treatment Options*. New York, Igaku-Shoin, 1995.
22. Sevick RJ et al: Cytotoxic brain edema: Assessment with diffusion-weighted MR imaging. *Radiology* 185:687–690, 1992.
23. Simonson T et al: MR imaging and HMPAO scintigraphy in conjunction with balloon test occlusion: Value in predicting sequelae after permanent carotid occlusion. *AJR* 59:1063–1068, 1992.
24. Tsai FY et al: MR staging of acute dural sinus thrombosis: Correlation with venous pressure measurements and implications for treatment and prognosis. *AJNR*. In press.
25. Wang AM et al: Intracranial magnetic resonance angiography. *Applied Radiol*. In press.
26. Wang AM et al: What is expected of CT in evaluation of stroke? *Neuroradiology* 30:54–58, 1988.
27. Yamada I et al: Moyamoya disease: Diagnosis with three-dimensional time-of-flight MR angiography. *Radiology* 184:773–778, 1992.
28. Yuh WTC et al: MR imaging of cerebral ischemia: Findings in the first 24 hours. *AJNR* 12:621–629, 1991.
29. Yuh WTC, Crain MR: Magnetic resonance imaging of acute cerebral ischemia. *Stroke* 2:421–439, 1992.
30. Yuh WTC et al: Venous sinus occlusive disease: MR findings. *AJNR* 15:309–316, 1994.

☐ QUESTIONS (True or False)

1. Hemorrhagic infarctions are usually
- **a.** Present immediately after the ictus.
- **b.** Located at the cortical ribbon and basal ganglia.
- **c.** Located at the cerebral white matter.
- **d.** More easily demonstrated on CT than MRI in the acute stage.
- **e.** More easily demonstrated on CT than MRI in the chronic stage.

2. Regarding hemodynamic factors for infarctions,
- **a.** The degree of ischemic infarction is related to anastomotic collateral circulation by arteries at the circle of Willis, intracranial to extracranial collaterals, and corticomeningeal anastomosis.
- **b.** Collateral circulation is generally inadequate if proximal internal carotid artery occlusion occurs.
- **c.** In general, thrombosis leads to sudden arterial occlusion.
- **d.** In general, emboli produce sudden and massive arterial occlusion.
- **e.** Migration or secondary fragmentation of the embolus is usually the cause of peripheral cortical hemorrhage.

3. Stroke
- **a.** Is the leading cause of death in the United States.
- **b.** Is hemorrhagic in 85 percent of cases.
- **c.** The incidence is higher in men than in women.
- **d.** Hypertension is the most important risk factor.
- **e.** Occurs 10 times more often in carotid/middle cerebral artery territory than in vertebrobasilar artery territory.

4. Computed tomography findings in hyperacute infarction are as follows:
- **a.** The hyperdense artery sign presents all the time.
- **b.** They are normal in half of the cases.
- **c.** There is slightly decreased density in the cerebral gray matter due to vasogenic edema.
- **d.** There is subtle mass effect with effacement of sulci.
- **e.** Loss of distinction between the densities of cerebral gray and white matter is seen.

5. On MRI, findings of contrast-enhanced T1-weighted images in stroke are as follows:
- **a.** Apparent early arterial enhancement is usually seen in patients with incomplete ischemia.
- **b.** Early demonstration of arterial enhancement may represent a slow blood flow and also inadequacy of collaterals.
- **c.** Parenchymal enhancement is usually seen during the acute stage of complete ischemia.
- **d.** Meningeal enhancement is usually seen within the first 3 days in large cortical infarcts and resolves after 1 week.
- **e.** Arterial enhancement usually persists through the chronic stage of complete stroke.

6. Parenchymal signal changes on T2-weighted images in stroke are as follows:
- **a.** There is absence of or minimal signal changes in the acute stage of complete ischemia.
- **b.** Presence of massive signal changes in the acute stage of incomplete ischemia.
- **c.** Resolution of signal changes in the subacute stage of complete ischemia.
- **d.** Persistence of massive signal changes in the subacute stage of incomplete ischemia.
- **e.** In watershed infarction, signal abnormalities are maximal at 2 to 3 days and persist into the chronic stage.

7. On MRI, findings of hemorrhagic infarctions are as follows:
- **a.** Oxyhemoglobin is initially present in hyperacute clots and appears isointense on both T1- and T2-weighted images.
- **b.** By 24 to 72 h, most intracerebral hematomas contain intracellular deoxyhemoglobin, which appears isointense on T1-weighted and hypointense on T2-weighted and gradient-refocused echo images.
- **c.** During the early subacute stage of an intracerebral hematoma, deoxyhemoglobin gradually converts to intracellular methemoglobin, which appears hyperintense on T1-weighted and hypointense on T2-weighted images.
- **d.** During the late subacute stage of an intracerebral hematoma, further hemoglobin oxidation and cell lysis occur; methemoglobin is released to the extracellular space and appears hyperintense on both T1- and T2-weighted images.
- **e.** In the early chronic stage of an intracerebral hematoma, the resolving clot consists of a relatively uniform pool of dilute extracellular methemoglobin surrounded by a vascularized wall that contains macrophages. These macrophages contain ferritin and hemosiderin; therefore the clot appears hyperintense on both T1- and T2-weighted images and does not have a pronounced low-signal rim on T2-weighted images.

8. The following questions are related to MR angiography (MRA).
- **a.** In spin-echo images, the flowing blood appears dark (flow-signal void).

b. In gradient-refocused echo images with flow compensation and phase contrast images, the flowing blood appears dark.
c. Time-of-flight MRA relies on the inflow of fully magnetized blood into the imaging plane and is encountered in flow-compensated gradient-echo MR images perpendicular to the axis of the blood vessel.
d. Phase-contrast MRA generates MR vascular images by detecting changes in the phase of blood's transverse magnetization as it moves along a magnetic field gradient.
e. The circle of Willis can be well evaluated noninvasively by time-of-flight MRA.

9. The following questions are related to nonatherosclerotic occlusive arterial disease.
a. Fibromuscular dysplasia affects middle-aged and older women; bilateral involvement is common.
b. Pseudoenlargement of the lumen of the internal carotid artery is a classic MRA finding in carotid dissection.
c. Takayasu's arteritis usually affects older women and typically involves the proximal portion of the brachiocephalic arteries.
d. Moyamoya disease is usually due to progressive bilateral stenosis or occlusion of the supraclinoid portion of the internal carotid artery, extending to the proximal portions of the anterior and middle cerebral arteries, with dilatation of the penetrating arteries to the basal ganglia and thalamus.
e. Cerebral hemorrhage in moyamoya disease is commonly seen in children.

10. The following questions are related to cerebral venous and dural sinus thrombosis.
a. The cord sign seen on noncontrast CT studies of the brain is a frequent finding.
b. The empty delta sign seen on contrast-enhanced CT studies is a pathognomonic sign for superior sagittal sinus thrombosis.
c. The severity of abnormal brain parenchymal MRI findings is related to the degree of elevation of the dural sinus pressure.
d. There is usually no abnormal parenchymal enhancement.
e. Venous MRA is reliable to demonstrate the occluded dural sinuses as well as the occluded cerebral veins and can replace cerebral angiography for screening venous occlusive disease.

☐ ANSWERS

1. **a.** F
b. T
c. F
d. T
e. F

2. **a.** T
b. F
c. F
d. T
e. F

3. **a.** F
b. F
c. T
d. T
e. F

4. **a.** F
b. T
c. F
d. T
e. T

5. **a.** F
b. T
c. F
d. T
e. F

6. **a.** F
b. F
c. F
d. F
e. T

7. **a.** T
b. T
c. T
d. T
e. F

8. **a.** T
b. F
c. T
d. T
e. T

9. **a.** T
b. T
c. F
d. T
e. F

10. **a.** F
b. T
c. T
d. T
e. T

CHAPTER

20 White Matter Disease

Benjamin C. P. Lee
Mukul Maheshwari
Chi S. Zee

☐ NORMAL MYELINATION

White matter fibers begin to myelinate around 16 weeks of fetal gestation. Approximately 90 percent of the myelination process takes place by the age of 2 years and the remainder continues up to early adulthood. Comparison of early childhood and early adulthood in myelination pattern is a matter of quality, not quantity. Myelin is produced by oligodendrocytes and is primarily composed of protein and lipid, which wrap around the axons. The composition of myelin is 70 to 80 percent lipid and 20 to 30 percent protein.

The process of myelination goes from caudal to cephalad, posterior to anterior, and central to peripheral. The sensory fibers myelinate earlier than motor fiber tracts (Table 20-1).

Magnetic resonance imaging (MRI) is utilized to evaluate the myelination pattern. However, MRI patterns of myelination vary with the magnetic field strength and pulse sequences.

The MRI changes that occur are due to varying water content of the gray and white matter and progression of white matter myelination. Beyond 2 years of age, the pediatric brain is similar to that of a young adult in terms of myelination. At birth, the water content of white matter is 87 percent and of gray matter is 89 percent. In the pediatric and young adult age groups, the water content diminishes, with 72 percent in white matter and 82 percent in gray matter.

The MRI pulse sequences used to study myelination are as follows:

1. *T1-weighted spin echo*: TR 500 to 800, TE 20 to 30 for evaluating immature and mature myelin. Myelination is always seen earlier in any white matter structure on T1-weighted images versus T2-weighted images. The myelination process predominates by 6 months on T1-weighted images. Myelinated white matter is hyperintense to gray matter. Unmyelinated white matter is hypointense to gray matter.
2. *T2-weighted spin echo*: TR 3000 to 4000, TE 100 to 120 for evaluating mature myelin formation and subtle changes in water content. The myelination process predominates T2-weighted images after 6 months. Myelinated white matter is hypointense to gray matter. Unmyelinated white matter is hyperintense to gray matter.
3. *Inversion recovery (IR) T1-weighted and T2-weighted images*: IR T1-weighted images, 2500 to 3000; T2-weighted images, 900 to 1200, TE 30. IR T2-weighted images, 2500 to 3000; T1-weighted images, 300 to 500, TE 40. Provides better resolution than routine spin-echo T1-weighted and T2-weighted sequences. There is a slight difference at which time myelination process occurs on IR versus SE sequences.

☐ LEUKODYSTROPHY

Leukodystrophy is the generic term for a white matter disorder other than demyelination. These disorders are often the result of dysmyelination in which there is defective myelination. They usually present in infancy or early childhood during the active stages of myelination. When such disorders present later than that, they probably result from defective maintenance of myelin and may be difficult to distinguish from demyelination. Dysmyelination is confined to the white matter and should be differentiated from metabolic disorders that affect cortical or deep gray matter. Many disorders are associated with elevation of specific biochemical products.

Table 20-1
NORMAL MYELINATION TIMETABLE

	T1-Weighted Images	T2-Weighted Images	IR T1-Weighted Images	IR T2-Weighted Images
INFRATENTORIAL				
Brainstem (dorsal medulla-midbrain)	Birth	Birth	Birth	Birth, mature by 6 months
CEREBELLAR PEDUNCLES				
Superior/Inferior	Birth	Birth to 6 months	Birth	Birth, mature by 6 months
Middle	Birth	2–3 months	Birth	1 month
Cerebellum, deep white matter (deep to peripheral)	1–3 months	3–18 months	1–3 months	1–3 months
SUPRATENTORIAL				
Thalamus	Birth	Birth	Birth	—
Internal capsule				
Posterior limb	Birth	Birth	Birth	Birth
Anterior limb	3 months	3–6 months	2 months	2 months
Corpus callosum				
Splenium	3 months	4 months	3 months	3 months
Genu	6 months	8 months	6 months	6–8 months
Postcentral gyrus	Birth	Birth	Birth	Birth
Precentral gyrus	Birth	2–3 weeks	Birth	Birth to 2 weeks
Centrum semiovale	Birth to 1 month	Birth to 2 months	—	Birth to 1 month
Optic nerves, tracts, radiation	Birth	1–2 months	Birth	1 month
Lobes: Occipital	6 months	6.5 to 15 months	6 months	6–8 months
Posterior frontal, temporal, parietal	6 months	6.5 to 15 months	6 months	6–8 months
Anterior frontal, parietal, and midtemporal lobes	8 months	6.5 to 15 months	8 months	—
Frontal and temporal pole	12 months	24 months	10 months	12–15 months

Modified from Byrd SE, Darling CR, Wilczynski NA: White matter of the brain: maturation and myelination on magnetic resonance in infants and children, *Neuroimaging Clin N Amer* 3:247–266, 1993.

Diagnosis of the specific enzyme defect is usually made by analysis of the blood or skin fibroblasts.

GENERAL MRI AND CT FEATURES

In general, MRI is more sensitive in evaluating white matter changes, but the changes are visible on computed tomography (CT) when the abnormalities are severe. However, CT is more specific in detecting calcification. Because myelination continues over a long time after birth, it is inadvisable to definitively diagnose white matter disorders until the brain is fully myelinated at 1 year to 18 months. The criteria for evaluating white matter changes in children are similar to those in adults.

It is seldom possible to be specific about the cause of dysmyelination on MRI and CT. The following features should be noted (Table 20-2):

Table 20-2
DISORDERS WITH CHARACTERISTIC MR IMAGING FEATURES

Macrocephaly: Krabbe's, Hurler's, Alexander's, Canavan's

Location of white matter changes:
- Posterior: X-linked adrenoleukodystrophy
- Anterior: Alexander's

Basal ganglia involvement: Fabry's, Leigh's, Kearn-Sayre's, glutaric acidemia I, methylmalonic acidemia, Wilson's, Cockayne's

Infarcts ± white matter involvement: MELAS, MERFF, Leigh's, homocystinuria, Fabry's

MELAS, mitochondrial myopathy encephalopathy lactic acidosis strokes; MERFF, myoclonic epilepsy with ragged red cell fibers.
With permission: Lee et al: Magnetic resonance imaging of metabolic and primary white matter disorders in children. *Neuroimaging Clin N Amer* 3:2, p 267–289, 1993.

Location of the changes
Involvement of the cortex and basal ganglia
Cavitations in the white matter
Shape and size of the cranium
Calcification or blood
Hydrocephalus

Cerebral atrophy and hypoplasia of the corpus callosum are nonspecific and are related to the severity and chronicity of the disorders. Contrast enhancement is an indication of acute changes and not generally indicative of specific types of disorder. The sex, age of onset, family history, and clinical course are also important considerations. Macrocephaly is an important consideration and is associated with Krabbe's, Canavan's, Hurler's, and Alexander's diseases.

CLASSIFICATION OF PEDIATRIC WHITE MATTER DISORDERS

White matter disorders are due to defects of peroxisomes, lysosomes, amino acid metabolism, or mitochondria. Those in which the cause is unknown are categorized as primary white matter disorders.

☐ PEROXISOMAL DISORDERS

Peroxisomes are cell organelles responsible for fatty acid metabolism. Single or multiple enzymes may be involved, leading to systemic accumulation of long and very long chain fatty acids. The disorders are autosomal recessive and may be sex-linked.

X-LINKED ADRENOLEUKODYSTROPHY

X-linked adrenoleukodystrophy is the most common peroxisomal disorder and involves a single enzyme. It presents as visual impairment, often with skin pigmentation. Diagnosis is made by detecting very long chain fatty acids in the blood and skin fibroblasts. Adrenomyeloneuropathy is a variant of this disorder that affects the spinal cord and peripheral nerves.

Age and Gender

- Presents in boys, usually between the ages of 4 and 8.

Magnetic Resonance Imaging and Computed Tomography

- Characterized by involvement of the posterior portion of the hemisphere: occipital lobes and visual pathways.
- The entire hemisphere is involved with progression of the disease.
- Best seen as nonspecific increased signal on T2-weighted images, decreased signal on T1-weighted images, and decreased attenuation on CT in more severe cases. Calcification may be seen (Fig. 20-1).

Differential Diagnosis

- Periventricular leukomalacia

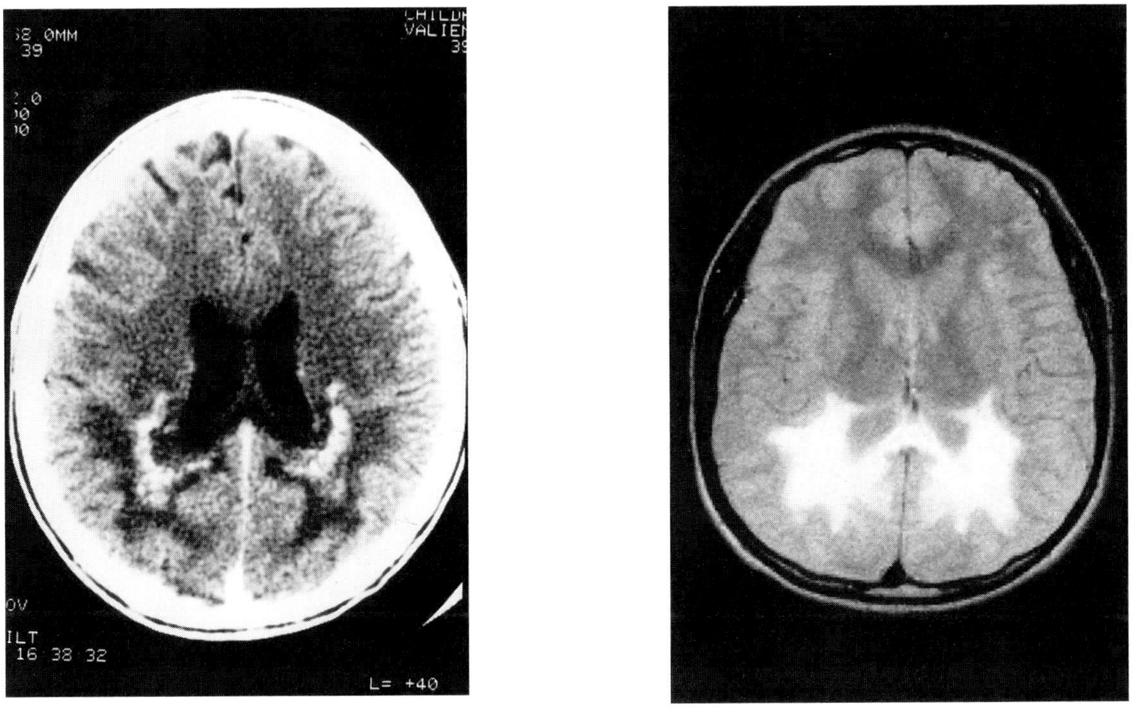

(A) (B)

Figure 20-1 Adrenoleukodystrophy. *A*. An axial CT scan shows low density in the periventricular white matter with irregular calcifications seen bilaterally around the lateral ventricle in the parietal region. *B*. An axial proton-density weighted image demonstrates irregular periventricular high signal intensity in both parietal regions.

NEONATAL ADRENOLEUKODYSTROPHY

Neonatal adrenoleukodystrophy is an autosomal recessive disorder involving multiple enzymes.

- It presents at birth.
- White matter changes are periventricular and global with no specific anatomic predisposition.

ZELLWEGER SYNDROME

Zellweger syndrome is a rare autosomal recessive disorder involving several enzymes and results in elevation of very long chain as well as several other fatty acids.

- It presents in infancy.
- Migrational defects are present.
- White matter changes are nonspecific.

☐ LYSOSOMAL DISORDERS

Lysosomes are involved with the synthesis of substrates for myelination. Lysosomal enzyme defects result in the accumulation of (1) phosphoglycolipids (lipidoses) and (2) mucopolysaccharides. These substances may be deposited systematically as well as in the cerebral white matter and result in defective function in various body organs.

LIPIDOSES

Phospho- and glycolipids are synthesized by various enzymes into ceramides, which are essential for myelination. The three groups of substrates involve (1) cerebrosides (Krabbe's disease) and sulfatides (metachromatic leukodystrophy), (2) sphingomyelin (Niemann-Pick and Fabry's disease) and (3) gangliosides (Tay-Sachs disease).

KRABBE'S DISEASE

Krabbe's disease (globoid-cell leukodystrophy) is an autosomal recessive disorder that is due to deficiency of the enzyme galactocerebroside.

Age and Gender

- It usually presents in early infancy and is rapidly progressive.
- A late-onset form that presents in later childhood and adolescence is less common.

Pathology

- Globoid cells are seen in the white matter.

Magnetic Resonance Imaging and Computed Tomography

- White matter involvement is nonspecific, with increased signal on T2-weighted images and decreased attenuation on CT. There is no specific anatomic preference.
- Macrocephaly is often present.
- The infantile form is rapidly progressive and results in severe dilatation of the lateral ventricle.

METACHROMATIC LEUKODYSTROPHY

Metachromatic leukodystrophy is an autosomal recessive disorder that is due to deficiency of arylsulfatase A (cerebroside sulfatase A); it results in the accumulation of sulfatides. The deficiency is systemic and affects other organs in addition to the nervous system.

Age and Gender

- The early infantile form is more common.
- Juvenile and adult forms also occur.

Magnetic Resonance Imaging and Computed Tomography

- There are nonspecific white matter changes in the cerebral hemispheres (Fig. 20-2).
- The cerebellar hemispheres are sometimes involved.
- Ventricular enlargement is generally less severe than in Krabbe's disease.

FABRY'S DISEASE

Fabry's disease (angiokeratoma corporis diffusum) is a rare disorder due to deficiency of the enzyme α-galactosidase A, which results in the accumulation of glycosphingolipids. This is a systemic disorder characterized by the presence of cutaneous and corneal lesions. Neurologic symptoms are the result of small strokes rather than white matter lesions. This is not strictly a dysmyelination disorder.

Pathology

- Small vessel thromboses and infarcts.

Magnetic Resonance Imaging and Computed Tomography

- Changes of basal ganglia infarcts.

TAY-SACHS DISEASE

Tay-Sachs disease is an uncommon disorder occurring in Ashkenazi Jews; it is due to a deficiency in the enzymes responsible for the breakdown of gangliosides and is characterized clinically by profound intellectual impairment.

- Nonspecific increase in white matter signal.

NIEMANN-PICK DISEASE

Niemann-Pick disease is due to a deficiency of the enzyme sphingomyelinase, which results in the accumulation of sphingomyelin.

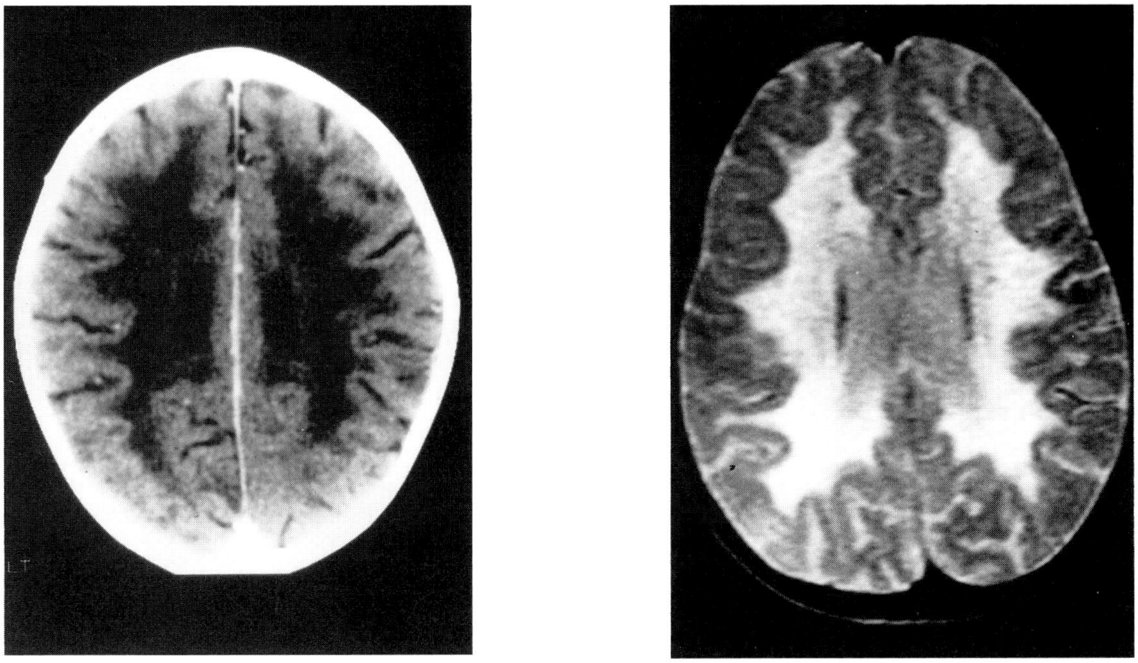

(A) (B)

Figure 20-2 Metachromatic leukodystrophy. *A*. An axial CT scan shows bilateral periventricular white matter of low density. *B*. Axial T2-weighted image shows extensive bilateral high signal intensity in the white matter.

- Diagnosis is usually made early because of systemic involvement. Cerebral involvement is uncommon and results in intellectual and motor impairment.

MUCOPOLYSACCHARIDOSES

Mucopolysaccharidoses are caused by deficiencies of enzymes involved in the degradation of heparan, dermatan, or keratan sulfate. Six major types of abnormalities that involve the skeletomuscular and nervous systems have been identified. Hurler's (type I) lesions cause severe cerebral abnormalities. Hunter's (type II), San Filippo (type III) affect the brain less severely and Maroteaux-Lamy (type VI) rarely. The clinical diagnoses of most mucopolysaccharidoses are obvious because of systemic involvement and the characteristic appearance of the cranium.

Pathology

- Cavities in the white matter are filled with mucopolysaccharide material. White matter myelination is less than normal.
- Hydrocephalus is secondary to occlusion of arachnoid granulations by mucopolysaccharides.

Magnetic Resonance Imaging and Computed Tomography

- Multiple lesions in the white matter and corpus callosum—with increased signal on T2-weighted images and decreased signal on T1-weighted images—are characteristic.
- Nonspecific increased signal in the periventricular and deep white matter on T2-weighted images and decreased signal on T1-weighted images may also be visible as decreased attenuation on CT.
- The head is macrocephalic and dolichocephalic.
- Severe dilatation of the ventricles is due either to hydrocephalus or atrophy of end-stage disease.
- Evidence of periventricular increased signal on T2-weighted images—due to transependymal CSF absorption—may be present with hydrocephalus.

☐ AMINO ACID AND ORGANIC ACID METABOLIC DISORDER

Amino acids are the substrates for the synthesis and maintenance of myelin. Defects in metabolism are all autosomal recessive: the amino acids may not be available for metabolism because of enzyme defects, or there may be failure of transportation to the appropriate sites. The MRI and CT appearances of these diseases are generally nonspecific, and it is rarely possible to diagnose the enzymatic defect.

Aminoacidemia with aminoaciduria is a deficiency of specific enzymes (aminoacidopathy) resulting in the systemic accumulation of the affected amino acids (aminoacidemia), which are excreted in excessive quantities in the urine (aminoaciduria). Examples of enzymatic aminoacidopathy include phenylketonuria, maple syrup disease, glutaricaciduria type I, and methylmalonic acidemia. Canavan's disease is representative of organic acid metabolic disorder due to enzyme deficiency.

PHENYLKETONURIA

Phenylketonuria is caused by a deficiency of phenylalanine 4-monooxygenase, which is required for the conversion of phenylalanine to tyrosine. Routine screening of blood reveals an incidence of 1 per 14,000. Patients are normal at birth but have failure of psychomotor development and may become severely mentally retarded. A defect of tyrosine hydrolase—which catabolizes tyrosine to dopa and catecholamines—results in tyrosinemia.

MAPLE SYRUP DISEASE

Maple syrup disease is due to failure to catabolize branched-chain amino acids (valine, leucine, and isoleucine) and has an incidence of 1 per 200,000. This disorder presents with severe, rapidly progressive neurologic defects. Unlike phenylketonuria, which is compatible with life without treatment, this disorder is usually fatal by 1 year.

HOMOCYSTINURIA

Homocystinuria is caused by one of several enzymes responsible for catabolism of this amino acid. Clinically, the disorder is characterized by systemic skeletomuscular and vascular abnormalities. The latter affect the intracranial vessels, resulting in arterial and venous thromboses and infarcts. Ocular abnormalities such as cataracts are also common.

Magnetic Resonance Imaging and Computed Tomography
- Arterial and venous infarcts may be seen.

METHYLMALONIC ACIDEMIA AND GLUTARIC ACIDEMIA TYPE I.

These disorders are interesting in that they are examples of aminoacidopathies affecting mitochondrial activity and thus have similarities to mitochondrial defects from other causes. Methylmalonic acidemia is a defect of methylmalonic coenzyme A mutase. Glutaric aciduria type I (GA I) is caused by defective glutaryl-CoA dehydrogenase.

Magnetic Resonance Imaging and Computed Tomography
- Abnormal signal is seen on MRI in the basal ganglia in both disorders:
- The globus pallidus is commonly affected in methylmalonic acidemia.
- The putamen and caudate nuclei are involved in GA I aminoaciduria.
- Frontotemporal atrophy is associated with GA I aminoaciduria.
- Nonspecific white matter changes may also be present.

CANAVAN'S DISEASE

Canavan's disease is caused by deficiency of aspartoacylase which results in the accumulation of *N*-acetylaspartic acid. It presents in infancy or early childhood and usually has a rapidly fatal course.

- Macrocephaly is pronounced.

Pathology The characteristic spongy appearance on histologic examination is due to vacuoles in the white matter and is responsible for the name *spongiform leukodystrophy*.

Magnetic Resonance Imaging and Computed Tomography
- Macrocephaly is pronounced in the initial stages of the disease.

AMINOACIDURIA WITHOUT AMINOACIDEMIA

In these disorders, metabolism is normal but there is a failure of the renal tubules to reabsorb urinary amino acids. Multiple instead of single amino acids are excreted.

OCULOCEREBRAL RENAL SYNDROME

Oculocerebral renal syndrome (Lowe's syndrome) is characterized by tubular acidosis, hypophosphatemic rickets , ocular abnormalities such as cataracts, and cerebral changes resulting in intellectual and motor deficits.

Magnetic Resonance Imaging and Computed Tomography
- Patchy increased signal on T2-weighted images in white matter.
- Multiple lacunar defects associated with these white matter changes.

☐ MITOCHONDRIAL DISORDERS

Mitochondrial disorders affect the oxidative respiratory cycle and result in lactic acidosis, sometimes with elevated systemic pyruvate. Often, several enzymes and coenzymes are involved: the smooth muscles of arteries and cerebral gray matter are affected. Radiologically, the changes are characterized by cortical and basal involvement. However, it is probably unwise to diagnose a specific biochemical defect based on MRI and CT appearances.

MELAS SYNDROME

The syndrome of mitochondrial myopathy, encephalopathy, lactic acidosis, and strokes (MELAS) is characterized by recurrent strokes and lactic acidosis. The strokes are probably caused by defective mitochondria of the metabolically active cortical and deep gray matter. Involvement of the larger cerebral arteries may be responsible for more extensive regions of infarct. A closely related disorder MERRF (myoclonic epilepsy with ragged red fibers) also affects cortical gray matter.

Magnetic Resonance Imaging and Computed Tomography

- Multiple cortical strokes are present. These show high signal during the acute stages on T2-weighted images.
- Basal ganglia may also be affected.
- Contrast enhancement is seen during the acute stages.

LEIGH'S DISEASE

Leigh's disease [subacute necrotizing encephalopathy (SNE)] is an autosomal recessive defect in pyruvate metabolism, involving deficiencies in pyruvate dehydrogenase, cytochrome-*c* oxidase, and related enzymes and is probably one of a number of mitochondrial disorders.

Pathology

- There are infarcts of the caudate, putamen, and tegmentum of the midbrain.
- The locations and pathologic changes are similar to those of Wernicke's encephalopathy, with sparing of the mamillary bodies.

Magnetic Resonance Imaging and Computed Tomography

- Increased signal on T2-weighted images in the putamen, caudate, and tegmentum.
- Other portions of the basal ganglia and brainstem as well as the cortical gray matter may also be involved.
- Contrast enhancement is seen during the acute stages.

KEARNS-SAYRE SYNDROME

Kearns-Sayre syndrome is an autosomal dominant defect with elevated serum pyruvate and pathologic and MRI changes similar to those of Leigh's disease.

WILSON'S DISEASE

Copper is an essential component of a number of coenzymes essential to mitochondrial activity and is transported by ceruloplasmin to the appropriate sites. In this disorder, there is defective transportation and copper is deposited in the putamen and caudate nuclei as well as systematically in the liver and other organs.

☐ PRIMARY WHITE MATTER DISEASES

These disorders do not cause any specific biochemical alterations and are diagnosed clinically and by histologic evaluation of brain biopsy specimens. The most common disorders are Alexander's, Cockayne's, and Pelizaeus-Merzbacher diseases.

ALEXANDER'S DISEASE

Alexander's disease is a rare disorder of unknown cause that presents in infancy or adolescence, has a progressive course, and is characterized by macrocephaly.

Pathology

- Astrocytic eosinophilic Rosenthal fibers are present in the white matter.

Magnetic Resonance Imaging and Computed Tomography

- Increased signal in the frontal lobes during the early stages of the disease.
- Eventually the entire brain is involved.
- Macrocephaly.
- Contrast enhancement has been described and probably indicates acute dys- and demyelination.

PELIZAEUS-MERZBACHER DISEASE

Pelizaeus-Merzbacher disease is an X-linked recessive disorder, with sporadic cases; it usually presents in infancy but may rarely occur in adults. Pathologic evidence suggests that this is a disorder of hypomyelination.

Pathology

- Patchy areas of demyelination with normal myelin in the perivascular regions giving rise to the typical "tigroid" appearance.

Magnetic Resonance Imaging and Computed Tomography

- Generalized increased signal in the white matter on T2-weighted images suggests hypomyelination.
- Scattered regions of hyperintensity on T2-weighted images may also be present.
- Decreased signal on T2-weighted images is sometimes seen in the basal ganglia and may represent iron.

COCKAYNE'S DISEASE

Cockayne's disease is a disorder of hypomyelination, similar to some cases of Pelizaeus-Merzbacher disease, with additional involvement of other organs. The disease presents in childhood with a characteristic facies and skin rash. It is autosomal recessive in some families.

Magnetic Resonance Imaging and Computed Tomography

- Diffuse increased signal on T2-weighted images due to hypomyelination.
- Calcification in the basal ganglia: increased density on CT, decreased signal on MRI.

☐ DEMYELINATING DISEASES

IDIOPATHIC

Multiple Sclerosis Multiple sclerosis (MS) is a demyelinating disorder that is characterized by multiple inflammatory plaques of demyelination involving the white matter of the central nervous system. These lesions characteristically cause waxing and waning symptoms with eventual disability. Multiple sclerosis is a clinical diagnosis that should never be made on the basis of imaging results alone.

Incidence

- Most common among northern Europeans or people of northern European extraction. Less common in Asians and almost unheard of in black Africans.
- In the United States, the incidence of MS varies, with incidence in the North being significantly more common than in the South.
- Average incidence in the United States 0.1 percent.

Age and Gender

- Female:male = 3:2.
- Between 18 and 50 years of age.

Location

- The majority of lesions occur at the periventricular white matter.
- Frequently affected areas are as follows in descending order:

1. Periventricular white matter adjacent to the trigones and bodies of the lateral ventricles
2. Corpus callosum
3. White matter adjacent to occipital horns
4. White matter adjacent to frontal horns
5. Brainstem
6. Along the floor of the fourth ventricle
7. Cerebellar hemisphere
8. Around the third ventricle
9. Basal ganglia
10. Internal capsule

Pathology

- *Acute phase*: Disintegration of the myelin with focal hypercellularity resulting from microglial infiltration and perivascular lymphocytic cuffing. The myelin sheath becomes fragmented, whereas the axons remain relatively preserved. Macrophages with foamy cytoplasms resulting from the phagocytosis of myelin breakdown products are seen.
- *Subacute phase*: The plaques become less cellular and show loss of both axons and oligodendrocytes. Reactive astrocytes may be seen.
- *Inactive phase*: Plaques are demarcated from the adjacent parenchyma. They show changes of hypocellularity, demyelination, and gliosis. No oligodendrocytes are seen in these lesions.

Imaging COMPUTED TOMOGRAPHY

- Hypointense to isointense white matter lesions.
- Contrast enhancement may or may not be seen.
- Some authors advocate double dose, delayed (30 min to 1 h) study to better demonstrate MS plaques.
- Large, masslike plaques or ringlike enhancing lesions can mimic neoplasms.

MAGNETIC RESONANCE IMAGING

- Magnetic resonance imaging is more sensitive than CT in demonstrating MS plaques on both pre- and post-contrast studies.
- Discrete, small, hyperintense foci in a transverse orientation in the periventricular white matter on proton-density and T2-weighted images (Fig. 20-3).
- Corpus callosum, subcortical U fibers, brainstem, and cerebellar white matter are also involved.
- The majority of lesions are hypointense to isointense on T1-weighted images and appear smaller than corresponding hyperintense lesions seen on T2-weighted images.
- The FLAIR (fluid attentuated inversion recovery) technique is superior to proton-density or T2-weighted images in demonstrating MS plaques.
- Confluent lesions in the periventricular white matter may be seen in long-standing cases.

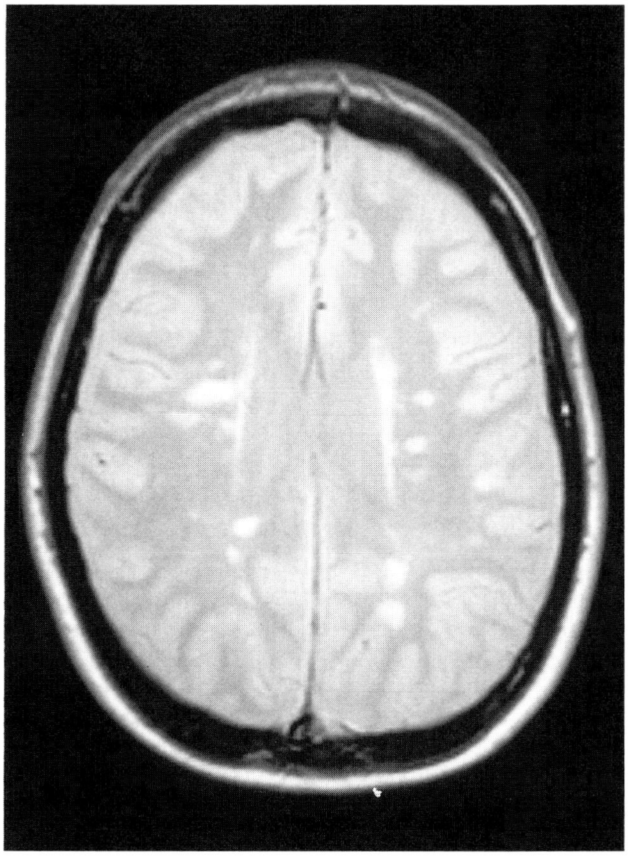

Figure 20-3 Multiple sclerosis. Axial proton-density and T2-weighted images demonstrate small areas of high signal intensity in the periventricular white matter bilaterally. These small areas of hyperintensity have a transverse orientation. Involvement of the subcortical U fibers is seen bilaterally.

- Contrast enhancement is variable.
- The MS lesions accumulate contrast such that signal intensity peaks at 30 min and remains elevated for up to 2 h.
- Diffuse atrophy, atrophy of corpus callosum.
- Occasionally, abnormal iron deposition in basal ganglia.
- Optic neuritis is best shown on gadolinium-enhanced, fat-suppressed MRI. Enhancement of the optic nerve may be seen.
- Spinal cord lesions may mimic neoplasm, with cord enlargement, hyperintensity on T2-weighted images, and contrast enhancement.

DIFFERENTIAL DIAGNOSIS

- Small-vessel white matter infarcts/ischemia—these lesions are seen in older age groups. Subcortical U fibers and the corpus callosum are usually spared.
- Vasculitis secondary to collagen vascular disease (systemic lupus erythematosus, Behçet's disease): these lesions are seen in similar age groups as multiple sclerosis.
- Encephalitis (acute disseminated encephalomyelitis, subacute sclerosing panencephalitis, etc.): ADEM is a monomorphic acute inflammatory demyelinating disease that rarely relapses.
- Trauma (diffuse axonal injury): the clinical history is obvious.
- Metastasis: enhancing lesions are seen at the gray-white junction.
- Sarcoidosis.
- Lyme disease.

Schilder's Disease (Myelinoclastic Diffuse Sclerosis)

- More virulent, childhood form of multiple sclerosis.
- Imaging shows more confluent areas of demyelination.
- Differential diagnosis is adrenoleukodystrophy.

POSTINFLAMMATORY

Acute Disseminated Encephalomyelitis

- An autoimmune response, ADEM follows a viral infection or vaccination.
- It is being diagnosed more frequently as a result of increased clinical awareness and the advent of MRI.
- It is more commonly seen in children than in adults.
- Pathologically, the lesions show perivenous demyelination. The demyelination is thought to represent an autoimmune response to a viral antigen mediated by antibody-antigen complexes.
- ADEM is a diagnosis of exclusion. Follow-up studies are necessary to exclude the possibility of multiple sclerosis.
- On MRI, there are hyperintense lesions in the white matter, which are often asymmetrical. Both cerebrum and cerebellum may be involved.
- Optic neuritis and spinal cord lesions are also frequently seen.

Subacute Sclerosing Panencephalitis (SSPE)

- SSPE is caused by measles virus and is seen primarily in children.
- SSPE is a progressive and fatal disease process.
- The MRI findings may be normal or show nonspecific white matter lesions or lesions involving the gray matter (cortex and basal ganglia) (Fig. 20-4).

Progressive Multifocal Leukoencephalopathy ***Incidence***
Progressive multifocal leukoencephalopathy (PML) is a devastating demyelinating disease that primarily affects immunocompromised patients, especially those with defective cell-mediated immunity. It is estimated that up to 4 percent of patients with acquired immunodeficiency syndrome (AIDS) have concomitant PML. Approximately 10 percent of patients with PML are transplant recipients. This condition is also seen in lymphoproliferative disease and other malignancies.

AGE AND GENDER

- More common in males than females.
- The peak incidence is in sixth decade of life, with an age range from 5 to 84 years.

PATHOLOGY

- The disease is caused by JC virus, a polyomavirus, which is a subgroup of papovavirus.
- PML is most likely due to activation of latent virus.
- Discrete, multifocal areas of demyelination involve the oligodendroglial cells and oligodendroglial nuclear enlargement with viral inclusion.

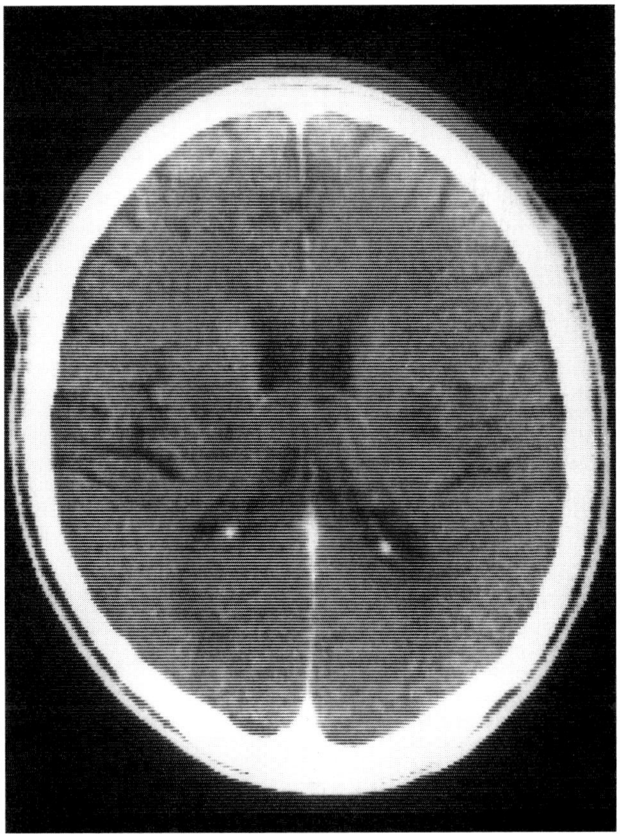

Figure 20-4 Subacute sclerosing panencephalitis. An axial CT scan demonstrates bilateral low-density lesions in both basal ganglia.

Imaging COMPUTED TOMOGRAPHY

- May be normal or show nonspecific hypodense areas.
- Usually does not demonstrate contrast enhancement of the lesions.

MAGNETIC RESONANCE IMAGING

- Multifocal, asymmetrical hyperintense lesions on T2-weighted images, which may be confluent.
- There is a predilection for the parietal and occipital lobes.
- The basal ganglia, corpus callosum, cerebellum, and brainstem are less commonly involved. The spinal cord is rarely involved.

Differential Diagnosis

- HIV infection
- Cytomegalovirus encephalopathy
- Multiple sclerosis
- White matter infarction/ischemia

TOXIC AND DEGENERATIVE

Central Pontine Myelinolysis Central pontine myelinosis (CPM) is related to rapid correction of hyponatremia in patients with alcoholism, liver disease, malnutrition, Addison's disease, renal failure, or diuretic usage.

Incidence

- Variable

Location

- Demyelination of the pons, which spreads outward from medial raffe.
- Areas of extrapontine myelolysis include the basal ganglia, thalamus, cerebral peduncles, cerebellum, brachium pontis, internal capsule, external capsule, and lateral geniculate bodies. Extrapontine myelinolysis may be seen in 10 percent of cases.

Pathology Grossly, the lesion may have a triangular shape. Microscopic examination shows destruction of myelin with relative sparing of neurons, axis cylinders, and blood vessels. There may be associated glial cytoplasmic swelling and nuclear pyknosis of the glial cells. Occasionally, neuronal shrinkage or neuronal death may be identified.

Imaging COMPUTED TOMOGRAPHY

- Abnormal area of low density in the mid pons without contrast enhancement or mass effect.
- May be normal.

MAGNETIC RESONANCE IMAGING

- Hypointense lesion in pons on T1-weighted images and hyperintense lesion on T2-weighted images. The tegmentum is usually spared.
- Extrapontine lesions may be seen.
- Gadolinium enhancement may be seen at the periphery of the lesion.

Differential Diagnosis

- Pontine infarct—may mimic CPM.
- Multiple sclerosis or other demyelinating disease—usually other white matter lesions are seen in addition to the pontine lesion.
- Brainstem gliomas—predominantly affect children but may be seen in adults. Asymmetrical lesion with exophytic growth and focal mass effect.
- Lymphoma—may be hypointense on T2-weighted images due to its high cellularity and high nuclear/cytoplasmic ratio.
- Inflammatory or infectious lesions—Lyme disease, tuberculosis, and fungal infection.

Marchiafava-Bignami Disease

- Marchiafava-Bignami disease (MBD) is an uncommon disorder associated with chronic alcoholism.
- Demyelination of the corpus callosum and less frequently demyelination of hemisphere white matter and other commissured fibers.
- Grossly, focal cystic necrosis of the corpus callosum in the middle layer is seen.
- On MRI, sagittal images show atrophy of the corpus callosum and focal areas of necrosis, which are hypointense on T1-weighted images and hyperintense on T2-weighted images.

POSTTHERAPY

Necrotizing Leukoencephalopathy

- In necrotizing leukoencephalopathy (NLE) there is a diffuse white matter injury that follows treatment with a chemotherapeutic agent (most often methotrexate), with or without associated radiation therapy. The latent period is 3 to 12 months.
- The pathologic findings in NLE consist of axonal swelling, multifocal demyelination, coagulation necrosis, and gliosis in the periventricular and centrum semiovale white matter (similar to radiation necrosis).
- Computed tomography shows low-density white matter lesions that may exhibit mass effect or ringlike enhancement.
- Magnetic resonance imaging shows hyperintense white matter lesions on T2-weighted images and ringlike enhancement on postcontrast images.
- Lesions may be focal or diffuse. When a focal lesion is seen, differentiation from recurrent neoplasm may be difficult. Dual-isotope single-photon emission computed tomography (SPECT) and positron emission tomography (PET) may be helpful in some cases.

Radiation Injury ***Early Delayed Radiation Injury***

- Occurs most frequently in the second month postradiation and usually improves within 6 weeks.
- Pathologic studies show diffuse demyelination.
- Computed tomography shows transient low-density areas in white matter, basal ganglia, and cerebral peduncles.

- On MRI, there is transient low signal intensity on T1-weighted images and high signal intensity on T2-weighted images in the same areas as on CT.

Late Radiation Injury

- The latent period between radiation therapy and development of radiation necrosis is from 1 to 10 years.
- Changes related to late radiation injury may be focal or diffuse.
- Microscopically, arteriolar hyalinization and fibrinoid necrosis, demyelination, and coagulation necrosis are seen.
- Computed tomography shows focal or diffuse low density in the white matter. Contrast enhancement and mass effect may be seen in focal lesions.
- On MRI, there is focal or diffuse high signal intensity in the white matter of T2-weighted images. Contrast enhancement and mass effect may be seen in focal lesions.

Age-Related White Matter Lesions *Perivascular Spaces (Virchow-Robin Spaces)*

- An invagination of the subarachnoid space that accompanies the penetrating vessel from subarachnoid space into the brain parenchyma.
- Perivascular spaces contain cerebrospinal fluid (CSF) and show similar signal intensity as CSF in all sequences. Proton-density-weighted sequences may be useful to distinguish perivascular spaces from lesions, which generally show higher signal intensity than CSF.
- Perivascular spaces are found in the inferior one-third of the basal ganglia and high convexity; they tend to be round or ovoid in shape.

Periventricular and Subcortical Hyperintensity on T2-Weighted Images

- The extent of periventricular hyperintensity on T2-weighted images may vary from a thin rim of high signal intensity to an almost sheetlike area of high signal intensity extending to the corticomedullary junction.
- There is poor correlation between neurologic function and the extent of such periventricular white matter disease.
- Periventricular hyperintensity is accentuated in patients with ischemic white matter disease.
- It can mimic subependymal resorption of CSF in hydrocephalus.
- Subcortical white matter lesions were more useful than periventricular white matter lesions in distinguishing multi-infarct dementia from Alzheimer's disease. Subcortical hyperintensities are seen in all the patients with multi-infarct dementia and only in half of the patients with Alzheimer's disease.
- Binswanger's disease (subcortical arteriosclerotic encephalopathy) is a slowly evolving dementia with focal defects, hypertension, and multifocal white matter lesions on MRI.
- Pathologic examination of the white matter lesions may range from myelin pallor, perivascular demyelination, axonal loss, and gliosis to frank infarction. The most severe pathologic changes are consistent with Binswanger's disease.
- Sone 30 percent of patients over age 60 show periventricular high-signal lesions in the white matter on T2-weighted images.

AIDS-RELATED WHITE MATTER DISEASES

Human Immunodeficiency Virus

- Neurologic manifestations associated with human immunodeficiency virus (HIV) in the absence of opportunistic infection or neoplasm include encephalopathy, myelopathy, peripheral neuropathy, and myopathy.
- Approximately one-third of AIDS autopsies show evidence of viral encephalopathy.
- Subacute encephalitis secondary to HIV virus is the most common neurologic complication seen in AIDS.
- The HIV virus is not only lymphotropic but also neurotropic. It is seen in multinucleated giant cells or macrophages and polymorphic microglia.
- Findings on CT include atrophy and low-density white matter lesions.

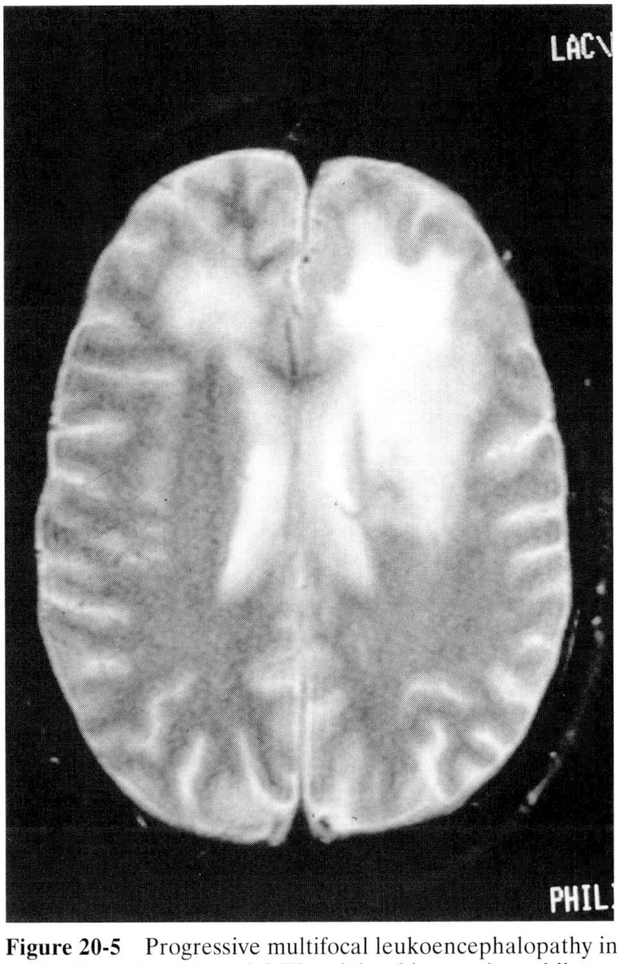

Figure 20-5 Progressive multifocal leukoencephalopathy in an AIDS patient. An axial T2-weighted image shows bilateral frontal periventricular areas of high signal intensity in the white matter, worse on the left side.

- Magnetic resonance imaging is more sensitive than CT in the evaluation of HIV encephalitis. High-signal-intensity lesions without mass effect are seen in the periventricular white matter diffusely or in a patchy pattern. Following administration of gadolinium, these lesions do not show enhancement.
- Cortical atrophy is the most common finding in AIDS encephalopathy on both CT and MRI.
- The clinical diagnosis of HIV encephalitis antedates significant radiologic findings of the disease.

Cytomegalovirus

- Cytomegalovirus (CMV) is latent in a large percentage of the adult population. Disseminated reactivation is seen in AIDS patients.
- Sites of reactivation include the respiratory, gastrointestinal, genitourinary, and hematopoietic systems in addition to the central nervous system.
- Neurologic manifestations of CMV infection include meningoencephalitis, cranial neuropathy, vasculitis, cerebral hemorrhage, subarachnoid hemorrhage, retinitis, myelitis, and peripheral neuropathy.
- White matter lesions related to CMV are seen in 15 to 30 percent of AIDS patients.
- Pathologically, intranuclear inclusions may be seen in ependymal cells, subependymal astrocytes, oligodendrocytes, endothelial cells, and neurons.
- The most common CT and MRI finding of CMV encephalitis is atrophy.
- Other CT findings include low-density white matter lesions, enhancing cortical nodules, and subependymal enhancement.
- On MRI, there are high-signal-intensity periventricular white matter lesions on T2-weighted images, which may be broad and nodular.
- Following gadolinium administration, MRI shows subependymal enhancement and periventricular enhancement.

Progressive Multifocal Leukoencephalopathy

- The etiologic agent is JC virus, a human polyomavirus.
- The JC virus is believed to infect up to 80 percent of the pediatric population without overt clinical symptoms.
- The latent JC virus is reactivated when the host is in an immunosuppressed state.
- The JC virus infects the oligodendrocytes, causing cytolytic destruction with resultant demyelination.
- Pathologically, swollen oligodendrocytes are seen at the periphery of demyelination. Intranuclear inclusion of JC virus can be identified on electron microscopy.
- Clinically, the disease is a progressive one with death commonly occurring within 9 months after the onset of symptoms.
- Computed tomography shows low-density lesions in the white matter, usually in the parietooccipital region. Scattered lesions may enlarge and become more confluent. Contrast enhancement or mass effect is not seen.
- Magnetic resonance imaging is more sensitive than CT in demonstrating white matter lesions.
- Magnetic resonance imaging shows high-signal-intensity lesions in the periventricular or subcortical white matter on T2-weighted images; this often progresses from small lesion(s) to larger extensive ones.
- Contrast enhancement is rare. When enhancement is seen, it is faint and in a ringlike pattern.
- White matter lesions are usually bilateral, but they may be unilateral and single.
- Parietooccipital and frontal locations are favored. The posterior fossa is involved in one-third of the cases.
- PML can also involve myelinated fibers in the deep gray matter, which could be detected on MRI.
- PML may be difficult to differentiate from HIV-related demyelination. White matter lesions in HIV-related encephalopathy are more diffuse and periventricular, whereas those in PML are more often multifocal, with a greater tendency for subcortical location.

SUGGESTED READINGS

Normal Myelination

1. Barkovich AJ et al: Normal maturation of the neonatal and infant brain: MR imaging at 1.5 T. *Radiology* 166:173–180, 1988.
2. Barkovich AJ et al: Formation, maturation, and disorders of white matter. *AJNR* 13:447–461, 1992.
3. Bird CR et al: MR assessment of myelination in infants and children: Usefulness of marker sites. *AJNR* 10:731–740, 1990.
4. Dietrich RB et al: MR evaluation of early myelination patterns in normal and developmentally delayed infants. *AJR* 150:889–896, 1988.
5. Holland BA et al: MRI of normal brain maturation. *AJNR* 7:201–208, 1986.

Pediatric White Matter Disease

1. Bewermeyer H et al: MR imaging in adrenoleukomyeloneuropathy. *J Comput Assist Tomogr* 9:793–796, 1985.
2. Bolthause E et al: MRI in Cockayne syndrome type I. *Neuroradiology* 31:276–277, 1989.
3. Borrett D, Becker LE: Alexander's disease. *Brain* 108:367–385, 1985.
4. Brismar J et al: Malignant hyperphenylalaninemia: CT and MR of the brain. *AJNR* 11:135, 1990.
5. Brismar J et al: Canavan disease: CT and MR of the brain. *AJNR* 11:805, 1990.
6. Geyer CA et al: Leigh disease (subacute necrotizing encephalopathy): CT and MR in five cases. *J Comput Assist Tomogr* 12:40, 1988.

7. Golden GS: Metabolic disorders, in Golden GS (ed): *Textbook of Pediatric Neurology*. New York, Plenum Press, 1987.
8. Goldfischer S et al: Peroxisomal defects in neonatal onset and X-linked adrenoleukodystrophies. *Science* 227:67–75, 1985.
9. Journel H et al: Magnetic resonance imaging in Pelizaeus-Merzbacher disease. *Neuroradiology* 29:403–405, 1987.
10. Lee BCP: Magnetic resonance imaging of metabolic and primary white matter disorders in children. *Neuroimaging Clin North Am* 3:267–289, 1993.
11. McAdams HP et al: CT and MR imaging of Canavan disease. *AJNR* 11:397, 1990.
12. Murata R et al: MR imaging of the brain in patients with mucopolysaccharidosis. *AJNR* 10:1165–1170, 1989.
13. Naidu S, Moser HW: Value of neuroimaging in metabolic disease affecting the CNS. *AJNR* 12:413–416, 1991.
14. Nowell MA et al: MR imaging of white matter disease in children. *AJNR* 9:503–509, 1988.
15. Silverstein AM et al: MR imaging of the brain in five members of a family with Peliazeus-Merzbacher. *AJNR* 9:493–499, 1990.
16. van der Knaap MS, Valk J: The reflection of histology in MR imaging of Pelizaeus-Merzbacher disease. *AJNR* 10:99, 1989.

Demyelinating and Other White Matter Diseases

1. Atlas SW et al: MR diagnosis of acute disseminated encephalomyelitis. *J Comput Assist Tomogr* 10:798–801, 1986.
2. Barkhof F et al: Quantitative MRI changes in gadolinium-DPTA enhancement after high dose intravenous methylprednisone in multiple sclerosis. *Neurology* 41:1219–1222, 1991.
3. Barnard RO, Triggs, M: Corpus callosum in multiple sclerosis. *J Neurol Neurosurg Psychiatry* 37:1259–1264, 1974.
4. Chrysikopoulos HS et al: Encephalitis caused by human immunodeficiency virus: CT and MR imaging manifestations with clinical and pathologic correlation. *Radiology* 175:185–191, 1990.
5. Drayer BP et al: Magnetic resonance imaging in multiple sclerosis: Decreased signal in thalamus and putamen. *Ann Neurol* 22:546–550, 1987.
6. Enzmann DR et al: CT of central nervous system infection in immunocompromised patients. *AJNR* 1:239–243, 1980.
7. Gean-Morton AD et al: Abnormal corpus callosum: A sensitive and specific indicator of multiple sclerosis. *Radiology* 180:215–221, 1991.
8. Giang DW et al: Multiple sclerosis masquerading as a mass lesion. *Neuroradiology* 34:150–154, 1992.
9. Grossman RI et al: Multiple sclerosis: Gadolinium enhancement in MR imaging. *Radiology* 161:721–725, 1986.
10. Guilleux MH et al: MR imaging in progressive multifocal leukoencephalopathy. *AJNR* 7:1033–1035, 1986.
11. Heinz ER et al: Computed tomography in white matter disease. *Radiology* 130:371–378, 1979.
12. Koch KJ, Smith RR: GD-DTPA enhancement in MR imaging of central pontine myelinolysis. *AJNR* 10:558, 1989.
13. Lee KH et al: Magnetic resonance imaging of the head in the diagnosis of multiple sclerosis: A prospective 2-year follow-up with comparison of clinical evaluation, evoked potentials, oligoclonal banding, and CT. *Neurology* 41:657–660, 1991.
14. Simon JH et al: Corpus callosum and subcallosal-periventricular lesions in multiple sclerosis: Detection with MR. *Radiology* 160:363–367, 1986.
15. Simon JH et al: Quantitative determination of MS-induced corpus callosum atrophy in vivo using MR imaging. *AJNR* 8:599–604, 1987.
16. Smith RR: Central pontine myelinolysis. *Neuroimaging Clin North Am* 3:319–329, 1993.
17. Whitman MLH et al: AIDS-related white matter diseases. *Neuroimaging Clin North Am* 3:331–359, 1993.

☐ QUESTIONS (True or False)

1. Regarding normal myelination,
   - **a.** Approximately 90 percent of the myelination process takes place by the age of 2 years.
   - **b.** The composition of myelin is 70 to 80 percent lipid and 20 to 30 percent protein.
   - **c.** The process of myelination goes from cephalad to caudad, anterior to posterior, and peripheral to central.
   - **d.** Myelin is produced by oligodendrocytes.
   - **e.** The sensory fibers myelinate earlier than motor fiber tracts.
2. Regarding adrenoleukodystrophy,
   - **a.** It is X-linked.
   - **b.** It is the most common disorder and involves multiple enzymes.
   - **c.** Diagnosis is made by detecting of very long chain fatty acids in the blood and skin fibroblasts.
   - **d.** It presents in boys between the ages of 4 to 8.
   - **e.** It characteristically involves the posterior portion of the hemisphere—the occipital lobes and visual pathway.
3. Metachromatic leukodystrophy
   - **a.** Is an autosomal recessive disorder due to deficiency of arylsulfatase A.
   - **b.** Is seen in two forms: the early infantile form and the juvenile/adult form.
   - **c.** Is associated with nonspecific white matter hyperintensity on T2-weighted images.
   - **d.** Includes cerebellar involvement.
   - **e.** Causes severe ventricular enlargement.
4. Leigh's disease
   - **a.** Is an autosomal recessive defect in pyruvate metabolism.
   - **b.** Involves a single enzyme.
   - **c.** Is associated with increased signal on T2-weighted images in the putamen, caudate, and tegmentum.
   - **d.** Shows contrast enhancement during the acute stages.
   - **e.** Causes pathologic changes similar to those of Wernicke's encephalopathy.
5. Regarding multiple sclerosis,
   - **a.** Most lesions occur at the periventricular white matter and corpus callosum.
   - **b.** Pathologically, macrophages with foamy cytoplasm resulting from the phagocytosis of myelin breakdown products are seen.
   - **c.** Atrophy of corpus callosum is not seen.

d. Enhancement of optic nerves may be seen on gadolinium-enhanced, fat-suppressed MRI images.
e. Spinal cord lesions may mimic neoplasm with cord enlargement.

6. Regarding acute disseminated encephalomyelitis,
a. It is a viral infection.
b. It is more commonly seen in children than in adults.
c. Optic neuritis can be seen.
d. Long-term follow-up is necessary to exclude multiple sclerosis.
e. Both cerebral and cerebellar white matter may be involved.

7. Regarding progressive multifocal leukoencephalopathy,
a. It is caused by JC virus.
b. It is more common in males than females.
c. Computed tomography frequently shows ringlike enhancement.
d. There is a predilection for the parietal and occipital lobes.
e. The spinal cord is rarely involved.

8. The differential diagnosis for central pontine myelinolysis on imaging includes:
a. Pontine infarct
b. Multiple sclerosis
c. Lyme disease
d. Brainstem glioma
e. Marchiafava-Bignami disease

9. Regarding HIV encephalopathy,
a. On postmortem studies, evidence of viral encephalopathy is found in one-third of AIDS patients.
b. HIV virus is not only lymphotropic but also neurotropic.
c. Atrophy is a common finding.
d. White matter lesions may show intense contrast enhancement.
e. It is underestimated by CT or MRI.

10. Macrocephaly is associated with
a. Canavan's disease
b. Alexander's disease
c. Neonatal adrenoleukodystrophy
d. Krabbe's disease
e. Mucopolysaccharidoses

☐ ANSWERS

1. **a.** T
b. T
c. F
d. T
e. T

2. **a.** T
b. F
c. T
d. T
e. T

3. **a.** T
b. T
c. T
d. T
e. F

4. **a.** T
b. F
c. T
d. T
e. T

5. **a.** T
b. T
c. F
d. T
e. T

6. **a.** F
b. T
c. T
d. T
e. T

7. **a.** T
b. T
c. F
d. T
e. T

8. **a.** T
b. T
c. T
d. T
e. F

9. **a.** T
b. T
c. T
d. F
e. T

10. **a.** T
b. T
c. F
d. T
e. T

CHAPTER

21

Degenerative, Toxic, and Metabolic Diseases

Lawrence N. Tanenbaum

☐ NORMAL AGING BRAIN

Changes characteristic of normal aging can be appreciated on imaging examinations. Many of these imaging features overlap with findings seen in neurodegenerative disorders.

BRAIN VOLUME

There is a mild to moderate progressive loss of brain volume, along with dilatation of the ventricles, cisterns, and sulci with aging.

WHITE MATTER SIGNAL

Some white matter hyperintense foci are physiologic and are found in young patients (terminal areas of myelination surrounding the trigones of the lateral ventricles) or in all ages (hyperintensity of the posterior internal capsule, ependymitis granularis, demyelination, gliosis, and increased interstitial fluid adjacent to the frontal horns of the lateral ventricles). Senescent white matter hyperintensities on intermediate (proton density) and T2-weighted magnetic resonance images (MRI) typically involve the periventricular white matter, optic radiations, basal ganglia, centrum semiovale, and brainstem, in decreasing order of frequency. The lesions are mildly hypointense on T1-weighted images and do not enhance. These areas of white matter signal alteration are seen in healthy elderly patients with normal cognitive function (25 to 50 percent of unselected patients over age 60), and prevalence increases with age. Similar areas of decreased attenuation are commonly seen on CT in the elderly. Neuropathologic studies indicate different processes in different individuals (e.g., incomplete to frank infarction, gliosis in association with vascular hyalinization, myelin pallor or Virchow-Robin (dilated perivascular) spaces.

IRON DEPOSITION

The extrapyramidal gray matter nuclei become hypointense on long TR/TE (repetition time/echo time) sequences with normal aging, in many neurodegenerative states, and in a variety of other pathologic processes including demyelinating and dysmyelinating processes and infarction. There is a progressive increase in brain ferric iron, most likely due to the deposition of ferritin, through childhood until adult levels are reached at about age 25, with relative hypointensity on T2-weighted MRI of the pallidum, red nucleus, and the pars reticulata of the substantia nigra. The dentate nuclei become hypointense more slowly and inconsistently, with only one-third of patients' nuclei being hypointense relative to white matter at age 25. With further aging, the striatum progresses in hypointensity and may match that of the pallidum by the eighth decade.

PHYSIOLOGY

With aging, little or no change in glucose utilization is evident on positron emission tomography (PET). There are no definitive MRI spectroscopic changes associated with aging. There have been controversial reports of alterations in cerebral blood flow on single photon emission computed tomography (SPECT).

☐ DEMENTIAS

In dementia, intellectual and higher integrative facilities are impaired, interfering with the activities of daily living. The prevalence of dementia in the elderly population is estimated to be approximately 15 percent, with an incidence rate of 187 new cases per 100,000 population per year. The prevalence of severe dementia increases with age, from 1 percent at 65 years to 15 percent at 85 years. Cortical dementias, including Alzheimer's and Pick's diseases, cause cortical symptoms such as agnosia, apraxia, amnesia, abnormal cognition, and abnormal affect—classically, disinhibition. Subcortical dementias, resulting from diseases producing dysfunction in the basal ganglia, thalamus, and brainstem, include the extrapyramidal syndromes, hydrocephalus, and white matter disorders. The subcortical dementias tend to manifest with motor symptoms, forgetfulness, slowing of cognition, and abnormal affect—classically, depression. Mixed dementias include conditions that involve cortical and subcortical structures. Examples include vascular dementia and Creutzfeld-Jakob disease. Neuroimaging should be performed in patients in whom a potentially treatable structural disorder is suspected, in whom neurologic signs or symptoms suggest other diseases causing or superimposed on dementia, or in whom there is an acute onset or abrupt deterioration of dementia.

ALZHEIMER'S DISEASE

Alzheimer's disease (AD) is a disorder characterized by insidious onset of cortical dementia with progressive deterioration of memory and global cognitive function. The biochemical pathogenesis is still unknown. Alzheimer's disease is the most common cause of dementia, with a prevalence of up to 6 percent among persons above age 65; it may account for one-half to three-quarters of dementias in the elderly. With an incidence rate of 123 new cases per 100,000 per year, AD has become the fourth leading cause of death in the United States. Men and women are affected equally. There is a familial form of early-onset AD that may be inherited in an autosomal dominant fashion. The course of illness usually extends over 5 or more years.

Neuropathology Autopsy diagnostic criteria for AD are based on the identification of neurofibrillary tangles and senile plaques in appropriate density and distribution in the hippocampus and neocortex, considering the age of the patient, in the setting of a clear clinical history of dementia. Amyloid B peptide deposition is seen in the brain parenchyma and meningeal blood vessels, along with extensive neuronal loss. Lower brain volumes, larger ventricles, and greater sulcal cerebrospinal fluid (CSF) volumes are seen in Alzheimer's disease than in age-matched populations.

Imaging

- Alzheimer's disease is characterized by central and cortical atrophy, particularly involving the hippocampus and anterior temporal lobe. The atrophy is more severe and more rapidly progressive than in normal aging.
- Also noted in AD is gyral hypointensity on T2-weighted MRI in the posterior frontal and anterior parietal cortex, possibly due to iron deposition.
- Some AD patients demonstrate T2 hyperintense sylvian and/or hippopcampal-uncal cortex. Periventricular white matter and, less commonly, subcortical lesions on CT and MRI occur more often than in elderly controls but probably less often than in multiple infarct dementia (MID) patients.
- In fact, the absence or mild extent of hyperintense white matter lesions on MRI in a demented individual favors the diagnosis of AD over MID.

Decreased *N*-acetylaspartate (NAA) and increased myoinositol have been reported on proton MRI spectroscopy in AD. An often striking pattern of hypometabolism on fluorodeoxyglucose (FDG) PET in the parietal, followed by temporal and, later, frontal lobes is commonly noted. Cerebral SPECT blood-flow studies show a characteristic reduction in flow in the same distribution as PET metabolic abnormalities. This can be useful in distinguishing Alzheimer's disease from multi-infarct dementia and pseudodementia due to depression. Positron emission tomography may be more sensitive than CT or MRI, and abnormalities may be observed before clinically significant cognitive defects appear.

MULTI-INFARCT DEMENTIA (VASCULAR DEMENTIA)

Multi-infarct dementia (MID) and AD are the most common causes of age-related dementia. Multi-infarct dementia is the cause of an estimated 10 percent of dementias, increasing in prevalence with advancing age. A recent U.S. study found dementia in 26 percent of ischemic stroke survivors over 60 years of age. Vascular dementia is classified as dementia resulting from ischemic and hemorrhagic brain lesions as well as from cerebral ischemic-hypoxic lesions such as those due to cardiac arrest. A wide spectrum of findings is seen in vascular dementia, including infarction, demyelination, myelin pallor, arteriolar hyalinization and sclerosis, lacunar infarcts, and dilated perivascular spaces (*etat crible*). Definitive diagnosis is complicated by the uncertainty of whether the presence of stroke in a demented patient is the cause of the dementia, a contributing factor to underlying degenerative dementia, or simply an unrelated event.

- There are no pathognomonic CT or MRI findings. There is significant overlap with the imaging appearance of the aging brain and AD.
- Extensive periventricular hyperintensity with subcortical lesions, cortical infarcts, and lacunar infarcts of the basal ganglia in a patient with dementia favors the diagnosis of MID over AD.

PICK'S DISEASE (LOBAR ATROPHY)

Pick's disease is a rare primary cortical dementia, 10 to 15 times less common than AD, and it may occur in a younger population. Women are probably more commonly affected than men. Pick's disease may be difficult to differentiate clinically from the cortical dementia associated with AD. Neuropathology reveals frontal and temporal atrophy with neuronal loss, gliosis, demyelination, swollen neurons, and Pick's bodies.

Computed tomography (CT) and MRI examinations demonstrate selective frontal and/or temporal lobe atrophy, often so severe that the lobes may appear icicle- or knifelike. There is usually sparing of the posterior two-thirds of the superior temporal gyrus, with striking atrophy anterior to this location and sparing posterior to it. Caudate atrophy, often noted in Pick's disease, may be useful in distinguishing this condition from AD. Magnetic resonance imaging also demonstrates mild hyperintensity on long-TR sequences within the cortex and adjacent white matter of the affected lobes, while FDG PET demonstrates hypometabolism in the caudate nucleus as well as the frontal and anterior temporal lobes with sparing of the posterior brain. Imaging by SPECT has shown frontal hypoperfusion.

NORMAL-PRESSURE HYDROCEPHALUS

Normal-pressure hydrocephalus (NPH) is thought to result most commonly from previous hemorrhage or meningeal infection resulting in interference with absorption of cerebrospinal fluid (CSF). In a second theory, ischemic damage to the periventricular white matter or edema decreases the tensile strength of the ventricular walls and leads to ventricular dilatation. Symptomatic NPH is uncommon before age 60 and increases in frequency thereafter. The classic clinical triad of normal-pressure hydrocephalus (NPH) is subcortical dementia, sphincteric incontinence, and a slowly progressive gait disorder. Symptoms may be progressive and can be reversible with shunting; therefore it is critical to distinguish patients who are likely to respond. Clinical improvement after lumbar puncture with CSF removal strengthens the diagnosis of NPH and favors the possibility that shunting will be beneficial.

The findings of reflux and stasis on isotope cisternography are insufficiently specific for NPH and are disappointing as predictors of positive outcome after ventricular shunting. Differentiation of atrophy due to aging or neurodegenerative processes from NPH on CT or MRI is difficult. The following MRI features may be helpful to diagnose hydrocephalus with or without concomitant atrophy in the elderly:

1. Ventricular enlargement dominant over sulcal enlargement
2. Rounding of the frontal horns
3. Prominence of the temporal horns
4. Thinning and elevation of the corpus callosum seen on sagittal images
5. Dilatation of the optic and infundibular recesses of the anterior third ventricle and downward displacement of the hypothalamus
6. Accentuation of the aqueductal and third ventricular flow void
7. Prominent periventricular hyperintensity on long-TR images

The combination of these findings with stasis and reflux on cisternography may improve the selection of patients who may benefit from shunt therapy.

CREUTZFELD-JAKOB DISEASE (SPONGIFORM ENCEPHALOPATHY)

Creutzfeld-Jakob disease is a transmissible disease caused by a small proteinaceous particle known as a prion, with an incidence of about one per million per year. The disease is characterized by a rapidly progressive mixed dementia associated with cerebellar ataxia, muscular rigidity, and myoclonus; it is invariably fatal, with an average course after symptoms develop of less than a year. The average age at onset is between 40 and 80 years. At pathology, there is diffuse cerebral atrophy without inflammation. Microscopically, widespread neuronal loss and gliosis accompanied by spongiform changes are seen.

Imaging

- Because the disease is rapidly progressive, CT and MRI are usually normal.
- Rarely, progressive severe atrophy may be seen.
- Occasionally, abnormal T2 hyperintensity can be seen in the gray matter of the striatum, thalamus, and cortex. The white matter is usually spared.
- Scans by FDG PET have shown severe diffuse hypometabolism when CT findings have been unremarkable.

☐ EXTRAPYRAMIDAL SYSTEM AND MOVEMENT DISORDERS

The most prominent responsibility of the extrapyramidal nuclei is mediation and control of the corticospinal tract. Lesions will therefore manifest as movement disorders such as impaired voluntary movements, abnormal muscle tone, and involuntary movements as well as abnormal postures and postural reflexes.

The striatum (caudate and putamen) plays a role in the activation and inhibition of certain voluntary and automatic muscle activity through a prefrontal cortico-striatal-pallidal-thalamic-motor cortical circuit. Removal of striatal influence causes choreoathetosis. Additional involvement of the pallidal and thalamic connections predisposes to rigidity and, when severe, to dystonia. Lesions of the globus pallidus can result in akinesia, rigidity, dystonia, and postural disorders. Selective pallidal necrosis is considered a hallmark of hypoxic-ischemic insults of various origins, such as carbon monoxide poisoning. Lesions of the subthalamic nucleus within the peduncular part of the internal capsule typically result in contralateral hemiballismus. The substantia nigra can be divided into the pars compacta, implicated in parkinsonian syndromes, and the pars reticulata, involved in Hallervorden-Spatz disease.

HUNTINGTON'S DISEASE

Huntington's disease is a neurodegenerative disease characterized by progressive choreoathetosis, psychological/behavioral changes, and subcortical dementia. It is an inherited disease with autosomal dominant transmission and complete penetrance, with the defective gene locus on chromosome 4. The disease occurs in approximately four to five per million people and the usual age of onset is the fourth to fifth decades. Once begun, the disease is relentless, with an average time from onset to death of 17 years.

Neuropathologic studies demonstrate caudate atrophy and neuronal loss, with less severe changes in the globus pallidus and putamen.

- Computed tomography and MRI demonstrate diffuse cortical atrophy as well as characteristic atrophy of the caudate and, somewhat less often, of the putamen (Fig. 21-1*A*).
- The bicaudate ratio (the ratio between the minimum distance between the caudate indentations of the frontal horns and the distance between the inner tables of the skull along the same line) has been shown to be a specific and sensitive tool in diagnosing Huntington's disease.
- The striatum may demonstrate gliosis-related increased signal on T2-weighted MRI, or decreased signal due to iron deposition.

Abnormalities on ^{31}P MR spectroscopy have been reported. FDG PET may show characteristic relative hypometabolism in the striatum, especially the caudate nucleus, which may or may not be associated with frontal lobe hypometabolism (Fig. 21-1*B*). The caudate hypometabolism is seen in patients with florid Huntington's disease and precedes the onset of clinically evident chorea in family members at risk.

HALLERVORDEN-SPATZ DISEASE

Hallervorden-Spatz disease is a rare metabolic neurologic disorder characterized clinically by progressive dystonia, choreoathetosis, dysarthria, dysphasia, mental deterioration, and retinal degeneration. Approximately 50 percent of cases are familial with autosomal recessive transmission. Onset is typically in the second decade. At neuropathology, there is deposition of iron in the basal ganglia with pallidal demyelination, neuronal loss, neuroaxonal dystrophy, and gliosis.

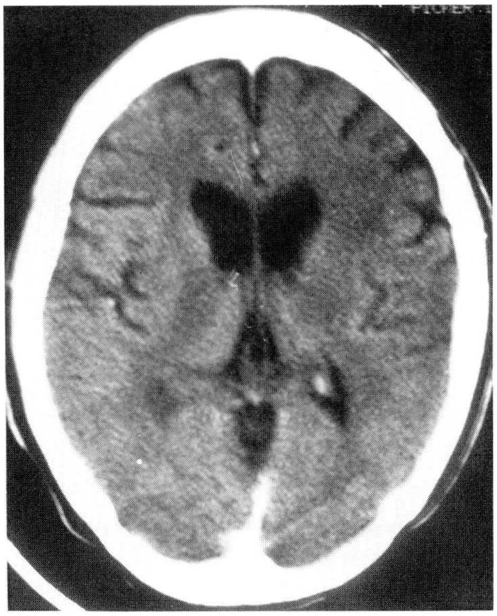

(A)

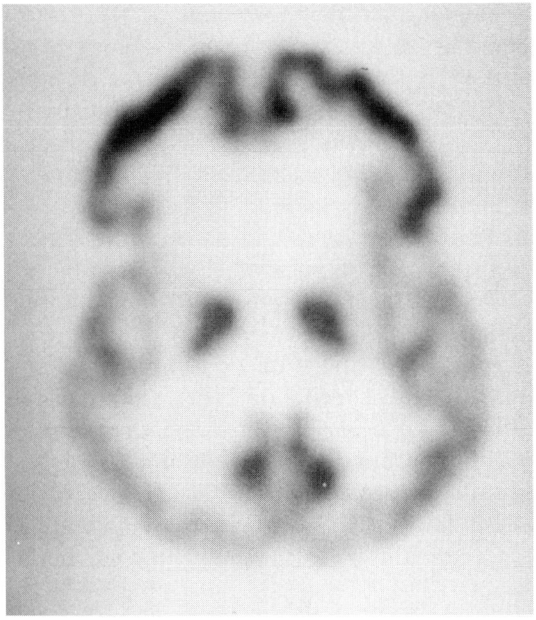

(B)

Figure 21-1 Huntington's disease. *A*. Axial CT scan shows atrophy of the head of the caudate nucleus bilaterally with focal dilatation of both frontal horns of the lateral ventricles. *B*. Axial FDG PET scan shows characteristic relative hypometabolism in the striatum, especially in the caudate nucleus. (Courtesy of Burton Drayer, MD.)

Diffuse hypointensity of the globus pallidus on T2-weighted MRI (due to iron deposition) is characteristic of Hallervorden-Spatz disease. A globus pallidus "target" or "eye of the tiger" sign has been described with gliosis related T2 high signal, surrounding a focus of hypointensity. A second subtype of this disease exists in which there is associated involvement of the red nucleus and pars reticulata of the substantia nigra. A similar appearance can be seen with hypothyroidism.

LEIGH'S DISEASE (SUBACUTE NECROTIZING ENCEPHALOMYELOPATHY)

Leigh's disease is a rare inherited neurodegenerative disease, usually transmitted in an autosomal recessive fashion, with an episodic or chronic, progressive clinical course. The age of onset of symptoms is typically less than 2 years, but juvenile and unusual adult forms exist. There is no known effective treatment. Death usually occurs within a few years after the onset of symptoms, typically from respiratory failure.

The defect is caused by a deficiency of either the mitochondrial enzyme cytochrome-*c* oxidase, pyruvate decarboxylase, or pyruvate dehydrogenase complex. Laboratory analysis shows metabolic acidosis with elevated blood and CSF lactate and pyruvate concentrations. Pathologic findings overlap with Wernicke's encephalopathy, with sparing of the mamillary bodies a key differentiating feature. The disease is characterized by capillary proliferation with bilaterally symmetrical gray and white matter necrosis, spongiform degeneration, and demyelination.

Imaging

- Nonenhancing hypodensities are identified on CT; MRI demonstrates T1 hypointensities and T2 hyperintensities. Some CT/MRI lesions may resolve over time.
- The most common lesion sites include the brainstem tegmentum, spinal cord, basal ganglia (particularly the putamen), and optic pathways, in descending order of frequency.

MITOCHONDRIAL ENCEPHALOMYELOPATHIES

The mitochondrial encephalomyelopathies are a group of disorders that have in common mitochondrial abnormalities resulting in multisystem disorders, including the central and peripheral nervous systems, skeletal muscles, heart, endocrine glands, gastrointestinal tract, hematopoietic system, and kidneys. These disorders include mitochondrial cytopathy, mitochondrial myopathy, Kearns-Sayre syndrome, MERRLA (myoclonus, epilepsy, ragged red fibers, and lactic acidosis), MERRF, and MELAS (mitochondrial myopathy, lactic acidosis, and stroke). There is heterogeneity and overlap with respect to clinical, pathologic, and imaging features.

Presentation is usually during childhood but may occur in adulthood. Typical clinical features include short stature, dementia, weakness, sensorineural hearing loss, and serum lactic acidosis. The MELAS syndrome can be differentiated by the presence of cortical blindness and hemiparesis and the absence of ophthalmoplegia, heart block, and nystagmus.

On imaging examinations, MELAS syndrome demonstrates bilateral infarctlike lesions that may not be strictly confined to vascular territories (Fig. 21-2). Common sites of involvement are the basal ganglia; parietal, occipital, and temporal lobes; and cerebellar hemispheres. The frontal lobes and brainstem are typically spared. Basal ganglia, cerebellum, brainstem, and spinal cord lesions are seen with MERRF.

WILSON'S DISEASE (HEPATOLENTICULAR DEGENERATION)

Wilson's disease is an autosomal recessive inherited condition resulting from defective genetic expression at a locus on chromosome 13. There is a prevalence of 1:30,000, with the age at presentation usually between 10 and 40 years and peak incidence between 8 and 16 years.

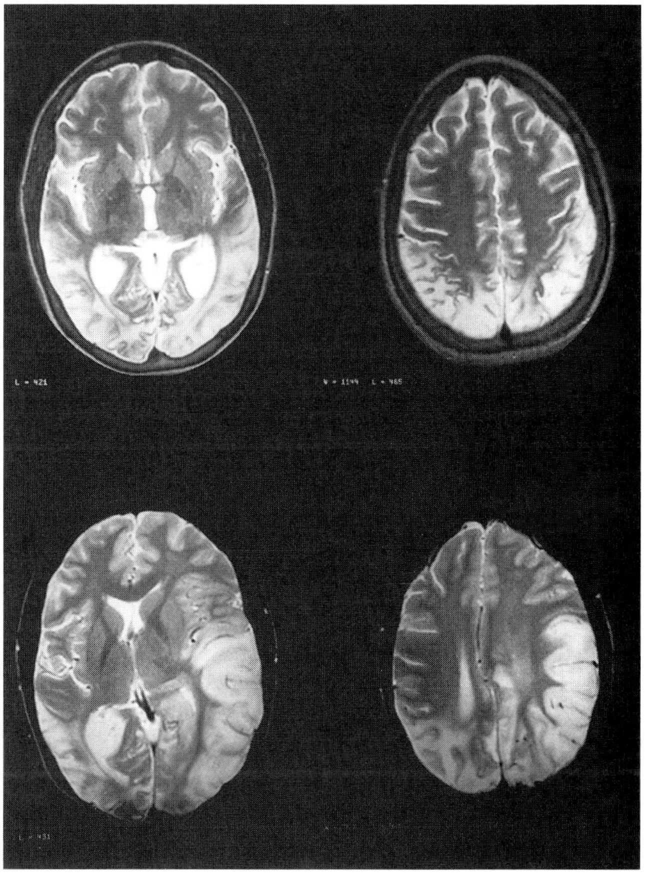

Figure 21-2 MELAS (mitochondrial myopathy, lactic acidosis, and stroke). T2-weighted axial images show bilateral infarctlike lesions involving the parietal, occipital, and temporal lobes. (Top row shows chronic change; bottom row shows acute change.)

Wilson's disease is characterized by a deficiency of ceruloplasmin, the serum transport protein for copper. As a result, copper is abnormally deposited in various tissues, with pronounced involvement of the brain (typically of the lentiform nucleus) and liver, with resultant toxicity to these organs (hence the term *hepatolenticular degeneration*). Typical neurologic signs of Wilson's disease are rigidity, tremor, dystonia, gait difficulty, incoordination, difficulty with fine motor tasks, and dysarthria. Hepatic encephalopathy, due to superimposed hepatic dysfunction, may influence neurologic signs. Ocular Kayser-Fleischer rings and copper deposits within the cornea are virtually diagnostic of Wilson's disease and are present in over 90 percent of patients. Definitive diagnosis is made biochemically with low levels of serum ceruloplasmin, increased rate of urinary copper excretion, and elevated hepatic copper levels. At neuropathology, atrophy, gliosis, edema, necrosis, and copper deposition are seen in the lentiform nuclei.

Imaging

- Early diagnosis is essential, since effective treatment with copper chelating agents can prevent disastrous neurologic damage.
- Low-density areas within the basal ganglia, cerebellar nuclei, brainstem, and white matter are often seen with CT.
- Both CT and MRI may show atrophy of the caudate nuclei and brainstem.
- Findings on MRI correlate well with clinical neurologic deficits. Symmetrical MRI T2 signal hyperintensity is present in the caudate, putamen, midbrain, and pons, presumably due to gliosis and edema. Asymmetrical areas of increased T2 signal can be seen in the white matter, most commonly in the frontal lobes.
- Characteristic irregular areas of T2 hypointensity are frequently seen within the caudate and putamen, most likely representing iron accumulation related to copper deposition. Copper itself is only minimally paramagnetic and does not contribute significantly to the signal changes on MRI (Fig. 21-3).

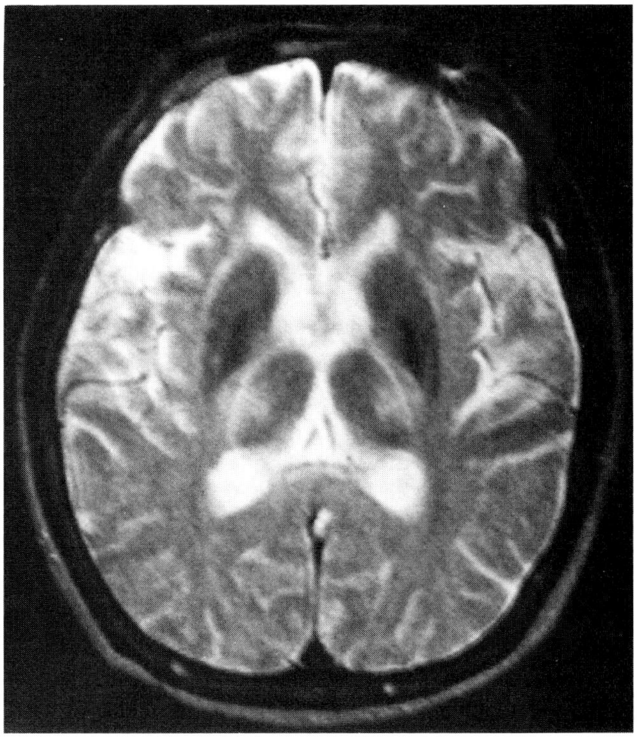

Figure 21-3 Wilson's disease. T2-weighted axial image shows predominantly hypointensity with small areas of hyperintensity in putamen and thalamus bilaterally.

PARKINSONISM

Parkinsonism is a clinical term for the neurologic abnormalities that result from malfunction of the major efferent projection of the substantia nigra (i.e., the nigrostriatal tract). The cell bodies of this dopaminergic system are in the pars compacta of the substantia nigra, and its axons ascend to the striatum. Primary parkinsonian syndromes include Parkinson's disease, progressive supranuclear palsy, and striatonigral degeneration. Secondary parkinsonism occurs as a result of brain injury by infarction, infection, or trauma; it can also be drug- or toxin-induced. The most important role of the imaging examination in parkinsonism is the exclusion of treatable causes of bradykinesia such as tumor, hematoma, or hydrocephalus.

PARKINSON'S DISEASE (PARALYSIS AGITANS)

Idiopathic Parkinson's disease is the most common movement disorder, affecting approximately 1 percent of the U.S. population over 50 years of age. The onset is typically between ages 50 and 60. The typical clinical presentation includes masked facies, cogwheel rigidity, shuffling gait, and a pill-rolling tremor. Dementia is commonly associated and can be identified in 20 to 90 percent of patients, increasing in prevalence with the severity and duration of the disease.

Parkinson's disease is a primary disorder of the pars compacta of the substantia nigra. Neuropathology demonstrates gliosis, Lewy body formation, and loss of neurons in the substantia nigra (especially the pars compacta), the locus ceruleus, the dorsal nucleus of the vagus, and the substantia innominata.

Imaging

- The most common MRI finding in individuals with Parkinson's disease is nonspecific, generalized enlargement of the cortical sulci and lateral ventricles, which overlaps with the normal changes of aging.
- In certain individuals with Parkinson's disease, characteristic narrowing of the pars compacta of the substantia nigra is seen, with indistinctness at the border between the substantia nigra and the red nucleus.

- The narrowing of the pars compacta, which is also seen in progressive supranuclear palsy and striatonigral degeneration, reflects neuronal loss of the pars compacta and iron deposition. The signal changes may be more prominent in patients who respond poorly to drug therapy, but they do not correlate with disease duration or severity.
- Classic idiopathic, L-dopa–responsive patients with Parkinson's disease, in contrast to other parkinsonian syndromes, do not have an increase in putaminal iron deposition (i.e., the globus pallidus is lower in signal on T2-weighted images than is the putamen).
- Examination by PET with ^{18}F-fluorodopa (FD) demonstrates decreased striatal uptake proportional to the number of dopaminergic neurons present and to the severity of clinical motor deficit. Since it has been shown that symptoms will not develop until 50 percent of dopaminergic neurons and 90 percent of striatal dopamine are lost, it may be possible to diagnose early or relatively asymptomatic Parkinson's disease with ^{18}F-FD PET.

PROGRESSIVE SUPRANUCLEAR PALSY

Progressive supranuclear palsy is a primary parkinsonian syndrome in which pseudobulbar symptoms are additionally present. The disease usually begins in the sixth or seventh decade with death occurring in 2 to 12 years. The clinical hallmark is paralysis of vertical gaze, especially downgaze (central ophthalmoplegia). Symptoms include axial rigidity with neck extension, pseudobulbar palsy, extrapyramidal symptoms, and occasional dementia. At pathology, there is neuronal loss with neurofibrillary tangles in the basal ganglia (particularly the pallidum), brainstem, and cerebellum. Nerve cell loss, gliosis, granulovacuolar changes, and atypical neurofibrillary tangles are present in the pontomesencephalic tegmentum, tectum, vestibular nuclei, striatum, and dentate nuclei.

Magnetic resonance imaging may demonstrate focal atrophy of the midbrain structures. Some patients may show T2 hypointensity and atrophy of the superior colliculi. Gliosis-related T2 hyperintensity may be seen in the periaqueductal region. As in other primary parkinsonian syndromes, there is evidence of excess iron deposition in the pars compacta of the substantia nigra, manifest as narrowing on T2-weighted images.

MULTIPLE SYSTEM ATROPHY (PARKINSON-PLUS DISORDERS)

Drug-unresponsive patients with parkinsonian symptoms are often classified as having multiple system atrophies (MSA) or Parkinson-plus disorders. Patients manifest parkinsonian features with involvement of additional systems (autonomic nervous system, extrapyramidal nuclei). The MSA syndrome is about one-fifth as common as Parkinson's disease. Three pathologic entities are generally classified as part of the multiple system atrophy grouping:

1. Olivopontocerebellar degeneration (OPCD)
2. Striatonigral degeneration (SND)
3. Shy-Drager syndrome (SDS)

Each entity can occur alone or in combination in MSA.

In SND there are prominent symptoms of rigidity. Pathology shows striatal atrophy due to neuronal loss, with greater involvement of the putamen. On MRI, generalized cortical atrophy along with putaminal hypointensity are demonstrated; the degree of these correlates with the severity of rigidity. The hypointensity is surrounded by high signal, presumably due to gliosis and/or cell loss. As in other primary parkinsonian syndromes, there is narrowing of the pars compacta of the substantia nigra, presumably reflecting neural loss and iron deposition.

Shy-Drager syndrome is characterized by autonomic system failure (orthostatic hypotension, urinary incontinence, and inability to sweat). Pathology shows neuronal loss and gliosis in the substantia nigra and intermediolateral column of the spinal cord. An MRI of pure SDS may be normal; however, in MSA there will be typical changes of SND and/or OPCD.

Prominent MRI T2 signal hypointensity, most likely related to abnormal iron accumulation, may be visualized in the putamen, and often the caudate nucleus, in 85 percent of individuals with MSA. As in other primary parkinsonian syndromes, there is narrowing of the pars compacta of the substantia nigra, presumably reflecting neuronal loss and iron deposition. Multiple system atrophies generally exhibit hypometabolism in the striatum and thalamus on PET, in association with generalized cerebellar hypometabolism. Less severe hypometabolism has been identified within the cerebral cortex. In straightforward Parkinson's disease, FDG PET is normal. Impaired nigrostriatal pathway function manifests as decreased ^{18}F-FD uptake in the striatum on PET in SND and SDS.

☐ SPINOCEREBELLAR DEGENERATION

The general term *spinocerebellar degeneration* describes a diverse group of heredofamilial disorders in which ataxia may be a prominent neurologic finding.

OLIVOPONTOCEREBELLAR DEGENERATION

Olivopontocerebellar degeneration (OPCD) occurs in inherited and sporadic forms. The onset varies between early childhood and old age, with a duration of illness of between 10 and 20 years. Manifestations common to all cerebellar atrophies include ataxia, which begins in the legs, followed by the arms and hands and bulbar musculature. The primary degeneration in OPCD centers in the pontine nuclei, leading to progressive anterograde myelin sheath loss and gliosis in the transverse pontocerebellar fibers and the cerebellar cortex. The cortical lesions cause retrograde degeneration of the inferior olives. Striatonigral degeneration and/or Shy-Drager syndrome may coexist with OPCD in MSA.

Imaging

- Neuroimaging findings are essential in the diagnosis of OPCD, since there is significant overlap of the clinical symptoms and signs with those of other cerebellar diseases.
- Atrophy is appreciable, involving the cerebellum, pons, and brachium pontis. Pontine atrophy is often so prominent that the anterior pons has a wedge shape. Olivary atrophy is appreciable as a loss of the normal contour bulge (Figure 21-4).
- Proton-density increased signal and T2 decreased signal intensity are observed in the transverse pontine fibers, cerebellum, and brachium pontis, sparing the adjacent uninvolved tegmentum, pyramidal tracts, and superior cerebellar peduncles.

FRIEDREICH'S ATAXIA

Friedreich's ataxia is the most common idiopathic cerebellar ataxia, inherited in autosomal recessive and dominant forms. The gene defect is located on chromosome 9. Symptoms—which develop from age 18 months to 24 years—consist of progressive gait ataxia, arm clumsiness,

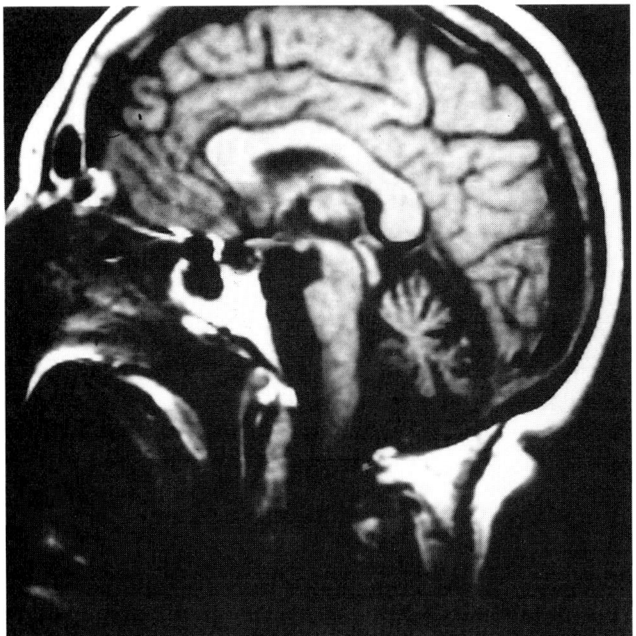

Figure 21-4 Olivopontocerebellar degeneration. Sagittal T1-weighted image shows severe atrophy of brain stem, especially the pons and cerebellum.

and dysarthria. Pes cavus, due to degeneration of the posterior columns, and kyphoscoliosis, a result of spinal muscular imbalance, are characteristic features. Ambulation is typically lost within 5 years of onset, and the mean age of death ranges from 25 to 40 years. Pathology and MRI reveal spinal cord atrophy due to demyelination and gliosis of the posterior columns and roots and of the spinocerebellar and corticospinal tracts. Cerebellar atrophy is variably present and mild, which may serve as a useful differentiating feature from primary cerebellar degenerative processes.

☐ MOTOR NEURON DISEASES

Motor neuron diseases are a heterogeneous group of syndromes in which the upper and/or lower motor neurons degenerate.

AMYOTROPHIC LATERAL SCLEROSIS

Amyotrophic lateral sclerosis (ALS) is the most frequent type of motor neuron disease, with an annual incidence rate of 0.4 to 17.6 per 100,000. Most patients are 40 years of age or older at the onset of symptoms and the incidence increases with age. About 10 percent of cases are familial, with autosomal dominant inheritance. Amyotrophic lateral sclerosis is a chronic, slowly or rapidly progressive degenerative disease of unknown etiology, characterized pathologically by progressive loss of motor neurons in the spinal cord, brainstem, and motor cortex. Patients present with upper or lower motor neuron symptoms and signs in bulbar or spinal innervated muscles, with most cases progressing to the characteristic clinical triad of atrophic weakness of the hands and forearms, slight spasticity of the legs, and generalized hyperreflexia. Prognosis is related to the onset of bulbar involvement, with death usually resulting from recurrent aspiration and respiratory insufficiency. Approximately 50 percent are dead within 3 years and 90 percent within 6 years.

The major role of imaging is to exclude a treatable abnormality of the cervical spine that might mimic the clinical manifestations of ALS, such as disk herniation, severe spondylosis, or tumor-related cord compression. The cervical cord is often normal in appearance in ALS, with anterior and lateral cord atrophy generally a late manifestation. The most common finding noted is hyperintensity on T2-weighted MRI in the posterior limbs of the internal capsule extending into the adjacent frontoparietal white matter, caused by secondary degenerative changes related to the spinal cord anterior horn cell abnormality. A gyral pattern of T2 hypointensity within the posterior frontal and anterior parietal lobes—similar to that seen in Alzheimer's disease—may be seen, presumably related to iron deposition. Less common forms of motor neuron disease include the following:

1. Juvenile amyotrophy of the distal upper extremity. This condition occurs most commonly in boys, and—in contrast to the relentlessly progressive course of ALS—stabilizes after a 1- to 3-year progressive course. Magnetic resonance imaging may show focal atrophy of the lower cervical cord, often limited to the anterior horn region.
2. Progressive spinal muscular atrophy.
3. Progressive bulbar palsy.

WALLERIAN DEGENERATION

Wallerian degeneration represents anterograde degeneration of axons and their myelin sheaths, which occurs along the usual direction of nerve conduction, secondary to proximal axonal injury or death of the axon's cell body. The most commonly associated etiology is infarction, occurring next most often with traumatic brain injury, although a variety of other processes—including neoplasm, hemorrhage, and primary white matter disease—may be causative.

On MRI, four stages of wallerian degeneration have been described, with signal changes evolving from normal (stage I), to T2 hypointense (stage II, 4 to 14 weeks), to T2 hyperintense (stage III, over 14 weeks). In the chronic stage (stage IV), volume loss and increased MRI T2 signal are appreciable, involving the ipsilateral cerebral peduncle, pons, and medullary pyramid. Computed tomography will demonstrate the atrophic changes in the brainstem. Wallerian degeneration does not demonstrate contrast enhancement.

☐ MISCELLANEOUS DISEASES (TOXIC, HYPOXIC, METABOLIC)

CENTRAL PONTINE MYELINOLYSIS

Central pontine myelinolysis is a demyelinating disorder in alcoholic, malnourished patients and others with electrolyte abnormalities, including children. The disorder is commonly associated with electrolyte disturbances, particularly rapid correction of hyponatremia. While many patients are asymptomatic, some demonstrate spastic quadriparesis, pseudobulbar palsy, and acute changes in mental status progressing to altered levels of consciousness, including coma and death.

The pontine lesion is central, with characteristic sparing of a peripheral rim of tissue. Extrapontine sites of myelinolysis may also occur. Histologically there is sharply demarcated myelinoclastic change displaying extensive loss of oligodendrocytes, infiltration with foamy macrophages, and reactive astrocytosis.

Imaging

- Low signal intensity on T1-weighted images and high signal intensity on T2-weighted images are seen on MRI most prominently within the central basis pontis (Fig. 21-5).
- Lesions are described as oval-shaped on sagittal, and batwing-shaped on coronal images; most of them do not demonstrate enhancement.
- The MRI findings are nonspecific and overlap with those of brainstem glioma, which typically presents

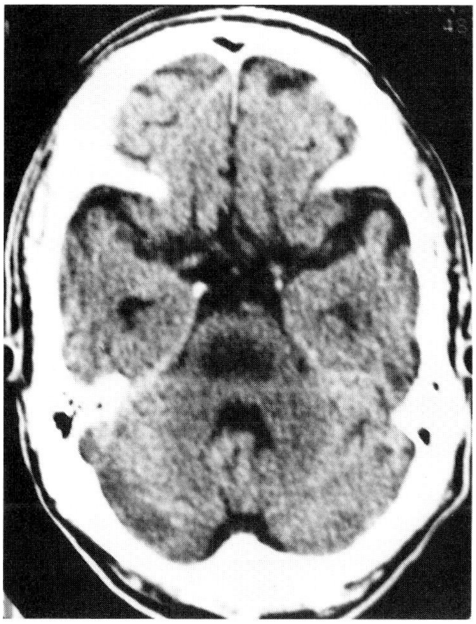

(A)

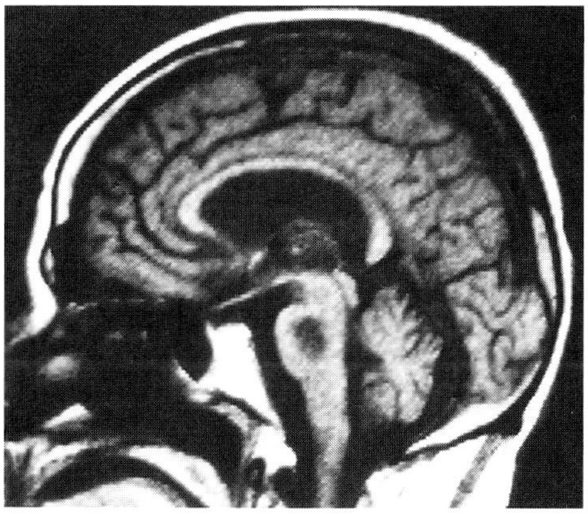

(B)

Figure 21-5 Central pontine myelinoysis. *A*. Axial CT scan shows a low-density area in the pons. *B*. Sagittal T1-weighted image shows a hypointense area in the pons.

clinically in a more insidious fashion. Differential diagnostic considerations include ischemia, multiple sclerosis, encephalitis radiation changes, and tumor.

MARCHIAFAVA-BIGNAMI SYNDROME

Marchiafava-Bignami syndrome is a rare demyelinating disease associated with excessive consumption of crude red wine, typically occurring in alcoholic, malnourished patients, and presenting clinically as a frontal lobe dementia. Pathologically, there is selective myelinolysis in the corpus callosum and, less commonly, in the deep white matter. Decreased attenuation of the corpus callosum is appreciable on CT. Magnetic resonance imaging demonstrates decreased T1 and increased T2 signal in the corpus callosum and deep white matter.

HYPOXIC ENCEPHALOPATHY

Both acute and chronic hypoxia can result in neuronal loss and dementia. There are numerous causes of acute hypoxic encephalopathy, including suffocation, carbon monoxide poisoning, acute exacerbations of respiratory-disease, and systemic hypoperfusion. Pathologically, several types of brain injury may be seen, including necrosis in the pallidum and hippocampus, white matter demyelination, and/or spongiform change and neuronal loss in the cortex.

Bilateral pallidal necrosis on CT or MRI is indicative of an acute hypoxic-ischemic insult and is seen most commonly with carbon monoxide poisoning. In acute carbon monoxide intoxication, findings on CT consist of symmetrical, diffuse hypodensity of the cerebral white matter and bilateral, symmetrical round hypodense lesions in the pallidum. Computed tomography may demonstrate mineralization of the basal ganglia years after the insult. Magnetic resonance imaging demonstrates bilateral pallidal high-signal lesions, cortical signal changes predominantly involving the hippocampi, and small or large, usually frontal white matter abnormalities. The white matter lesions can be reversible and correspond pathologically to demyelination. On T2 weighted images, increased signal, reflecting gliosis, and low signal, due to iron deposition, can be identified in the thalamus and putamen.

Table 21-1
IMAGING HALLMARKS SIGNAL INTENSITY (SI)

	Atrophy	Signal Intensity (SI) Changes on T2 Weighted Images	Functional
Dementias			
Alzeheimer's	Hippocampus, anterior temporal lobe		Temporal and parietal hypometabolism
Pick's	Frontal lobe, caudate		Frontal, anterior temporal, caudate hypometabolism
Creutzfeld-Jakob	Diffuse	Increased SI putamen, caudate	Diffuse hypometabolism
Marchiafava-Bignami		Increased SI corpus callosum	
Wernicke's	Mamillary bodies	Increased SI thalami, colliculi	
Hypoxic		Increased SI pallidum, WM	
Movement disorders			
Huntington's	Caudate		Striatal hypometabolim
Hallervorden-Spatz		Pallidum "target" sign	
Parkinson's	Generalized, PCSN	Decreased SI PCSN	FDG normal, F-dopa hypometabolism
Multiple system atrophy	PC substantia nigra	Deceased SI putamen, PCSN	Striatal hypometabolism
Wilson's		Increased and decreased SI putamen	Basal ganglia hypometabolism
Motor diseases			
Amyotrophic lateral sclerosis	Cord (late)	PL internal capsule, adjacent WM	
Ataxia			
OPCD	Brainstem, cerebellum	Decreased SI putamen	
Friedreich's	Cerebellum—absent or mild		

Abbreviations: PCSN = Pars compacta of substantia nigra; WM = white matter; PL = posterior limb; FDG = Fluorodeoxyglucose.

METABOLIC DISORDERS

Dementia related to metabolic disorders can be difficult to differentiate on clinical examination from primary degenerative dementias.

WERNICKE ENCEPHALOPATHY

Wernicke-Korsakoff syndrome is the most common deficiency syndrome related to chronic alcoholism. Wernicke syndrome is the acute phase of the triad of oculomotor disturbance (nystagmus, ophthalmoplegia, gaze palsy), cerebellar ataxia, and confusion. Korsakoff syndrome is a more chronic condition, which includes anterograde amnesia. Both syndromes are attributed to thiamine deficiency. Microscopically, typical features include neuronal loss, edema, gliosis, and vascular proliferation. Computed tomography may show bilateral thalamic hypodensity. Magnetic resonance imaging reveals increased signal intensity in the collicular and medial thalamic regions, with associated atrophic changes in the mamillary bodies.

HYPOTHYROIDISM

In hypothyroidism, irritability, diminished awareness, and paranoia with auditory hallucinations may be seen. In the elderly, the cognitive dysfunction may resemble a dementia. On MRI, there is characteristic prominent signal hypointensity in the normally iron-containing areas of the brain in addition to prominent decreased signal in the dentate nuclei of the cerebellum and the putamen.

SUGGESTED READINGS

Aging Brain—Dementia

1. Atlas SE (ed): *Magnetic Resonance Imaging of the Brain and Spine*. New York, Raven Press, 1991.
2. Ball MJ et al. A new definition of Alzheimer's disease: A hippocampal dementia. *Lancet* vol. 1 14–16, 1985.
3. Bonner JS, Bonner JJ (eds): *The Little Black Book of Neurology*. St Louis, Mosby-Year Book, 1991.
4. Bonte FJ et al: Brain blood flow in the dementias: SPECT with histopathologic correlation. *Radiology* 186:361–365, 1993.
5. Bottomley PA et al: Alzheimer dementia: Quantification of energy metabolism and mobile phosphoesters with P-31 NMR spectroscopy. *Radiology* 183:695–699, 1992.
6. Bowen BC et al: MR signal abnormalities in memory disorder and dementia. *AJNR* 11:283–290, 1990.
7. Brown JJ et al: MR and CT of lacunar infarcts. *AJR* 151:367–372, 1988.
8. Caselli RJ et al: Asymmetric cortical degenerative syndromes: Clinical and radiologic correlations. *Neurology* 42:1462–1468, 1992.
9. Dahlbeck SW et al: The interuncal distance: A new MR measurement for the hippocamapal atrophy of Alzheimer disease. *AJNR* 12:931–932, 1991.
10. DeCarli C et al: Longitudinal changes in lateral ventricular volume in patients with dementia of the Alzheimer type. *Neurology* 42:2029–2036, 1992.
11. deLeon MJ et al: The radiologic prediction of Alzheimer disease: The atrophic hippocampal formation. *AJNR* 14:897–906, 1993.
12. deLeon MJ et al: Alzheimer's disease: Longitudinal CT studies of ventricular change. *AJR* 152:1257–1262, 1989.
13. Drachman DA: Editorial: New criteria for the diagnosis of vascular dementia: Do we know enough yet? *Neurology* 43:243–245, 1993.
14. Drayer BP: *Syllabus: Special Course in Neuroradiology: Degenerative Disorders of the Central Nervous System*. Chicago, RSNA, 1994, pp 165–177.
15. Drayer BP et al: Magnetic resonance imaging of brain iron. *AJNR* 7:373–380, 1986.
16. Drayer BP: Imaging of the aging brain: I. Normal findings. *Radiology* 166:785–796, 1988.
17. Falcone S et al: Creutzfeld-Jakob disease: Focal symmetrical cortical involvement demonstrated by MR imaging. *AJNR* 13:403–406, 1992.
18. Fazekas F et al: Comparison of CT, MR, and PET in Alzheimer's dementia and normal aging. *J Nucl Med* 30:1607–1615, 1989.
19. Fazekas F et al: MR signal abnormalities at 1.5T in Alzheimer's dementia and normal aging. *AJR* 149:351–356, 1987.
20. George AE et al: CT diagnostic features of Alzheimer disease: Importance of the choroidal/hippocampal fissure complex. *AJNR* 11:101–107, 1990.
21. Hallgren B, Sourander P: The effect of age on the nonheam in iron in the human brain. *J Neurochem* 3:41–51, 1958.
22. Hesselink JR: *Syllabus: Special Course in Neuroradiology: White Matter Diseases*. RSNA, 1994, pp 157–159.
23. Holman BL et al: The scintigraphic appearance of Alzheimer's disease: A prospective study using technetium-99m-HMPAO. *J Nuclear Med* 33:181–185; 1992.
24. Hyman BT et al: Alzheimer's disease: Cell specific pathology isolates the hippocampal formation. *Science* 225:1168–1170, 1984.
25. Jack CR et al: MR imaging–based volume measurements of the hippocampal formation and anterior temporal lobe: Validation studies. *Radiology* 176:205–209, 1990.
26. Jack CR: Brain and cerebrospinal fluid volume: Measurement with MR imaging. *Radiology* 178:22–24, 1991.
27. Johnson DW et al: Stable xenon CT cerebral blood flow imaging: Rationale for and role in clinical decision making. *AJNR* 12:201–213, 1991.
28. Kabawata K et al: A comparative I-123 IMP SPECT study in Binswanger's disease and Alzheimer's disease. *Clin Nuclear Med* 18:329–336, 1993.
29. Kido DK et al: Temporal lobe atrophy in patients with Alzheimer disease: A CT study. *AJNR* 10:551–555, 1989.

30. Mazziotta JC et al: The use of positron emission tomography in the clinical assessment of dementia. *Semin Nuclear Med* 22:233–246, 1992.
31. Miller BL et al: Alzheimer disease: Depiction of increased cerebral myo-inositol with proton MR spectroscopy. *Radiology* 187:433–437, 1993.
32. Ohnishi T et al: Regional cerebral blood flow study with 123 I-IMP in patients with degenerative dementia. *AJNR* 12:513–520, 1991.
33. Osborn AG (ed): *Handbook of Neuroradiology*. St Louis, Mosby-Year Book, 1991.
34. Pirtilla T et al: Brain atrophy In neurodegenerative diseases: Quantitative and qualitative CT analysis. *Acta Radiol* 34:296–302, 1993.
35. Roman GC et al: Vascular dementia: Diagnostic criteria for research studies. Report of the NINDS-AIREN International Workshop. *Neurology* 43:250–260, 1993.
36. Rusinek H et al: Alzheimer disease: Measuring loss of cerebral gray matter with MR imaging. *Radiology* 178:109–114, 1991.
37. Sackeim HA et al: Regional cerebral blood flow in mood disorders: II. Comparison of major depression and Alzheimer's disease. *J Nucl Med* 34:1090–1101, 1993.
38. Sappey-Marinier D et al: Alterations in brain phosphorus metabolite concentrations associated with areas of high signal intensity in white matter at MR imaging. *Radiology* 183:247–256, 1992.
39. Schlenska GK, Walter GF: Serial computed tomography findings in Creutzfeld-Jakob disease. *Neuroradiology* 31:303–306, 1989.
40. Tanna NK et al: Analysis of brain and cerebrospinal fluid volumes with MR imaging: Impact on PET data correction for atrophy. Part II. Aging and Alzheimer dementia. *Radiology* 178:123–130, 1991.
41. Tien RD et al: The dementias: Correlation of clinical features, pathophysiology, and neuroradiology. *AJR* 161:245–255, 1993.
42. Van Heertum RL, O'Connell RA: Functional brain imaging in the evaluation of psychiatric illness. *Semin Nuclear Med* 21:24–39, 1991.
43. Wippold FJ et al: Senile dementia and healthy aging: A longitudinal CT study. *Radiology* 179:215–219, 1991.
44. Wyper D et al: Abnormalities in rCBF and computed tomography in patients with Alzheimer's disease and in controls. *Br J Radiol* 66:23–27, 1993.

Extrapyramidal System and Movement Disorders

1. Abdollah A et al: Wilson's disease: Computed tomography and magnetic resonance imaging findings. *J Assoc Can Radiol* 42:130–134, 1991.
2. Ambrosetto P et al: Late onset familial Hallervorden-Spatz disease: MR findings in two sisters. *AJNR* 13:394–396, 1992.
3. Antonini A et al: T2 relaxation time in patients with Parkinson's disease. *Neurology* 43:697–700, 1993.
4. Atlas SE (ed): *Magnetic Resonance Imaging of the Brain and Spine*. New York, Raven Press, 1991.
5. Bonner JS, Bonner JJ (ed): *The Little Black Book of Neurology*. St Louis, Mosby-Year Book, 1991.
6. Braffman BH et al: MR imaging of Parkinson disease with spin-echo and gradient-echo sequences. *AJNR* 9:1093–1099, 1988.
7. Chen JC et al: MR of human postmortem brain tissue: Correlative study between T2 and assays of iron and ferritin in Parkinson and Huntington disease. *AJNR* 14:275–281, 1993.
8. Clark RG (ed): The basal ganglia and related structures, in *Manter and Gatz's Essentials of Clinical Neuroanatomy and Neurophysiology*. Philadelphia, Davis, pp 160–166, 1992.
9. Drayer BP: *Syllabus: Special Course in Neuroradiology: Degenerative Disorders of the Central Nervous System*. RSNA, 1994, pp 165–177.
10. Drayer BP et al: Magnetic resonance imaging of brain iron. *AJNR* 7:373–380, 1986.
11. Gray F et al: Adult form of Leigh's disease: A clinico pathological case with CT scan examination. *J Neurol Neurosurg Psychiatry* 47:1211–1215, 1984.
12. Heckmann JM et al: Leigh disease (subacute necrotizing encephalomyelopathy): MR documentation of the evolution of an acute attack. *AJNR* 14:1157–1159, 1993.
13. Hoshi H et al: 6-(18-F)Fluoro-L-dopa metabolism in living human brain: A comparison of six analytical methods. *J Cereb Blood Flow Metab* 13:57–69, 1993.
14. Imiya M et al: MR of the base of the pons in Wilson disease. *AJNR* 13:1009–1012, 1992.
15. Jackson JA et al: Progressive supranuclear palsy: Clinical features and response to treatment in 16 patients. *Ann Neurol* 13:273–278, 1983.
16. Mutoh K et al: MR imaging of a group I case of Hallervorden-Spatz disease. *JCAT* 12:851–853, 1988.
17. Nazer H et al: Magnetic resonance imaging of the brain in Wilson's disease. *Neuroradiology* 35:130–133, 1993.
18. Nygaard TG et al: Seizures in progressive supranuclear palsy. *Neurology* 38:138–140, 1989.
19. Osborn AG (ed): *Handbook of Neuroradiology*. St Louis, Mosby-Year Book, 1991.
20. Park BE et al: Pathogenesis of pigment and spheroid formation in Hallervorden-Spatz syndrome and related disorders. *Neurology* 25:1172–1178, 1975.
21. Prayer L et al: Cranial MRI in Wilson's disease. *Neuroradiology* 32:213–214, 1993.
22. Savoiardo M et al: Hallervorden-Spatz disease: MR and pathologic findings. *AJNR* 14:155–162, 1993.
23. Savoiardo M et al: MR imaging in progressive supranuclear palsy and Shy-Drager syndrome. *JCAT* 13:555–560, 1989.
24. Sener RN: Wilson's disease: MRI demonstration of cavitations in basal ganglia and thalami. *Pediatr Radiol* 23:157, 1993.
25. Simmons JT et al: Magnetic resonance imaging in Huntington disease. *AJNR* 7:25–28, 1986.
26. Starosta-Rubinstein S et al: Clinical assessment of 31 patients with Wilson's disease—Correlations with structural changes on magnetic resonance imaging. *Arch Neurol* 44:365–370, 1987.
27. Thuomas KA et al: Magnetic resonance imaging of the brain in Wilson's disease. *Neuroradiology* 35:134–141, 1993.
28. Wardlaw JM et al: Measurement of caudate nucleus area—A more accurate measurement for Huntington's disease? *Neuroradiology* 33:316–319, 1991.
29. Zetusky WJ et al: The heterogeneity of Parkinson's disease: Clinical and prognostic implications. *Neurology* 35:522–526, 1985.

Miscellaneous, Motor and Spinocerebellar Degenerative Diseases

1. Atlas SE (ed): *Magnetic Resonance Imaging of the Brain and Spine*. New York, Raven Press, 1991.
2. Bonner JS, Bonner JJ (ed): *The Little Black Book of Neurology*. St Louis, Mosby-Year Book, 1991.
3. Drachman DB, Kuncl RW: Amyotrophic lateral sclerosis: An unconventional autoimmmune disease? *Ann Neurol* 26:269–274, 1989.

4. Drayer BP: *Syllabus: Special Course in Neuroradiology: Degenerative Disorders of the Central Nervous System*. Chicago, RSNA, 1994, pp 165–177.
5. Drayer BP et al: Magnetic resonance imaging of brain iron. *AJNR* 7:373–380, 1986.
6. Ho VB et al: Resolving MR features in osmotic myelinolysis (central pontine and extrapontine myelinolysis). *AJNR* 14:163–167, 1993.
7. Korogi Y et al: MR findings in two presumed cases of mild central pontine myelinolysis. *AJNR* 14:651–654, 1993.
8. Kuhn MJ et al: Wallerian degeneration: Evaluation with MR imaging. *Radiology* 168:199–202, 1988.
9. Mascalchi M et al: Case report: MRI demonstration of pontine and thalamic myelinolysis in a normonatremic alcoholic. *Clin Radiol* 47:137–138, 1993.
10. Miller GM et al: Central pontine myelinolysis and its imitators: MR findings. *Radiology* 168:795–802, 1988.
11. Osborn AG (ed): *Handbook of Neuroradiology*. St Louis, Mosby-Year Book, 1991.
12. Rowland LP: Editorial: Looking for the cause of amyotrophic lateral sclerosis. *N Engl J Med* 311:979–981, 1984.
13. Wullner U et al: Magnetic resonance imaging in hereditary and idiopathic ataxia. *Neurology* 43:318–325, 1993.
14. Yokote K et al: Wernicke encephalopathy: Follow-up study by CT and MR. *JCAT* 15:835–838, 1991.

☐ QUESTIONS

1. Pick's disease (T or F):
- **a.** Hallmark is striking frontal lobe atrophy.
- **b.** Involved brain structure hypometabolism is detected by FDG PET.
- **c.** Is far more common than Alzheimer's disease.
- **d.** Is best characterized as a cortical dementia.

2. Dementias (T or F):
- **a.** White matter sparing may be useful in differentiating Creutzfeld-Jakob disease.
- **b.** An abnormal cisternogram is definitive in selecting patients with NPH who are likely to respond to shunting.
- **c.** Multi-infarct dementia is the most common form of dementia.
- **d.** The imaging findings in vascular dementia are pathognomonic.

3. Aging brain (T or F):
- **a.** White matter hyperintensities can be seen in young, normal patients.
- **b.** Progressive iron deposition in the brain may be associated with normal aging.
- **c.** Diminished glucose utilization with normal aging is demonstrated by PET.
- **d.** The prevalence of white matter hyperintensities increases with age.

4. Alzheimer's disease (T or F):
- **a.** The most common cause of dementia.
- **b.** More common in women than men.
- **c.** Imaging hallmark is atrophy disproportionately affecting the hippocampus.
- **d.** Associated with iron deposition in the hippocampus.

5. Best associated (mix and match):

a. Huntington's disease	**1.** Ceruloplasmin deficiency
b. Hallervorden-Spatz disease	**2.** Enzyme defect
c. MELAS syndrome	**3.** Pallidum target sign
d. Wilson's disease	**4.** Strokelike syndrome
e. Leigh's disease	**5.** Caudate hypometabolism

6. Parkinson's disease (T or F):
- **a.** Most common movement disorder.
- **b.** Primary disorder of the pars reticulata.
- **c.** Atrophy and iron deposition in the substantia nigra.
- **d.** Iron deposition in the putamen.

7. Multiple system atrophies (T or F):
- **a.** Excess iron in putamen characteristic of Parkinson's plus.
- **b.** May present as drug-unresponsive parkinsonism.
- **c.** Approximately twice as common as Parkinson's disease.
- **d.** Hypometabolism on FDG PET.

8. Motor neuron diseases (T or F):
- **a.** Key imaging examination in ALS is MRI of the cervical spine.
- **b.** Infarction most common etiologic factor in wallerian degeneration.
- **c.** ALS is generally self-limited.
- **d.** Hallmark of WD is anterograde degeneration with atrophy and signal alteration.

9. Spinocerebellar degeneration (T or F):
- **a.** Hallmark of OPCD is atrophy of pontocerebellar pathway.
- **b.** OPCD may occur with SDS and/or SND in MSA.
- **c.** Hallmark of Friedreich's ataxia is severe cerebellar atrophy.
- **d.** Pes cavus and scoliosis associated with OPCD.

10. Toxic, metabolic disorders (mix and match):

a. Central pontine myelinolysis	1. Thiamine deficiency
b. Marchiafava–Bignami syndrome	2. Carbon monoxide
c. Wernicke syndrome	3. Electrolyte disturbance
d. Pallidal necrosis	4. Tainted Chianti

☐ ANSWERS

1. a. T
   b. T
   c. F
   d. T

2. a. T
   b. F
   c. F
   d. F

3. a. T
   b. T
   c. F
   d. T

4. a. T
   b. F
   c. T
   d. F

5. a. 5
   b. 3
   c. 4
   d. 1
   e. 2

6. a. T
   b. F
   c. T
   d. F

7. a. T
   b. T
   c. F
   d. T

8. a. T
   b. T
   c. F
   d. T

9. a. T
   b. T
   c. F
   d. F

10. a. 3
    b. 4
    c. 1
    d. 2

CHAPTER

22

Developmental Spine Abnormalities

Hervey D. Segall
Marvin D. Nelson, Jr.
Jamshid Ahmadi
Chi S. Zee

Severe anomalies affecting the spinal cord and spine have traditionally been grouped together under the term *spinal dysraphism*. Spinal dysraphism has been defined as a group of lesions in which there is imperfect developmental fusion of neural, mesenchymal, and osseous structures in the median dorsal plane. More recently *neural tube defect* has been used to categorize these anomalies. These neural tube defects can be subsequently subdivided into two groupings—namely, open and closed defects. The open form of neural tube defect is described in a subsequent section (myelomeningocele). The closed (occult) form includes abnormalities that are covered by skin, so that meninges and neural tissue are not exposed; there may be, however, in this group of lesions, subcutaneous lipomas or cutaneous abnormalities. Lesions in this closed category include split-notochord syndrome (including neurenteric cysts), dermoids, epidermoids, dorsal dermal sinus, lipomatous masses, tight filum or other lesions causing tethering of the spinal cord, and diastematomyelia. Hydromyelia has also been classified along with these lesions. It should also be mentioned here that 20 percent of adults and an even larger percentage of children may be found to have an isolated minor midline lumbar osseous defect termed *spina bifida occulta*. In the absence of neurologic deficits or associated anomalies, this is considered an incidental radiologic finding.

Imaging studies should be performed in a neonate who presents with a superficial midline hairy tuft, hemangioma, lipoma, dimple, or sinus. This is because such superficial lesions may herald the presence of an underlying dysraphic lesion. In many of these occult dysraphic lesions, early surgical intervention may well be necessary to prevent progressive neurologic or orthopedic defects. Spinal dysraphic lesions may produce neurologic deficits by a variety of mechanisms, including spinal cord tethering and mass effect. Neurologic deficits may be present at birth, or they may appear later in childhood. Neuroradiologic workup for an occult dysraphic lesion may also be necessitated by orthopedic deformities or progressive scoliosis.

Imaging studies may also be required to elucidate the cause of scoliosis (lateral curvature of the spine). Although vertebral fusion and segmentation anomalies may be the cause of congenital scoliosis, intraspinal lesions must be ruled out in a young child with scoliosis even when the clinical neurologic examination is otherwise normal. Idiopathic scoliosis is virtually nonexistent in children under the age of 6, and a progressive idiopathic curve in children under the age of 11 is unusual in the United States. Because of this, magnetic resonance imaging (MRI) is performed routinely at the Children's Hospital of Los Angeles in children below age 11 who have progressive scoliotic curves, regardless of the pattern of the scoliotic curve or the presence of a normal neurologic examination.

Congenital lesions such as hydromyelia with Chiari I or lipoma with cord tethering have been found in such cases, as well as intramedullary, extramedullary, and paraspinal tumors. The possibility of an underlying diastematomyelia must always be considered before beginning corrective treatment for congenital scoliosis. In such cases prior diagnosis and excision of the spur can prevent the tragedy of paraplegia, a possible complication resulting from a corrective procedure in the patient with an unrecognized diastematomyelia spur.

It is not uncommon to have more than one spinal anomaly in the same patient with a dysraphic spine abnormality. This must be always kept in mind in imaging such patients; an incomplete neuroradiologic study that fails to define the full extent of the disease, leading to ineffective surgical repair, is to be avoided.

Imaging and related morphologic findings and clinical considerations in dysraphic and other congenital spine anomalies will be considered in this review. Currently MRI is the ideal method for studying such patients, while plain radiographs and computed tomography (CT) remain useful in delineating osseous and complex vertebral abnormalities. Ultrasound may also be informative in experienced hands when there is a suitable sonographic window.

☐ EMBRYOLOGY

The development of the spinal cord and osseous spine commences as early as the second embryonic week. The spinal cord begins to develop in the embryo through the processes of gastrulation, neurulation, disjunction, and canalization and retrogressive differentiation. These processes, however, will not be described in this practical review.

Rudimentary vertebral bodies are derived from mesoderm via several processes. This occurs by the fourth embryonic week. Cartilage forms at 6 weeks of gestation, while ossification starts at 9 weeks. Fundamentally, the nucleus pulposus develops from the embryonic notochord.

A malfunction in the above-mentioned processes leads to development of the anomalies considered in this chapter. There may be a variety of theories as to how some of these anomalies originate. However, it is beyond the scope of this review to detail the presumed mechanisms for the genesis of these spinal anomalies.

☐ MYELOMENINGOCELE

Myelomeningocele is an open dysraphic lesion. This anomaly is discovered at birth, at which time raw, exposed neural tissue is found protruding through midline vertebral arch defects as well as through deficient dura and skin. This neural placode projects along with the meningeal sac beyond the skin surface. The terms *myeloschisis* and *myelocele* have been used to designate cases in which this placode is flush with the skin surface. Most cases involve the thoracolumbar or lumbar region.

Prenatal diagnosis of myelomeningocele has been made possible by using blood and amniotic fluid alpha-fetoprotein levels and fetal ultrasound or MRI. A variety of factors—including hereditary, genetic, teratogenic, environmental, or dietary causes—have been invoked. Hydrocephalus is present in roughly 90 percent of such cases in children, and the Chiari II malformation has almost invariably been associated with myelomeningocele.

Imaging plays a minor role in evaluating such lesions shortly after birth, although cranial ultrasound to detect hydrocephalus is worthwhile. Basically the emphasis in the early stage is in the direction of performing aggressive neurosurgical treatment for myelomeningocele (to diminish the risk of infection and minimize additional trauma to the exposed placode and nerve roots). During surgery, the placode is dissected away from surrounding tissues and, by proper closure of dura and overlying skin, normal anatomic barriers are reconstructed.

Later on, imaging can play an important role in the patient with myelomeningocele. Neurologic dysfunction or accelerated progression of scoliosis may necessitate prompt radiologic evaluation. This workup may reveal treatable conditions such as hydromyelia or, rarely, diastematomyelia. Scoliosis can also be related to cord retethering, but it is debatable whether or not this is a common cause of neurologic dysfunction toward the end of the first decade of life, a period of rapid growth. Scoliosis might also be accounted for by congenital vertebral anomalies. Late neurologic deterioration is most frequently explained by shunt malfunction but might also be accounted for by changes associated with the Chiari II malformation. In such cases, imaging studies may also demonstrate cystic lesions and assorted bands and adhesions, often lying rostral to the defect.

Studies by MRI or ultrasound following meningomyelocele repair normally depict a low-lying cord terminating in a placode that is not clearly separable from the posterior thecal sac at the operative site. Nelson and coworkers (see "Suggested Readings"), based on their experience with almost 200 patients with repaired myelomeningocele, found that 98 percent showed attachment at the site of surgical closure. Thus, these authors contend that clinical diagnosis is paramount in determining whether or not treatment for retethering should be performed, since virtually all are technically "tethered."

☐ HYDROMYELIA

Hydromyelia frequently coexists with myelomeningocele. Both of these entities have a well-known association with the Chiari malformations. Hence this is a point at which to discuss hydromyelia.

The central canal is normally closed at birth. In hydromyelia, the central canal of the spinal cord is patent and dilated. It is partially or completely lined by ependyma. There are a variety of theories (including those by Gardner and Williams) designed to explain the persistent dilatation of the hydromyelia channel. Dilatation of some portion of the central canal can be found in at least one-half of the cases of myelodysplasia at autopsy.

Frequently there is early rupture of the dilated central canal into the spinal cord parenchyma. Thus, in cases of hydromyelia, syringomyelic cavities may be created within cord tissue that are not ependyma-lined. Thus, the more inclusive term *syringohydromyelia* has been commonly used for this disorder. Reactive gliosis may be found pathologically in the area around syringomyelic and hydromyelic cavities. Syringobulbia occurs when there is upward dissection of the process into the brainstem.

Syringomyelia can be a primary idiopathic process, but syringes can be secondary to other processes such as trauma and infection. These causes will not be considered further in this discussion of congenital spine anomalies.

Magnetic resonance imaging of the entire spine and head is encouraged to provide the most detailed and informative studies in patients with hydromyelia. This will enable demonstration of the extent of the cord channel as well as the association of other lesions. Usually at least two or three segments are involved, but occasionally the process extends throughout the entire cervical and thoracic cord. When initial images suggest hydromyelia, it is worthwhile to obtain multiplanar demonstration, which adds to the diagnostic confidence level. In some instances, on sagittal images, one may be dealing with a truncation artifact having a syrinx-like appearance. In such cases a normal axial scan can be helpful in confirming that one is indeed dealing with an artifact. On the other hand, one might identify a small channel only on transverse images, a channel that might, however, be missed on sagittal images. T1-weighted spin-echo images are optimal for depicting hydromyelia because they give good contrast between cavity and cord. Such images can be obtained quickly. Since the protein content of hydromyelia cavities tends to be similar to that of cerebrospinal fluid (CSF), imaging studies usually show the hydromyelia cavity to be isointense with CSF.

The eccentric component of syringohydromyelic cavities are related to rupture of hydromyelia with dissection into adjacent cord tissue. This can be readily observed on axial images, which nicely display the eccentric component. A beaded configuration of hydromyelia channels and multiple septations within them are frequently shown on sagittal images. Circumferential gliotic bands account for these septations. T2-weighted images may display flow voids within a spinal cord cyst, representing pulsations. Reduction of such flow voids on serial images may be an indicator of a successful shunt procedure. Although MRI is the most valuable noninvasive method, one can employ CT in the uppermost cervical region or ultrasound (in children less than 8 months of age and in those with large dorsal bone defects) to depict a hydromyelia cavity.

There is a great variety of treatment options available in patients with hydromyelia and Chiari malformation; selection of the location for surgery and the type of procedure will be aided by obtaining optimal imaging information.

☐ MENINGOCELE

Posterior meningocele is the simplest form of open neural defect. These meningoceles consist of meninges but contain no neural tissue and occur more frequently in the occipital and lumbar regions. This entity is much less frequent than meningomyelocele and is rarely associated with hydrocephalus or Chiari II.

In *anterior sacral meningocele*, the dura and arachnoid extend out of the sacral canal via a sacral bony defect into the pelvis anteriorly. The bony defect may be merely an enlarged intervertebral foramen, or it may consist of a complete agenesis of the lower sacrum and coccyx. A lateral "scimitar" defect in the lower sacrum is a typical appearance. The meningocele may enlarge gradually as a result of the hydrostatic pressure of CSF within it, but it may not produce symptoms until adulthood. This condition may result in symptoms of a pelvic-abdominal mass, including those related to compression of sacral nerves. Water-tight closure of the meningocele pedicle is the treatment of choice for anterior meningocele.

Thoracic meningoceles are morphologically similar to sacral meningoceles. They may project laterally or anteriorly from the spinal canal. Two-thirds or more of lateral thoracic meningoceles are associated with neurofibromatosis. Occasionally a neurofibroma may be found within the wall of a meningocele. Even more rare are anterior meningoceles that project through the dorsal vertebral bodies. These are not associated with neurofibromatosis, but they may be found in conjunction with other congenital anomalies. Thoracic meningoceles may also enlarge with time and may cause pulmonary and neural compression. They may also be associated with myelopathy and abnormalities of spinal curvature. Surgical closure of the communicating pedicle is the optimum treatment.

Lateral and anterior meningoceles in the cervical and lumbar regions are even rarer than lesions in the abovementioned locations.

☐ INTRASPINAL CYSTS, DIVERTICULA, AND SINUSES

Occult intrasacral meningoceles consist of a fluid-filled sac *within* the spinal canal, which communicates with the tip of the thecal sac by a narrow or broad aperture that transmits CSF. This so-called meningocele has an inner lining of arachnoid and a fibrous wall resembling dura. Such a lesion is not strictly a meningocele because there is no herniation of meninges and no vertebral defect related to the cystic lesion in question. In this condition there may be back pain and radiating leg pain (in the sciatic distribution) or other neurologic findings.

Root sleeve and sheath cysts are usually clinically insignificant but may be seen relatively frequently on imaging studies. *Meningeal diverticula* are arachnoid-lined outpouchings that communicate freely with the subarachnoid space and thus are found related to nerve root sleeves when water-soluble myelography is performed. *Root sheath cysts* (perineural, Tarlov cysts) arise between the perineurium (arachnoid) and endoneurium (pia) of the nerve roots, with walls composed of those elements. Surgical excision may be required in the rare instances (with radicular pain and nerve root compression) where the perineural cyst enlarges and communication with the subarachnoid space has been interrupted. On the other hand, meningeal diverticula are virtually always incidental and do not require treatment.

Congenital extradural spinal cysts are posteriorly situated collections that communicate with the subarachnoid space by way of a narrow pedicle. These rare lesions enlarge by hydrostatic pressure and CSF pulsations, and contrast may enter them at myelography. Depending on their location, they can cause progressive spastic paraparesis or quadriparesis. Lumbar cysts can present with pain, especially of a radicular nature. Once they are promptly diagnosed by imaging studies, successful treatment may be rendered. Complete excision along with closure of the dural defect is the treatment of choice.

Congenital spinal intradural cysts include arachnoid cysts, ependymal cysts, neurenteric cysts, epidermoid cysts, and dermoid cysts.

Arachnoid cysts of developmental origin are most commonly found in the thoracic region dorsal to the spinal cord. These can cause spinal cord compression but are amendable to surgery. They are sharply marginated, contain CSF-like fluid, and have a wall of slightly thickened arachnoid.

Ependymal cysts, on the other hand, tend to be ventrally situated. These may also produce spinal cord compression.

Neurenteric cysts tend to be unilocular. The simplest neurenteric cysts are differentiated from ependymal cyst pathologically because their epithelial lining includes at least some cells that contain mucin (Fig. 22-1). More complex neurenteric cysts have, in addition to this type of lining, other gastrointestinal or tracheobronchial elements as well. Neurenteric cysts are but one type of anomaly grouped together with the numerous anomalies of the "split-notochord syndrome." In the severest form of this syndrome, the entire tract between the gut and the skin remains open. This extreme variant is called dorsal enteric fistula. When portions of this fistula become obliterated, less severe anomalies arise (diverticula, sinuses, cysts). Osseous and central nervous system (CNS) malformations of this type tend to occur in the cervical and upper thoracic region.

Spinal neurenteric cysts may enlarge the spinal canal with pedicular thinning, and there may be vertebral anomalies including anterior or posterior spina bifida. The cyst is sharply marginated and the differing fluid contents within (mucin, blood, etc.) may result in variable MRI signals. These cysts are usually anterior or anterolateral to the cord (Fig. 22-1). Magnetic resonance imaging may show low-intensity bands running through fat representing fibrous fistula remnants.

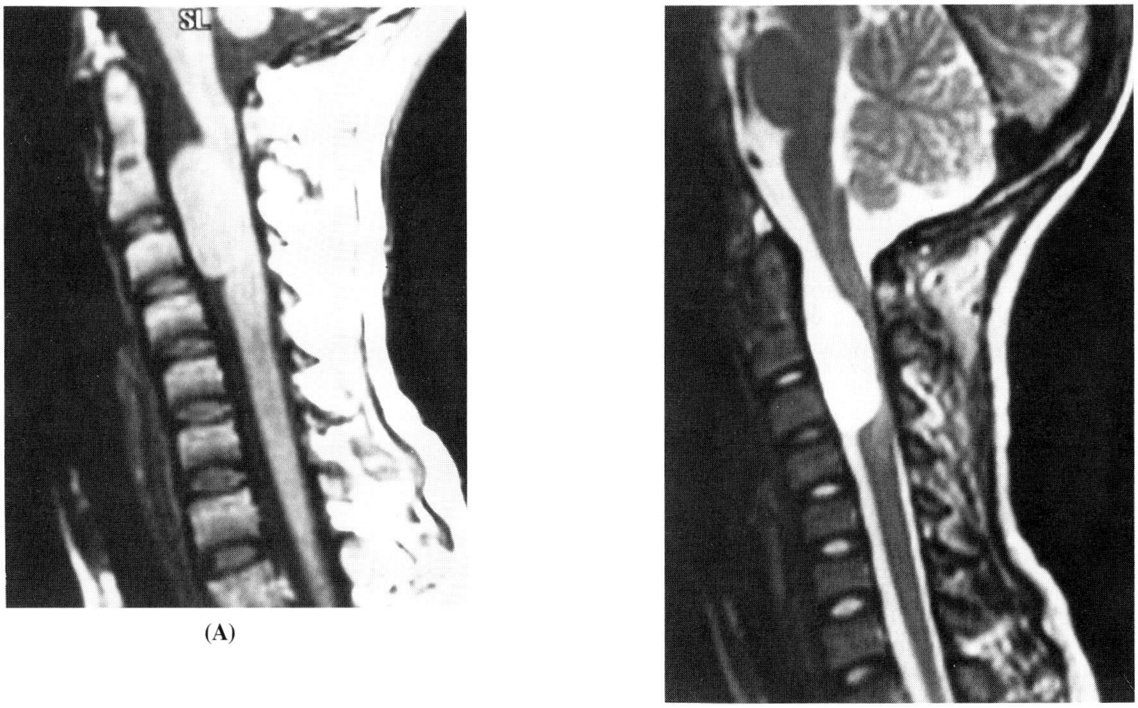

(A)

(B)

Figure 22-1 Neuroenteric cyst at the C2-3 level with cord compression. Sagittal MRI: (*A*) SE 483/17; (*B*) FSE 4000/17. Note that the signal intensity of the cyst exceeds that of CSF on both sequences. Pathologically the cyst wall had gastric-type columnar epithelium and, in another area, respiratory-type epithelium with cilia. Mucous-secreting cells were also observed.

Epidermoid and dermoid cysts are developmental lesions composed of skin elements. These do not have neoplastic growth and are not true tumors. Some epidermoidomas are formed from retained epidermal tissue following spinal puncture or surgery. Hence, some epidermoidomas are not congenital.

Epidermoid cysts are ectodermal in origin and characteristically have a bright "pearly" appearance. Dermoids, on the other hand, arise from ectodermal and related tissues and contain debris from sloughed epithelium as well as dermal appendages such as sebaceous material and hair.

Ten percent of spinal tumors in patients under 15 years of age are developmental lesions of this sort. Clinically, they may appear as a mass lesion. Leakage of the contents of these cysts can cause local meningeal and radicular irritation and can lead to a dense, chronic arachnoiditis. These cysts are commonly associated with cutaneous abnormalities and 20 percent are associated with dermal sinus. The majority of these lesions are found in the lumbar or lumbosacral area, although occasionally they may be found in the dorsal or cervical area.

These intradural extramedullary cysts can lie posteriorly in the spinal canal. Epidermoids may have a substantial protein content with a signal intensity exceeding that of CSF. The signal intensity of dermoids is dependent on the amount of epithelial debris or sebaceous material. Signal intensities in the latter type of lesion may occasionally approach those of subcutaneous fat. Bone changes of spina bifida are frequent and pedicular erosion and scalloping may also be seen.

Congenital dermal sinus may be suspected clinically because of the presence of a skin dimple on the back. This skin opening may be small and very difficult to see. Debris or purulent material may be found draining from the skin opening and there may be protruding hairs and other cutaneous stigmata on the surface associated with dermal sinus. Most congenital dermal sinuses are found in the lumbosacral region. On MRI, studies of patients with congenital dermal sinus may show a low-intensity band that traverses the subcutaneous fat, best seen on T1-weighted images. A study utilizing several planes may be most effective in delineating the course of this lesion. Studies in such cases should, of course, be evaluated for tumors within underlying spinal structures. Abscesses may develop with dermal sinuses that become infected, and these may be demonstrated within underlying spinal structures on MRI. In studying these sinuses radiologically, it is important to avoid injecting contrast material into the sinus tract, as this may provoke infection.

Treatment for congenital dermal sinus involves complete removal of the entire sinus tract which may include extension of the tract intraspinally and even deeply upward to the conus medullaris region of the spinal cord. Removal of this dermal sinus tract in its entirety and removal of coexisting dermoid cysts is also warranted. Once these sinuses are discovered it is important to perform surgery on them to avoid the complication of infection and resultant neurologic deficit.

☐ CONGENITAL LIPOMATOUS SPINAL LESIONS

Congenital lipomas within the spinal canal (Fig. 22-2) are not neoplastic and grow very slowly relative to a patient's

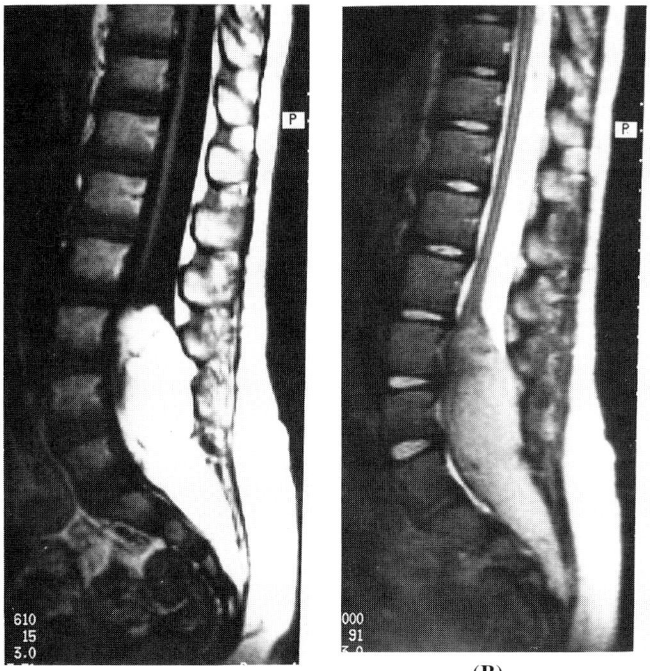

(A) (B)

Figure 22-2 Lumbosacral lipoma with tethered cord. Sagittal images: (*A*) SE 610/15; (*B*) SE 4000/91. Note that the MRI signals from the lipomatous mass are characteristic for fat with high signal on T1-weighted images and with signal drop-off on the T2-weighted images.

general growth pattern. They have normal adipose tissue histologically but may also contain abundant fibrous tissue within the lesion.

Lipomyelomeningocele implies fatty tissue that is tightly adherent to a myeloschisic plate and extends through a spina bifida defect into more superficial subcutaneous tissues. At birth, this appears as a lumbosacral lipoma and, as a rule, there is no neurologic deficit at that time. However if these lesions remain untreated by 2 years of age, there is a 90 percent incidence of neurologic deficit related to spinal cord tethering and neural impingement by fibrous band and perhaps fatty mass. Characteristically lipomyelomeningoceles are not associated with hydrocephalus, Chiari malformations, or other CNS anomalies. However, other cutaneous stigmata may be present.

The morphology of lipomyelomeningocele features a lipoma firmly adherent to the placode at the level of the spina bifida. This primitively shaped placode is draped over the lipoma and the placode and lipoma are tightly joined by a thick connective tissue layer, which is reinforced by fibrous tissue projecting into both placode and lipoma. The lumbosacral lipoma appears as a mass above the intergluteal cleft, as opposed to sacrococcygeal teratoma, which is usually found caudad to the intergluteal cleft.

Magnetic resonance imaging reveals typical lipomatous tissue signals on T1- and T2-weighted images (Fig. 22-2). The fat, which is largely dorsal to the neural tissue, may be associated with a chemical shift artifact in the direction of the frequency-encoding gradient. The dense fibrous connective tissue described above appears on MRI as a discrete low-signal band at the liponeural junction. The distal cord is tethered and thinned, while the neural placode has a flattened configuration instead of having the usual rounded shape of the conus. Characteristically, there is an enlargement of the ventral subarachnoid space. Spina bifida; vertebral scalloping; small, thin pedicles and laminae—in addition to other osseous changes—are characteristically present.

Early surgical treatment is advised following diagnosis, since untreated lipomyelomeningocele can progress and cause paraplegia, other neurologic deficits, and serious orthopedic deformities.

Intradural lipomas are usually found in the cervical or thoracic canal. Characteristically these do not have cutaneous markers for dysraphism, and they may be found incidentally. However, they may tether or compress the spinal cord, causing symptoms and findings in some cases. Minor fusion defects or bony erosions may be found, but the bony canal is often normal.

Filum terminale lipomas can be seen in up to 5 percent of normal individuals. The small collection of fat within the filum terminale can be considered a benign incidental finding when there is no cord tethering and there are also no osseous or superficial abnormalities clinically. However, the lipoma has greater clinical significance when it thickens the filum and is associated with conus tethering.

☐ TIGHT FILUM TERMINALE SYNDROME

A short, thickened filum terminale can tether the conus in an abnormally low position. Symptoms and findings may occur as a result of stretching of the cord, which may become evident at times of rapid growth when the spine elongates more than the cord. Added tension on the cord can also be associated with exercise.

One-fourth of patients with tight filum terminale also have filum lipomas. Imaging studies in these cases show a filum thicker than 2 mm and a low conus. Routinely, there is a spina bifida in the tight filum terminale syndrome, and MRI occasionally demonstrates cord myelomalacia or syrinx. Untethering of the spinal cord by division of the filum terminale is the definitive treatment in these cases.

☐ TERATOMAS

Spinal teratomas are very rare; hence they will be considered here only very briefly. These tumors can occur anywhere along the spinal axis, but they are most common in the cervical or lumbodorsal region. Imaging studies may show osseous changes. Magnetic resonance imaging studies will show inhomogeneous signals related to the presence of lipid, calcific, hemorrhagic, cystic, and osseous components within the intradural extramedullary tumor.

Sacrococcygeal teratomas are initially benign tumors that are firmly attached to the coccyx. Clinically they may present externally, and they are situated much lower than lumbosacral myelomeningoceles and lipomas. Their solid portions enhance on imaging studies. In 60 percent, the solid components calcify.There may also be cystic areas within these lesions. The lesion occurs in the region of the coccyx, which may appear abnormal or absent on imaging studies. Immediate surgical excision is recommended upon discovery because of the malignant potential of these initially benign tumors.

☐ CAUDAL REGRESSION SYNDROME

The caudal regression syndrome involves a spectrum of anomalies in which there is failure of development of the distal spine and corresponding spinal cord segments. The mildest form consists only of solitary coccygeal absence. Extreme cases may involve agenesis of the sacrum, lumbar spine, and even some dorsal segments as well. Anomalies of the limbs, anal atresia, and genitourinary malformations may coexist.

The cause of caudal regression syndrome is probably multifactorial, with extrinsic teratogenic factors appearing to be a requirement. In up to 20 percent of cases, there is an association with maternal diabetes.

Isolated coccygeal agenesis is usually asymptomatic, but the more severe anomalies are accompanied by significant neurologic deficits associated with cord and root dysplasia. The caudal regression syndrome by itself leaves a static deficit. Thus, when there is a progressive neurologic deficit in the afflicted patient, a workup is indicated to find associated treatable lesions. There are many other anomalies that can coexist and account for a worsening condition.

Sacral agenesis may be shown to be partial or complete on one or both sides on imaging studies. Ultrasound or MRI can show hypoplasia and dysplasia of the cord in the area ordinarily occupied by the lumbodorsal enlargement; this results in an appearance of a squared-off terminus. Imaging studies may also reveal associated treatable lesions such as hydromyelia, diastematomyelia, or spinal stenosis with neural compression, or a variety of other conditions causing cord tethering such as lipomas, dermoids, thick filum, or adhesive arachnoidal bands. Such lesions may account for progressive deficits in patients with caudal regression syndrome.

☐ SPLIT SPINAL CORD

Cases in which there is splitting of the spinal cord have traditionally been grouped together by the term *diastematomyelia*. On imaging studies the two hemicords are frequently somewhat rotated, and they are separated by an intervening cleft. A fibrous septum or bony or cartilaginous spur may traverse the area of the cleft. This septum or spur is most frequently situated between T-12 and L-5. On the other hand, cervical diastematomyelia is very rare. In most cases the hemicords reunite caudal to the septum.

On MRI, sections in all planes are helpful in delineating the split cord and cleft. Coronal and axial planes are the most useful for MRI depiction. Occasionally, the cleft may not extend through the full thickness of the cord. This is termed *partial diastematomyelia*.

Vertebral osseous abnormalities are seen in virtually all patients with diastematomyelia (Fig. 22-3). However, plain radiographs are less effective than CT for showing a bony septum. Scoliosis, vertebral body segmentation anomalies, and anomalies of the posterior elements are seen in up to 90 percent of cases; spina bifida and abnormal or fused laminae are also common. Generally one observes widening of the interpediculate distance in the region of the septum (Fig. 22-3).

Many other conditions can exist with diastematomyelia, and these can account for clinical problems. Imaging studies may show entities such as thick filum and low conus, hydromyelia, meningocele, dermal sinus, lipoma, Klippel-Feil syndrome, and Chiari malformations.

Hypertrichosis may be present on the midline back in 50 percent or more of patients with diastematomyelia. Other cutaneous abnormalities may also present. Two-thirds of patients may develop scoliosis, and there may be a variety of neurologic manifestations with paraplegia a possible consequence if there is not proper identification and removal of a spur or septum. Upon identification, the median spur or septum is removed to give the spinal cord free mobility within the thecal sac; this makes possible normal growth of the spine as well as prevention of injury to the cord by offending spurs or septum with resultant loss of function or neurologic deterioration.

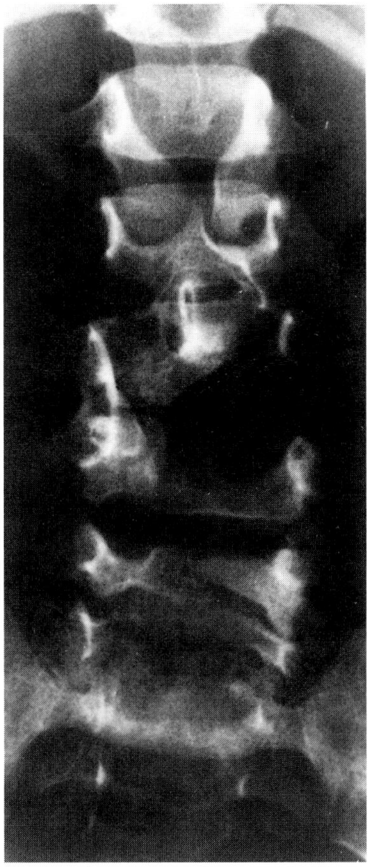

Figure 22-3 Diastematomyelia. Anteroposterior lumbar x-ray showing bony spur, widened interpediculate distance, and numerous osseous anomalies.

☐ DEVELOPMENTAL OSSEOUS SPINAL ABNORMALITIES

Spinal stenosis is common. Some cases are directly related to specific syndromes, but most have no such relationship. When spinal stenosis is pronounced, relatively small degenerative or other superimposed changes can be sufficient to cause neural impingement.

In achondroplasia, there may be stenosis of the entire spinal canal and constriction of the foramen magnum. Short, thick pedicles and reduction of the interpediculate distance may be associated with narrowing of the spinal canal. In patients with achondroplasia, early degenerative changes may provoke symptoms of cord compression. Spinal stenosis may also be found in patients with mucopolysaccharidosis (Morquio's syndrome, Hurler's syndrome, etc). Patients with caudal regression syndrome may also have constriction of the lower spinal canal.

Many *occipitoatlantoaxial anomalies* and variants exist. Most of these do not produce symptoms, but sometimes their radiologic appearance may suggest a serious anomaly when, in fact, the abnormality is quite benign. A case in point is congenital absence of the posterior arch of the atlas. Symptoms rarely occur with such an arch defect. In this anomaly, the articulating parts of the occipital condyles, the lateral masses of C-1, and the lateral masses of C-2 are still intact. The dens and the transverse ligament are still intact. Thus, craniocervical structures are stable.

Some bony anomalies at the craniovertebral junction, however, may lead to instability with resulting serious symptomatology and neurologic handicap. One may use plain radiographs in flexion and extension to determine whether or not there is instability associated with a particular lesion involving the craniovertebral bony structures and ligaments.

Stability may be lost with abnormalities of the dens. Thus, anomalies of this structure can be very important. When the dens is intact (and when it is held solidly by the transverse ligament against the anterior arch of the atlas), stability is ensured. When these structures are intact, this enables the cranium and upper cervical vertebrae to move freely as a stable unit.

We discourage the use of the term *os odontoideum*, since it is controversial and also because it adds very little to the clinical care of patients. We prefer *congenitally separate and dysplastic dens* as a term for such anomalies. In these cases there may be a decidedly abnormal configuration of the dens, and it may be seen to be unquestionably attached to the basiocciput or the anterior arch of C-1. Such appearances indicate a congenital rather than a posttraumatic lesion. Patients with conditions such as Down's or Morquio's syndrome may also have anomalies of the dens. Dens anomalies (including absent dens) and atlantoaxial subluxation can also occur in achondroplasia.

Patients with atlantooccipital fusions may have excessive movement at the atlantoaxial joint because the head does not flex or extend at the atlantooccipital joint. Therefore, atlantoaxial subluxation is a threat in such patients. Furthermore, there may be additional stress at the atlantoaxial joint in these cases because of additional associated fusion of C-2 and C-3. Thus, if the transverse ligament has become stretched or degenerated in these patients, atlantoaxial dislocation may occur in flexion.

Coexisting Chiari I malformations can occur in some patients with atlantooccipital and atlantoaxial fusions. Atlantooccipital fusions and Chiari I malformations can coexist with the Klippel-Feil syndrome.

Many *vertebral segmentation anomalies* are known. Plain radiographs and other imaging studies may reveal specific osseous abnormalities such as congenital absence of the pedicles and other vertebral parts, block vertebrae, butterfly vertebrae, and hemivertebrae. Patients with Klippel-Feil syndrome will show vertebral fusion anomalies. Multiple bizarre vertebral anomalies may be seen with spinal dysraphia. There are also other conditions associated with various skeletal and visceral anomalies.

Spondylolysis probably results from stress fractures of the pars interarticularis; in most cases, it is caused by repeated minor trauma. It does not appear to be developmental in origin, since the incidence of pars defects is extremely low on imaging studies in young children. Pars defects have rarely been identified in children as young as 5½ to 6½ years of age. On the other hand, spondylolysis may be identified in up to 5 percent of the adult population.

☐ SPINAL VASCULAR MALFORMATIONS

Spinal vascular malformations are reviewed elsewhere in this text.

SUGGESTED READINGS

1. Anderson FM: Occult spinal dysraphism: A series of 73 cases. *Pediatrics* 55:826–835, 1975.
2. Anderson FM: Occult spinal dysraphism: Diagnosis and management. *J Pediatr* 73:163–177, 1968.
3. Barkovich AJ, Raghavan N: MR imaging of the caudal regression syndrome. *AJNR* 10:1223–1231, 1989.
4. Barnes PD et al: Magnetic resonance imaging in infants and children with spinal dysraphism. *AJNR* 7:465–472, 1986.
5. Brunberg JA et al: Magnetic resonance imaging of spinal dysraphism. *Radiol Clin North Am* 26:181–205, 1988.
6. Cheung G et al: Spinal dysraphism, in Cohen MD, Edwards MK (eds): *Magnetic Resonance Imaging of Children*. Philadelphia, Decker, 1990, pp 421–462.
7. DeLaPaz RL: Congenital anomalies of the spine and spinal cord, in Enzmann D et al (eds): *MR of the Spine*. St Louis, Mosby-Year Book, 1991, pp 176–236.

8. Fitz CR, Harwood-Nash DC: The tethered conus. *AJR* 125:515–523, 1975.
9. Gardner WJ, McMurry FG: "Non-communicating syringomyelia": A non-existent entity. *Surg Neurol* 6:251–256, 1976.
10. Geremia GK et al: MR imaging: Characteristics of a neurenteric cyst. *AJNR* 9:978–980, 1988.
11. Gilmor RL, Batnitzky S: Diastematomyelia—Rare and unusual features. *Neuroradiology* 16:87–88, 1978.
12. Heinz ER et al: Tethered spinal cord following meningomyelocele repair. *Radiology* 131:153–160, 1979.
13. Hilal SK et al: Diastematomyelia in children: Radiographic study of cases. *Radiology* 112:609–621, 1974.
14. Hori A et al: Dimyelia, diplomyelia, and diastematomyelia. *Clin Neuropathol* 1:23–30, 1982.
15. Kaplan JO, Quencer RM: The occult tethered conus syndrome in the adult. *Radiology* 137:387–391, 1980.
16. Lee BCP et al: MR imaging of the craniocervical junction. *AJNR* 6:209–213, 1985.
17. Lewonowski K et al: Routine use of magnetic resonance imaging in idiopathic scoliosis patients less than eleven years of age. *Spine* 117:109–117, 1992.
18. McComb JG: Personal communication, 1995.
19. Menkes JH et al: Malformation of the central nervous system, in Menkes J (ed): *Textbook of Child Neurology*, 4th ed. Philadelphia, Lea & Febiger, 1990, pp 209–283.
20. Naidich TP et al: A new understanding of dorsal dysraphism with lipoma (lipomyeloschisis): Radiologic evaluation and surgical correction. *AJNR* 4:103–116, 1983.
21. Naidich TP et al: Spinal dysraphism, in Newton TH, Potts DG (eds): *Modern Neuroradiology*: Vol 1. *Computed Tomography of the Spine and Spinal Cord*. San Anselmo, CA, Clavadel, 1983, pp 299–353.
22. Nelson M et al: The natural history of repaired myelomeningocele. *Radiographics* 8:695–706, 1988.
23. Page LK: Occult spinal dysraphism and related disorders, in Wilkins RH, Rengachary SS (eds): *Neurosurgery*. Vol 3. New York: McGraw-Hill, 1985.
24. Pojunas K et al: Syringomyelia and hydromyelia: Magnetic resonance evaluation. *Radiology* 153:679–683, 1984.
25. Post MJD et al: Radiologic evaluation of spinal cord fissures. *AJNR* 7:329–335, 1986.
26. Raghavan N et al: MR imaging in the tethered spinal cord syndrome. *AJNR* 10:27–36, 1989.
27. Rothman SLG, Glenn WV: Spondylolysis and spondylolisthesis, in Newton TH, Potts DG (eds): *Modern Neuroradiology*: Vol 1. *Computed Tomography of the Spine and Spinal Cord*. San Anselmo, CA, Clavadel, pp 267–280, 1983.
28. Sarwar M et al: Experimental cord stretchability and the tethered cord syndrome. *AJNR* 4:641–643, 1983.
29. Sarwar M et al: Primary tethered cord syndrome: A new hypothesis of its origin. *AJNR* 5:234–242, 1984.
30. Scatliff JH et al: Closed spinal dysraphism: Analysis of clinical, radiological and surgical findings in 104 consecutive patients. *AJNR* 10:269–277, 1989.
31. Segall HD et al: Craniovertebral junction pathology, in Taveras JM, Ferrucci J (eds): *Radiology: Diagnosis/Imaging/Intervention*: Vol 3. Philadelphia, Lippincott, 1988, pp 1–27.
32. Sherman JL et al: The MR appearance of syringomyelia: New observations. *AJNR* 7:985–995, 1986.
33. Smoker WRK et al: Intradural spinal teratoma: Case report and review of the literature. *AJNR* 7:905–909, 1986.
34. Sostrin R et al: Occult spinal dysraphism in the geriatric patient. *Radiology* 125:165–169, 1977.
35. Tadmor R et al: Importance of early radiologic diagnosis of congenital anomalies of the spine. *Surg Neurol* 23:493–501, 1985.
36. Williams B: Simultaneous cerebral and spinal fluid pressure recordings: II. Cerebrospinal dissociation with lesions at the foramen magnum. *Acta Neurochir (Wien)* 59:123–142, 1981.
37. Wolpert SM et al: Computed tomography in spinal dysraphism. *Surg Neurol* 8:199–206, 1977.
38. Zimmerman RA, Bilaniuk LT: Applications of magnetic resonance imaging in diseases of the pediatric central nervous system. *MRI Pediatr* 4:11–24, 1986.

☐ QUESTIONS (True or False)

1. Regarding progressive scoliosis,
- **a.** Idiopathic progressive scoliosis is not common in children under age 6.
- **b.** Intraspinal lesions must be ruled out in a young child with scoliosis.
- **c.** When clinical neurologic examination is normal, progressive scoliosis need not be evaluated in children.
- **d.** Magnetic resonance imaging is the imaging modality of choice for evaluating patients with progressive scoliosis.
- **e.** Scoliosis in children may be associated with tethered cord, diastematomyelia, Chiari I malformation, etc.

2. Regarding myelomeningocele,
- **a.** Myelomeningocele is an open dysraphic lesion.
- **b.** Chiari II malformation is not associated with myelomeningocele.
- **c.** Hydrocephalus is present in 90 percent of cases in children.
- **d.** Imaging plays a minor role in evaluating such lesions shortly after birth, although cranial ultrasound to detect hydrocephalus is worthwhile.
- **e.** Studies by MRI following meningocele repair normally depict a low-lying cord terminating in a placode that is not clearly separable from the posterior thecal sac at the operative site.

3. Regarding diastematomyelia,
- **a.** Plain spine x-rays are frequently normal.
- **b.** On imaging studies, the two hemicords are frequently somewhat rotated, and they are separated by an intervening cleft.
- **c.** Hydromyelia may be associated with diastematomyelia.
- **d.** Hypertrichosis may be present on the midline back in 50 percent of cases.
- **e.** A fibrous septum or bony cartilaginous spur may traverse the area of the cleft.

4. Regarding congenital intradural cysts,
- **a.** Arachnoid cysts of developmental origin are most commonly found in the thoracic region dorsal to the spinal cord.
- **b.** Ependymal cysts tend to be dorsally situated.
- **c.** Neurenteric cysts are differentiated from ependymal cysts pathologically.
- **d.** Neurenteric cysts are usually anterior or anterolateral to the cord.
- **e.** Spinal neurenteric cysts may enlarge the spinal canal.

5. Regarding meningocele,
- **a.** Posterior meningocele is the simplest form of open neural defect.
- **b.** In anterior sacral meningocele, the dura and arachnoid extend out of the sacral canal via a sacral bony deficit into the pelvis anteriorly.
- **c.** Thoracic meningocele may project laterally or anteriorly from the spinal canal.
- **d.** Thoracic lateral meningoceles are not associated with neurofibromatosis.
- **e.** Thoracic meningoceles may enlarge and cause pulmonary and neural compression.

☐ ANSWERS

1. **a.** T
b. T
c. F
d. T
e. T

2. **a.** T
b. F
c. T
d. T
e. T

3. **a.** F
b. T
c. T
d. T
e. T

4. **a.** T
b. F
c. T
d. T
e. T

5. **a.** T
b. T
c. T
d. F
e. T

CHAPTER

23 Bone Lesions

Patrick M. Colletti
William D. Boswell

Diseases of the bony spine can be divided into diseases of the marrow space, diseases of the marrow space with associated bony involvement, diseases of the bone with associated marrow involvement, diseases of bone, epidural lesions, and ligamentous abnormalities.

Magnetic resonance imaging (MRI) is an excellent imaging modality for diseases of the bony spine, particularly the evaluation of diseases of bone marrow. Computed tomography (CT) is useful in the evaluation of the bony cortex of the vertebral bodies, particularly fracture of the bony spine. Plain radiography remains an important imaging modality for the evaluation of the bony spine. Several well recognized radiographic changes are discussed in this chapter.

☐ MARROW REPLACEMENT ABNORMALITIES

While spinal bone marrow abnormalities can be demonstrated with CT, MRI is clearly the examination of choice in the evaluation of abnormalities confined to the bone marrow. The appearance of the bone marrow depends upon the relative amounts of fat and cellularity that are present, and this varies with age and physiologic state. In the newborn, the bone marrow is entirely cellular. There is progressive fatty change within the bone marrow, and the elderly patient may have predominately fatty marrow. Most bone marrow abnormalities have a relatively low signal on T1-weighted images and high signal on T2-weighted images (Fig. 23-1). Very high signal on T1-weighted images is seen with fatty replacement of the marrow. This occurs most commonly with radiation therapy (Fig. 23-1), chemotherapy, or steroid administration. One may also see high signal within bone marrow on T1-weighted images when there is hemorrhage, as, for example, after trauma, where the shortened T1 of methemoglobin can be demonstrated. Very low signal on both T1- and T2-weighted images may be identified in bone marrow in patients that are iron-loaded from multiple transfusions. Relatively low signal within bone marrow may be seen in patients receiving large amounts of iron supplementation. The signal characteristics of bone marrow in a variety of medical conditions are summarized in Table 23-1.

The most sensitive way to evaluate bone marrow abnormalities is with fat-suppressed images. A variety of techniques including chemical saturation and short Tao inversion (inversion time) recovery imaging may be used. Occasionally, the administration of contrast may be useful.

- Marrow replacement abnormalities—such as metastasis, myeloma, or lymphoma—characteristically show bony cortical involvement and are frequently associated with epidural masses.
- Marrow replacement abnormalities such as anemia, myelosclerosis, and radiation change characteristically do not involve bony cortex.
- Total fatty replacement of marrow is seen as very high signal intensity (higher than that of the normal marrow) on T1-weighted images; this may be seen with radiation therapy, chemotherapy, or steroid administration.
- Very low signal within the marrow on both T1- and T2-weighted images is seen in patients who are iron-loaded from multiple transfusions.

METASTASIS

- Metastatic disease is the most common malignant tumor of bone.

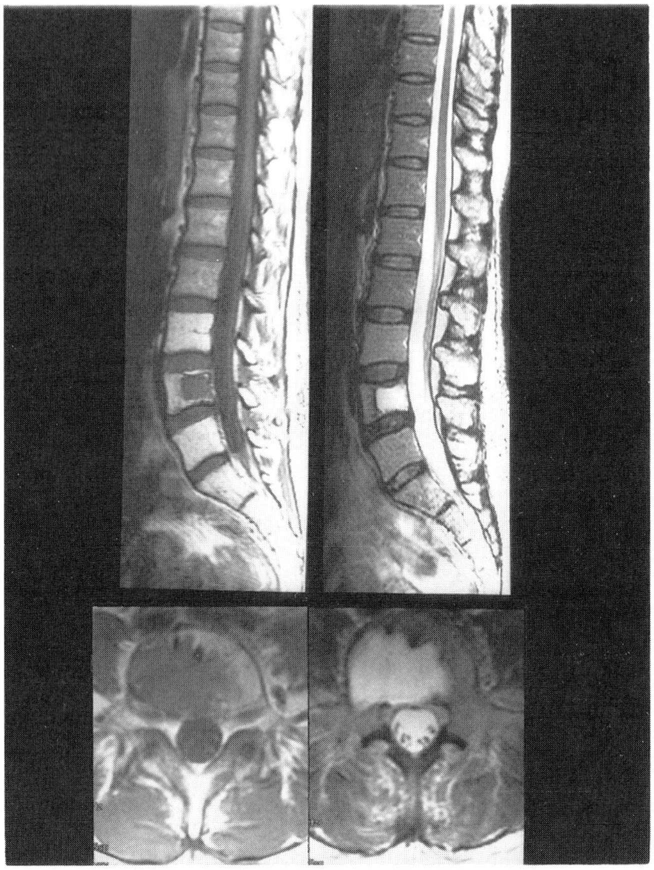

Figure 23-1 A 65-year-old woman with a history of L4 plasmacytoma was studied by MRI. Sagittal T1-weighted image shows increased signal in the bone marrow from L3 through the sacrum from prior radiation. The L4 lesion shows low signal on T1-weighted images (*upper and lower left*) and increase signal on T2-weighted images (*upper and lower right*). This patient's images show the effects of radiation on the bone marrow with fatty replacement within the port of radiation. As is typical with most bone marrow abnormalities primarily manifested by increased tissue water, the primary lesion in any L4 vertebra shows low signal on T1-weighted images and high signal on T2-weighted images.

- Spinal metastatic disease most frequently involves the vertebral bodies, followed by the pedicles and neural arch.
- Metastases to the spine are most frequently seen in the thoracic spine, followed by lumbar spine.
- Primary neoplasms include carcinoma of breast, lung, prostate, kidney, and lymphoma, melanoma.

Table 23-1
MRI SIGNAL CHARACTERISTICS IN BONE MARROW REPLACEMENT ABNORMALITIES

Abnormality	T1-Weighted Images	T2-Weighted Images
Metastases	Low signal	Intermediate/high signal
Myeloma	Low signal	High signal
Lymphoma	Low signal	High signal
Anemia	Low signal	Low signal
Myelosclerosis	Low signal	Low signal
Leukemia	Low signal	Intermediate/high signal
Radiation change	High signal	Intermediate/high signal
Chemotherapy	High signal	Intermediate/high signal
Iron loading	Low signal	Low signal

- Most metastases are osteolytic.
- Osteoblastic lesions are seen in metastatic prostatic carcinoma, or, less likely, in breast carcinoma.
- Spinal metastasis begins with the replacement of fatty trabeculae.
- Magnetic resonance imaging is more sensitive than plain x-ray, CT, or radionuclide bone scan in detecting early bony involvement in the spine.
- Metastases show hypointensity on T1-weighted images, compared to the hyperintensity of normal bone marrow, and hyperintensity on T2-weighted images.
- Variable degrees of contrast enhancement are seen in bony metastases. Contrast enhancement may masquerade the lesion, making it isointense to normal bone marrow.
- Metastatic disease is the most common epidural neoplasm.

MYELOMA

- Myeloma is a malignant tumor of bone marrow plasma cells.
- Male:female ratio = 3:1.
- The age of onset is usually in the fifth or sixth decade.
- The thoracic and lumbar spine are more frequently affected than the cervical spine and sacrum.
- Involvement of multiple vertebral bodies is common.

- On imaging studies, multiple myeloma resembles metastatic disease.

LYMPHOMA

- Osseous lymphoma may involve the bone marrow of the spine without significant epidural mass.
- Epidural lymphoma may result from osseous lymphoma or nonosseous lymphoma (from retroperitoneal lymph nodes).
- Intradural lymphoma probably results from hematogenous spread or spread via perineural lymphatics.

☐ PRIMARY MARROW LESIONS WITH BONY INVOLVEMENT

Spinal lesions with both bone marrow and bone involvement are typically metastases, myeloma, lymphoma, hemangioma, and eosinophilic granuloma. These will be seen as well with CT as with MRI; occasionally, CT may be useful for characterization—as, for example, in identifying the vertical spiculations in spinal hemangioma. Again, these lesions typically have relatively low signal on T1-weighted images and higher signal on T2-weighted images. Hemangiomas, however, often contain fat or hemorrhage and may show relatively high signal on T1-weighted images. All of the lesions tend to enhance somewhat with contrast agent.

HEMANGIOMA

- Two histologic types are described, cavernous and capillary. Cavernous hemangiomas are commonly found in the vertebrae.
- The incidence of spinal hemangioma is about 10 percent at autopsy.
- Usually a single vertebral body is involved, but two or more vertebral bodies may be involved.
- Usually the body of the vertebra is involved, but posterior arch involvement may also be seen.
- Vertical striped orientation of the bone is seen on plain x-ray or CT. The vertebral body may be enlarged.
- High signal intensity is seen within the marrow on T1-weighted MRI due to the presence of fat and/or hemorrhage.
- The cortical margin is usually intact. Occasionally, an aggressive hemangioma may be seen, with cortical destruction and associated epidural mass.
- The differential diagnosis of an enlarged vertebral body on plain x-ray includes myeloma, lymphoma, Paget's disease, metastasis, and hemangioma.

LANGERHANS' HISTIOCYTOSIS

- The disease causes destructive changes involving the vertebral body or pedicle.
- Collapse of the vertebral body results in vertebra plana.
- An associated paraspinal mass may be seen.
- The differential diagnosis includes fracture, hemangioma, metastasis, myeloma, fracture secondary to steroid therapy, and Ewing's sarcoma.

SICKLE-CELL DISEASE

- Loss of bone density and a coarsening of the trabecular pattern are seen on plain x-ray and CT.
- The spine exhibits a uniform biconcave contour of all the vertebral bodies—fish-mouth vertebrae.
- The differential diagnosis includes Cushing's syndrome and steroid therapy.
- The spine in sickle-cell patients is vulnerable to *Salmonella* osteomyelitis.

☐ PRIMARY BONE LESIONS WITH MARROW INVOLVEMENT

A number of benign and malignant bony tumors of the spine occur. Computed tomography and plain radiographs are quite useful for detection and characterization of these lesions; MRI is only occasionally necessary for further evaluation. Osteoid osteoma may be difficult to identify within the spine and occasionally bone scintigraphy is required to locate the lesion. Once the proper level is identified, CT will always show the radiodense nidus, which is most common in the posterior elements. Clinically, these lesions are characterized by rather significant pain. By contrast, osteoblastoma, osteochondroma, aneurysmal bone cysts, and giant-cell tumor all cause a certain amount of expansion of bone and are easier to identify on plain radiographs. Osteoblastoma tends to be more destructive, while aneurysmal bone cysts and giant cell tumor may produce typical bubbly-type lesions. Aneurysmal bone cysts in the spine may actually extend across the facet joints to involve adjacent vertebrae. Giant-cell tumors may also appear to be relatively aggressive. Identification of fluid fluid levels by magnetic resonance imaging is most typical of aneurysmal bone cysts. Secondary aneurysmal bone cysts may occur with other lesions, including giant cell tumor. Osteochondroma of the spine is relatively uncommon. Sclerotic spicules of bone in osteochondroma can be shown to contain marrow by MRI.

The most common malignant tumor of the spine is metastatic disease. This most commonly occurs in the vertebral bodies and pedicles and is generally destructive except in cases of prostatic carcinoma and treated metastatic breast carcinoma. Occasionally other metastatic lesions demonstrate sclerosis. This includes some gastrointestinal malignancies and lymphoma.

The primary malignant bone lesions of the spine may be characterized to some extent radiographically with the use of CT along with clinical history and the patient's age. Chordoma of the spine most commonly occurs in the sacrum and may appear to be rather destructive, with amorphous calcification. Ewing's sarcoma tends to be more permeative and may involve a periosteal reaction. Chondrosarcoma most commonly involves posterior elements, with expansion and stippled calcification. Osteogenic sarcoma may also involve posterior elements and although the vertebral body may be involved. Cortical destruction with zones of osteosclerosis are typically seen. The primary bone lesions with marrow involvement are summarized in Table 23-2.

BENIGN LESIONS

Osteoid Osteoma

- Uncommon.
- Occurs in patients between 5 to 25 years of age.
- Classic x-ray appearance is that of a small radiolucent intracortical nidus surrounded by a large sclerotic area of cortical thickening.
- The neural arch, spinous process, and transverse process may be involved in the spine.

Osteoblastoma

- Rare.
- The most common location is in the vertebral arch, mainly in the transverse and spinous processes.
- About 50 percent of cases have vertebral body involvement as well.
- A well-circumscribed, expansile bone lesion.

Aneurysmal Bone Cyst

- Predilection for cervical and thoracic spine.
- A bone lesion characterized by a "blown out" cortical appearance.
- May involve the body, arch, and spinous or transverse processes of the spine.
- Vertebral involvement exhibits an expanding trabeculated lesion.
- The lesion may extend along the spine to involve several adjacent vertebral bodies with a large soft tissue mass.
- Computed tomography is better in the demonstration of a thin shell of expanded bone.

Table 23-2
RADIOGRAPHIC FINDINGS IN BENIGN PRIMARY BONE LESIONS WITH MARROW INVOLVEMENT

Lesion	Patient's Age	Radiographic Finding
Osteoid osteoma	5 to 25 years	Radiodense lesion typically involving posterior elements.
Osteoblastoma	20 to 40 years	Lytic lesion with cortical destruction and bony shell involving the posterior elements. Half show epidural mass.
Osteochondroma	10 to 40 years	Asymptomatic sclerotic spicule, contains marrow
Aneurysmal bone cyst	10 to 20 years	Expansile bony lesion typically involving posterior elements. May show fluid fluid levels on MRI. May extend across to involve posterior elements of adjacent vertebra.
Giant cell tumor	20 to 40 years	Expansile lesion involving posterior elements. May appear to be aggressive.
Hemangioma	Any	CT—reduced density, vertical striation. MRI—high-signal vertebral body on T1-weighted images. Lesion may focal or may involve entire body.

RADIOGRAPHIC FINDINGS IN MALIGNANT PRIMARY BONE LESIONS WITH MARROW INVOLVEMENT

Lesion	Patient's Age	Radiographic Finding
Chordoma	30 to 70 years	Solid tumor with cystic area primarily involving the sacrum, skull base, or spinal axis. Osteolytic with midline mass with amorphous calcification and peripheral sclerosis.
Ewing's sarcoma	5 to 25 years	4% occur in spine. Permeative changes with periosteal reaction and expansion with associated mass.
Chondrosarcoma	Over 40 years	Posterior element involvement with expansion, destruction, and stippled calcification.
Osteogenic sarcoma	15 to 35 years	Vertebral body or posterior elements. Cortical destruction with associated osteosclerotic zone.
Metastatic disease	Any	Located in vertebral body and pedicles. Primarily destructive except with prostate, treated breast, occasionally others.

- Both CT and MRI can demonstrate the soft tissue mass, which is usually of mixed hypo- and hyperintensity on both T1- and T2-weighted images.
- MRI shows multiseptated mass with fluid-fluid level with hemorrhage.

Giant-Cell Tumor
- Giant-cell tumors of the spine are rare (3 percent).
- Approximately half of spinal giant-cell tumor occur in the sacrum.
- Spinal giant-cell tumors tend to occur earlier than those at other sites and have a peak incidence in the second and third decades.
- Female:male ratio = 2:1 for spinal lesions.
- Involvement of the spine occurs at the vertebral body, neural arch. A paravertebral mass may be seen.
- Radiographically, they can mimic aneurysmal bone cyst.

MALIGNANT LESIONS

Chordoma
- Rare, slow-growing, locally invasive malignant bone tumors.
- Common locations include:
  Sacrococcygeal, 50 percent
  Clivus, 35 percent
  Vertebral body, 15 percent
- Bone destruction with soft tissue mass.
- Intervertebral disk may or may not be involved.
- Amorphous calcification and residual bone are better seen on CT.
- Chordomas have low signal intensity on T1-weighted images and high signal intensity on T2-weighted images.
- Chordomas enhance with gadolinium.

Ewing's Sarcoma
- Ill-defined, permeative destruction of vertebral bodies associated with paraspinal mass.
- Collapse of the vertebral body may be seen.
- The differential diagnosis includes osteomyelitis, Langerhans' histiocytosis.
- Primary Ewing's sarcoma of the spine is rare; most spinal Ewing's sarcomas are metastatic in nature.

Chondrosarcoma
- Osteolytic expansile lesions with amorphous calcification.
- Spine is only occasionally involved.
- Posterior elements may be involved.
- Chondrosarcoma may develop in a preexisting cartilaginous lesion or in association with Paget's disease or previous radiation.

Osteogenic Sarcoma
- Cortical destruction associated with sclerotic change and soft tissue invasion.
- The vertebral body or neural arch may be involved.
- May be associated with preexisting osteochondroma, Paget's disease, or previous radiation.

☐ PRIMARY BONE LESIONS

The primary bone lesions of the spine are best detected and characterized with plain radiography and CT. Lesions with increased bony density include osteopetrosis, osteoblastic metastases (prostate, breast, gastrointestinal malignancy), lymphoma, osteoid osteoma, Paget's disease, myelosclerosis, and fluorosis. Primarily lucent changes occur with osteoporosis, most metastases, myeloma, and infections.

Fractures of the bony spine are more conspicuous on CT, although they may be seen on MRI (Fig. 23-2). Fractures of the spine may be either stable or unstable depending upon the extent and location of the trauma. Injuries to the cervical spine are summarized in Table 3. Vertebra plana may be associated with fractures, but eosinophilic granuloma, hemangioma, tumor, and infection must also be considered. "Fish-mouth"-shaped vertebrae may be seen in sickle cell anemia (Fig. 23-3).

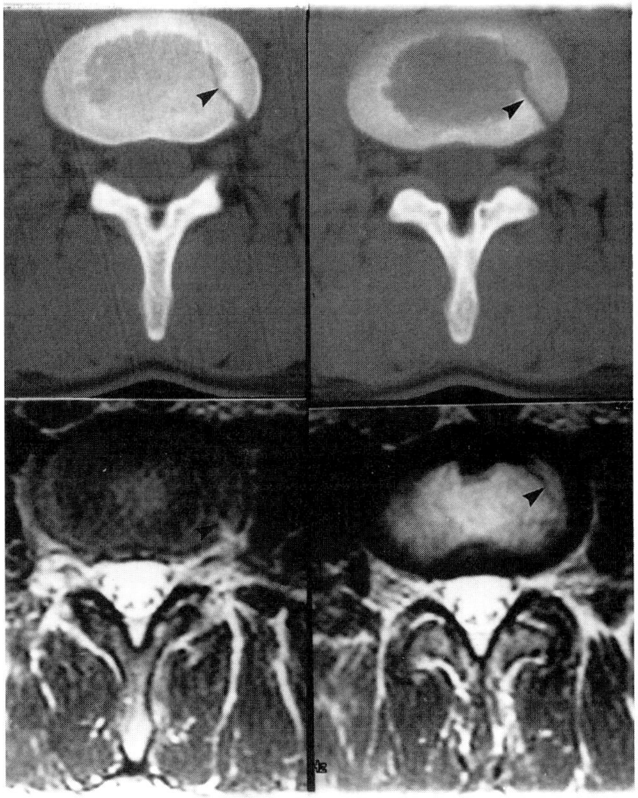

Figure 23-2 This 20-year-old woman presented with back pain after an automobile accident. Computed tomography (*upper row*) better shows the minimally displaced fracture of the vertebral body as compared to T2-weighted axial MRI (*lower row*). The arrowhead points to the fracture line. This case demonstrates that fractures and other primary lesions of cortical bone may be demonstrated with MRI but are much more conspicuous with CT.

Table 23-3
CLASSIFICATION OF INJURIES OF THE CERVICAL SPINE

Type	Subtype	Findings	Stability
Flexion	Subluxation	Soft tissue swelling with increased distance between spinal processes.	Stable
	Bilateral interfacetal dislocation	Soft tissue swelling. Incidental fractures. Anterior dislocation with respect to inferior vertebrae.	Unstable (do not flex/extend)
	Simple wedge fracture	Anterior compression fracture.	Stable
	Flexion teardrop fracture	Triangular fracture fragment anteriorly with severe comminution of body and posterior dislocation	Very dangerous, associated with anterior cord injury (do not flex/extend)
	Clay shoveler's fracture	Fracture of spinous processes (C-6, C-7).	Stable
Flexion/Rotation	Unilateral interfacetal dislocations	Perched vertebrae, anterior dislocation.	Stable (do not flex/extend)
Vertical compression	Jefferson's C-1 fracture	Anterior and posterior fracture of C-1 with bilateral displacement.	Unstable (do not flex/extend)
	Other bursting fractures	Comminuted fracture.	Stable (do not flex/extend)
Extension	Posterior neural arch	Nondisplaced fractures.	Stable
	Extension teardrop	Usually anterior chip fracture of C-2.	Stable in flexion, unstable in extension
	Hangman's fracture	Fracture dislocation, C-2 anterior dislocation, fractured pedicles.	Unstable (do not flex/extend)

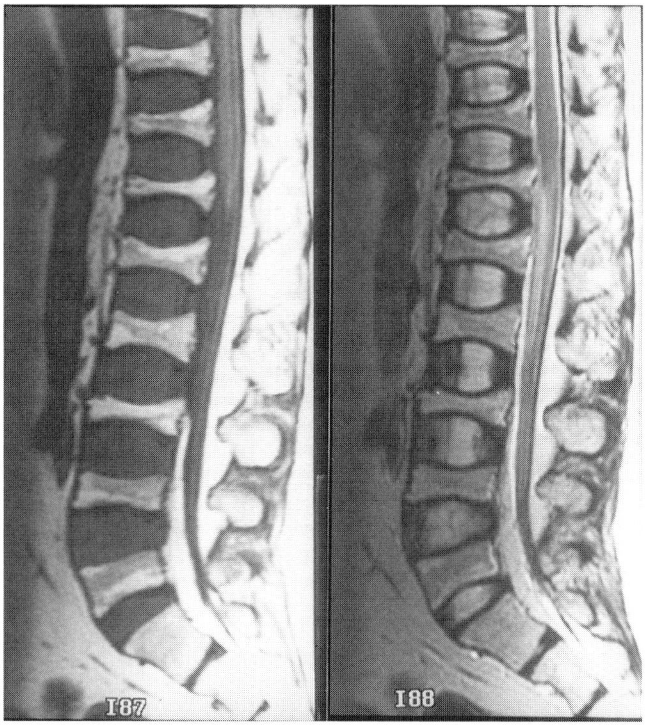

Figure 23-3 This 24-year-old woman had a history of sickle cell anemia and presented with back pain. Sagittal T1- (*left*) and T2-weighted images (*right*) show fish-mouth vertebrae. In this case the bone marrow has relatively high signal. However, in most cases of sickle cell anemia, the signal in the bone marrow is relatively low secondary to a combination of increased cellularity, infarction, and iron loading.

Fractures of the thoracolumbar junction are typically related to compressive and flexion injuries. These may cause a variety of deformities depending upon the amount of structural damage to the three columns of the spine. The three columns of the spine include the anterior vertebral body and anterior longitudinal ligament, the posterior vertebral body and posterior longitudinal ligament, and the posterior elements and the interspinous ligaments. When more than one column is involved in trauma, instability occurs (Fig. 23-4).

Ossification of the posterior longitudinal ligament is discussed in Chapter 24.

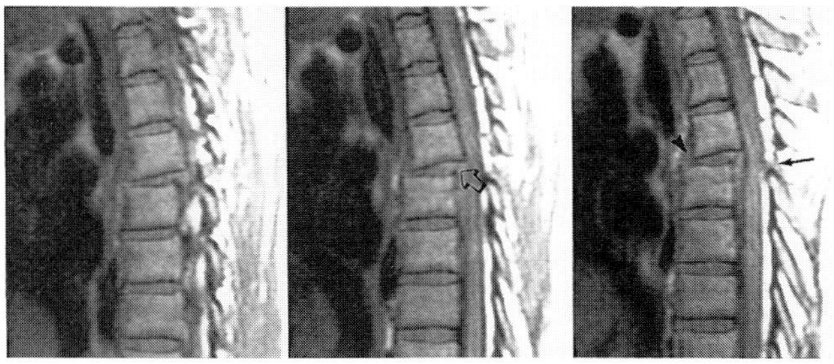

Figure 23-4 A 21-year-old woman received a flexion injury in an automobile accident. She presented with weakness in both legs. On MRI, sagittal T1-weighted images show disruption of the anterior longitudinal ligament (*arrowheads*), posterior longitudinal ligament (*open arrow*), and interspinous ligament (*arrow*). Disruption of two of the three columns of the spine results in instability. All three columns are disrupted in this case.

SUGGESTED READINGS

1. Algra PR et al: Detection of vertebral metastases: Comparison between MR imaging and bone scintigraphy. *RadioGraphics* 11:219–232, 1991.
2. Colletti PM et al: Spinal MR imaging in suspected metastases: Correlation with skeletal scintigraphy. *Magn Reson Imaging* 9:349–355, 1991.
3. Krandsorf MJ et al: Imaging of bone and soft tissue tumors. *Radiol Clin North Am* 31:359–372, 1993.
4. Munday TL et al: Musculoskeletal causes of spinal axis compromise: Beyond the usual suspects. *RadioGraphics* 14:1225–1245, 1994.
5. Remedios PA et al: Magnetic resonance imaging of bone after radiation. *Magn Reson Imaging* 6:301–304, 1988.
6. Steiner RM et al: Magnetic resonance imaging of bone marrow: Diagnostic value in diffuse hematologic disorders. *Magn Reson Q* 6:17, 1990.
7. Vogler JB, Murphy WA: Bone marrow imaging. *Radiology* 168:679, 1988.
8. Weinreb JC: MR imaging of bone marrow: A map would help. *Radiology* 177:23, 1990.
9. Yuh WT et al: Vertebral compression fractures: Distinction between benign and malignant causes with MR imaging *Radiology* 172:215–218, 1989.

☐ QUESTIONS

1. Regarding MRI of bone marrow abnormalities, which of the following are true?
- **a.** Lesions with increased cellularity have low signal on T1-weighted images and intermediate to high signal on T2-weighted images.
- **b.** Lesions with edema have low signal on T1-weighted images and high signal on T2-weighted images.
- **c.** Iron overload within the bone marrow causes low signal on all sequences.
- **d.** Radiation change causes high signal on T1-weighted images in bone marrow secondary to fatty replacement.
- **e.** Sclerotic lesions give low signal on all pulse sequences.

2. Regarding benign primary bone lesions, which of the following is true?
- **a.** In general, CT may be more useful in characterizing lesions than MRI.
- **b.** Osteoid osteoma typically presents in the spine as a focal radiodense lesion involving the posterior elements.
- **c.** Aneurysmal bone cysts may be difficult to differentiate from giant-cell tumor by imaging.
- **d.** Hemangioma of the spine often contains vertically oriented striations surrounded by fat.

3. The following are true regarding malignant bone lesions of the spine:
- **a.** Generally, CT is more useful for characterization as compared with MRI.
- **b.** The most common malignant bone lesion of the spine is osteogenic sarcoma.
- **c.** The most common location for chordoma in the spine is in the sacrum.
- **d.** Chordoma, chondrosarcoma, and osteogenic sarcoma are more likely to demonstrate calcifications as compared with Ewing's sarcoma.

4. Which of the following cervical spine injuries are unstable?
- **a.** Flexion subluxation
- **b.** Bilateral interfacetal dislocation
- **c.** Simple wedge fracture
- **d.** Flexion teardrop fracture
- **e.** Clay shoveler's fracture
- **f.** Jefferson's C-1 fracture
- **g.** Bursting fracture
- **h.** Extension teardrop fracture
- **i.** Hangman's fracture

☐ ANSWERS

1.
- **a.** T
- **b.** T
- **c.** T
- **d.** T
- **e.** T

2.
- **a.** T
- **b.** T
- **c.** T
- **d.** T

3.
- **a.** T
- **b.** F (Metastatic disease is the most common malignant bone lesion of the spine)
- **c.** T
- **d.** T

4.
- **a.** stable
- **b.** unstable
- **c.** stable
- **d.** very unstable
- **e.** stable
- **f.** unstable
- **g.** stable (do not flex/bend)
- **h.** stable in flexion/unstable in extension
- **i.** unstable

CHAPTER

24

Disk Space Disease, Spondylosis, and Related Disorders

Michael R. Terk
D. M. Forrester

☐ ANATOMY

The intervertebral disk is part of a three-joint complex that provides controlled motion to the spinal columns. The disks account for 20 to 30 percent of the length of the spine in humans. There are four relatively distinct anatomic zones that form the anatomic unit of the intervertebral disk.

ANNULUS FIBROSUS

- There is no clear anatomic distinction between the nucleus pulposus and the annulus in adults.
- The annulus is composed of, on average, 12 lamellae, which form a tube enclosing the nucleus pulposus.
- The water content is 60 to 70 percent by weight.
- Collagen accounts for 60 to 70 percent of the dry weight.
- Type I collagen predominates in the peripheral zone of the annulus (Sharpey's fibers). This type of collagen is more resistant to radial tension. More centrally and in the nucleus pulposus, there is an increasing proportion of type II collagen, which is thought to be more hydrated than type I and more resistant to compressive forces.
- Sharpey's fibers attach to the vertebral body's end plates at the ring apophysis.
- Pain-sensitive nerve fibers are located in the outer fibers of the annulus.

NUCLEUS PULPOSUS

- The nucleus represents the definitive remnant of the embryonal notochord.
- Histochemically, the nucleus is composed of 30-Å collagen fibrils in a dense proteoglycan matrix, producing a gellike consistency.
- The collagen content is 5 percent of the total weight or 15 to 20 percent dry weight.
- Proteoglycans make up to 50 percent of the dry weight, decreasing with age.
- The water content is 90 percent in infants, reducing to 70 percent with maturity. Among the commonly encountered proteoglycans are chondroitin-6-sulfate, keratan sulfate, hyaluronic acid, and chondroitin-4-sulfate.
- Type II collagen fibers, which resist compression, predominate in the nucleus and in the more central portions of the annulus.

TRANSITION ZONE

- The blending of nuclear and annular fibers.
- The zone becomes very indistinct with increasing age, as the distribution of collagen types changes.

HYALINE CARTILAGE END PLATES

- While only 1 mm thick, these form an effective barrier to the diffusion of large molecules, thereby limiting nutrition. Although the newborn end plates contain numerous blood vessels, vascularity is lost during childhood, and the end plates become avascular in adulthood.

☐ DISK DISEASE

Back pain is a problem of major magnitude. Some 80 percent of adults have back pain at some point in their lives, and 31 million Americans have back pain at any one time. While pain is not necessarily related to disk disease and the relationship is unclear, the prevalence of disk abnormality is extremely high (up to 64 percent) even in patients who are asymptomatic at the time of examination. This incidence increases with age, such that by age 50, some 85 to 95 percent of autopsies show evidence of degenerative disk disease.

NOMENCLATURE

The nomenclature applied to these common disk abnormalities is at times confusing and ambiguous. An emotionally neutral but anatomically specific classification follows:

Normal: No disk extension beyond the interspace.
Bulge: Circumferential symmetrical extension with an intact annulus.
Protrusion: Focal or asymmetrical extension, with the base in contact with the disk of origin contained by the posterior longitudinal ligament.
Extrusion: More extreme extension with narrow communication with the disk of origin. The disk may or may not be contained by the posterior longitudinal ligament. There may be migration of the fragment caudal or less commonly cephalad.
Free disk fragment: A free fragment has no communication with the disk of origin. The disk fragment may migrate in any direction. Rarely, a free fragment may be seen intradurally.

- Cervical disk herniations most commonly (90 percent) occur at the C5–6 of C6–7 levels, whereas lumbar disk herniations most commonly (90 percent) occur at L4–5 and L5–S1 levels.
- Disk protrusion, disk extrusion, and free disk fragment are considered by some to be equivalent to disk herniation. In the majority of cases, they are associated with pain caused by direct mechanical compression of the nerve roots.

IMAGING

Plain Radiographs

- Narrowing of disk space
- Vacuum disk
- Disk calcification

Contrast Myelography

- Provides definition of the thecal sac and indicates the extent of extradural disk compression on the nerve roots or the central sac.
- Correlation of 80 to 90 percent with surgical findings at L4–5 but less sensitive at L5–S1 because of the width of the thecal sac.
- Less sensitive for lateral disks, where epidural venography has been historically helpful.

Computed Tomography

- Accuracy of 90 percent or higher in the diagnosis of disk displacements.
- More sensitive than myelography to lateral and L5–S1 herniations.
- Presently the most sensitive modality for bone and foraminal disease.

Diskography

- Direct injection into the area confined by the annulus.
- The normal disk will accommodate 1 to 1.5 mL of contrast.
- Reproduction of the patient's pain is important in evaluating the significance of annular leak of contrast. When pain and contrast leak are present, the examination is thought to be very accurate.

Magnetic Resonance Imaging

- Of at least equal sensitivity to CT but offering the additional capabilities of multiplanar imaging, better contrast resolution, direct visualization of the spinal cord, and a larger field of view more suited to screening.
- With disk degeneration, marrow changes adjacent to the end plates has been categorized into three types by Modic (see "Suggested Readings"):

Type I: Low signal on T1-weighted and increased signal on T2-weighted images (edematous phase)
Type II: Increased signal on T1-weighted images, iso- or slightly hyperintense on T2-weighted images (fatty marrow-replacement phase)
Type III: Decreased signal on T1-weighted images, decreased signal on T2-weighted images (diskogenic sclerosis)

- With MRI, the disk protrusion or extrusion is demonstrated by the disk fragment obliterating the epidural fat, compressing the nerve roots, and displacing the thecal sac or epidural veins.
- On T1-weighted images, the disk fragment is similar to the disk in signal intensity. However, on T2-weighted images, the disk fragment is typically hyperintense as compared to the degenerating portion of the disk.
- In the cervical spine, disk herniation is often associated with an engorged epidural vein. On sagittal T1-weighted images, the "disk fragment" looks larger than it really is due to the engorged veins seen along the posterior margins of the vertebral bodies. However, the disk fragment can generally be separated from engorged epidural veins on T2-weighted images. Furthermore, the posterior longitudinal ligament is seen as a dark band on T2- or T2*-weighted images.

Operative treatment may be considered in patients with signs and symptoms that persist beyond 6 weeks. It is interesting to note the following about nonoperative treatment of extruded disk fragments:

- In 11 percent, there was a decrease in size to less than 50 percent
- In 36 percent, there was a 50 to 75 percent decrease
- In 46 percent, there was a 50 to 100 percent decrease

☐ DEGENERATIVE DISEASES OF THE SPINE

Degenerative diseases of the spine are among the most common afflictions of humanity. Because these conditions can occur at any joint, clinical signs are likely to be distributed as defined by anatomic relationships, and symptomatology is governed by the level of involvement. The most common levels of degenerative or aging changes occur at C5–C6 in the cervical spine and L5–S1 in the lumbar spine.

DISK DEGENERATION

- Disk degeneration is most commonly due to chronic or acute trauma, although metabolic and genetic factors may also play a role.
- There may be thinning, fissuring, and hyalinization of the end plate.
- Desiccation of the nucleus pulposus (decreased signal on T2-weighted MRI) with increase in type II collagen and increased ratio of keratan sulfate to chondroitin sulfate resulting in reduced water-binding capacity.
- Development of annular radial fissures, of which the following three types have been described by Yu and coworkers: concentric, radial, and transverse. (See Suggested Readings.)
- As disk degeneration progresses, the disk collapses and gas forms within the disk. This gas is seen as an area of low signal intensity on T2-weighted images.

COMBINED DEGENERATIVE DISORDERS

Degenerative changes of the spine may be categorized as follows:

Intervertebral Osteochondrosis Injury to the nucleus pulposus. The radiographic features are as follows:

Vacuum disk phenomenon centrally
Disk space narrowing
Osteophyte formation
Marginal eburnation of the vertebral bodies

Spondylosis Deformans Injury at the attachment of the disk to the end plate.

Asymmetrical vacuum disk near end-plate attachment
Normal height of disk space
Osteophyte formation

Arthrosis
- Uncovertebral arthrosis occurring in the lower four cervical vertebral bodies (C3–C7)
- Osteoarthrosis of the following joints, any or all of which may be involved: apophyseal, costovertebral, transitional or median atlantoaxial

Ligamentous Degeneration and Hyperostosis
- Ligamentous degeneration of the ligamentum flavum, interspinous ligaments, or capsular ligaments
- Diffuse idiopathic skeletal hyperostosis (DISH)

☐ INFECTION

PRIMARY INFECTION OF THE DISKS (DISKITIS)

Because of differences in vascularity at the end plate, infection in children and adults differs slightly in appearance and clinical manifestations.

Children
- Occurs at the disk because of the vascularity of the end plate.
- Occurs most commonly in the lumbar spine.
- Infection is presumed to be bacterial in origin; however, frequently no organism can be recovered.
- Disk involvement is frequently associated with preexisting infections, such as otitis media.

Adults
- Diskitis in adults is uncommon and is usually secondary to hematogeneous spread from infections of the adjacent vertebral bodies. Rarely, it can occur from direct violation of the disk space, which most commonly is iatrogenic.

Causes of iatrogenic diskitis:

- Surgery
- Diskography
- Myelography
- Chemonucleolysis

PRIMARY INFECTIONS OF THE VERTEBRAL BODY (INFECTIOUS SPONDYLITIS) (Table 24-1)

Pyogenic vertebral osteomyelitis (Fig. 24-1)
- The most common pathogen is *Staphylococcus aureus*.
- Disk involvement occurs earlier than with *Mycobacterium tuberculosis*.
- Disk destruction is proportional to bone involvement.
- Contiguous spread associated with bone infarction occurs characteristically.
- Contiguous spread to adjacent vertebral bodies may occur via Batson's plexus or transdiskally.
- Smaller paraspinous masses are seen in pyogenic infection than in tuberculosis.

Table 24-1
FEATURES OF INFECTIOUS VERTEBRAL SPONDYLITIS

Type of Infection	Amount of Disk Involvement	Likelihood of Paraspinal Involvement	Location	Amount of Deformity
Pyogenic	+ + + + +	+	Anywhere	+
Tuberculosis	+	+ + + +	Thoracic	+ + + +
Coccidiomycosis	+/−	+ + +	Anywhere	+/−
Blastomycosis	+ + +	+ + +	Thoracolumbar	+ + + +
Brucellosis	+	+ + +	Lumbar	+ + +

- Replacement of marrow by inflammatory tissue is usually seen as abnormally low signal intensity within the vertebral body on T1-weighted images and high signal intensity on T2-weighted images.
- Gadolinium-enhanced MRI with fat-suppression technique is the most sensitive technique for detecting vertebral spondylitis.

Tuberculous spondylitis (Fig. 24-2)

- The source of infection is typically a pulmonary lesion that is often clinically silent.
- Begins in the anteroinferior portion of the vertebral body and then through the disk to the adjacent vertebral body.
- There is a tendency for a midthoracic or lower thoracic distribution.
- Extensive bony destruction is seen.
- Gibbous deformity is a common complication (Pott's disease).
- Lack of proteolytic enzymes in mycobacterial infection confers limited protection to the disk relative to pyogenic infections.

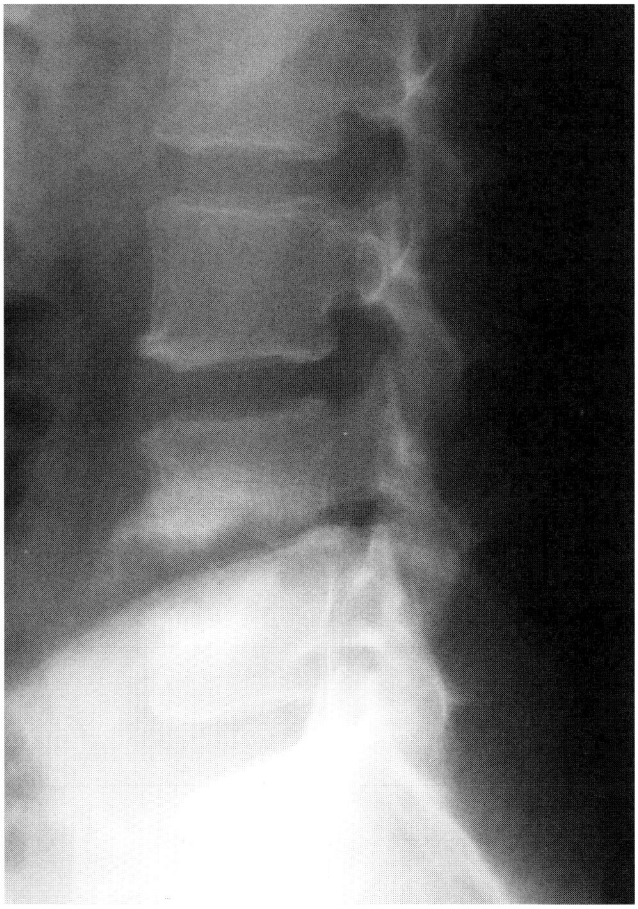

(A)

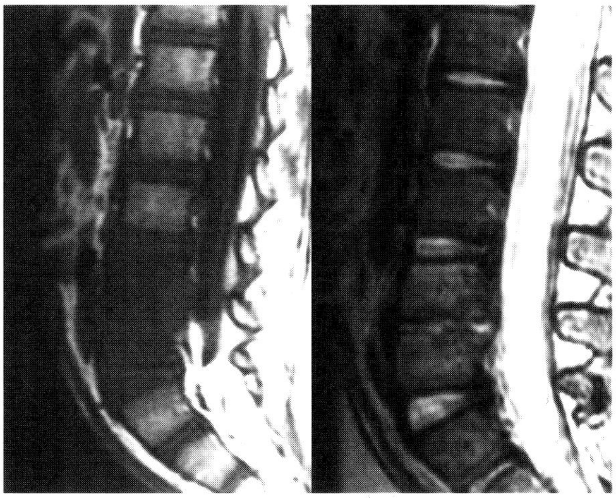

(B) (C)

Figure 24-1 Pyogenic vertebral osteomyelitis. *A*. Lateral radiograph of a patient with pyogenic vertebral osteoymyelitis at L4–5 level. End plate destruction is evident, with narrowing of the disk space. Contiguous involvement of adjacent vertebral bodies is evident. *B* and *C*. T1-weighted (*B*) and T2-weighted fast spin-echo (*C*) sagittal image of a patient with pyogenic osteomyelitis at L4–5 level. There is altered signal in the vertebral body marrow and indistinct visualization of the end plates. Notice the signal alteration and destruction of the contours of the intervertebral disk.

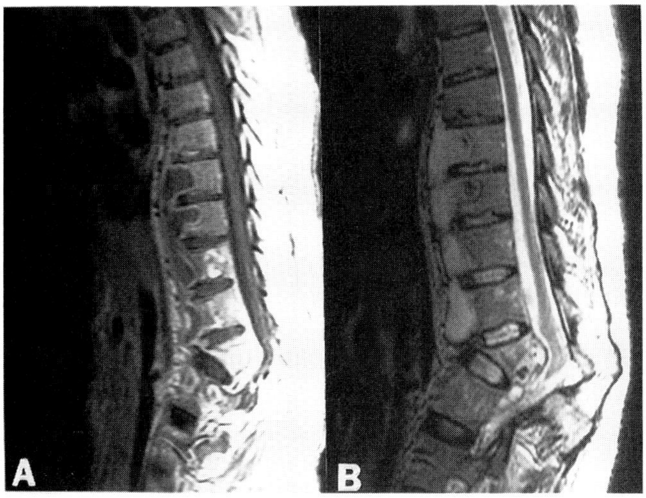

Figure 24-2 Tuberculous spondylitis. *A* and *B*. Gadolinium-enhanced T1-weighted (*A*) and T2-weighted fast spin-echo (*B*) sagittal images of a patient with proven tuberculous spondylitis. There is a prominent gibbous deformity and extensive anterior paraspinous mass. The vertebral body destruction is primarily anterior, with relative preservation of the end plates. The intervertebral disks retain relatively normal morphology.

- Infection tends to spread beneath the longitudinal ligaments to involve adjacent vertebral bodies.
- Posterior element and posterior body involvement is more common than in pyogenic osteomyelitis.
- Frequently associated with psoas abscess.
- Rarely, significant vertebral sclerosis may mimic blastic metastases.
- Magnetic resonance imaging is useful in demonstrating the extent of bony destruction and the degree of cord compression.
- Posterior element involvement and multiplicity of vertebral body involvement make differentiation of tuberculous spondylitis from metastatic disease difficult in some instances; MRI is useful in this regard by demonstrating abnormal high signal in the disk on T2-weighted images.

Coccidiomycosis
- Single vertebral or two adjacent vertebral bodies involved.
- Intervertebral disk often relatively spared.
- Vertebral body collapse uncommon.
- Frequently associated with paraspinous mass.
- Rarely, significant vertebral body sclerosis may mimic blastic mestastases.

Blastomycosis
- Resembles tuberculous spondylitis.
- Thoracolumbar predilection.
- Anterior vertebral erosion.
- Collapse of vertebral body with gibbous deformity.
- Posterior element involvement.
- Paraspinous mass may erode adjacent ribs.
- Disk destruction.

Brucellosis
- Tendency for lumbar involvement.
- Vertebral body may be morphologically intact.
- Less severe deformity than with tuberculosis.
- Otherwise has an appearance similar to that of tuberculosis.

POSTOPERATIVE DISKITIS

Postoperative diskitis occurs with a frequency of 0.075 to 2.8 percent. The most common pathogen is *Staphylococcus aureus*, although at times no organism can be recovered. Following diskectomy, immediate pain relief may be experienced; postoperative diskitis is suspected when pain returns 7 to 28 days after surgery.

Imaging PLAIN FILM
- Demineralization, decreased disk height, and end-plate destruction appearing at 4 to 6 weeks.
- Sclerosis and fusion may occur 6 months to 2 years after surgery.

COMPUTED TOMOGRAPHY
- Findings on CT are similar to those on plain films. Appearance differs slightly because of the axial plane.

RADIONUCLIDE IMAGING
- May be negative until end-plate changes occur, positive but not significant thereafter.

MAGNETIC RESONANCE IMAGING
- Magnetic resonance imaging is the most sensitive imaging modality. Typically low signal is seen on T1-weighted images and high signal on T2-weighted images. Specificity may be increased by the use of gadolinium with T1-weighted fat-suppressed images, which enhances the marrow, disk space, and posterior annulus.

INFECTIONS OF THE EPIDURAL SPACE

- Typically results from hematogeneous spread of infection elsewhere, as in the respiratory or urinary tracts or inoculation via the intravenous route, as with intravenous drug abuse.
- *Staphylococcus aureus* is the most common organism.
- Associated with diskitis or osteomyelitis in 80 percent of cases.
- Phlegmonous material precedes frank abscess.
- Multiple segment involvement (two to six) is common.
- Spinal block is common on myelography or CT myelography.
- Magnetic resonance imaging directly demonstrates the mass and associated bone and disk involvement. Gadolinium-enhanced MRI shows homogeneous enhancement of the epidural abscess in most cases.
- Thrombophlebitis of the epidural venous plexus may cause venous infarction of the cord.

THE POSTOPERATIVE SPINE

The incidence of failed back syndrome is variously reported to be between 11 and 40 percent. The syndrome is ill defined and may result from a variety of causes:

- Insufficient removal of the offending disk
- Formation of scar
- Displacement or extrusion of remaining disk material subsequent to surgery
- Lateral or ventral spinal stenosis
- Mechanical instability
- Arachnoiditis
- Psychological or societal factors

Reoperation in patients with failed back is generally undesirable, offering relief in approximately 30 percent of cases. It is useful to distinguish between the presence of scar with retained/recurrent material, since only patients with retained/recurrent disk displacement are likely to benefit from surgery. The incidence of recurrent disk as a cause of symptoms was 6 percent in a recent series, with 33 percent of disk recurrence in the first year after surgery.

There are morphologic criteria that suggest scar on unenhanced MRI: anterior location, lack of mass effect, lack of continuity with the parent disk, and slightly higher signal than disk.

Because these criteria are of limited usefulness, current practice relies on the paramagnetic contrast (gadolinium chelate) enhancement characteristics of the scar versus the disk material.

The method of examining these patients consists of axial and sagittal T1-weighted images both before and after the administration of gadolinium-containing paramagnetic contrast material. Scar material tends to enhance uniformly and intensely, while disk material will remain low in signal. Peripheral enhancement of a recurrent or retained disk fragment is typical and represents unavoidable scar formation secondary to vascularization and attempts at healing; centrally, however, the disk remains low in signal. It is important to perform the postcontrast examination within 20 min following the administration of the contrast, since delay may allow for diffusion of contrast into the otherwise low-signal disk.

Scar enhancement results from the presence of neovascularity and a rich capillary network in the epidural space. These changes are dynamic and protect against the formation of fibrosis. Because of the immediate postoperative hypervascularity and extravascular fluid accumulation, MRI examination is thought to be less reliable in the first 6 weeks postoperatively. The most intense enhancement is thought to occur prior to 9 months postoperatively. While there is some reduction in signal intensity with time, when or whether enhancement disappears entirely remains unclear.

SPINAL STENOSIS

There exists a congenital predisposition to spinal stenosis resulting from a specific anatomic alteration (i.e., congenitally short pedicles).

Cervical spinal stenosis produces clinical symptoms dependent on and predictable from the anatomic involvement.

- Central stenosis—myelopathic signs and symptoms. Upper motor neuron.
- Foraminal stenosis—radiculopathic signs and symptoms. Postganglionic, lower motor neuron.

Because the spinal cord itself may be compressed in central stenosis, ischemic injury may occur, with the resultant complication of myelomalacia and central cord syndrome, wherein there is upper extremity neurologic deficit with normal extremity function.

Lumbar spinal stenosis can best be understood as a clinical syndrome associated with an anatomically abnormal spinal canal. The symptoms may result from compression of the vascular supply.

Clinical Syndrome

- Lower extremity pain resembling claudication.
- Pain associated with walking.
- Pain relieved by rest, squatting, and bending forward.

Spinal stenosis may occur as a result of congenital spondylodysplasias such as achondroplasia.

ANATOMIC FEATURES

There are three loosely defined sites for stenosis.

Central The central portion of the canal medial to the facets. The normal round or oval configuration becomes trefoil. Some causes of central stenosis are:

- Bulging or protrusion of disk material.
- Osteoarthritis of the apophyseal joints.
- Calcification, ossification, thickening or redundancy of the ligamentum flavum.
- Vertebral body osteophytes.
- Postoperative hypertrophy of bone grafts or scar.

Lateral Recess (Subarticular) The region of the canal between the central portion and the foramen medial to the pedicle. This is generally understood as being at the level of the facet joints, from which the descriptive term *subarticular* derives. The following may be causes of lateral recess stenosis:

- Hypertrophy of redundancy of the ligamentum flavum.
- Hypertrophy of the facet joints may produce lateral recess stenosis.
- Congenitally short pedicles.

Foraminal The foramen is the bony canal lateral to the lateral recess that contains the exiting nerve root. The following may be causes of foraminal stenosis:

- Spondylolisthesis, either degenerative, traumatic, or congenital.
- Lateral disk displacement (Fig. 24-3)
- Osteophytosis originating from the vertebral body or articular processes.
- Focal inflammatory changes.
- Tumors.
- Synovial cysts.
- Proximal placement of the dorsal root ganglia.
- Postoperative fibrosis.

OTHER CAUSES OF SPINAL STENOSIS

Ossification of the Posterior Longitudinal Ligament (OPLL) Originally reported to be most common in the Asian population, it is now recognized as occurring throughout the world. The process is most common in the cervical spine and can result in myelopathy. Associated entities are:

- Diffuse idiopathic skeletal hyperostosis (DISH)
- Ossification of the ligamentum flavum (OLF)
- Ankylosing spondylitis

Suggested etiologies include:

- Fluoride intoxication
- Abnormal calcium and glucose metabolism
- Abnormalities in growth hormone
- Infection

Imaging PLAIN FILM By plain-film findings, OPL is classified into four types, as follows:

- Segmental
- Continuous
- Mixed
- Circumscribed

COMPUTED TOMOGRAPHY A CT classification characterizes the axial appearance as follows:

- Mushroom
- Square
- Hill

Ossification of the posterior longitudinal ligament in evolution (OEV) is a variant of OPLL found in younger patients. It is characterized by the presence of focally hypertrophied OPLL with or without punctate calcifications at the level of the interspaces. It can be distinguished from a disk or osteophyte by its enhancement with gadolinium.

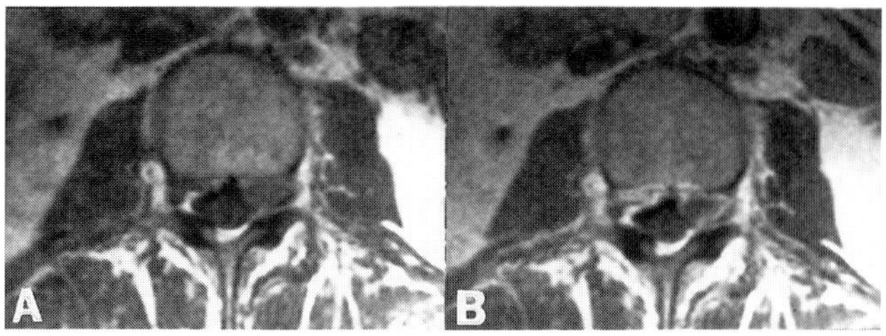

Figure 24-3 Extruded disk fragment in neural foramen. *A* and *B*. T1-weighted (*A*) and gadolinium-enhanced (*B*) T1-weighted axial images through the L2 vertebral body in a patient with left-sided radiating pain. An extruding disk fragment is present in the left neural foramen. Peripheral enhancement is noted even in the absence of prior surgery.

Ossification of Ligamentum Flavum (OLF) This is among the most common causes of stenosis resulting in compression of the posterior thoracic cord in the Orient. It commonly results in myelopathy, particularly if associated with OPLL or spondylosis.

Both OPLL and OLF have CT findings of thickened ligament with bone attenuation either anteriorly, in the location of the posterior longitudinal ligament (OPLL), or posteriorly and posterolaterally in the ligamentum flavum location (OLF). On MRI, high-signal structures may be encountered on T1-weighted sequences histologically consisting of fat, probably within marrow.

The above causes of spinal stenosis may occur separately or in combination. They are much more likely to result in clinically significant spinal stenosis when associated with congenitally short pedicles.

☐ SPONDYLOLYSIS AND SPONDYLOLISTHESIS

SPONDYLOLYSIS

- Spondylolysis is an abnormality of the spine in which a defect is found in the pars interarticularis.
- The incidence of pars interarticularis defects is 3 to 10 percent.
- Plain-film classification of pars defects in spondylolysis:

Type 0—Normal
Type 1—Irregular lucent line
Type 2—Sclerosis, narrowing, or both may be present
Type 3—Nonunited fracture with wide lucent defect

SPONDYLOLISTHESIS

Spondylolisthesis may be classified by degree:

- First degree: Up to one-quarter vertebral body displacement
- Second degree: One-quarter to one-half vertebral body displacement
- Third degree: One-half to three-quarters vertebral body displacement

- Fourth degree: Three-quarters to complete vertebral body displacement

Spondylolisthesis occurs secondary to spondylolysis, which is thought to be a result of trauma. These defects usually occur between the ages of 5 and 18 years. There may be a congenital predisposition to stress fracture as a result of weakness of a narrow pars interarticularis. The width of the spinal canal will be increased in sagittal imaging.

First-degree spondylolisthesis may occur in the absence of spondylolysis as a result of disk degeneration, causing laxity in the annulus and longitudinal ligaments. In this instance the slippage occurs at the apophyseal facet joints. The spinal canal will be unchanged or narrowed on sagittal imaging in this situation.

Degenerative retrolisthesis occurs in relation to disk degeneration and loss of height, resulting in laxity of the stabilizing ligaments.

☐ SYNOVIAL CYSTS

Synovial cysts (Fig. 24-4) may be continuous with the synovium, representing "true" cysts or they may be juxtaarticular or lacking in synovial attachment. Some believe that the juxtaarticular variety or "ganglion" cysts represent true synovial cysts that have lost their connection. Some 75 percent occur at L4–5, with most of the remainder at L3–4 or L5–S1. Lesions are always adjacent to degenerative facets. Pathologically, cyst walls are composed of several layers of fibrous tissue of variable thickness and cellularity.

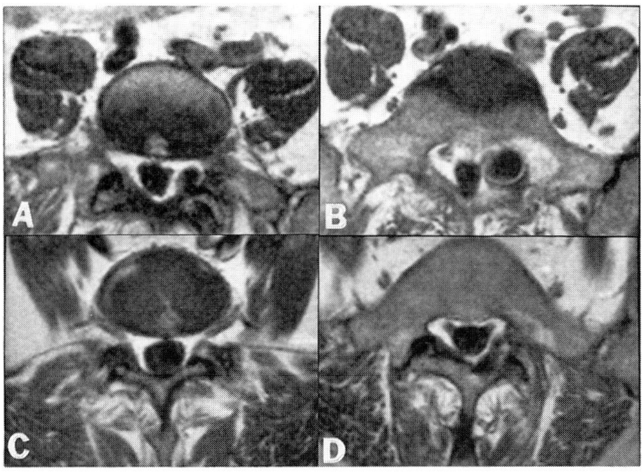

Figure 24-4 Synovial cyst. *A* and *B*. Gadolinium enhanced T1-weighted axial images of the L5–S1. A mass is seen on the left beneath the abnormal L5–S1 facet. Note the apparent peripheral enhancement. *C* and *D*. The same patient imaged 14 months later at approximately the same levels. The mass has almost completely disappeared with no therapy.

VARIATIONS

- Hemorrhagic— because of the sudden enlargement, myelopathy has been reported when synovial cysts occur in the cervical spine.
- Pneumatized—these may occur because of communication with an air-containing degenerating disk. When present, this appearance is thought to be pathognomonic of a juxtaarticular synovial cyst.

COMMON SYMPTOMS OF A SYNOVIAL CYST

- Intermittent pain with or without radiculopathy.
- Radicular symptoms because of mass effect on dorsal aspect of adjacent spinal root.
- Nonradicular symptoms of facet arthropathy because of association with facet arthritis.
- If the cyst communicates with the joint, it may resolve spontaneously.
- Both the symptoms and appearance may simulate those of disk disease.

The diagnosis of synovial cysts may be made by CT or MRI by demonstration of an epidural mass adjacent to the degenerative facet. Air-filled cysts may be more difficult to detect by MRI; however, uncomplicated or hemorrhagic cysts are far better characterized by a combination of T1- and T2-weighted or gradient-echo imaging sequences. Calcification of the synovial cyst wall is better shown on CT.

DIFFERENTIAL DIAGNOSIS

- Schwannoma
- Perineural cyst
- Epidural hematoma
- Migrated disk fragments

SUGGESTED READINGS

1. Boden SD et al: Postoperative diskitis: Distinguishing early MR imaging findings from normal postoperative disk space changes. *Radiology* 184:765–771, 1992.
2. Davis RA: A long-term outcome analysis of 984 surgically treated herniated lumbar discs. *J Neurosurg* 80:415–421, 1994.

3. Epstein NE: Ossification of the posterior longitudinal ligament in evolution in 12 patients. *Spine* 19:673–681, 1994.
4. Flannigan BD et al: MR imaging of the cervical spine: Neurovascular anatomy. *AJR* 148:785–790, 1987.
5. Glickstein MF, Sussman SK: Time-dependent scar enhancement in magnetic resonance of the postoperative lumbar spine. *Skeletal Radiol* 20:333–337, 1991.
6. Jackson DE et al: Intraspinal synovial cyst: MR imaging. *Radiology* 170:527–530, 1989.
7. Jensen MC et al: Magnetic resonance imaging of the lumbar spine in people without back pain. *N Engl J Med* 331:69–73, 1994.
8. McAfee PC, Yuan HA: Computed tomography in spondylolisthesis. *Clin Orthop* 166:62–71, 1982.
9. Modic MT et al: Imaging of degenerative disk disease. *Radiology* 168:177–186, 1988.
10. Modic MT et al: Degenerative disk disease: Assessment of changes in vertebral body marrow with MR imaging. *Radiology* 166:193–199, 1988.
11. Osborn A: *Diagnostic Neuroradiology*. St Louis, Mosby-Year Book, 1994.
12. Pennell RG et al: Stress injuries of the pars interarticularis: Radiologic classification and indications for scintigraphy. *AJR* 145:763–766, 1985.
13. Reinsel TE, Andersson BJ: Ossification of the posterior longitudinal ligament. *AJNR* 13:1068–1070, 1992.
14. Resnick D: *Diagnosis of Bone and Joint Disorders*. Philadelphia, Saunders, 1995.
15. Resnick D: Degenerative diseases of the spinal column: Annual oration. *Radiology* 156:3–14, 1985.
16. Ross JS et al: MR imaging of the postoperative lumbar spine: Assessment with gadopentetate dimeglumine. *AJNR* 11:771–776, 1990.
17. Saal JA et al: The natural history of lumbar intervertebral disc extrusion treated nonoperatively. *Spine* 15:683–686, 1990.
18. Sharif HS et al: Brucellar and tuberculous spondylitis: Comparative imaging features. *Radiology* 171:419–425, 1989.
19. Silbergleit R et al: Lumbar synovial cyst: Correlation of myelographic, CT MR and pathologic findings. *AJNR* 11:777–779, 1990.
20. Smith AS et al: MR imaging characteristics of tuberculous spondylitis vs vertebral osteomyelitis. *AJNR* 10:619–625, 1989.
21. Sugimura H et al: MRI of ossification of ligamentum flavum. *JCAT* 16:73–76, 1992.
22. Thornbury JR et al: Disk-caused nerve compression in patients with acute low back pain: Diagnosis with MR, CT myelography, and plain CT. *Radiology* 186:731–738, 1993.
23. Ulmer JL et al: Distinction between degenerative and isthmic spondylolisthesis on sagittal MR images: Importance of increased anteroposterior diameter of the spinal canal ("wide canal sign"). *AJR* 163:411–416, 1994.
24. Yu S et al: Tears of the annulus fibrosis: Correlation between MR and pathologic findings in cadavers. *AJNR* 9:367–370, 1988.

☐ QUESTIONS

1. Blastomycosis most resembles
a. Tuberculosis
b. Pyogenic vertebral osteomyelitis
c. Coccidiomycosis

2. The most common organism isolated from epidural abscess is
a. *Mycobacterium tuberculosis*
b. *Staphylococcus aureus*
c. *Pseudomonas*

3. Intervertebral osteochondrosis is associated with injury to the
a. End plate
b. Annulus fibrosus
c. Posterior longitudinal ligament
d. Nucleus pulposus

4. Spondylosis deformans is associated with injury to the
a. End plate
b. Annulus fibrosus
c. Posterior longitudinal ligament
d. Nucleus pulposus

5. The most common cause of posterior thoracic cord compression in the Orient is
a. Ossification of the posterior longitudinal ligament (OPLL)
b. Ossification of the ligamentum flavum (OLF)
c. Diffuse idiopathic skeletal hyperostosis (DISH)
d. Ossification of the posterior longitudinal ligament in evolution (OEV)

☐ ANSWERS

1. a. T
b. F
c. F

2. a. F
b. T
c. F

3. a. F
b. F
c. F
d. T

4. a. T
b. F
c. F
d. F

5. a. T
b. F
c. F
d. F

CHAPTER 25

Lesions Involving the Spinal Cord and Nerve Roots

James S. Teal

Pathology involving the spinal cord and nerve roots can be divided into three major categories regarding location. These are intramedullary, intradural extramedullary, and extradural locales. Intramedullary lesions are enveloped completely within the cord parenchyma or filum terminale. However, lesions such as subpial-juxtamedullary lipomas are actually extramedullary in location but are usually considered for imaging purposes to be intramedullary lesions. Intramedullary lesions may grow in exophytic fashions to involve both the intramedullary and extramedullary compartments. Intramedullary lesions of the filum terminale usually behave as intradural extramedullary lesions by myelography. Intradural extramedullary lesions are located within the dura but are not invested within the cord parenchyma. Extradural lesions, for the purpose of this chapter, consist of lesions external to the dural compartment not involving the osseous spine. Lesions involving the nerve roots are usually located in either the intradural extramedullary and/or extradural compartments but are rarely intramedullary in location.

☐ INTRAMEDULLARY LESIONS

NEOPLASMS

Intramedullary tumors (Table 25-1) comprise 6 to 10 percent of central nervous system (CNS) neoplasms in children and overall approximately 20 percent of intraspinal neoplasms.

Ependymoma ***Incidence*** Ependymoma (Fig. 25-1), while the second most common spinal glioma of childhood, is overall the most common spinal glioma. In a large series of 273 spinal intramedullary gliomas, Slooff and colleagues (see "Suggested Readings") found 169 or 61.9 percent to represent ependymomas of the spinal cord and filum terminale.

Age and Gender Approximately 68 percent of ependymomas occur between the ages of 30 and 60 years and only about 10 percent occur before the age of 19 years. A male preponderance in a ratio of 3:2 or 60/40 percent has been reported in multiple series.

Location Most are located in the lower thoracic cord, conus, and filum terminale. Of the 169 spinal ependymomas reported by Slooff and coworkers, 99 or 58.6 percent were located in the filum.

Pathology The vascular myxopapillary ependymoma is the predominant variant found in the regions of the conus medullaris and filum terminale. These sites are the location of 95 percent of this variant. However, the more classic epithelial, cellular, and papillary types are also seen in these sites. Microscopic evidence of previous hemorrhage is often identified in myxopapillary ependymomas.

Ependymomas are an occasional source of subarachnoid hemorrhage (SAH). Only 5 of the 169 (3 percent) intramedullary spinal ependymomas reported by Slooff and associates demonstrated malignant change, and only 2 (1 percent) subependymomas were noted.

Imaging RADIOGRAPHY Occasionally localized expansion of the spinal cord is manifest by widening of the interpediculate distance and increased anteroposterior (AP) diameter of the spinal canal at the involved levels.

MYELOGRAPHY Ependymomas located within the spinal cord proper cause fusiform widening of the

Table 25-1
INTRAMEDULLARY LESIONS

Neoplasms	Inflammatory
Ependymoma	Transverse myelitis
Astrocystoma	AIDS myelopathy
Hemangioblastoma	Sarcoidosis
Cavernous hemangioma	Tuberculosis
Lipoma	Abscess
Epidermoid	
Dermoid	
Teratoma	
Oligodendroglioma	**Vascular**
Melanoma	Vascular malformations
Ganglioglioma	Capillary telangiectasia
Nerve sheath tumor	Infarction
Meningioma	Aneurysm
Metastasis	
Miscellaneous	**Traumatic**
Multiple sclerosis	Contusion
Syringohydromyelia	Hematomyelia
Atrophy	Cord compression
Acute disseminated encephalomyelitis	
Radiation myelitis	
Subacute necrotizing myelopathy	

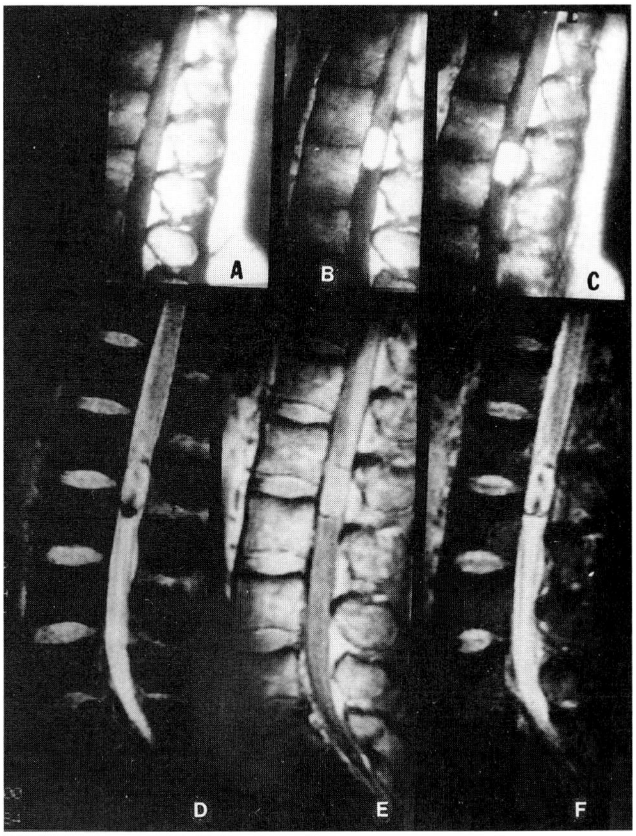

Figure 25-1 Filar ependymoma. *A*.T1-weighted (T1W) (683/20) image demonstrates a mass occupying most of the spinal canal, from mid-L1 to mid-L2, which is isointense to the cord. *B* and *C* T1W (683/20) images demonstrate intense, homogeneous contrast enhancement of the tumor in midline (*B*) and 4 mm to right (*C*) of midline. *D* to *F*. These demonstrate the tumor on gradient echo (GE) [19° flip angle (FA), 1000/15], spin-density weighted (SDW) (1350/20), and T2-weighted (T2W) (1350/100) images respectively. Note the areas of lesion hypointensity on the GE and T2W images, probably representing hemosiderin deposition secondary to prior hemorrhages.

cord and decrease in width of the adjacent subarachnoid space in all directions; this may result in block of passage of the contrast.

Ependymomas of the filum terminale and conus medullaris may demonstrate a sharply delineated, rounded defect at the interfaces of the lesion and contrast medium, simulating an intradural, extramedullary mass and frequently a block of the subarachnoid space, since those lesions may go unrecognized until late. Magnetic resonance imaging (MRI) has rendered myelography seldom necessary to diagnose tumors of the spinal canal.

COMPUTED TOMOGRAPHY Computed tomography (CT) without intrathecal contrast usually provides minimal additional information from that provided by radiography, including conventional tomography. Computed tomography/myelography demonstrates focal widening of the cord or filum and thinning of the adjacent subarachnoid space. Reformatted sagittal and coronal images demonstrate findings similar to those noted by conventional myelography.

MAGNETIC RESONANCE IMAGING Ependymomas demonstrate focal enlargement of the cord or filum and, relative to the cord, are typically hypointense or isointense on T1W (spin-echo short TR, short TE), iso- or hyperintense on SDW (spin-echo long TR, short TE) and hyperintense on T2W (spin-echo long TR, long TE) images. In the presence of subacute or early chronic hemorrhage, they tend to demonstrate T1W hyperintensity and T2W hyperintensity, possibly with associated peripheral hypointensities secondary to hemosiderin deposition. Marked, homogeneous contrast enhancement typically occurs. Associated cystic cavitation of the cord or syringohydromyelia is common (50 percent).

Astrocytoma *Incidence* Astrocytomas account for approximately 25 to 30 percent of cord intramedullary gliomas overall but account for 50 to 60 percent of these tumors in the pediatric age group.

Age and Gender Overall, astrocytomas are more common in adults. Nearly 60 percent of 86 spinal astrocytomas reported by Slooff and colleagues were in patients 30 years of age and older. The sexual predilection favors males in a 3:2 ratio, as with spinal ependymomas.

Location Over 80 percent of spinal astrocytomas are located in the cervical and upper thoracic spine. Long segments of the cord may be involved. The filum terminale is a rare site for astrocytomas.

Pathology Cord astrocytomas are usually of low grade and of the fibrillary type, with common conversion to the pilocytic variety. Malignant astrocytomas comprise approximately 7 percent of spinal intramedullary gliomas and approximately 24 percent of spinal intramedullary astrocytomas.

Imaging Except for location preferences and a tendency of less intense, inhomogeneous MRI contrast enhancement, the imaging characteristics of astrocytomas are indistinguishable from those of ependymomas utilizing all modalities. Cyst formation is common (25 to 38 percent).

Hemangioblastoma *Incidence* Hemangioblastomas represent approximately 3 percent of spinal intramedullary tumors. Approximately 13 percent of hemangioblastomas are within the spinal canal. Approximately 60 percent are intramedullary, 11 percent both intramedullary and intradural extramedullary, 21 percent intradural extramedullary, and 8 percent extradural in location.

Age and Gender Hemangioblastomas may occur in any age group. Occurrence is unusual in children. The overwhelming majority occur between the ages of 25 and 50 years. There is no apparent sexual predilection.

Location Approximately 90 percent of spinal intramedullary hemangioblastomas are located from the cervical to the middle third of the thoracic spine. They tend to occur in the dorsal aspect of the cord.

Pathology Approximately 80 percent of spinal intramedullary hemangioblastomas are solitary. Approximately 67 percent of intramedullary hemangioblastomas are cystic. Microscopically, reticular (common) and cellular variants are noted and both variants may be noted in the same tumor. The adjacent pia, which may be quite vascular, is usually attached to the tumor. There is a strong (50 to 70 percent) association with syringohydromyelia.

Imaging Radiographic, myelographic, and CT findings are generally indistinguishable from those of ependymomas. However, myelography may demonstrate serpentine filling defects on the cord surface manifesting meningeal varicosities. Contrast-enhanced CT will usually demonstrate dense contrast enhancement of the solid component of the lesion.

MAGNETIC RESONANCE IMAGING Noncontrast T1W images demonstrate cord enlargement and heterogeneous areas of hypointensity, isointensity, and sometimes hyperintensity. T2W images show homogeneous hyperintensity secondary to tumor, cyst, and edema. Contrast-enhanced T1W images show marked hyperintensity of the entire tumor if solid and of the tumor nodule if cystic.

ANGIOGRAPHY Spinal angiography demonstrates intense tumor staining and dilated feeding arteries and draining veins.

Cavernous Hemangioma *Incidence* The incidence of spinal intramedullary cavernous hemangioma is unknown but is probably less than 1 percent of spinal intramedullary tumors. Technically, these lesions are vascular hamartomas. Spinal intramedullary cavernous hemangiomas are sometimes associated with those located in the brain.

Age and Gender The usual age of presentation of cavernous hemangiomas is between the ages of 20 and 60 years, frequently with an associated long history of symptoms. Most series have reported a male preponderance of approximately 67 percent; however, no definite sexual predilection was observed upon case reviews of several reports.

Location No known preferential site has been reported. Prior to MRI, diagnosis was frequently difficult because nonexpansion of the cord is common. Review of the recent (1987 to 1994) English-language literature revealed reports of 20 cases from the spinomedullary junction to the T11–12 level. However, 50 percent of the lesions were between C6 and T4.

Pathology Cavernous hemangiomas are nonencapsulated lesions consisting of multiple contiguous blood-filled spaces of varying sizes lined by a single layer of epithelium with little or no interspersed parenchyma. These lesions have a propensity for intramedullary hemorrhage and have been reported to occasionally cause massive hematomyelia. Associated enlargement of leptomeningeal arteries and veins does not occur. There has been at least one case reported of cavernous hemangioma of a cauda equina nerve root.

Imaging RADIOGRAPHY There are usually no associated abnormal radiographic findings.

COMPUTED TOMOGRAPHY AND MYELOGRAPHY There has been at least one report of slight contrast enhancement following intravenous contrast best demonstrated on sagittal reformatted images. However, contrast enhancement does not usually occur and conventional myelography may be normal or demonstrate the typical findings of an intramedullary mass depending upon the size of the lesion and the extent of associated hemorrhage.

MAGNETIC RESONANCE IMAGING The appearance on MRI is dependent upon the presence of previous hemorrhage and the time sequence relative to the hemorrhage. The typical appearance following subacute or early chronic hemorrhage is that of an intramedullary lesion with variable cord expansion and T1W and T2W hyperintensity with peripheral T1W hypointensity and marked T2W hypointensity. Edema external to the lesion may be seen with recent hemorrhage. During the subacute phase with respect to hemorrhage, peripheral contrast enhancement may be noted. The MRI appearance months to years following the most recent hemorrhage may be that of a hypointense area in a region of normal width or expanded cord on T1W images, which becomes markedly hypointense on T2W images.

Lipoma *Incidence* Intradural intramedullary lipomas consist of subpial-juxtamedullary lipomas and fibrolipomas of the filum terminale. Subpial-juxtamedullary lipomas comprise approximately 4 percent of spinal lipomas. Fibrolipomas of the filum terminale have been noted in about 6 percent of normal adults; in the absence of neurologic symptoms and cord tethering, this should be considered as a normal variant. Approximately 30 percent of patients with the tight filum terminale syndrome have associated fibrolipomas of the filum. Fibrolipomas of the filum terminale associated with neurologic dysfunction represent about 12 percent of spinal lipomas. Excluding the normal variant fibrolipomas of the filum terminale and spinal lipomas associated with spinal dysraphism, spinal lipomas account for approximately 1 percent of all primary spinal tumors. Subpial-juxtamedullary spinal lipomas are generally referred to as intradural lipomas.

Age and Gender Symptomatic subpial-juxtamedullary lipomas may present as monoparesis, paraparesis, sensory loss, and sphincter dysfunction from early childhood to late adulthood. However, approximately 80 percent present by the age of 30 years, with about 25 percent presenting during the first 5 years of life. There is no sexual predilection for this type of spinal lipoma. Patients with neurologic dysfunction associated with fibrolipomas of the filum terminale usually present by the age of 20 years. Sexual predilection has not been confirmed.

Location The location of filar fibrolipomas is obvious; however, they may involve the conus superiorly and the epidural space inferiorly. Subpial lipomas most commonly occur in the thoracic and cervical regions, where approximately 67 percent have been identified.

Pathology Technically, neither subpial-juxtamedullary lipomas nor filar fibrolipomas are intramedullary, since neither is completely surrounded by the spinal cord. Subpial-juxtamedullary lipomas arise in the dorsal midline cleft of the cord. These lipomas are posterior in 67 percent, posterolateral in 23 percent, lateral in 5 percent, anterolateral or anterior in 2 percent, and occupying virtually the entire cord cross section in 3 percent. Cord rotation is present when these lipomas are in anterior and anterolateral positions. The outer surface of these lipomas is covered by pia. Approximately 45 percent have been noted to be partially exophytic at the superior or inferior end. These lipomas consist of mature fat cells containing variable amounts of collagen with variable degrees of penetration of neural tissue by the collagen. Malignant degeneration occurs in about 1 percent.

Imaging RADIOGRAPHY Intradural lipomas may be associated with spina bifida, but in most cases spine radiography is normal. Localized expansion of the spinal canal is occasionally present. Spina bifida is usually present when filar fibrolipomas are associated with neurologic dysfunction. Hyperlucency of the spinal canal is occasionally noted in the presence of large subpial and filar lipomas.

MYELOGRAPHY The myelographic findings are indistinguishable from those previously mentioned for ependymomas of the cord and filar ependymomas.

COMPUTED TOMOGRAPHY Computed tomography and CT/myelography can identify the lipomatous lesions by their characteristic −50 to −150 HU of fat density.

MAGNETIC RESONANCE IMAGING The high signal intensity of fat identifies the lesions in their appropriate locations on T1W sagittal and axial images. Fat-suppression techniques render the fat hypointense. The fat displays decreased signal intensity on T2W images, and the intensity is usually similar to that of subcutaneous fat. The fat-water chemical-shift artifact may be used to identify the lesion as fat.

Oligodendroglioma *Incidence* Oligodendrogliomas represent approximately 3 percent of spinal gliomas.

Age and Gender Most spinal oligodendrogliomas present between the ages of 10 and 50 years (63 percent); however, 34 percent have presented between the ages of 6 and 20 years. There is no sexual predilection.

Location Intramedullary oligodendrogliomas have been reported from C1 to the filum terminale, with approximately 26 percent located each from C1–T2, T4–T10, and T11–L2, and about 12 percent in the filum and 6 percent involving the entire cord.

Pathology The typical microscopic picture of oligodendroglioma is that of honeycomblike compact masses of swollen cells containing clear cytoplasm and rather uniform round to oval nuclei interspersed within a scanty, delicate supporting structure of blood vessels and collagen.

Imaging RADIOGRAPHY, MYELOGRAPHY, AND COMPUTED TOMOGRAPHY The findings by these modalities are indistinguishable from those of astrocytoma and ependymomas.

MAGNETIC RESONANCE IMAGING There are no known reports of MRI of spinal oligodendrogliomas, but the findings would most likely be indistinguishable from ependymoma and astrocytoma.

Ganglioglioma ***Incidence*** Gangliogliomas of the spinal cord represent about 1 percent of spinal tumors.

Age and Gender Neither an age nor sexual predilection is known. Cases have been known to present from the age of 2 to 69 years.

Location The most common site is the cervical cord, but cases have been reported in all areas, including the conus. Involvement of the entire cord has been reported. Involvement of long segments of the cord appears to be more common in the pediatric age group.

Pathology Gangliogliomas in the cord, like gangliogliomas in the brain, are mixed neurogliogenic tumors with participation of adult ganglion cells and relatively mature glial tumor cells. The usual glial component consists of pilocytic or gemistocytic astrocytes, but oligodendrocytes may be involved. Microscopic calcifications have been noted in oligodendroglial components of spinal gangliogliomas.

Imaging RADIOGRAPHY Except for some reports of associated kyphoscoliosis, plain-film studies are usually negative. However, in view of the prolonged course of the process, both focal and generalized widening of the spinal canal are possible.

MYELOGRAPHY AND COMPUTED TOMOGRAPHY The findings are those of other intramedullary masses.

MAGNETIC RESONANCE IMAGING The MRI findings in the only two known reported cases studied by this modality were expansion of the cord associated with T1W hypointensity and T2W hyperintensity, simulating the appearance of astrocytoma or ependymoma with associated syrinx. However, at surgery, the suspected cystic areas were noted to be solid. Neither patient received MRI contrast media.

Melanoma ***Incidence*** Primary melanoma of the spinal cord represents less than 1 percent of spinal tumors. As of 1989, there had been 31 reported cases in the literature.

Age and Gender Spinal melanoma is primarily a disease of adulthood, with multiple cases having presented between the ages of 60 and 73 years. There is no known sexual predilection.

Location The most frequent locations have been the middle and lower portions of the thoracic cord.

Pathology Primary melanoma of the cord consists of a black or dark blue, poorly marginated mass usually located eccentrically in the thoracic cord. Exophytic extension has been common.

Imaging RADIOGRAPHY AND COMPUTED TOMOGRAPHY Radiographic and CT studies without intrathecal contrast are usually noncontributory.

MYELOGRAPHY AND CT/MYELOGRAPHY The findings are those indistinguishable from other intramedullary masses.

MAGNETIC RESONANCE IMAGING The only known reported case with MRI findings demonstrated a T1W heterogeneous, hyper-/isointense mass with adjacent decreased signal, T2W decreased signal intensity, associated syrinx cavities above and below the lesion, and homogeneous, dense contrast enhancement. The signal intensities were comparable to those that occur in the brain with nonhemorrhagic melanoma metastases.

Neurolemmoma ***Incidence*** Intramedullary neurolemmomas comprise about 1 percent of spinal neurolemmomas and about 0.3 percent of spinal tumors. As of 1991, there had been 28 reported cases without physical evidence and family history of neurofibromatosis.

Age and Gender The median age of presentation has been 43 years, with ages ranging from 12 to 75 years. About 80 percent have presented between the ages of 30 and 69 years. There has been a 2:1 male preference.

Location Sites from C1 to L2 have been reported; however, approximately 65 percent have been cervical and cervicothoracic in location.

Pathology These tumors are the same as those of extramedullary origin, described later in this chapter.

Imaging RADIOGRAPHY, MYELOGRAPHY, AND COMPUTED TOMOGRAPHY The findings are generally the same as for other intramedullary masses. Exophytic components may be present.

MAGNETIC RESONANCE IMAGING The two known cases with reported MRI findings demonstrated cord enlargement by T1W hypointense and T2W hyperintense intramedullary masses. One of the cases had contrast medium administration, which resulted in T1W dense homogeneous enhancement of the lesion.

Meningioma ***Incidence*** As of 1992, only four cases had been reported.

Age and Gender The mean age of the four cases was 53.5 years. As in meningiomas elsewhere, a female preference is likely.

Location All four cases involved the cervical cord.

Pathology The psammomatous variety was present in two cases and one each was of the papillary and fibroblastic types.

Imaging RADIOGRAPHY, MYELOGRAPHY, AND COMPUTED TOMOGRAPHY The findings are the nonspecific findings of intramedullary masses in general.

Magnetic Resonance Imaging The only reported case with MRI findings demonstrated an intramedullary mass hypointense to CSF and isointense to cord on T2W images and isointense to cord on T1W images. Intravenous contrast medium apparently was not given.

Teratoma *Incidence* Intramedullary teratomas comprise about 0.7 percent of intramedullary tumors. Except for the sacrococcygeal variety, which are usually discovered shortly after birth, spinal teratomas are very rare and may be intra- or extradural in location.

Age and Gender Too few cases have been reported to determine an age or sexual predilection; however, one report of two cases involved males aged 20 and 67 years.

Location There appears to be a predilection for the lower thoracic cord.

Pathology Teratomas are masses composed of a mixture of mature tissues derived from all three germ layers, which together do not resemble any recognizable organ despite being composed of adult tissue elements. The more common congenital sacrococcygeal teratomas are covered elsewhere in this text.

Imaging Radiography, Myelography, and Computed Tomography These findings are the same as for other intramedullary masses, with the additional possibility of detecting calcifications and fat within the lesion.

Magnetic Resonance Imaging The only known reported MRI findings were an intramedullary lower thoracic mass demonstrating increased signal secondary to fat and decreased signal felt to be secondary to calcium on T1W images.

Dermoid and Epidermoid *Incidence* Dermoids and epidermoids each represent about 1 percent of intramedullary tumors. Dermoids and epidermoids together comprise about 10 percent of spinal tumors in patients less than 15 years of age.

Age and Gender There is no definite sexual predilection. Dermoids usually cause symptoms before the age of 20 years. Epidermoids usually produce symptoms in the 20- to 50-year age group.

Location Only about 20 percent of dermoids occur above the level of the cauda equina. Intramedullary epidermoids most commonly occur between T5 and T8, with the remainder being distributed between the upper and lower thoracic and lumbar regions.

Pathology Dermoids are usually cystic masses composed of dermal elements consisting of squamous epithelium, hair follicles, sweat glands, sebaceous glands, and their products. Epidermoids are cystic masses lined by a membrane of superficial (epidermal) layers of the skin. Some epidermoid cysts are felt to be secondary to spinal surgery, lumbar puncture, or other penetrating injuries to the spine.

Imaging Radiography Bony anomalies such as spina bifida or block vertebrae may be present.

Myelography and Computed Tomography The myelographic and CT findings are usually the same as with other intramedullary masses but with the possibility of demonstration of fat density within the mass by CT.

Magnetic Resonance Imaging The MRI signal of dermoid cysts is variable and dependent upon the fat content and other chemical composition of the cyst fluid. The T1W signal may vary from isointense to hyperintense with respect to CSF while the T2W signal is isointense to CSF. The MRI signal of epidermoids is variable but typically isointense to CSF in both T1W and T2W imaging. Contrast enhancement usually does not occur with either lesion.

Metastases *Incidence* The incidence is unknown but has been reported to be less than 3 percent in cancer patients, at autopsy. As the length of survival increases in cancer patients, the incidence of intramedullary metastases may increase.

Age and Gender The peak ages are 40 to 70 years. The distribution is weighted by primary tumor type rather than by sex per se.

Location Approximately 50 percent involve the thoracic cord and approximately 35 percent involve the cervical cord.

Primary Site Lung carcinoma accounts for almost 66 percent, with the breast being the second most common site. Other occasionally known primary sites are the skin (melanoma), kidney, and colon/rectum. Lymphoma may also represent a primary lesion. The primary site is unknown in about 5 percent.

Imaging Radiography Radiographs may demonstrate associated bony metastases.

Myelography, Computed Tomography, and Magnetic Resonance Imaging Findings are nonspecific. The degree of cord enlargement is variable, from imperceptible to gross enlargement. The MRI findings are T1W lesions isointense to hypointense relative to the cord, T2W hyperintense to cord, and marked contrast enhancement.

INFLAMMATORY

Transverse Myelitis *Incidence* The etiology and incidence of transverse myelitis are unknown. Its diagnosis is one of exclusion and the imaging findings are nonspecific. The set of diagnostic criteria established by Berman and coworkers are as follows:

1. Acute development of paraparesis affecting motor and sensory systems; also sphincter disturbances.
2. Complete spinal segmental level sensory disturbance (exclusion of patients with cord hemisection syndromes and patchy sensory deficits).
3. Stable, nonprogressive clinical course.
4. No clinical, laboratory, or imaging evidence of cord compression.
5. Absence of any known neurologic disease, including trauma, syphilis, metastatic malignancy, encephalitis, and prior spinal radiation therapy.

A preceding viral infection or vaccination has commonly been associated in children. Preceding viral infections reported include varicella, rubeola, influenza, mumps, varicella-zoster, herpes simplex type II, and polio. Preceding vaccinations include smallpox, polio, tetanus, and variola. In adults, AIDS, collagen vascular disease, sarcoidosis, multiple sclerosis, and paraneoplastic syndrome have been associated.

Neuromyelitis optica or Devic's syndrome consists of paraplegia, induced by transverse myelitis, and blindness. Disorders associated with Devic's syndrome—in addition to those already noted for transverse myelitis—include infectious mononucleosis, acute disseminated encephalomyelitis, systemic lupus erythematosus, pulmonary tuberculosis, and clioquinol intoxication.

Location The cord levels below which all sensory functions were lost were cervical, 10 percent; high thoracic, 42 percent; low thoracic, 38 percent; and lumbar, 10 percent.

Pathology Histopathology demonstrates distortion of normal cord architecture, with hemorrhage, necrosis, perivascular inflammation, and demyelination. The length of cord involvement is variable but usually at least one to three segments in length.

Imaging **RADIOGRAPHY** There are no associated radiographic findings.

MYELOGRAPHY AND COMPUTED TOMOGRAPHY Myelography and CT/myelography may vary from normal to the nonspecific findings of intramedullary masses.

MAGNETIC RESONANCE IMAGING The MRI appearance of transverse myelitis is variable and ranges from normal to T2W focal or diffuse cord hyperintensity and focal contrast enhancement.

AIDS Myelopathy The history of acquired immunodeficiency syndrome (AIDS) in association with the presence of clinical findings of myelopathy combined with the absence of intrinsic cord neoplasia/inflammation and extrinsic cord compression lead to the diagnosis of AIDS myelopathy. Approximately 20 to 30 percent of patients dying from AIDS demonstrate a vacuolar myelopathy characterized histopathologically by vacuolation in the spinal white matter, predominantly in the lateral and posterior columns of the thoracic cord, in association with lipid-laden macrophages. The vacuoles are surrounded by a thin myelin sheath and appear to arise from swelling within myelin sheaths. Axonal disruption may be present in areas of severe vacuolation. Axons without myelin sheaths are usually not found. These histologic findings closely resemble the pathologic findings of subacute combined degeneration due to vitamin B_{12} deficiency. The clinical manifestations of vitamin B_{12} deficiency closely resemble those of AIDS myelopathy. The imaging findings are the same as for transverse myelitis.

Sarcoidosis Neurosarcoidosis of the spinal cord is much less common than cerebral involvement. Sarcoid granulomas produce localized cord enlargement, usually of the cervical cord. The imaging findings are nonspecific and demonstrate the typical finding of intramedullary masses secondary to neoplasms and inflammation. The MRI enhancement pattern is sometimes less intense and more patchy than is typical for tumors. Associated meningeal enhancement increases the likelihood of sarcoidosis.

Tuberculosis Tuberculomas of the spinal cord occur in association with tuberculosis elsewhere in the body. Because of the prevalence of AIDS, it is likely that the incidence of cord tuberculomas will increase. Unlike sarcoid granulomas of the cord, tuberculomas have shown no predilection for the cervical cord and have been noted to be fairly well distributed throughout the cord. The imaging characteristics are nonspecific and—except for absence of predilection for the cervical cord—are indistinguishable from those of intramedullary sarcoid granuloma.

Abscess Intramedullary abscesses are extremely rare, with most diagnoses having been previously made during surgery or autopsy. However, the nonspecific findings of an intramedullary mass have been demonstrated by myelography. One would expect MRI to show an intramedullary mass that is hypointense on T1W images and hyperintense on T2W images, with hyperintense T2W surrounding edema. Contrast enhancement should range from nodular to ringlike, depending upon the stage of the abscess.

VASCULAR

Arteriovenous Malformation ***Incidence*** Spinal vascular malformations are rare. Intramedullary arteriovenous malformations (AVMs) of the cord consist of type II (glomus AVMs) and type III (juvenile-type AVMs) spinal vascular malformations. The juvenile-type AVMs usually have both intramedullary and extramedullary components.

Age and Gender Intramedullary AVMs present with symptoms at a mean age of approximately 20 years, with nearly all presentations by the age of 40 years. There is no known sexual preference.

Location Approximately 57 percent occur in the thoracic region, with most of the others occurring in the cervical region.

Pathology Glomus AVMs are made up of compact vascular nidi buried within a relatively short segment of cord parenchyma fed by one or more branches of the anterior or posterior spinal arteries and drained by enlarged, tortuous, arteriolized veins. Associated aneurysms of the feeding arteries are present in approximately 20 percent. The juvenile-type AVMs tend to occur in children and adolescents, are generally larger than the glomus AVMs, and are usually both intramedullary and extramedullary in location. Juvenile AVMs are the rarest type of spinal vascular malformations.

Imaging RADIOGRAPHY AND COMPUTED TOMOGRAPHY Radiography and CT are noncontributory.

MYELOGRAPHY Myelography demonstrates the presence of serpentine filling defects secondary to dilated vessels. If hematomyelia is present, cord enlargement may be noted.

MAGNETIC RESONANCE IMAGING Flow voids may be noted within the cord parenchyma and on the surface in both T1W and T2W images.

ANGIOGRAPHY Spinal angiography demonstrates the typical findings of one or more dilated feeding arteries to an intraparenchymal nidus of tangled blood vessels associated with one or more dilated, tortuous, early draining veins.

Capillary Telangiectasia Capillary telangiectasia represents the most common spinal vascular malformation. However, these lesions are seldom of clinical interest and are usually incidental autopsy findings. Pathologically, capillary telangiectasia is similar to cavernous hemangioma, but with neural tissue present between the dilated capillaries.

Cavernous Hemangioma Previously discussed under "Neoplasms."

Infarction Spinal cord infarction apparently represents approximately 1 percent of cases of central nervous system ischemic infarction. In the absence of associated pathology—such as necrosing myelopathy due to vascular malformations, systemic lupus erythematosus, cord phlebothrombosis, radiation therapy, and so on—spinal cord infarctions are probably secondary to compromised flow in the anterior spinal artery. Because of the limited supply of anastomotic channels to the single anterior spinal artery, with its extensive vascular territory, and the much more plentiful supply of anastomotic channels to the paired posterior spinal arteries, with their somewhat limited vascular territories, spinal cord infarction is much more likely to result from insults to the anterior spinal artery flow insults than from posterior spinal artery involvement. Prior to the advent of MRI, the sequelae of acute and subacute infarction could not be directly imaged in vivo. The MRI findings in ischemic cord infarction are analogous to those in ischemic brain infarction. Acute and subacute infarcts demonstrate T1W hypointense/isointense regions of cord that become hyperintense on T2W images. During the middle and late subacute phases, contrast enhancement is common. During the chronic phase, cord atrophy and myelomalacia (well-demarcated T1W hypointense and T2W hyperintense regions in the cord) are noted. Some causes of flow compromise in the anterior spinal artery are atherosclerosis, compression by herniated disk, osteophytes, displaced vertebral body fragment, aortic dissection, and aortic aneurysmal surgery that disrupts intercostal arteries with radicular branches to the anterior spinal artery.

Aneurysm Nearly all spinal aneurysms are associated with vascular malformations. Approximately 20 percent of intramedullary AVMs have associated aneurysms involving the feeding arteries. This presence of aneurysms results in a statistically significant increased incidence of spontaneous hemorrhage compared to intramedullary AVMs without associated aneurysms.

TRAUMATIC

Only since the advent of MRI has the direct in vivo imaging of intramedullary cord injuries been available. The spectrum of the MRI findings of cord injuries ranges from normal to edema to hemorrhage to transection. Cord injuries can be typed in categories analogous to brain injuries—i.e., edematous contusion, hemorrhagic contusion, hematomyelia, and laceration (transection is the highest degree of laceration). Kolkarni and coworkers have typed these categories as follows:

Type I—Hematomyelia, poor prognosis, with no recovery of function
Type II—Edematous contusion, best recovery of function
Type III—Hemorrhagic contusion, mixture of edema and blood, intermediate recovery of function

This classification scheme is somewhat confusing, since the least degree of injury, associated with the best prognosis, is called type II; the greatest degree of injury, associated with the worst prognosis, is called type I; and the intermediate degree of injury, associated with an intermediate prognosis, is called type III. Obviously, complete cord injuries carry a poor prognosis. Partial cord injuries are classified relative to clinical findings, as follows:

1. Anterior cord syndrome—caused by flexion injuries and central disk herniations.
2. Central cord syndrome—caused by hyperextension injuries.
3. Brown-Séquard's syndrome—caused by cord injury to lateral half of cord.
4. Posterior cord syndrome—rare; caused by dorsal column injury.
5. Conus medullaris syndrome—caused by compression fracture of T12 or L1.

Imaging RADIOGRAPHY Plain films may demonstrate the results of an associated bony injury. Good correlation between the extent of bony and soft tissue injury and the extent of cord injury does not exist in most cases.

MYELOGRAPHY AND COMPUTED TOMOGRAPHY Conventional and CT/myelography may demonstrate the presence of localized cord enlargement or cord laceration.

MAGNETIC RESONANCE IMAGING Sagittal and coronal images demonstrate the cord contour and thus demonstrate the presence or absence of cord swelling and transection. The findings of edema and blood in the cord are analogous to those involving the brain. Cord edema is hypointense/isointense on T1W images and hyperintense on T2W images. The appearance of blood is primarily dependent upon the age of the clot and secondarily upon the volume of the clot. During the acute (deoxyhemoglobin) phase, blood appears hypointense/isointense on T1W images and very hypointense on T2W images. During the early subacute (intracellular methemoglobin) phase, blood appears hyperintense on T2W images and very hypointense on T2W images. During the later subacute (extracellular methemoglobin) phases, blood is hyperintense in both T1W and T2W images. During the early chronic (extracellular methemoglobin/hemosiderin) phase, blood is hyperintense with peripheral hypointensity on T1W images and hyperintense with peripheral marked hypointensity on T2W images. During the intermediate chronic phase, the areas of hemorrhage are T1W hypointense and T2W hyperintense with peripheral marked hypointensity secondary to hemosiderin deposition. During the late chronic (hemosiderin/ferritin) phase, the sites of increased hemosiderin deposition are hypointense on T1W images and markedly hypointense on T2W and low-flip-angle gradient-echo images; however, regions of myelomalacia and cystic cavitation will remain T1W hypointense and T2W hyperintense. Small hematomas complete these phases faster than large hematomas because the hemoglobin changes take place from outward toward the center.

Cord Compression Obviously, cord compression results in varying degrees of intramedullary injury to the spinal cord. The spectrum of injuries includes the previously described contusional types in addition to necrosis, gliosis, and demyelination. The contour abnormalities of cord compression are best noted by MRI obtained in planes in the direction of and perpendicular to the compressing force, which usually means sagittal and axial images. Occasionally, coronal, sagittal oblique, and coronal oblique images are needed in addition to axial images to optimally delineate the compressed cord. Optimal imaging of the contours of a compressed cord typically shows cord narrowing in the plane parallel to the direction of the compressive force and cord widening in the perpendicular plane. The intramedullary signal abnormalities depend upon the nature of the parenchymal injury and time of imaging with regard to time of injury.

MISCELLANEOUS

Multiple Sclerosis ***Incidence*** Multiple sclerosis (MS) is the most common demyelinating disease of the spinal cord. Patients with known MS and spinal cord symptoms have been reported to have MRI-detectable cord lesions in 55 to 75 percent of cases. Less than 10 percent of MS patients have cord involvement only.

Age and Gender The clinical onset of the disease is usually between the ages of 20 and 50 years. The overall sexual preponderance favors females in a 2:1 ratio. In the pediatric age group, the female preponderance is approximately 10:1.

Location Approximately 67 percent of spinal MS plaques are located in the cervical cord, with most of these being in the mid- and lower cervical cord. This has been noted in both autopsy and imaging studies.

Pathology Spinal MS plaques are similar to those in the brain, which involve areas of selective demyelination with axonal sparing and a tendency toward perivenous locations. Most plaques involve the lateral columns of the cord and abut the lateral pial surface. The second most common site involves the posterior columns of the cord, and these lesions tend to lie in the midline. The etiology of MS remains unknown, but the most favored theory is that of an autoimmune etiology and the second most favored theory is that of a response to a low-grade viral infection.

Imaging The only current imaging modality having a role in the evaluation of MS of the cord is MRI. The cord is occasionally noted to be mildly enlarged during an acute phase. Cord atrophy is noted in about 10 percent of all patients with MS. The typical MRI findings of spinal MS are vertically elongated regions of hyperintensity involving the lateral or posterior aspect of the cord on T2W and low-flip-angle gradient-echo images, which sometimes demonstrate homogeneous contrast enhancement.

Associated edema with T2W hyperintensity is noted in the minority of cases. Contrast enhancement is claimed to relate to the acuteness of plaques. Contrast enhancement is rare in the presence of normal T2W images. Brain MRI has been reported to be abnormal in 10 to 50 percent of patients manifesting only spinal symptoms. The imaging findings of MS are nonspecific and must be correlated with clinical and laboratory findings in order to make the definite diagnosis.

Syringohydromyelia The term *syringohydromyelia* refers to cystic cavitation of the cord, representing either classic hydromyelia or classic syringomyelia. Since frequently neither imaging studies nor histopathologic examinations can clearly differentiate between hydromyelia and syringomyelia, it is felt appropriate to use either the term *syringohydromyelia* or *hydrosyringomyelia*. Syringohydromyelia may be either congenital or acquired. The congenital form is usually associated with the Chiari I and II malformations as well as other congenital lesions such as diastematomyelia. Acquired syringohydromyelia is usually related to trauma, spinal cord neoplasms, spontaneous intramedullary hemorrhage, ischemia, and arachnoiditis.

Incidence The incidence is unknown.

Age and Gender Syringohydromyelia presents from childhood through adulthood, but an adult presentation is more common. There is no known sexual preference.

Location There may be segmental involvement of any part of the cord, or the entire cord may be involved.

Pathology There is cystic cavitation of the cord. In classic hydromyelia, which is the result of dilatation of the central canal of the cord, the cyst should be lined by ependyma, whereas a syrinx cyst should be lined by reactive glial tissue. However, this distinction cannot be made by imaging studies and is commonly not made by histology, especially in instances where the wall of a hydromyelic cavity splits and the fluid dissects into the cord parenchyma and when the reverse process occurs with syringomyelia. Both of these processes would lead to cavities, each lined partially by ependyma and partially by reactive glial tissue.

Imaging Magnetic resonance imaging is the modality of choice. Sagittal and axial T1W images show hypointense cystic cavitation within a dilated cord. Motion-compensated sagittal and coronal T2W images demonstrate rather uniform hyperintensity of the cord cavity. Non-motion-compensated sagittal and coronal T2W images show hypointensities within the hyperintense cord cavity indicative of CSF flow within the cavity. The absence of central hypointensities in T2W images obtained without motion-compensating techniques indicates slow or no flow of fluid within the cord.

Atrophy Atrophy of the cord, like atrophy of the brain, has multiple etiologies, including trauma, ischemia, MS, degenerative disorders, etc. The imaging modality of choice is MRI, which demonstrates a small spinal cord with variable intrinsic signal characteristics dependent somewhat upon the underlying etiology.

Acute Disseminated Encephalomyelitis Acute disseminated encephalomyelitis is usually a monophasic demyelinating disease affecting children after a recent vaccination or viral infection. The histopathologic findings of foci of perivenous white matter inflammation accompanied by perivenous and subpial demyelination are indistinguishable from those of MS. Likewise, the imaging findings are indistinguishable from those of MS.

Radiation Myelitis Radiation myelitis is usually a self-limited disorder that produces symptoms starting a few weeks or months following radiation therapy during which included the spinal cord within the treatment ports. However, a progressive myelopathy may commence several months to years following therapy and progress to permanent paralysis. During the first few months after the onset of symptoms, MRI, the imaging modality of choice, may demonstrate a normal or slightly swollen cord with T1W hypointensity, T2W hyperintensity, and nonspecific, somewhat eccentric focal cord enhancement. Patients studied by MRI more than 3 years following the onset of symptoms usually demonstrate cord atrophy without associated signal abnormality. The vertebral bodies included in the radiation ports demonstrate marked T1W hyperintensity due to fatty replacement of the irradiated marrow.

Subacute Necrotizing Myelopathy ***Incidence*** Subacute necrotizing myelopathy (SNM) is characterized clinically by progressive deterioration. This is in contrast to the stable and commonly improving clinical course of transverse myelitis. The etiology of SNM is uncertain, but the leading current theory is cord ischemia secondary to local venous hypertension, which causes impaired spinal cord perfusion, and venous drainage produced by the presence of a spinal dural arteriovenous fistula (AVF). The end stage of SNM in this setting is termed the Foix-Alajouanine syndrome. Other etiologies of SNM have been reported (see "Pathology," below). It is an uncommon disorder, the incidence of which is uncertain. The progressive deterioration can sometimes be halted or even reversed by surgical resection and/or therapeutic embolization when the condition is secondary to the presence of dural AVF.

Age and Gender The Foix-Alanjouanine syndrome affects men more commonly than women, with peak incidence between the ages of 50 and 70 years.

Location Most spinal dural AVFs are located at or below the midthoracic level; therefore, SNM related to this entity should produce cord lesions in similar locations. However, ischemia above the level of the AVF does commonly occur.

Pathology The histopathologic findings of SNM are variable, but the end result is necrosis. When SNM is related to AVF, it demonstrates hyalinization and mural thickening within the venocapillary network of the cord. Paraneoplastic-related SNM and idiopathic SNM have demonstrated striking necrosis with a paucity of inflammatory cells.

Imaging **RADIOGRAPHY, MYELOGRAPHY, COMPUTED TOMOGRAPHY, AND MAGNETIC RESONANCE IMAGING** These modalities produce findings indistinguishable from those of transverse myelitis.

ANGIOGRAPHY Selective or superselective spinal angiography may demonstrate the presence of an associated dural AVF.

☐ INTRADURAL EXTRAMEDULLARY LESIONS (TABLE 25-2)

NEOPLASMS

More than half of all primary spinal tumors are classified as intradural extramedullary neoplasms. The overwhelming majority of these lesions are nerve sheath tumors and meningiomas.

Table 25-2
INTRADURAL EXTRAMEDULLARY LESIONS

Neoplasms	Inflammatory
Nerve sheath tumors	Arachnoiditis
Neurolemmoma	Subdural empyema
Neurofibroma	
Meningioma	
Lipoma	
Epidermoid and dermoid cysts	**Traumatic**
Teratoma	Nerve root/sheath avulsion
Ependymoma	Arachnoid cyst
Astrocytoma	Postsurgical meningocele
Cavernous hemangioma	Subdural hematoma
Capillary hemangioma	
Paraganglioma	
Leptomeningeal metastases	
Vascular	**Miscellaneous**
Arteriovenous fistula	Arachnoid cyst
Arteriovenous malformation	Conjoined nerve root sheaths

Nerve Sheath Tumors Nerve sheath tumors consist of schwannomas (neurolemmomas) and neurofibromas. Even though schwannomas and neurofibromas are distinctly different histologically, they have often not been classified separately in the literature and in general their radiologic characteristics are indistinguishable. Therefore, distinctly separate data for them are not readily available.

Incidence Nerve sheath tumors have been reported to comprise approximately 15 to 30 percent of primary spinal tumors. Neurofibromatosis type 1 is associated with neurofibromas and neurofibromatosis type 2 is associated with schwannomas.

Age and Gender These tumors are most commonly seen in patients between the ages of 20 and 50 years with no predilection for either sex.

Location Nerve sheath tumors usually involve the dorsal nerve roots and may be located anywhere in the spine, but the most common site is the thoracic spine (43 percent), followed by the lumbar spine (34 percent). Approximately 70 percent are intradural extramedullary, about 15 percent each extradural and combined extradural/intradural, and less than 1 percent intramedullary in location.

Pathology Schwannomas are firm, circumscribed, and encapsulated lesions. Schwannomas arise from Schwann cells and are comprised mostly of compact cellular Antoni type A tissue intermingled with less prevalent, less compact Antoni type B tissue. Cyst formation is common. Malignant schwannomas are rare.

Neurofibromas are soft, elastic, and nonencapsulated lesions. Neurofibromas also arise from Schwann cells and consist of loosely textured mixtures of Schwann cells and fibroblasts with wide separation of nerve fibers by poorly cellular tissue lacking orderly architecture. The plexiform variant commonly undergoes malignant transformation. The major distinction between neurofibromatosis types 1 and 2 is that acoustic schwannomas are present in type 2 and are rare in type 1.

Imaging **RADIOGRAPHY** Large tumors may show evidence of localized enlargement of the spinal canal.

MYELOGRAPHY In the cervical and thoracic regions, well-circumscribed, sharply marginated filling defects causing displacement of the spinal cord are noted. Displacement of the spinal cord results in the subarachnoid space near the lesion being widened on one side and narrowed on the opposite side. Blockage of the subarachnoid space may be present. In the lumbar area, the lesions produce changes indistinguishable from filar ependymomas. A small lesion arising from a lumbosacral nerve root may appear as a solitary grapelike filling defect attached to a nerve root. Multiple nerve roots may be involved.

COMPUTED TOMOGRAPHY The bony changes resulting from localized expansion of the spinal canal may be noted in the presence of large masses. CT/myelography demonstrates a soft tissue mass producing findings similar to those of conventional myelography.

MAGNETIC RESONANCE IMAGING The MRI appearance is variable. However, typically, both schwannomas and neurofibromas are isointense/hypointense to cord on T1W sequences and hyperintense to the cord on T2W sequences. When located in the cervical or thoracic region, displacement of the cord is frequently obvious. When located in the lumbar region, the lesion may be difficult to detect when it is hypointense to cord on T1W images without the use of contrast. Both lesions typically demonstrate homogenous, intense contrast enhancement, but due to cyst formation within schwannomas, ring enhancement is not unusual.

Meningioma *Incidence* Meningiomas (Fig. 25-2) have been reported to comprise 25 to 45 percent of intraspinal tumors.

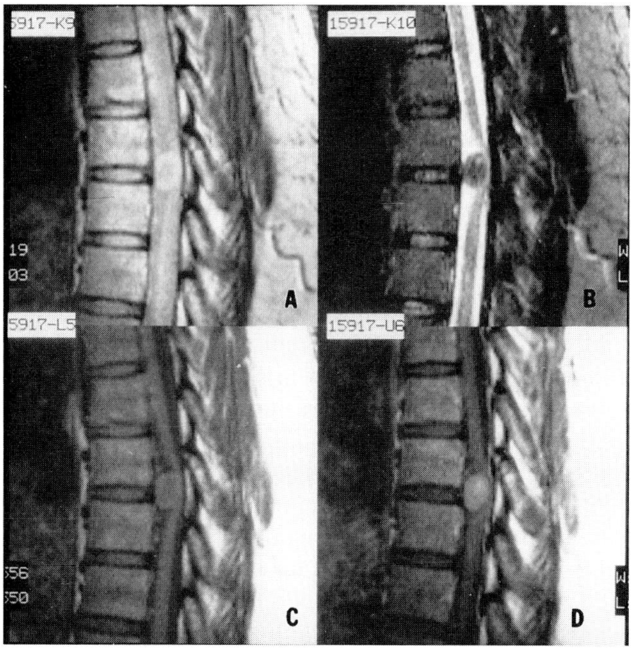

Figure 25-2 Meningioma. *A* and *B*. SDW (1900/20) and T2W (1900/100) images, respectively, show a mass at T8–9, which is peripherally hyperintense on SDW and isointense on T2W to cord, causing posterior displacement and marked thinning of the cord. *C* and *D*. Pre- and postcontrast T1W (667/20) images, respectively, show the mass relative to the cord to be peripherally isointense and centrally slightly hypointense on the precontrast image (*C*) and essentially homogeneously contrast-enhancing on the postcontrast image (*D*). Note that the contrast enhancement is shown by an apparent decrease in the signal intensity of the intervertebral disks and spinal cord, a phenomenon commonly noted in spinal neoplastic and inflammatory disorders.

Age and Gender Meningiomas typically present between the ages of 40 and 60 years and demonstrate an 80 percent female preponderance. Meningiomas account for about only 3 percent of pediatric spinal tumors.

Location Approximately 80 percent of spinal meningiomas occur in the thoracic region, 15 percent are cervical, 3 percent are lumbar, and 2 percent are located at the foramen magnum. Thoracic meningiomas tend to be located posterior or lateral to the cord. Cervical meningiomas tend to be located anterior to the cord.

Pathology Pathohistologically, spinal meningiomas are the same as cranial meningiomas. The most common type of spinal meningioma is the psammomatous variety. Multiple spinal meningiomas are usually associated with neurofibromatosis type 2.

Imaging RADIOGRAPHY Localized widening of the spinal canal may be present. Calcifications within the spinal canal are occasionally seen; when noted, they increase the likelihood of meningioma as opposed to nerve sheath tumor.

MYELOGRAPHY AND COMPUTED TOMOGRAPHY The myelographic and CT findings are similar to those for nerve root tumors except that the mass may be hyperdense, possibly secondary to psammomatous calcifications or dense tumor tissue.

MAGNETIC RESONANCE IMAGING The MRI appearance is variable. However, the typical findings are those of a somewhat broad dura-based mass demonstrating signal findings of isointensity to the cord on both T1W and T2W sequences. Occasionally, meningiomas may be T1W-hypointense or T2W-hyperintense lesions. Following contrast administration, homogeneous, intense contrast enhancement is the rule.

Lipoma For imaging purposes, intradural extramedullary lipomas are exophytic components of subpial-juxtamedullary lipomas; they have been discussed earlier. As previously mentioned, subpial lipomas are technically intradural extramedullary lesions, since they are not completely encompassed by the cord.

Epidermoid and Dermoid Cysts Approximately 60 percent of both epidermoids and dermoids are extramedullary in location. These lesions were previously discussed under "Intramedullary Lesions." The myelographic, CT, and MRI findings would be the same as previously discussed but applied to the intradural extramedullary compartment.

Teratoma Teratomas were previously discussed under "Intramedullary Lesions." The imaging findings are the same as previously discussed but applied to the intradural extramedullary compartment.

Ependymoma and Astrocytoma Scloff and associates reported finding intradural extramedullary ependymomas (3.4 percent) and astrocytomas (2.7 percent) among 301 intraspinal gliomas. These were felt to be secondary to the presence of heterotopic glial tissue. The MRI findings of an encapsulated extramedullary thoracic ependymoma were reported as essentially T1W isointense and T2W hyperintense, which is typical for intramedullary ependymomas.

Cavernous Hemangioma Cavernous hemangiomas are usually intramedullary lesions. The rare extramedullary spinal hemangiomas usually involve the cauda equina but have been reported in the cervical and thoracic regions. The lesions may cause SAH. Cavernous hemangiomas have been previously discussed under "Intramedullary Lesions."

Capillary Hemangioma Capillary hemangiomas of the spinal canal are very rare. Most spinal hemangiomas are of the cavernous variety. At myelography and CT/myelography, extramedullary intradural blockage of the lumbar subarachnoid space was noted in a reported capillary hemangioma of the cauda equina. Magnetic resonance imaging demonstrated a mass that was T1W hyperintense to CSF and isointense to the cord and exhibited intense homogeneous contrast enhancement.

Paraganglioma More than fifty intraspinal paragangliomas have been reported, with a slight male preponderance (55 to 60 percent). In a report of 31 patients ranging in age from 30 to 71 years (mean age, 51 years), 29 of these lesions were of filar origin, 2 originated from caudal nerve roots, and 1 involved the conus. At least 1 intradural thoracic paraglioma has been reported. These are usually firm, encapsulated masses attached to the filum terminale, which can be completely resected. Conventional and CT/myelography demonstrate the typical findings of a lumbar intradural extramedullary mass, often with blockage of the subarachnoid pathway and dilated intradural vessels. Spinal angiography shows these to be highly vascular lesions exhibiting an intense angiographic tumor stain. The reported MRI findings have been those of T1W isointensity to the cord, T2W hyperintensity to the cord and at times to CSF, and dense contrast enhancement.

Leptomeningeal Metastases Leptomeningeal metastases (LMM) usually occur from either "seeding" of the CSF from CNS neoplasms or from hematogenous spread from systemic tumors. Lymphatic spread via perineural, perivascular, and endoneural lymphatics and spread from direct extension are probably less common routes.

Incidence The incidence is unknown because the entire spinal axis is not closely scrutinized during autopsies.

Age and Gender Obviously LMM are more common past the age of 50 because of the higher incidence of malignant neoplasms in that age group. However, because primary brain tumors are rather common in children, leptomeningeal spread is not uncommon in this age group. Sexual predilection is dependent upon the predilection of the primary tumor.

Location The lumbosacral region is involved in nearly 75 percent of LMM. In the cervical and thoracic regions, involvement is mainly posterior in location, probably because the CSF flow dynamics involve flow away from the brain primarily dorsal to the cord and return to the brain primarily ventral to the cord. Gravity probably accounts for the lumbosacral preponderance.

Pathology Leptomeningeal metastases have a variable appearance and may lead to localized or diffuse involvement. Coating of the nerve roots and cord with nodules or sheets of tumor cells and diffuse thickening of the thecal sac are the more common patterns of gross anatomic and histopathologic changes of LMM. Those arising from primary CNS tumors are referred to as "drop" metastases. The usual sources of origin of such metastases are medulloblastoma (48 percent), glioblastoma multiforme (14 percent), ependymoma (12 percent), oligodendroglioma (12 percent), astrocytoma (7 percent), and retinoblastoma (5 percent). Other less common sites of origin are germinoma, pineoblastoma, and choroid plexus papilloma. The two most common systemic sources are carcinomas of the breast and lung, followed by melanoma, non-Hodgkin's lymphoma, leukemia, and carcinomas of the genitourinary tract, gastrointestinal tract, and head/neck region.

Imaging Radiography Although conventional radiography is very useful in the evaluation of osseous metastatic disease, it is seldom helpful in evaluating intradural metastatic disease.

Myelography and Computed Tomography

Conventional and CT/myelography are quite useful in the evaluation of LMM. Myelographic findings include nerve root irregularity, nodular filling defects involving the cord and nerve roots, crowding together of thickened nerve roots, an irregular streaky appearance simulating arachnoiditis, irregular narrowing of the subarachnoid space by thickening of the thecal sac, and varying degrees of blockage of the subarachnoid space.

Magnetic Resonance Imaging Leptomeningeal metastases are best seen by MRI as T1W contrast-enhancing nodules, irregularly thickened nerve roots, and irregularly thickened meninges. Noncontrast images demonstrate nodules or irregular masses hyperintense to CSF on T1W and hypointense to CSF on T2W. Contrast enhancement occurs and usually presents as focal, nodular areas of enlargement and/or an enhancing coat on the surface of the cord and nerve roots. Conventional and CT/myelography are probably as effective as MRI in the detection of LMM.

Vascular Malformations ***Incidence*** The true incidence is unknown; however, symptomatic vascular malformations (VMs) are responsible for about 10 percent of spinal pathology among the combined group of symptomatic patients with neoplasms and VMs. Type II to IV VMs outnumber type I VMs in an approximate 2:1 ratio.

Age and Gender Patients with dural AVFs present at a mean age of approximately 50 years, whereas patients with intramedullary VMs present at a mean age of approximately 23 years. Men outnumber women at a ratio of 3 or 4 to 1.

Location Nearly all intradural type I and type IV spinal VMs occur at or below the midthoracic level.

Pathology Intradural extramedullary VMs are of the type I (dural AVF), type III (juvenile type AVMs), and type IV (intradural extramedullary AVFs) varieties. Type III VMs, as previously discussed, are large and located in both the intramedullary and extramedullary compartments. Type IV VMs are AVFs, in which typically the anterior spinal artery feeds directly into a draining vein on the anterior surface of the cord without an interposed nidus of vessels. Occasionally type IV VMs involve posterior spinal arteries and veins. Type I VMs are AVFs in which arteries located on the cord surface or within nerve root sleeves feed directly into perimedullary veins and may eventually produce cord edema secondary to perimedullary venous hypertension.

Imaging RADIOGRAPHY Conventional radiography rarely contributes significantly.

MYELOGRAPHY AND COMPUTED TOMOGRAPHY Conventional and to a lesser degree CT/myelography remain extremely useful in the demonstration of the presence of abnormal serpentine filling defects indicating the probable presence of enlarged vessels.

MAGNETIC RESONANCE IMAGING Nonspecific associated cord edema may be shown by T1W hypointensity and T2W hyperintensity. Dilated perimedullary veins are best visualized as areas of hypointensity within high-intensity CSF representing flow void on T2W images. Occasionally contrast-enhancing perimedullary veins may be seen, indicating the possibility of slow flow.

ANGIOGRAPHY Spinal angiography is the only reliable way to demonstrate the site of an AVF. This demonstrates direct arteriovenous shunting without an intervening nidus of vessels or other tissue.

TRAUMATIC

Direct trauma to the dura is caused by nerve root/sheath avulsions; severe spinal dislocation injury, which could result in cord and dural transection; and penetrating injuries due to surgery, needle puncture, stab wound, gunshot wound, bone splinter, etc. Nerve root sheaths may be avulsed without an accompanying nerve root avulsion. Each mechanism of injury could result in the formation of some type of pseudomeningocele. Penetrating injuries have been known to result in the formation of posttraumatic arachnoid cysts. The incidence of postsurgical pseudomeningocele is quite high and is frequently seen following lumbar laminectomy and/or lumbar disk surgery. Most nerve root/sheath avulsion injuries involve the brachial plexus; however, avulsion injuries of the lumbosacral region do occur.

Dural trauma may be imaged equally effectively by conventional or CT/myelography and MRI. Postsurgical pseudomeningoceles usually appear as posterior bulging of the thecal sac in the cervical and lumbar spine at sites of previous laminectomy. The myelographic and MRI appearances are obvious. Nerve root/sheath avulsions usually demonstrate bulbous or cylindrical, somewhat irregular collections of CSF or intrathecally introduced contrast at the sites of origin of nerve roots/sheaths of CSF intensity by MRI studies and of contrast density by myelographic studies. Posttraumatic subarachnoid cysts may present as intradural defects initially which may eventually fill with contrast by myelography. However, failure to fill with contrast will result in failure to differentiate them from solid intradural lesions.

Posttraumatic arachnoid cysts are more readily detected by MRI as intradural regions of T2W hyperintensity (usually hyperintense to CSF) frequently associated with a thin line of hypointense border separating it from the CSF and not usually causing significant mass effect.

Spinal subdural hematomas are rare lesions usually associated with blunt or penetrating trauma, anticoagulation therapy, bleeding diasthesis, vascular malformations, or vasculitis. Magnetic resonance imaging is the only reliable imaging technique with the ability to both detect and identify the nature of the subdural mass. Identification of a mass situated between the hypointense dura and the adjacent subarachnoid space allows for localization within the subdural space. The previously described imaging characteristics of hematoma would apply, but restricted to a location within the subdural space. Spinal subdural and epidural hematomas may coexist.

INFLAMMATORY

Arachnoiditis *Arachnoiditis* is a general term for arachnoidal inflammation associated with arachnoidal adhesions. The arachnoidal adhesions result in the adherence of nerve roots, variable degrees of obliteration of the subarachnoid space, intradural cyst formation, and intramedullary cavitation presumably secondary to ischemia. Among the reported causes of arachnoiditis are

(1) infection, (2) trauma, (3) SAH, (4) surgery, (5) lumbar puncture, (6) intraspinal neoplasms, (7) tuberculosis, (8) sarcoidosis, (9) idiopathic, (10) hereditary, and (11) intrathecal injections, including contrast agents, anesthetics, steroids, and other therapeutic agents.

Incidence The incidence is unknown and at least 50 percent of cases are of unknown cause.

Age and Gender Since many cases probably take years to produce clinical manifestations, this is primarily an adult disorder. There is apparently no sexual predilection.

Location Arachnoiditis most commonly occurs in the thoracic (67 percent) region, with the lumbar region being the next most common site.

Pathology Following the acute presence of a fibrinous exudate and vascular response, the fibrin-covered nerve roots and thecal sac become adherent. With this adherence and the reparative production of collagen adhesions, multiple loculations of CSF occur, resulting in intradural cyst formation. These processes lead to varying degrees of obliteration of the subarachnoid space and changes in CSF flow patterns. Neurologic symptoms may be produced secondary to the direct cord or nerve root pressure by the intradural cysts or from the generalized fibrosis producing venous stasis or possibly arterial occlusion resulting in cord ischemia.

Imaging CONVENTIONAL AND CT/MYELOGRAPHY Myelographic findings are variable and are most striking in the lumbar region, where thickened, matted nerve roots, absence of filling of nerve root sleeves, irregular collections of contrast, irregular contour of the subarachnoid space, and an empty thecal sac apparently devoid of nerve roots may be noted. The empty appearance of the thecal sac is due to the adherence of the nerve roots to the walls of the thecal sac; they can be demonstrated as peripheral filling defects by CT. Cystic filling defects may be noted in the thecal sac; some of these may fill with contrast in a delayed fashion. Variable degrees of blockage and narrowing of the subarachnoid space may be seen. The combination of conventional and CT/myelography probably is the most definitive method of confirming the diagnosis of arachnoiditis.

MAGNETIC RESONANCE IMAGING T1W images are the most useful where thickened nerve roots may be noted clumped together centrally within the thecal sac or adherent to the walls of the thecal sac as structures hyperintense to CSF. Soft tissue masses hyperintense to CSF may be noted obliterating the subarachnoid space. Contrast enhancement is not usually present. Associated intramedullary cavitation is best demonstrated by MRI in sagittal and coronal planes.

Subdural Empyema Spinal subdural empyema, usually the result of meningitis, is extremely rare, and its MRI findings may not have been reported. However, the MRI findings should be similar to those of epidural abscess but with the abscess subdural in location.

MISCELLANEOUS

Arachnoid Cyst Arachnoid cysts are defined as diverticula of the subarachnoid space, usually with a communication through a relatively narrow neck. They may be primarily intradural, extradural, or combined intradural/extradural in location.

Incidence Arachnoid cysts comprise approximately 1.3 percent of intraspinal mass lesions excluding Tarlov cysts, which are found in about 14 percent of autopsies. Extradural arachnoid cysts are more common than the intradural variety.

Age and Gender Since most arachnoid cysts are felt to be of congenital origin, they may produce symptoms from childhood through late adulthood. However, only a few of either type produce symptoms. Extradural arachnoid cysts are more common in males. Intradural arachnoid cysts have no sexual predilection and may be of the congenital type or the acquired type secondary to arachnoiditis.

Pathology Nabors' classification of arachnoid cysts is as follows (see Suggested Readings).

1. Type I: Arise directly from the dura and contain no nerve tissue; extradural cysts.
2. Type II: Consist of Tarlov cysts (usually sacral in location, contain neural tissue in cyst wall, and arise at or distal to dorsal root ganglion) and meningeal diverticula (arise proximal to dorsal root ganglion, nerve tissue within cyst but not in cyst wall); extradural cysts.
3. Type III: Intradural cysts.

Location Excluding Tarlov cysts, approximately 65 percent of extradural cysts are thoracic in location, 20 percent are lumbosacral, 10 percent are thoracolumbar, and 5 percent are cervical. Approximately 85 percent are posterior or posterolateral and about 15 percent are lateral to the thecal sac. Intrasacral extradural arachnoid cysts, often called intrasacral meningoceles, are Nabors' type I cysts. Approximately 67 percent of both congenital and acquired intradural arachnoid cysts occur in the upper to midthoracic region. Congenital intradural arachnoid cysts (Fig. 25-3) are usually posterior to the cord, whereas the acquired cysts are commonly anterior in location.

Imaging RADIOGRAPHY Plain films frequently demonstrate bony erosion of the spinal canal and neural foramina with extradural cysts. Plain-film findings are infrequent with intradural cysts; when present, they usually demonstrate widening of the spinal canal.

CONVENTIONAL AND CT/MYELOGRAPHY Congenital intradural and extradural arachnoid cysts demonstrate filling of smoothly marginated diverticula in

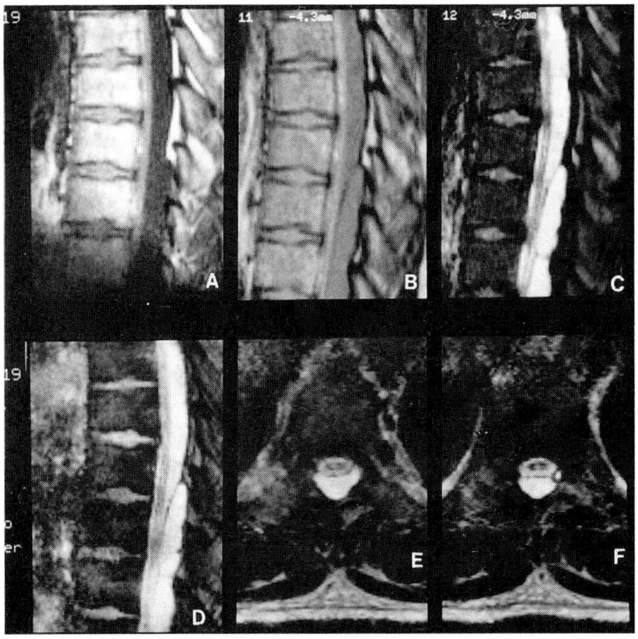

Figure 25-3 Intradural arachnoid cyst. *A* to *D*. T1W (500/20), SDW (2000/20), T2W (2000/100), and GE (18° FA, 783/18) sagittal images, respectively, of the lower thoracic spine demonstrating a mass isointense to CSF on all sequences, with a linear hypointensity separating the mass from the CSF in *B* through *D*. Note the abrupt paucity of the posterior epidural fat, starting at the apex of the cyst. *E* and *F*. T2W (2200/100, axial plane) images show the cord and surrounding subarachnoid space separated from the cyst by a linear hypointensity, which is felt to represent apposed arachnoidal membranes.

the appropriate locations. Often this filling is delayed and perhaps not demonstrated until delayed CT exams are performed. Tarlov cysts are usually noted as root sleeve diverticula of sacral nerve roots measuring up to 3 cm in diameter. Acquired intradural arachnoid cysts are usually associated with arachnoiditis and demonstrate the findings previously described under arachnoiditis.

MAGNETIC RESONANCE IMAGING Arachnoid cysts are usually T1W isointense and T2W isointense/hyperintense lesions compared to CSF in the appropriate locations. As with CT, the congenital varieties demonstrate smooth margination, whereas irregularity is usually present in the acquired forms. Magnetic resonance imaging is the imaging modality of choice for demonstration except for Nabors' type II variants.

Conjoined Nerve Rooth Sheaths When two nerve roots share a common dural root sleeve, the condition of conjoined nerve root sheath exists.

Incidence The incidence noted at surgery is approximately 1 percent and the myelographic incidence is approximately 4 percent.

Age and Gender Obviously this is a lesion present at birth. However, most are detected in life during adulthood, in the evaluation of back pain. In the absence of superimposed abnormalities, these lesions are felt to be asymptomatic.

Location The most common site involves the L5 and S1 roots, although conjoined L3–4 and L4–5 root sleeves are not uncommon. This anomaly is rare above L3.

Pathology The nerve roots usually exit through their respective foramina; occasionally however, they exit through the same foramen. When this happens, the nerve roots may exit through either the superior or inferior foramen.

Imaging COMPUTED TOMOGRAPHY Computed tomography without intrathecal contrast may demonstrate obliteration of extradural fat in a lateral recess, suggesting the presence of a disk fragment. However, the distinction can usually be made by CT density determinations, since the thecal sac and conjoined roots should be in the range of 10 to 20 HU and disk material should be σ 40 HU.

MAGNETIC RESONANCE IMAGING T1W images may show partial absence of extradural fat in a lateral recess combined with predominantly isointense to CSF thickened nerve root/sheath or two distinct normal predominantly isointense to CSF nerve roots/sheaths in a neural foramen. On T2W images, these regions remain essentially isointense to CSF. Occasionally, it will be necessary to resort to conventional and/or CT/myelography for definitive identification.

CONVENTIONAL AND CT/MYELOGRAPHY

Conventional myelography usually clearly identifies the presence of two linear hypolucencies within and paralleling the course of a contrast-filled, enlarged nerve root sleeve. Frequently by CT, the division of a single root sleeve into two separate root sleeves on contiguous thin slices can be identified.

☐ EXTRADURAL (NONOSSEOUS) LESIONS (TABLE 25-3)

NEOPLASMS

Extraosseous epidural tumors consist mostly of lipomatous lesions, lymphomas, hemangioblastomas, meningiomas, cavernous hemangiomas, sarcomas, neuroblastomas, nerve sheath tumors (Fig. 25-4), and paragangliomas. Extradural extramedullary hematopoiesis associated with betathalassemia and myelofibrosis, which, although not neoplastic, can present with compression, usually of the thoracic cord, and imaging findings indistinguishable from those of neoplasms in the same location.

Lipomatous lesions consist of lipomas, angiolipomas, and lipomatosis. Approximately 40 percent of spinal lipomas have been reported to be extradural in location;

Table 25-3
EXTRADURAL NONOSSEOUS LESIONS

Neoplasms	Traumatic/Degenerative
Lipoma	Herniated disk
Lipomatosis	Epidural hematoma
Angiolipoma	Bony dislocation
Hemangioblastoma	Bony fragment
Meningioma	Foreign body
Cavernous hemangioma	
Nerve sheath tumor	**Infectious**
Paraganglioma	Epidural abscess
Lymphoma	
Neuroblastoma	**Miscellaneous**
Sarcoma	Extramedullary hematopoiesis

however, it is not clear that a distinction between the three named types of lipomatous lesions were made. The distinction between these lesions frequently cannot be made by imaging. Epidural lipomatosis and lipomas are most common in the posterior aspect of the thoracic spinal canal. Involvement in the lumbar area often results in circumferential narrowing of the thecal sac by the surrounding fat. The frequency of symptomatic epidural lipomatosis is unclear. Epidural lipomatosis is frequently associated with steroid therapy; however, in the author's experience, it is most commonly associated with obesity without an accompanying history of steroid use. Significant reduction in epidural fat has been noted to accompany weight loss. Angiolipomas are usually located in the thoracic region (80 percent) and are differentiated from lipomas and lipomatosis by the presence of vascular elements. Even though epidural lipomas, epidural lipomatosis, and angiolipomas are frequently asymptomatic, the entire spectrum of neurologic symptoms ranging from nonspecific back pain to paraplegia can be present. The imaging findings are the same as those previously discussed for lipomatous lesions but they are located in an extradural site.

Hemangioblastomas, meningiomas, cavernous hemangiomas, nerve sheath tumors, and paragangliomas have previously been discussed for intradural sites. The imaging characteristics are the same but with a change of site to an extradural location. Except for nerve sheath tumors, extradural locations of these lesions are uncommon; however, approximately 8 percent of spinal hemangioblastomas are extradural in location.

Nonosseous lymphoma with involvement of the extradural compartment most likely results from spread from retroperitoneal lymph nodes. Intradural lymphoma probably results from hematogenous spread or spread via perineural lymphatics. Extradural lymphomas present as small or large masses that are T1W hypointense to isointense and T2W hyperintense relative to the spinal cord. These lesions usually demonstrate moderate contrast enhancement.

Neuroblastoma accounts for approximately 10 percent of all pediatric neoplasms. Approximately 15 percent of neuroblastomas extend into the spinal canal through one or more neural foramina. Extension of neuroblastomas through abdominal and thoracic neural foramina is well demonstrated by MRI without the need for CT or myelography. Calcifications are frequently (> 25 percent) noted on plain films. Neuroblastomas demonstrate low to intermediate signal on T1W images and high signal on T2W images and exhibit heterogeneous contrast enhancement. Sarcomatous lesions tend to demonstrate similar MRI signals to neuroblastomas, with fairly homogeneous contrast enhancement.

HERNIATED DISKS

Herniated disks are treated more extensively elsewhere in this text; they are treated only superficially here.

Lumbar Lumbar disk herniations are the most common type of disk herniation. Most occur in males, and they are unusual in the pediatric age group.

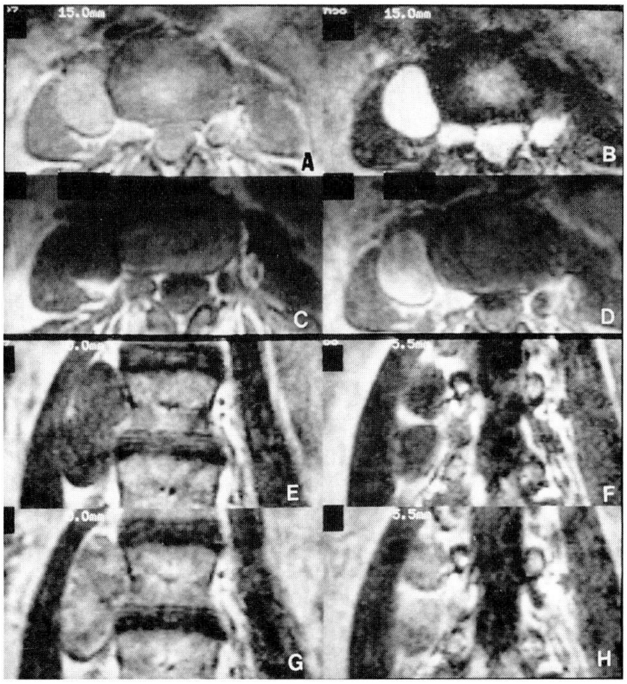

Figure 25-4 Extradural neurofibroma in patient with neurofibromatosis type 1. *A* and *B*. SDW (2700/20) and T2W (2700/80) axial images demonstrate a large right neurofibroma, hyperintense to the psoas muscle, extending from the neural foramen to an area between the spine and psoas muscle. Patulous root sleeves were noted in multiple foramina. *C* and *D*. T1W (567/20) axial pre- and postcontrast axial images showing significant contrast enhancement of the lesion, which was isointense to the psoas prior to contrast. *E* and *F* (precontrast), *G* and *H* (postcontrast). T1W (667/20) coronal images demonstrate lateral displacement of the right psoas muscle and similar findings as in *C* and *D*.

Location Approximately 95 percent of lumbar herniated disks occur at the L4–5 and L5–S1 levels.

Thoracic Thoracic disk herniations (Fig. 25-5) are the least common type of disk herniation and are symptomatic in about 0.3 percent of the total of symptomatic disk herniations. There is a male predominance but no particular age predilection.

Location Most are located at the T9–10, T10–11, and T11–12 levels, where there is greater mobility of the thoracic spine. Thoracic herniated disks have the greatest propensity for calcification among herniated disks.

Cervical Cervical disk herniations tend to occur in males from 20 to 40 years of age and are often associated with trauma.

Location Almost 95 percent occur at the C6–7, C5–6, and C4–5 levels.

Pathology Disk herniations are associated with defects in the annulus fibrosus, allowing herniation of nuclear material through the defects. The annular defects are most commonly posterior or posterolateral, where the annulus is thinner and the restraining vertebral ligament (posterior longitudinal ligament) is weaker than its anterior counterpart. In bulging disks, the annulus fibrosus is intact. Herniated disks are of three types, as follows:

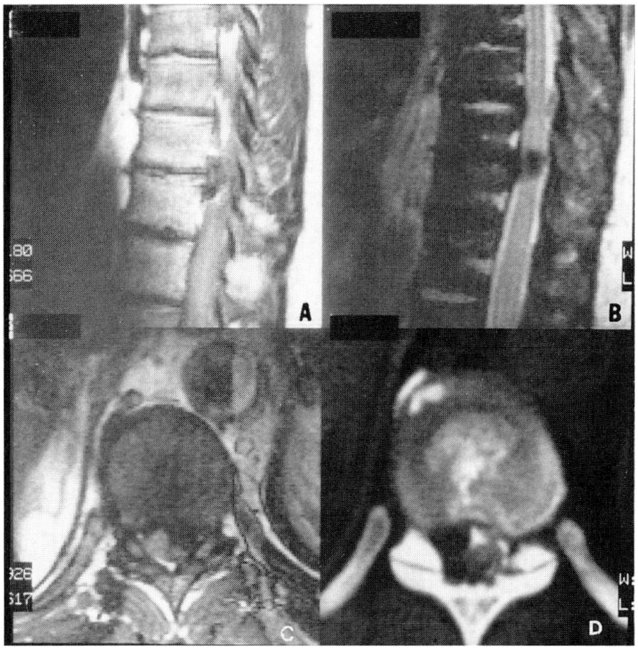

Figure 25-5 Calcified, herniated thoracic disk. *A* and *B*. T1W (550/20) and T2W (1350/100) sagittal images 4 mm to the left (*A*) of and in the midline (*B*), respectively, demonstrating the hypointense calcified T10–11 herniated disk. *C* and *D*. Axial T1W (600/20) MRI and CT images, respectively, demonstrating that virtually the entire left half of the spinal canal is occupied by this surgically proven herniated disk. Note that the CT image clearly demonstrates differentiation between the ventral calcified and dorsal noncalcified aspects of the herniated disk.

1. Protrusion: The nuclear material remains attached to nucleus pulposus and herniates through the annular defect but is contained by the posterior longitudinal ligament and presents as a small anterior epidural mass.
2. Extrusion: A more advanced protrusion produces a larger anterior epidural mass but is still contained to some degree by the posterior longitudinal ligament.
3. Sequestration or free fragment: The nuclear material becomes detached from the parent nucleus pulposus and herniates through the annular defect to a position anterior or posterior to the posterior longitudinal ligament; migration of herniated nuclear material to a location posterior to the posterior longitudinal ligament indicates ligamentous disruption; free fragments may rest considerable distances above or below the affected disk space.

Imaging ***Myelography*** Myelography usually demonstrates either compression of a nerve root, compression of a nerve root and thecal sac, or compression of the thecal sac. Myelography in the cervical and thoracic regions may demonstrate cord compression. Currently, myelography is seldom indicated for the diagnosis of herniated disks.

Computed Tomography Computed tomography in the lumbar area demonstrates displacement of the anterior epidural and foraminal fat in posterolateral and lateral foraminal herniations by soft tissue masses, which may also result in obscuring of a nerve root sheath. Computed tomography in the thoracic area may demonstrate obscuring of epidural fat, as in the lumbar area when sufficient fat is present. Calcification of herniated disks is more common in the thoracic region than in the cervical and lumbar areas. Little epidural fat is present in the cervical region; thus cervical herniations are not usually outlined by displaced fat but by subtle soft tissue encroachment upon the spinal canal. Computed tomography without intrathecal contrast has been reported to be about as effective as MRI in detecting lumbar herniations. Frequently, CT/myelography is needed to definitively detect thoracic and cervical herniations; it may result in an additional 1 to 3 percent detection rate in lumbar herniations.

Magnetic Resonance Imaging The preferred method of most neuroradiologists in the evaluation of disk herniations is MRI, because of the superb anatomic detail that can be obtained directly in multiple planes by a noninvasive technique. Also, much larger segments of the spine can be imaged by MRI than can be practically imaged by CT. However, the role of spiral CT in the evaluation of disk disease has not yet been established.

Herniated disk material is usually of relatively low or intermediate signal on T1W images and either low, intermediate, or high on T2W images. On both low- and high-flip-angle gradient-echo images, disk material tends to be of high signal.

TRAUMATIC

The extradural manifestations of trauma consist primarily of epidural hematomas, disk herniations (especially cervical), encroachment by parts of the osseous spine, and residual foreign bodies (usually metallic fragments from gunshot wounds).

Spinal epidural hematomas have been reported to be associated with approximately 1 to 8 percent of spinal fractures. Because of the large number of sizable veins in the epidural space, their disruption is an enticing etiology; however, because of the frequently rapid onset of cord compression symptoms, many think that bleeding may be more likely from the higher-pressure small and delicate arterial system. Myelography and CT demonstrate nonspecific varying degrees of extradural compression of the thecal sac not necessarily associated with fractures or dislocations. Magnetic resonance imaging is the imaging modality of choice where long segments of the spinal canal can be imaged in the sagittal plane, thereby expediting localization of the lesion. As previously noted and described, the MRI appearance of hemorrhage is time- and volume-dependent. The MRI appearance of an epidural hematoma may vary, from an extradural mass ranging from slightly hypointense to markedly hyperintense in reference to the cord on T1W images, to markedly hypointense to the cord, or to isointense to CSF on T2W images, depending on the age of the hematoma and the relative proportions of hemoglobin break-down products present.

Disk herniations have previously been discussed. However, at least one report associates 25 percent of acute cervical disk herniations with motor vehicle accidents. Traumatic lumbar disk herniations are less common than similar lesions in the cervical region; however, lumbar disk herniations are not uncommon among weight lifters, which probably is a manifestation of trauma.

The presence of bony encroachment upon the epidural space may result in pressure upon the spinal cord and/or nerve roots, producing myelopathy and/or neuropathy. The imaging of bony encroachment or foreign-body residue may demonstrate the obvious anatomic findings by radiography, CT, or MRI.

INFECTIOUS

Epidural abscesses have been reported to account for approximately 1 case per 10,000 admissions to large tertiary hospitals with increases noted in recent years secondary to increased intravenous drug abuse and the increased sensitivity of detection by modern imaging modalities. Epidural abscesses may result from hematogenous spread or direct spread from paraspinal, osseous spinal, and disk space infections. The average age reported has been in the middle of the sixth decade with a range from childhood to the elderly. In view of the increased incidence of intravenous drug abuse, the mean age is likely to drop. The most common causative organism is *Staphylococcus aureus* (62 percent). Tuberculous epidural abscesses are usually associated with tuberculous spondylitis (Fig. 25-6), but cases do occur where tuberculous spondylitis is not initially noted (Fig. 25-7). MRI exceeds CT in the evaluation of epidural abscesses, but associated bony destruction is best evaluated by CT. Myelography and CT/myelography may show blockage of the subarachnoid space or cord compression by an epidural mass at the level of the abscess. Noncontrast T1W and T2W images usually demonstrate epidural abscesses to be isointense to slightly hyperintense to CSF on both sequences. Contrast-enhanced T1W images demonstrate peripheral enhancement, diffuse homogeneous enhancement, or a combination of the two patterns.

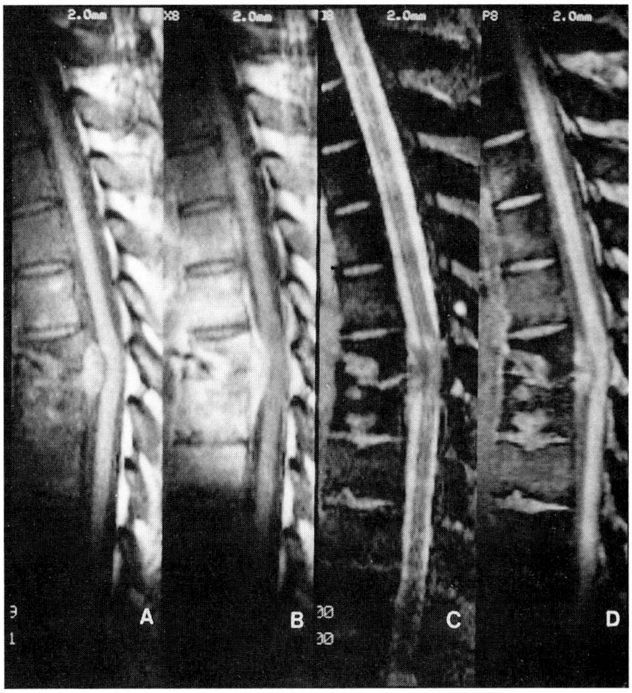

Figure 25-6 Thoracic tuberculous epidural abscess and spondylitis. Sagittal pre- (*A*) and postcontrast (*B*) T1W (667/20) and noncontrast GE [(*C*), 18° FA, 783/18; (*D*), 90° FA, 533/13] images demonstrate obvious anterior epidural tuberculous abscess at T6–7 associated with tuberculous spondylitis and intraosseous abscesses. Note that the epidural abscess on the noncontrast images demonstrates heterogeneous but mostly isointense signal as compared to the cord. Contrast enhancement of the epidural and intraosseous abscesses is noted by the cord and intervertebral disks changing from isointense to the abscesses precontrast to hypointense to the abscesses postcontrast.

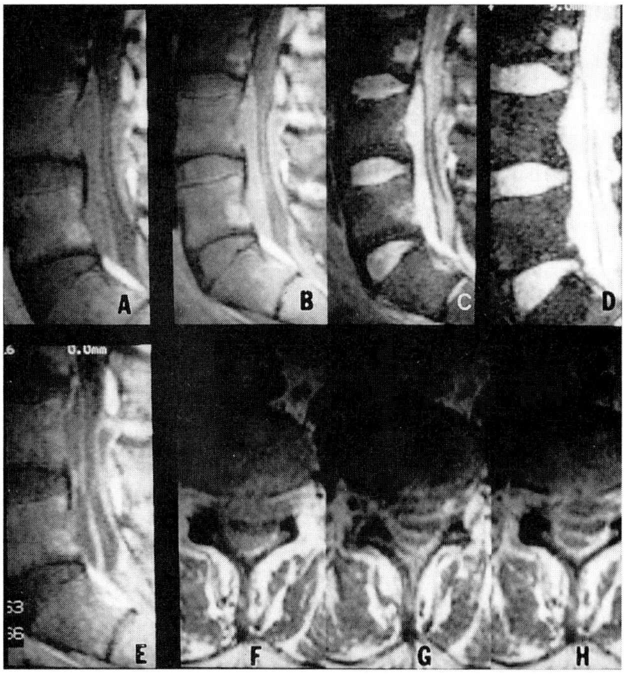

Figure 25-7 Lumbar tuberculous epidural abscess. *A* to *D*. Sagittal T1W (667/20), SDW (1350/20), T2W (1350/80), and GE (20° FA, 1000/18) images respectively that demonstrate hyperintense (*A* to *C*) and isointense (*D*) to CSF epidural abscess anterior and posterior to the thecal sac. *E*. T1W (667/20) image demonstrates marked contrast enhancement about the periphery of the abscess and other intensity changes that render the interior of the abscess isointense to CSF. *F* to *H*. Axial pre- (*F*) and postcontrast (*G*, *H*) T1W (900/20) images showing findings similar to those of *A* and *E*. Note the possible intraosseous abscess in the third lumbar vertebral body.

MISCELLANEOUS

As previously discussed under "Neoplasms," extradural extramedullary hematopoiesis in certain hematologic disorders can be confused with extradural neoplasms.

SUGGESTED READINGS

Neoplasms

1. Augenstein HM et al: Imaging of spinal meningiomas, in Al-Mefty O (ed): *Meningiomas*. New York, Raven Press, 1991, pp 603–613.
2. Awwad EE et al: The imaging of an intraspinal cervical dermoid tumor by MR, CT and sonography. *Comput Radiol* 11:169, 1987.
3. Barkovich AJ: *Pediatric Neuroimaging*, 2d ed. New York, Raven Press, 1995, pp 541–568.
4. Bourgouin PM et al: Multiple occult vascular malformations of the brain and spinal cord. *Neuroradiology* 34:110, 1992.
5. Brotchi J et al: A survey of 65 tumors within the spinal cord: Surgical results and the importance of preoperative magnetic resonance imaging. *Neurosurgery* 29: 651,1991.
6. Byrd SE et al: Developmental disorders of the pediatric spine. *Radiol Clin North Am* 29:711, 1991.
7. Carmody RF et al: Spinal cord compression due to metastatic disease: Diagnosis with MR imaging versus myelopathy. *Radiology* 173:225, 1989.
8. Cheung Y et al: MRI features of spinal ganglioma. *Clin Imaging* 15:109, 1991.
9. Cohen LM et al: Benign schwannomas: Pathologic basis for CT inhomogeneities. *AJR* 147:141, 1986.
10. Corr P, Beningfield SJ: Magnetic resonance imaging of an intradural spinal lipoma: A case report. *Clin Radiol* 40:216, 1989.
11. Dillon WP et al: Intradural spinal cord lesions: Gd-DTPA-enhanced MR imaging. *Radiology* 170:229, 1989.
12. Dorwart RH et al: Tumors, in Newton TH, Potts DG (eds): *Modern Neuroradiology*: Vol 1. *Computed Tomography of the Spine and Spinal Canal*. San Anselmo, CA, Clavadel Press, 1983, pp 115–147.
13. Egelhoff JC et al: Spinal MR findings in neurofibromatosis types 1 and 2. *AJNR* 13:1071, 1992.
14. Emery JL, Lendon RG: Lipomas of the cauda equina and other fatty tumors related to neurospinal dysraphism. *Dev Med Child Neurol* 11(suppl 20):62, 1969.
15. Enzman DR, De La Paz RL: Tumors, in Enzman DR et al (eds): *Magnetic Resonance of the Spine*. St Louis, Mosby, 1990, pp 327–339.
16. Fincher EF: Spontaneous subarachnoid hemorrhage in intradural tumors of the lumbar sac: A clinical syndrome. *J Neurosurg* 8:576, 1951.

17. Fontaine S et al: Cavernous hemangiomas of the spinal cord: MR imaging. *Radiology* 166:839, 1991.
18. Fredericks RK et al: Gadolinium-enhanced MRI: A superior technique for the diagnosis of intraspinal metastases. *Neurology* 39:734, 1989.
19. Friedman DP et al: Intradural schwannomas of the spine: MR findings with emphasis on contrast enhancement characteristics. *AJR* 158:1347, 1992.
20. Graham DV et al: Intramedullary dermoid tumor diagnosed with the assistance of magnetic resonance imaging. *Neurosurgery* 23:765, 1988.
21. Halliday AL et al: Benign spinal nerve sheath tumors: Their occurrence sporadically and in neurofibromatosis types 1 and 2. *J Neurosurg* 74:248, 1991.
22. Herregodts P et al: Solitary dorsal intramedullary schwannoma: Case report. *J Neurosurg* 74:816, 1991.
23. Hodges SC: Neoplastic diseases of the spine, in St. Amour TF et al (eds): *MRI of the Spine*. New York, Raven Press, 1994, pp 299–542.
24. Kaffenberger DA et al: MR imaging of spinal cord hemangioblastoma associated with syringomyelia. *J Comput Assist Tomogr* 12:495, 1988.
25. Kamholtz R, Sze G: MRI of spinal metastases. *MRI Decisions* 4:2, 1990.
26. Lapointe JS et al: Value of intravenous contrast enhancement in the CT evaluation of intraspinal tumors. *AJNR* 6:939, 1985.
27. Larson TC et al: Primary spinal melanoma. *J Neurosurg* 66:47, 1987.
28. Li, MH, Holtas S: MR imaging of spinal neurofibromatosis. *Acta Radiol* 32:279, 1991.
29. Li, MH, Holtas S: MR imaging of spinal intramedullary tumors. *Acta Radiol* 32:502, 1991.
30. Masaryk TJ: Neoplastic disease of the spine. *Radiol Clin North Am* 29:829, 1991.
31. McCormick PC et al: Intradural extramedullary tumors in adults. *Neurosurg Clin North Am* 1:591, 1990.
32. McCormick PC, Stein BM: Intramedullary tumors in adults. *Neurosurg Clin North Am* 1:609, 1990.
33. Nemoto Y et al: Intramedullary spinal cord tumors: Significance of associated hemorrhage at MR imaging. *Radiology* 182:793, 1992.
34. Neumann HPH et al: Hemangioblastomas of the central nervous system. *J Neurosurg* 70:29, 1989.
35. Osborn AG: *Diagnostic Neuroradiology*. St Louis, Mosby-Year Book, 1994, pp 876–918.
36. Palkovic S et al: Angiolipomas of the spinal cord: Magnetic resonance imaging and microsurgical management. *Surg Neurol* 29:243, 1988.
37. Penisson-Besnier I et al: Intramedullary epidermoid cyst evaluated by computed tomographic scan and magnetic resonance imaging: Case report. *Neurosurgery* 25:955, 1989.
38. Quencer RM et al: Syringomyelia associated with intradural extramedullary masses of the spinal canal. *AJNR* 7:143, 1986.
39. Roscoe MWA, Barrington TW: Acute spinal hematoma: A case report and review of the literature. *Spine* 9:672, 1984.
40. Ross DA et al: Intramedullary neurolemmomas of the spinal cord: Report of two cases and review of the literature. *Neurosurgery* 19:458, 1986.
41. Roux A et al: Intramedullary epidermoid cysts of the spinal cord. *J Neurosurg* 76:528, 1992.
42. Russell DS, Rubinstein LJ: *Pathology of Tumors of the Nervous System*, 5th ed. Baltimore, Williams & Wilkins, 1989, pp 83–350, 421–808, 945–974.
43. Salvati M et al: Intramedullary meningioma: Case report and review of the literature. *Surg Neurol* 37:42, 1992.
44. Scotti G et al: Magnetic resonance diagnosis of intramedullary tumors of the spinal cord. *Neuroradiology* 29:139, 1987.
45. Shapiro R: *Myelography*, 4th ed. Chicago, Year Book, 1984, pp 183–197, 345–421.
46. Slasky BS et al: MR imaging with gadolinium-DTPA in the differentiation of tumor, syrinx and cyst of the spinal cord. *J Comput Assist Tomogr* 11:845, 1987.
47. Slooff JL et al: *Primary Intramedullary Tumors of the Spinal Cord and Filum Terminale*. Philadelphia, Saunders, 1964.
48. Swann KW et al: Spontaneous spinal subarachnoid hemorrhage and subdural hematoma: Report of two cases. *J Neurosurg* 61:975, 1984.
49. Sze G et al: Multicenter study of gadopentetate dimeglumine as an MR contrast agent: Evaluation in patients with spinal tumors. *AJNR* 11:967, 1990.
50. Sze G, Twohig M: Neoplastic disease of the spine and spinal cord, in Atlas SW (ed): *Magnetic Resonance Imaging of the Brain and Spine*. New York, Raven Press, 1991, pp 921–965.
51. Takemoto K et al: MR imaging of intraspinal tumors—Capability in histological differentiation and compartmentalization of extramedullary tumors. *Neuroradiology* 30:303, 1988.
52. Wagle WA et al: Intradural extramedullary ependymoma: MR-pathologic correlation. *J Comput Assist Tomogr* 12:705, 1988.
53. Wang A-M et al: Cavernous hemangioma of the thoracic spinal cord. *Neuroradiology* 30:261, 1988.
54. Weil SM et al: Concurrent intradural and extradural meningiomas of the cervical spine. *Neurosurgery* 29:629, 1990.
55. Wood BP et al: Intradural spinal lipoma of the cervical cord. *AJNR* 6:452, 1985.
56. Yamasaki T et al: Primary spinal intramedullary malignant melanoma: Case report. *Neurosurgery* 25:117, 1989.
57. Zimmerman RA, Bilaniuk LT: Imaging of tumors of the spinal canal and cord. *Radiol Clin North Am* 26:965, 1988.

Inflammatory

1. Barakos JA et al: MR imaging of acute transverse myelitis and AIDS myelopathy. *J Comput Assist Tomogr* 14:45, 1990.
2. Bates DJ: Inflammatory diseases of the spine. *Neuroimaging Clin North Am* 1:231, 1991.
3. Berman M et al: Acute transverse myelitis: Incidence and etiologic considerations. *Neurology* 31:966, 1981.
4. Chang KH et al: Tuberculous arachnoiditis of the spine: Findings on myelography, CT and MR imaging. *AJNR* 10:1255, 1989.
5. Delamater RB et al: Diagnosis of lumbar arachnoiditis by magnetic resonance imaging. *Spine* 15:304, 1990.
6. Friedman DP: Herpes zoster myelitis: MR appearance. *AJNR* 13:1404, 1992.
7. Gero B et al: MR imaging of intradural inflammatory disease of the spine. *AJNR* 12:1009, 1991.
8. Hodges SC: Differential diagnosis of intramedullary tumors, in St. Amour TE et al (eds): *MRI of the Spine*. New York, Raven Press, 1994, pp 351–360.
9. Johnson CE, Sze G: Benign lumbar arachnoiditis. *AJNR* 11:763, 1990.
10. Jorgensen J et al: A clinical and radiological study of lower spinal arachnoiditis. *Neuroradiology* 9:139, 1975.
11. Laakman RW: Arachnoiditis, thoracic arachnoiditis with syrinx formation, in St. Amour TE et al (eds): *MRI of the Spine*. New York, Raven Press, 1994, pp 263–276.
12. Kricun R et al: Epidural abscess of the cervical spine: MR findings in five cases. *AJR* 158:1145, 1992.

13. Mark AS: Nondegenerative, non-neoplastic diseases of the spine and spinal cord, in Atlas SW (ed): *Magnetic Resonance Imaging of the Brain and Spine*. New York, Raven Press, 1991, pp 967–1011.
14. Malhern ER, Wang H: Intramedullary spinal cord tuberculoma in a patient with AIDS. *AJNR* 13:986, 1992.
15. Nussbaum ES et al: Spina epidural abscess: A report of 40 cases and review. *Surg Neurol* 38:225, 1992.
16. Osborn AG: *Diagnostic Neuroradiology*. St. Louis, Mosby-Year Book, 1994, pp 820–875.
17. Petito CK et al: Vacuolar myelopathy pathologically resembling subacute combined degeneration in patients with acquired immunodeficiency syndrome. *N Engl J Med* 312:874, 1985.
18. Post MJD et al: Gadolinium-enhanced MR in spinal infection. *J Comput Assist Tomogr* 14:721, 1990.
19. Ross JS et al: MR imaging of lumbar arachnoiditis. *AJNR* 8:885, 1987.
20. St. Amour TE: Spinal infections, in St. Amour TE et al (eds): *MRI of the Spine*. New York, Raven Press, 1994, pp 593–668.
21. Sandhu FS, Dillon WP: Spinal epidural abscess: evaluation with contrast-enhanced MR imaging. *ANJR* 12:1087, 1991.
22. Shabas D et al: MR imaging of AIDS myelitis. *AJNR* 10:551, 1989.
23. Shapiro R: Inflammatory lesions, in Shapiro R (ed): *Myelography*, 4th ed. Chicago, Year Book, 1984, pp 282–317.
24. Sharit HS: Role of MR imaging in the management of spinal infections. *AJR* 158:1333, 1992.
25. Simmons JD, Newton TH: Arachnoiditis, in Newton TH, Potts DG (eds): *Modern Neuroradiology*: Vol 1. *Computed Tomography of the Spine and Spinal Cord*. San Anselmo, CA, Clavedel Press, 1983, pp 223–229.
26. Toshiro K et al: MR imaging of spinal cord in Devic's disease. *J Comput Assist Tomogr* 11:516, 1987.

Miscellaneous

1. Bernini PM et al: Metrizamide myelography and the identification of anomalous lumbosacral nerve roots: Report of two cases and review of the literature. *J Bone Joint Surg* 62A:1203, 1980.
2. Blaser SI, Modic MT: Herniation of the intervertebral disc. *Top Magn Reson Imaging* 1:25, 1988.
3. Bouchard JM et al: Preoperative diagnosis of conjoined roots anomaly with herniated discs. *Surg Neurol* 10:229, 1978.
4. Edwards MK et al: Cranial MR in spinal cord MS: Diagnosing patients with isolated spinal cord symptoms. *AJNR* 7:1003, 1986.
5. Helms CA et al: The CT appearance of conjoined nerve roots and differentiation from a herniated nucleus pulposus. *Radiology* 144:803, 1982.
6. Hoddick WK, Helms CA: Bony spinal canal changes that differentiate conjoined nerve roots from herniated nucleus pulposus. *Radiology* 154:119, 1985.
7. Hodges SC: Arachnoid (meningeal) cysts, in St. Amour TE et al (eds): *MRI of the Spine*. New York, Raven Press, 1994, pp 793–808.
8. Kadish LJ, Simmons EH: Anomalies of the lumbosacral nerve roots: An anatomical investigation and myelographic study. *J Bone Joint Surg* 66B:411, 1984.
9. Larson E-M et al: GD-DTPA-enhanced MR of suspected spinal multiple sclerosis. *AJNR* 10:1071, 1989.
10. Lee H-J et al: MRI of the spine in multiple sclerosis. *J Neuroimaging* 2:61, 1992.
11. Maravilla KR et al: Magnetic resonance demonstration of multiple sclerosis plaques in the cervical cord. *AJNR* 5:685–689, 1984.
12. McElvenny RT: Anomalies of the lumbar spinal cord and nerve roots. *Clin Orthop* 8:61, 1956.
13. Modic MT: Degenerative disorders of the spine, in Modic MT et al (eds): *Magnetic Resonance Imaging of the Spine*. Chicago, Year Book, 1989, pp 75–119.
14. Nabors MW et al: Updated assessment and current classification of spinal meningeal cysts. *J Neurosurg* 68:366, 1988.
15. Naidich TP et al: Arachnoid cysts, paravertebral meningoceles and perineurial cysts, in Newton TH, Potts DG (eds): *Modern Neuroradiology*: Vol 1. *Computed Tomography of the Spine and Spinal Cord*. San Anselmo, CA, Clavadel Press, 1983, pp 383–396.
16. Peyster RG et al: Computed tomography of lumbosacral conjoined nerve root anomalies: Potential cause of false-positive reading for herniated nucleus pulposus. *Spine* 10:331, 1985.
17. St. Amour TE: Degenerative diseases of the spine, in St. Amour TE et al: *MRI of the Spine*. New York, Raven Press, 1994, pp 51–210.
18. St. Amour TE: Multiple sclerosis, in St. Amour TE et al (eds): *MRI of the Spine*. New York, Raven Press, 1994, pp 731–740.
19. Shapiro R: Congenital lesions, in Shapiro R (ed): *Myelography*, 4th ed. Chicago, Year Book, 1984, pp 198–246.
20. Shapiro R: The herniated intervertebral disc, in Shapiro R (ed): *Myelography*, 4th ed. Chicago, Year Book, 1984, pp 422–496.
21. Williams AL, Haughton VM: Disc herniation and degenerative disc disease, in Newton TH et al (eds): *Modern Neuroradiology*: Vol 1. *Computed Tomography of the Spine and Spinal Cord*. San Anselmo, CA. Clavadel Press, 1983, pp 231–249.

Vascular

1. Anson JA, Spetzler RF: Classification of spinal arteriovenous malformations and implications for treatment. *Barrow Neurol Inst Q* 8:2, 1992.
2. Avrahami E et al: MR demonstration of spontaneous acute epidural hematoma of the thoracic spine. *Neuroradiology* 31:90, 1989.
3. Brown E et al: Clinical images: MR imaging of cervical spinal cord infarction. *J Comput Assist Tomogr* 13:920, 1989.
4. Criscuolo, GR et al: Reversible acute and subacute myelopathy in patients with dural arteriovenous fistulas: Foix-Alajouanine syndrome reconsidered. *J Neurosurg* 70:354, 1989.
5. Djindjian R: Vascular malformations, in Shapiro R (ed): *Myelography*, 4th ed. Chicago, Year Book, 1984, pp 318–344.
6. Dormont D et al: MRI study of spinal arteriovenous malformations. *J Neuroradiol* 14:351, 1987.
7. Elksnis SM et al: MR imaging of spontaneous spinal cord infarction. *J Comput Assist Tomgr* 15:228, 1991.
8. Gundy CR, Heithoff KB: Epidural hematoma of the lumbar spine: 18 surgically confirmed cases. *Radiology* 187:427, 1993.
9. Larson EM et al: Venous infarction of the spinal cord resulting from dural arteriovenous fistula: MR imaging findings. *AJNR* 12:739, 1991.
10. Maravilla KR, Cohen WA: *MRI Atlas of the Spine*. New York, Raven Press, 1991, pp 302–339.

11. Mark AS: Nondegenerative, non-neoplastic diseases of the spine and spinal cord, in Atlas SW (ed): *Magnetic Resonance Imaging of the Brain and Spine*. New York, Raven Press, 1991, pp 967–1011.
12. Masaryk TJ et al: Radiculomeningeal vascular malformations of the spine: MR imaging. *Radiology* 164:845, 1987.
13. Mawad ME et al: Spinal cord ischemia after resection of thoracoabdominal aortic aneurysms: MR findings in 24 patients. *AJNR* 11:987, 1990.
14. Mirich DR et al: Subacute necrotizing myelopathy: MR imaging in four pathologically proven cases. *AJNR* 12:1077, 1991.
15. Mirkovik S, Melany M: A thoracolumbar epidural hematoma simulating a disc syndrome. *J Spinal Disord* 5:112, 1992.
16. Rosenblum B et al: Spinal arteriovenous malformations: A comparison of dural arteriovenous fistulas and intradural AVMs in 81 patients. *J Neurosurg* 67:795, 1987.
17. Rothfus WE et al: MR imaging in the diagnosis of spontaneous spinal epidural hematomas. *J Comput Assist Tomogr* 11:851, 1987.
18. St. Amour TF: Spinal cord infarction, vascular malformations, intraspinal hemorrhage, in St. Amour TF et al (eds): *MRI of the Spine*. New York, Raven Press, 1994, pp 755–786.
19. Sandson TA, Friedman JH: Spinal cord infarction. *Medicine* 68:282, 1989.
20. Symon L et al: Dural arteriovenous malformations of the spine: Clinical features and surgical results in 55 cases. *J Neurosurg* 60:238, 1984.
21. Vincent FM: Anterior spinal artery aneurysm presenting as a subarachnoid hemorrhage. *Stroke* 12:230, 1981.
22. Vinters HV et al: Subdural hematoma of the spinal cord and widespread subarachnoid hemorrhage complicating anticoagulant therapy. *Stroke* 11:459, 1980.
23. Wirth EP et al: Foix-Alajouanine disease: Spontaneous thrombosis of a spinal cord arteriovenous malformation: A case report. *Neurology* 170:1114, 1970.
24. Wrobel CJ et al: Myelopathy due to intracranial dural arteriovenous fistulas draining intrathecally into spinal medullary veins: Report of three cases. *J Neurosurg* 69:934, 1988.
25. Zuccarello M et al: Spontaneous spinal extradural hematoma during anticoagulant therapy. *Surg Neurol* 14:411, 1980.

Trauma

1. Brant-Zawadzki M, Post MJD: Trauma, in Newton TH, Potts DG (eds): *Modern Neuroradiology*: Vol 1. *Computed Tomography of the Spine and Spinal Cord*. San Anselmo, CA, Clavadel Press, 1983, pp 149–186.
2. Freedy RM et al: Traumatic lumbosacral nerve root avulsion evaluation by MR imaging. *J Comput Assist Tomogr* 13:1052, 1989.
3. Gupta RK et al: MR evaluation of brachial plexus injury. *Neuroradiology* 31:377, 1989.
4. Hackney DB et al: Hemorrhage and edema in acute spinal cord injury: Demonstration by MR imaging. *Radiology* 161:387, 1987.
5. Kolkarni MV et al: Acute spinal cord injury: MR imaging at 1.5T. *Radiology* 164:837, 1987.
6. Kerslake RW et al: Magnetic resonance imaging of spinal trauma. *Br J Radiol* 64:386, 1991.
7. Maravilla KR, Cohen WA: *MRI Atlas of the Spine*. New York, Raven Press, 1991, pp 302–339.
8. Mark AS: Nondegenerative, non-neoplastic diseases of the spine and spinal cord, in Atlas SW (ed): *Magnetic Resonance Imaging of the Brain and Spine*. New York, Raven Press, 1991, pp 967–1011.
9. Matsumura AA et al: Magnetic resonance imaging of spinal cord injury without radiologic abnormality. *Surg Neurol* 33:281, 1990.
10. Mendelsohn DB et al: MR of cord transection. *J Comput Assist Tomogr* 14:909, 1990.
11. Oller DW, Boone S: Blunt cervical spine Brown-Sequard injury: A report of three cases. *Am Surg* 57:361, 1991.
12. Osburn AG: *Diagnostic Neuroradiology*. St Louis, Mosby-Year Book, 1994, pp 820–875.
13. Pratt ES et al: Herniated intervertebral disks associated with unstable spine injuries. *Spine* 15:662, 1990.
14. Quencer RM: The injured cord. *Radiol Clin North Am* 26:1025, 1988.
15. Quencer RM et al: Acute traumatic central cord syndrome: MRI-pathological correlation. *Neuroradiology* 34:85, 1992.
16. Raynor RB: Cervical cord compression secondary to acute disk protrusion in trauma. *Spine* 2:39, 1977.
17. Rizzolo SJ et al: Intervertebral disc injury complicating cervical spine trauma. *Spine* 16:S187–S189, 1991.
18. Tamas DE: Trauma, in St. Amour TE et al (eds): *MRI of the Spine*. New York, Raven Press, 1994, pp 543–592.
19. Viraponse C, Kier EL: Trauma to the spinal cord and nerve roots, in Shapiro R (ed): *Myelography*, 4th ed. Chicago, Year Book, 1984, pp 247–281.
20. Yamashita V et al: Chronic injuries of the spinal cord: Assessment with MR imaging. *Radiology* 177:25, 1990.

☐ QUESTIONS (True or False)

1. Regarding spinal ependymoma,
- **a.** Considering all age groups, it is the most prevalent spinal glioma.
- **b.** The most common site is the lower thoracic cord.
- **c.** A female preference of 3:2 exists.
- **d.** The most common type is the myxopapillary variant.
- **e.** About 20 percent demonstrate malignant change.

2. Regarding spinal ependymoma,
- **a.** Evidence of previous hemorrhage is common.
- **b.** By myelography, filar ependymomas may be indistinguishable from cauda equina nerve sheath tumors.
- **c.** Rare instances of primary location in the intradural extramedullary compartment have been reported.
- **d.** The typical MRI presentation is that of a mass T1W hypo-/isointense and T2W hyperintense relative to CSF.
- **e.** Associated syringohydromyelia is unusual.

3. Regarding spinal astrocytoma,
- **a.** This is the most common pediatric spinal glioma.
- **b.** The most common site is in the lower thoracic cord.
- **c.** Frequently demonstrate less intense MRI contrast enhancement than ependymomas.
- **d.** Commonly occur in the filum terminale.
- **e.** Occasionally are of the fibrillary type.

4. Regarding spinal hemangioblastoma,
- **a.** Most are intradural extramedullary in location.
- **b.** They are commonly present in the spectrum of pediatric spinal tumors.
- **c.** Most are cystic when intramedullary in location.
- **d.** Spinal angiography is of little use in their detection.
- **e.** Myelography may aid in differentiating them from astrocytoma.

5. Regarding spinal cavernous hemangioma,
- **a.** They probably represent less than 1 percent of intramedullary tumors.
- **b.** A male predilection exists.
- **c.** Associated subarachnoid hemorrhage is common.
- **d.** Normal study by conventional and CT/myelography would be unusual.
- **e.** T2W marked hypointensity is a commonly associated MRI finding.

6. Regarding spinal lipoma,
- **a.** Filar fibrolipomas are usually associated with tethering of the cord.
- **b.** Filar fibrolipomas are present in about 80 percent of patients with the tight filum terminale syndrome.
- **c.** Subpial-juxtamedullary lipomas are usually in the ventral aspect of the cord.
- **d.** The conus medullaris is the favored site of subpial lipomas.
- **e.** Malignant degeneration is uncommon.

7. Spinal oligodendrogliomas have a greater propensity for the filum terminale than astrocytomas.

8. Spinal gangliogliomas have a propensity for the cervical cord.

9. Primary melanoma of the cord may present as a T1W mixed iso-/hyperintense and T2W hypointense intramedullary mass.

10. Intramedullary neurolemmomas in the absence of neurofibromatosis have not been reported.

11. Most spinal teratomas are congenital sacrococcygeal teratomas.

12. Most spinal dermoids are in the lower thoracic cord.

13. The midthoracic cord is the site of most intramedullary epidermoids.

14. Hair follicles and sweat glands are typical components of epidermoids.

15. Some spinal epidermoids are felt to result from previous lumbar punctures.

16. Typically, epidermoids are isointense to the cord on both T1W and T2W sequences.

17. Regarding metastases,
- **a.** Intramedullary metastases have been noted at autopsy in about 10 percent of cancer patients.
- **b.** Lung carcinoma is the most frequent cause of intramedullary metastases.
- **c.** The typical MRI findings in intramedullary metastases are lesions T1W hypo-isointense and T2W hyperintense exhibiting intense contrast enhancement.
- **d.** Thoracic leptomeningeal metastases are usually ventral to the cord.
- **e.** Glioblastoma multiforme is the most common CNS source of "drop" metastases.

18. Regarding transverse myelitis
- **a.** Is often difficult to differentiate clinically from the Brown-Séquard's syndrome.
- **b.** Has frequently been associated with preceding viral infections and vaccinations.
- **c.** Transverse myelitis accompanied by blindness is called Devic's syndrome.
- **d.** Most commonly involves the cervical cord.
- **e.** May have associated normal MRI study.

19. AIDS myelopathy results in symptoms and pathologic findings similar to those of amyotrophic lateral sclerosis.

20. Sarcoid granulomas of the cord usually involve the thoracic cord.

21. Tuberculous granulomas of the cord usually involve the cervical cord.

22. Intramedullary abscesses have most frequently been detected by myelography and/or CT/myelography.

23. Except for location preferences, sarcoid and tuberculous granulomas present indistinguishable imaging findings.

24. Regarding vascular malformations,
- **a.** The most common type of spinal vascular malformation usually does not produce clinical symptoms.
- **b.** The cervical cord is the most common site of intramedullary AVM.
- **c.** More than 50 percent of cord AVMs have associated aneurysms.

d. Juvenile AVMs are the rarest group of the spinal vascular malformations.
e. Spinal angiography and myelography usually contribute little in the detection of spinal vascular malformations.

25. Regarding the vascular system,
a. Spinal cord infarctions represent approximately 1 percent of ischemic infarctions of the CNS.
b. Aneurysms associated with spinal AVMs increase the likelihood of spontaneous hemorrhage.
c. Clinical symptoms are more likely to result from occlusion of a posterior spinal artery occlusion than from anterior spinal artery occlusion.
d. Imaging of ischemic infarction of the spinal cord presents similar findings to those for ischemic brain infarcts.
e. Subacute necrosing myelopathy is felt usually to be the result of cord ischemia produced by an intramedullary glomus AVM.

26. Regarding trauma,
a. The anterior cord syndrome is usually caused by hyperextension injuries.
b. The Brown-Sequard syndrome is usually caused by flexion injuries.
c. The conus medullaris syndrome is usually caused by compression fracture of L1 and/or T12.
d. The central cord syndrome is usually caused by dorsal column injury.
e. The extent of cord injury usually correlates well with the extent of accompanying bony and soft tissue injury.

27. Regarding multiple sclerosis,
a. About 20 percent of MS patients have solely cord involvement.
b. A female preponderance exists.
c. Most plaques involve the lateral columns.
d. Contrast enhancement is not unusual when T2W images are normal.
e. The thoracic cord is the predominant site of cord involvement.

28. Regarding neurofibromatosis,
a. Acoustic tumors are associated with neurofibromatosis type 1.
b. Multiple spinal meningiomas are associated with neurofibromatosis type 2.
c. Cyst formation is more common in schwannomas than in neurofibromas.
d. Neurofibromas tend to be encapsulated whereas schwannomas tend to be nonencapsulated.
e. In the absence of associated cyst formation neurofibromas and schwannomas are indistinguishable by imaging.

29. Regarding nerve sheath tumors,
a. Nerve sheath tumors usually involve the ventral roots.
b. The thoracic and lumbar spine are the favored sites for nerve sheath tumors.
c. Nerve sheath tumors have no sexual predilection.
d. Plexiform neurofibromas frequently undergo malignant transformation.
e. At myelography nerve sheath tumors typically present as well circumscribed, sharply marginated filling defects.

30. Regarding meningioma,
a. Approximately 80 percent involve females.
b. Cervical and thoracic locations occur at approximately equal frequencies.
c. The typical MRI appearance is that of a lesion isointense to the cord on T1W and T2W images with marked, homogeneous contrast enhancement.
d. The identification of calcifications increases the likelihood of an extramedullary intradural mass being a meningioma compared to a nerve sheath tumor.
e. Most thoracic meningiomas are ventral to the cord.

31. Type I vascular malformations typically are arteriovenous fistulas in which the anterior spinal artery feeds directly into a draining vein on the anterior surface of the cord.

32. Type IV vascular malformations typically are arteriovenous fistulas in which arteries located on the cord surface feed directly into perimedullary veins.

33. Most type I vascular malformations occur at or below the midthoracic spine.

34. Root sleeve avulsion injuries sometimes occur without accompanying nerve root avulsions.

35. The most common site of arachnoiditis is the cervical region.

36. Myelography is probably more specific than MRI in the evaluation of arachnoiditis.

37. Tarlov cysts represent the most common type of arachnoid cyst.

38. Nabors' type I arachnoid cysts have nerve tissue in the cyst walls.

39. Meningeal diverticula arise at or distal to dorsal root ganglia.

40. Neuroblastomas are frequently accompanied by calcifications identifiable by plain radiography.

☐ ANSWERS

1. a. T
b. F
c. F
d. T
e. F

2. a. T
b. T
c. T
d. F
e. F

3. a. T
b. F
c. T
d. F
e. F

4. a. F
b. F
c. T
d. F
e. T

5. a. T
b. T
c. F
d. F
e. T

6. a. F
b. F
c. F
d. F
e. T

7. T

8. T

9. T

10. F

11. T

12. F

13. T

14. F

15. T

16. F

17. a. F
b. T
c. T
d. F
e. F

18. a. F
b. T
c. T
d. F
e. T

19. F

20. F

21. F

22. F

23. T

24. a. T
b. F
c. F
d. T
e. F

25. a. T
b. T
c. F
d. T
e. F

26. a. F
b. F
c. T
d. F
e. F

27. a. F
b. T
c. T
d. F
e. F

28. a. F
b. T
c. T
d. F
e. T

29. a. F
    b. T
    c. T
    d. T
    e. T

30. a. T
    b. F
    c. T
    d. T
    e. F

31. F

32. F

33. T

34. T

35. F

36. T

37. T

38. F

39. F

40. T

APPENDIX

1 MRI Physics

George Magre

Magnetic resonance imaging (MRI) is dependent on the existence of atoms whose nuclei contain an odd number of protons and neutrons, possess angular momentum, act as dipoles (tiny bar magnets with north and south poles), and therefore tend to align themselves when placed in an external magnetic field. Atoms such as ^{19}F, ^{23}Na, ^{31}P, ^{39}K, and ^{1}H fulfill these criteria. The atom in most abundance, of practical use in MRI, is hydrogen (^{1}H).

Hydrogen atoms (protons, spins) in the body placed in a strong magnetic field, the MRI unit, tend to align themselves predominantly along the direction of the field (B_0). This is the "parallel" or low-energy condition. A net magnetic vector (M_z) representing the vector sum of magnetic moments of individual protons, results. This vector is oriented in the Z axis, paralleling the main magnetic field (B_0) generated by the MRI unit (Fig. A1-1). Additionally, these protons, since they are not precisely aligned parallel to the main magnetic field, begin to wobble (precess) at a specific frequency. All protons precess at the same frequency, which is proportional to the strength of the magnetic field and a constant specific for each type of nucleus (*Larmor frequency*). (Refer to the glossary at the end of this appendix for definitions of the italicized terms.)

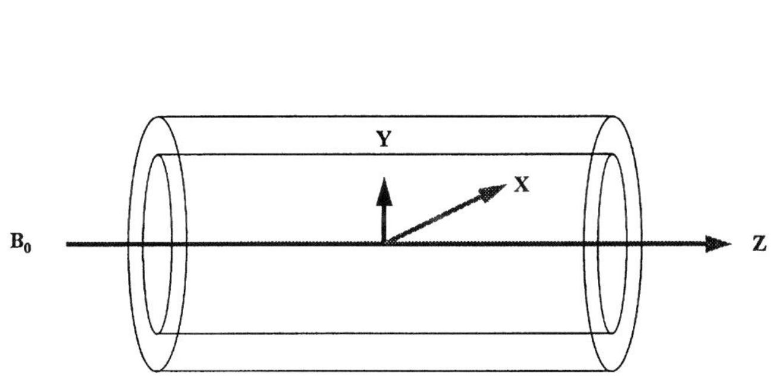

Figure A1-1 Orientation of the main magnetic field (B_0) and the various reference axes (X, Y, Z) within the magnet used to describe events occurring in image formation.

Electromagnetic radiation, in the form of a radiofrequency (RF) pulse of a specific frequency (the Larmor frequency) and duration, is then applied in order to displace the net magnetic vector from its longitudinal (M_z) or resting state onto the transverse plane (M_{xy}). (See Figure A1-2).

The RF is applied by loops of wire placed within the magnet acting as transmitters. The passage of an alternating current through these coils induces the electromagnetic (RF) radiation used to displace these protons from their original orientation (*Faraday's law*). With time, the deflected net magnetization vector will return to its original longitudinal orientation. This return to, or regrowth of, longitudinal magnetization is referred to as *T1 relaxation* (Fig. A1-3). The T1 of a tissue, in milliseconds, is the time required for it to recover 63 percent of its longitudinal magnetization. Occurring simultaneously with the regrowth of longitudinal magnetization is a second process. The initial RF pulse, in addition to displacing the net magnetization vector into the transverse plane, forces the majority of the precessing protons to precess together (in phase). Immediately after cessation of the RF pulse, the various component magnetization vectors that form the net vector in the transverse plane begin to be affected by the variations in magnetic field lines of flux that are present inherently in the imaging system as well as in the tissues themselves. This results in different protons beginning to precess at varying rates. In time, more and more protons fall out of phase from each other, and the net magnetization vector in the transverse plane begins to decrease in magnitude. This is *T2 relaxation* (Fig. A1-4).

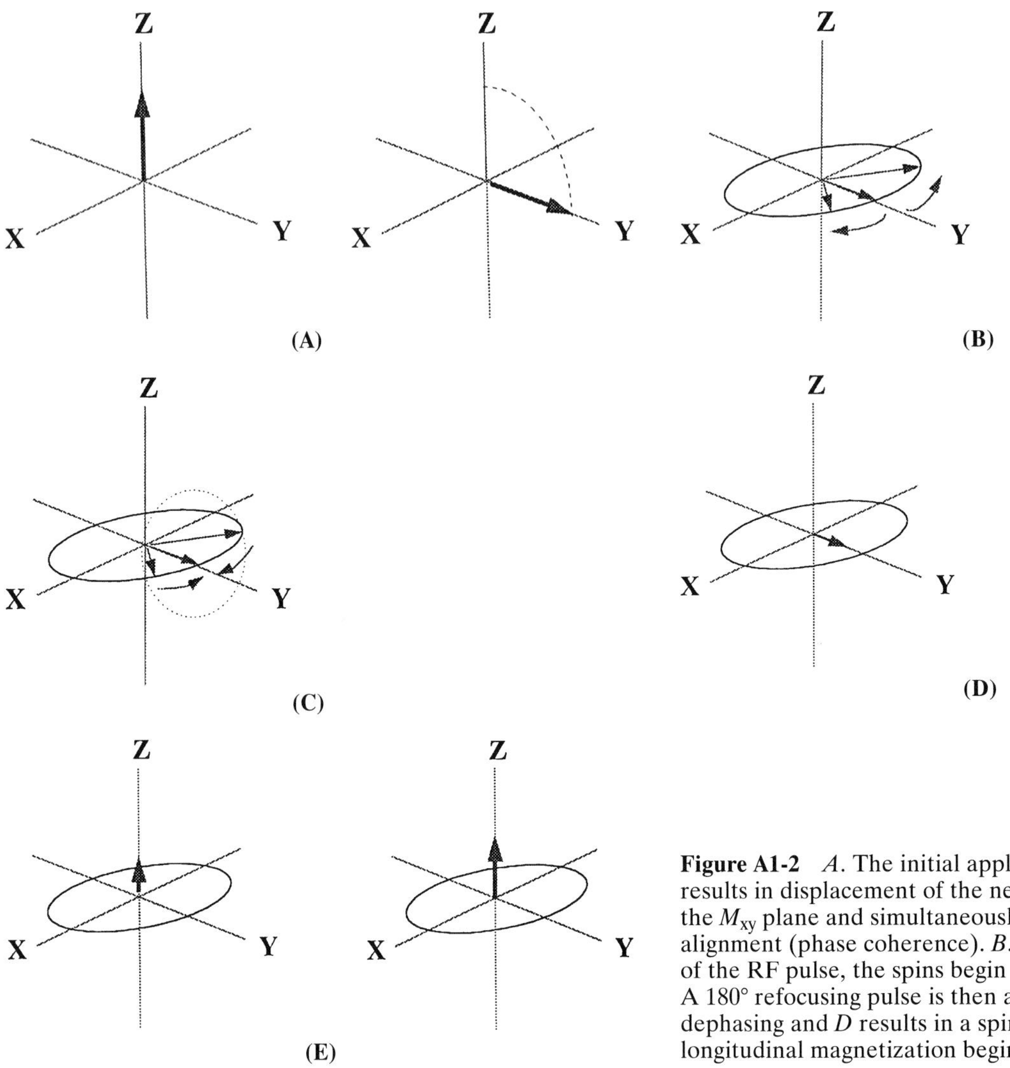

Figure A1-2 *A*. The initial application of a 90° RF pulse results in displacement of the net magnetization vector into the M_{xy} plane and simultaneously places all of the spins into alignment (phase coherence). *B*. Immediately after cessation of the RF pulse, the spins begin to lose phase coherence. *C*. A 180° refocusing pulse is then applied, which reverses the dephasing and *D* results in a spin echo. *E*. At the same time, longitudinal magnetization begins to regrow.

The time in milliseconds required to decrease a tissue's transverse magnetization to 37 percent of its peak value after the administration of an RF pulse is a tissue's T2 relaxation time.

The loss of transverse-phase coherence results in a decreasing RF signal emanating from the patient called a *free induction decay* (FID). Magnetic vectors precessing in the transverse plane induce a current in MRI coils (Faraday's law). These coils therefore act as RF receivers or antennas. The FID decays at a rate that is different (faster) than T2 called *T2** ("T-two-star"). *T2* more correctly refers to the rate of spin-echo decay (Fig. A1-5).

T1 and T2 effects as well as proton density work together to determine final image contrast. The signal characteristics of different tissues imaged using sequences that highlight either T1 or T2 effects are summarized in Table A1-1.

Selection of an imaging plane, identification of slices to be imaged, and spatial localization of the information returned from the excitation of the volume of interest require specialized techniques. In MRI, this is accomplished by using magnetic field gradients (weak magnetic fields of progressively changing intensity) to increase or decrease the precessional frequency of spins in a linear fashion. These gradients are superimposed upon the uniform main magnetic field. The end result is a range of precessional frequencies. This range of frequencies can be used to select a slice to image as well as to define the location of a signal returned after an excitation. This is accomplished by the application of gradients in the *Z*, *X*, and *Y* axes (slice-select, frequency, and phase-encoding directions). One gradient coil is used to select a slice and the remaining two gradient coils are used to localize the returned RF signal. Any gradient coil can perform any of these functions, making multiplanar imaging possible.

Advanced computer software and hardware techniques are then used to transform the RF energy being returned from the imaged volume into phase/frequency data matrices that are then further transformed into a format which can be displayed on a screen, manipulated, and subsequently captured on film.

Magnetic resonance imaging requires that imaging parameters be preset in order to generate an image with the

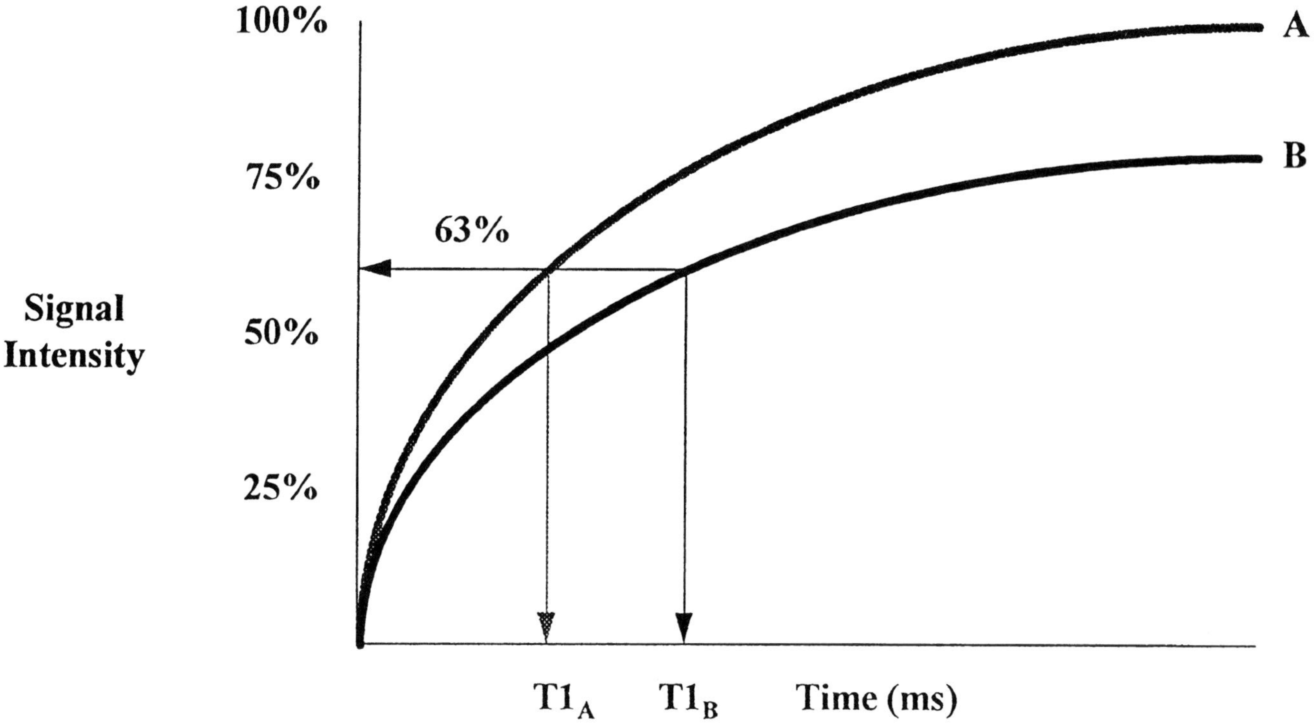

Figure A1-3 Longitudinal relaxation.

properties and attributes that best characterize the anatomy to be viewed or the disease process to be evaluated. The operator must first select the body part to be evaluated, then the plane of orientation in which the image will be acquired, and finally the overall imaging strategy, called the *pulse sequence* (see below). The operator must next decide upon the specific parameters (*TR, TE, flip angle, field of view,* slice thickness, and number of *phase and frequency encodings*) to be used. Each parameter chosen can affect image quality. The amount of signal returned for image generation relative to the amount of noise returned is an important consideration. This signal to noise ratio has many determinants that affect the overall image in quantifiable ways (Fig. A1-6). Changing imaging parameters also affects image contrast (Table A1-3) as well as imaging time (Fig. A1-7).

Commonly used pulse sequences include conventional spin echo, gradient-echo technique, inversion recovery, and newer fast-scan techniques including fast spin echo, fast gradient echo, and echo planar imaging.

Conventional spin echo (CSE) technique (Fig. A1-5) consists of the initial application of a 90° RF pulse of a specific frequency range and duration that displaces the net magnetization vector in the slice or slab of interest into the transverse plane (M_{xy}). Subsequently, a second 180° RF pulse is applied to rephase the component vectors in the transverse plane. A signal is then generated (the spin echo) that can be detected by a receiver coil. The time in milliseconds between two successive 90° pulses is the *repetition time (TR)*. The time in milliseconds between the 90° RF pulse and the time the spin echo is generated is the *echo time (TE)* (Fig. A1-5).

Newer **fast-spin-echo (FSE)** techniques follow the initial 90° RF pulse with a series of 180° RF pulses, each of which generates a separate spin echo. Imaging time is therefore decreased by a factor equal to the number of 180° pulses used (echo train length or turbo factor). Fast spin echo is traditionally used in neuroimaging to produce heavily T2-weighted images that are of high signal-to-noise ratio and high resolution in acceptable time.

Table A1-1
TYPICAL SIGNAL INTENSITY OF VARIOUS TISSUES IN IMAGES THAT ARE ACQUIRED USING PRIMARILY T1- OR T2-WEIGHTED SEQUENCES

	T1-Weighted Sequence	T2-Weighted Sequence
Fat	+	Int
Water (urine, CSF, edema)	−	+
Air	− −	− −
Muscle	Int	Int
Cortical bone, calcification	− −	− −
Fibrous tissue	−	−
Proteinaceous fluid	+	+ +
Melanin	+ +	+
Gadolinium	+ +	+
Iron	− −	− −

Abbreviations: + = bright; + + = very bright; Int = intermediate signal intensity; − = dark; − − = very dark; − − − = extremely dark.

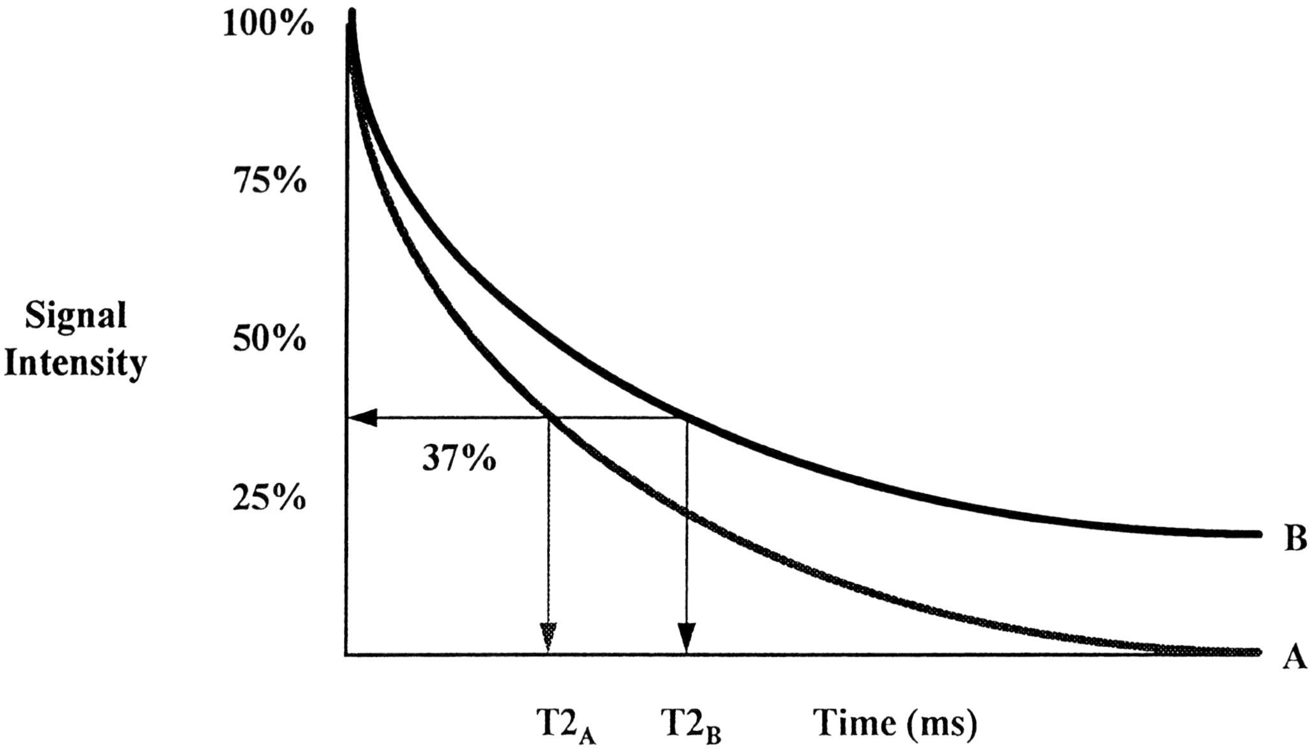

Figure A1-4 Transverse relaxation.

Fast-spin-echo imaging is less sensitive to the presence of blood products than conventional spin-echo or gradient-echo techniques.

Gradient echo (GRE) technique consists of the application of an RF pulse that displaces the longitudinal magnetization vector (M_z) less than 90° (alpha pulse). The amount the longitudinal vector that is displaced into the transverse plane, in degrees, is called the *flip angle*. Subsequently, a magnetic field gradient reversal rather than a 180° RF pulse is used to rephase the magnetization vectors in the transverse plane. The echo produced is called a gradient echo. The principal advantage of gradient-echo over spin-echo technique is shorter TRs and TEs and therefore greater imaging speed. Greater speed minimizes artifacts due to motion, thereby improving image quality. Gradient-echo technique also renders flowing blood consistently bright, permitting the localization and characterization of vascular structures. Additionally, gradient-echo techniques are more sensitive to magnetic susceptibility effects. This results in an increased sensitivity for the detection of blood products as well as subtle areas of calcification compared to other MRI strategies.

Table A1-2
TYPICAL TECHNOLOGIST-ADJUSTED PARAMETERS USED TO OBTAIN IMAGES THAT ARE PREDOMINANTLY T1- OR T2-WEIGHTED

	T1-Weighted	T2-Weighted
TR	<500 ms	>2000 ms
TE	<20 ms	>30 ms
Flip angle	Large	Small

Image contrast can be controlled by tailoring pulse sequences to highlight tissues with short or long T1 or T2 relaxation times. This is done by adjusting external parameters such as TR, TE, and flip angle or by using alternative pulse sequences. For example, the TR of a pulse sequence can be shortened in order to maximize the difference in signal intensities due to tissues' T1 relaxation times. The contrast between the tissues will then reflect primarily their differences in T1. Such a short TR pulse sequence would therefore be considered "T1-weighted." The TE, and in gradient echo sequences the flip angle, are also adjusted to control the image's appearance (Table A1-2).

The application of RF prepulses prior to the start of a standard pulse sequence is also used. **Inversion recovery (IR)** is just such an imaging strategy (Fig. A1-8). Here a 180° inverting prepulse is applied prior to the start of a spin-echo sequence. Longitudinal magnetization is placed in the $-M_z$ plane and then is allowed to regrow. The timing between the initial prepulse and the subsequent 90° pulse initiating the spin-echo portion of the sequence (TI or inversion time) can be adjusted so that imaging begins at the point where the longitudinal vector of fat is zero and therefore has no component in the transverse plane. At this point, no fat signal is generated.

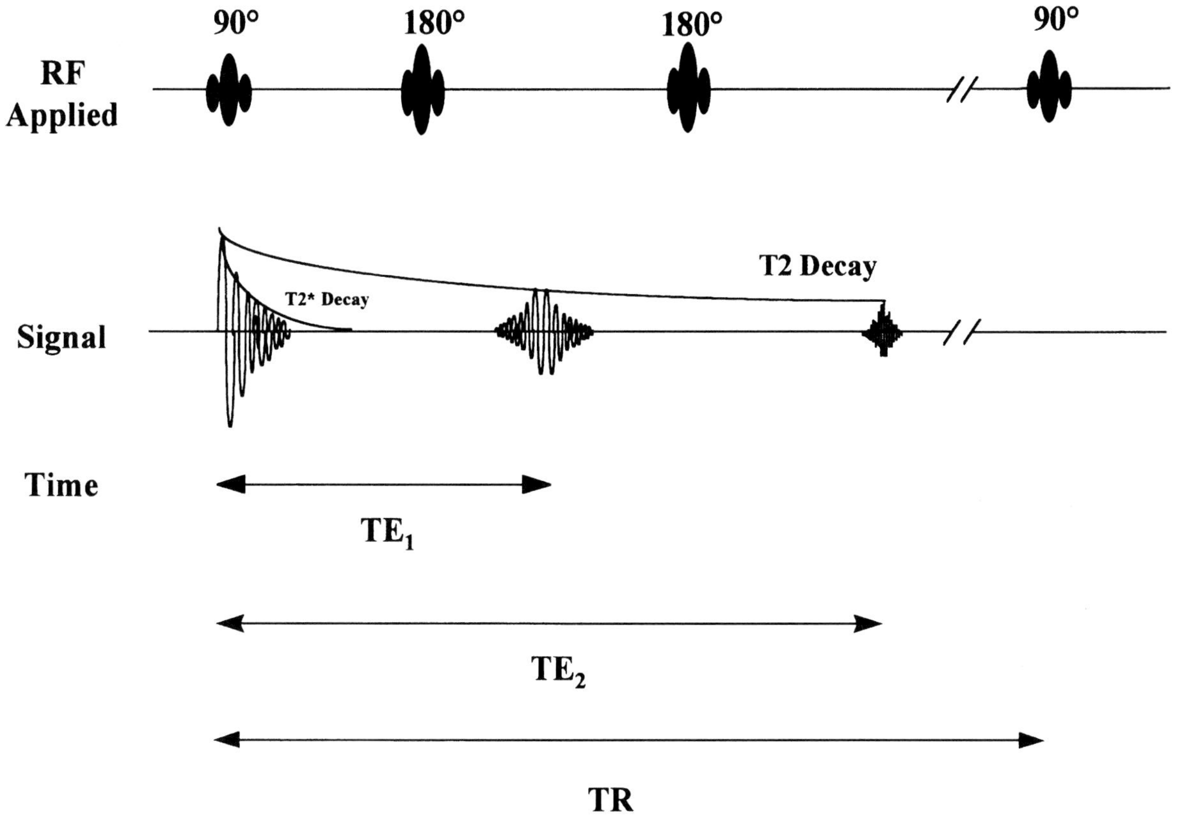

Figure A1-5 Abbreviated pulse-sequence diagram. TE_1 = time to first echo; TE_2 = time to second echo.

This method of fat suppression is used widely to enhance the conspicuity of edema or neoplasms.

Magnetization transfer contrast (MTC) represents another form of background suppression used primarily in conjunction with cerebral MR angiography (MRA). The application of RF prepulses prior to the start of imaging results in the destruction of longitudinal magnetization in protons in close proximity to large macromolecules (bound water). This population is in equilibrium with free-water protons (unbound water), which are largely unaffected. An exchange between these two populations of protons results in a decrease in the signal-generating capability of the background. This makes vessels seen during MRA (MRA/MRV) as well as lesions enhancing after intravenous gadolinium administration considerably more conspicuous.

Imaging time is dependent on many factors (Fig. A1-7). Whether or not images are acquired as two- or three-dimensional (volume) data sets also greatly affects acquisition time. Three-dimensional data sets typically require more time to acquire and are much more sensitive to patient motion. Three-dimensional (volume) acquisitions permit the imaging of smaller structures in great detail (increased spatial resolution) and, through postprocessing, the retrospective division of the image into slices of various orientations. Three-dimensional acquisitions suffer from greater imaging times and marked degradation by motion.

$$S/N = k \frac{FOV_{Freq} \times FOV_{Phase} \times SL \times \sqrt{NSA}}{\sqrt{(N_{Freq} \times N_{Phase} \times BW)}}$$

Figure A1-6 Determinants of signal-to-noise ratio. S/N = signal to noise ratio. FOV = field of view, SL = slice thickness, NSA = number of signal averages, N_{Freq} = number of frequency encodings, N_{Phase} = number of phase encodings, BW = bandwidth.

$$T_S = TR \times N_S \times N_P \times NSA$$
(A)

$$T_S = TR \times N_P \times NSA$$
(B)

$$T_S = (TR \times N_P \times NSA)/ETL$$
(C)

$$T_S = TR \times N_S \times N_P \times NSA$$
(D)

Figure A1-7 Determinants of imaging time under various image-acquisition strategies. (A) 2D Conventional spin echo single slice technique (B) 2D Conventional spin echo multi-slice technique (C) 2D Fast spin echo multi-slice technique (D) 3D Volumetric acquisition T_S = overall imaging time; TR = time to repetition; N_S = number of slices; N_P = number of phase-encoding steps; NSA = number of signal averages; ETL = echo-train length (= turbo factor).

Table A1-3 lists the MRI strategies used at our institution to image various portions of the neuraxis.

☐ MAGNETIC RESONANCE ANGIOGRAPHY

In MRA, techniques are broadly separated into two basic categories, those that depend on bulk flow of spins into and out of the area being imaged (time-of-flight MRA) and those that capitalize on the difference in phase between moving and stationary spins (phase-contrast MRA).

Time-of-flight (TOF) methods are particularly useful in evaluating vessels demonstrating fast flow. In these vessels, there exists a continuous inflow of *unsaturated*, fully relaxed spins from outside the imaging plane that will yield high signal in response to RF stimulation. The signal intensity within these vessels will then be particularly prominent in contrast to the diminished signal returned from the partially saturated tissues in the imaging

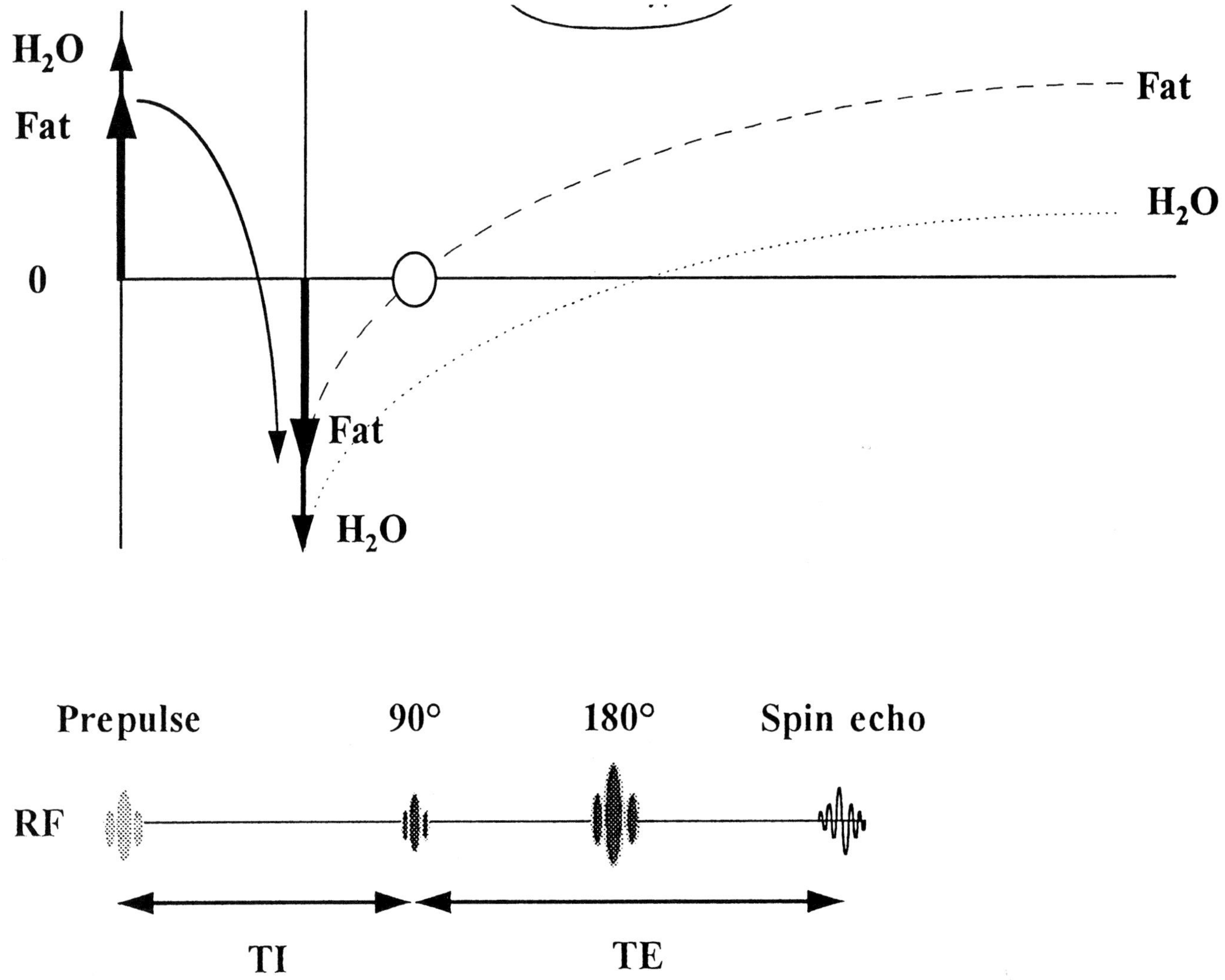

Figure A1-8 Short tau inversion recovery (STIR). TE = time to echo. TR = time to repetition. TI = inversion time.

Table A1-3
MAGNETIC RESONANCE IMAGING PROTOCOLS (GE SIGNA 1.5T/5X)

EXAM	PROJECTION	TECHNIQUE	TE	TR	FLIP	NSA	MATRIX	SLICE THICK	GAP	FOV	ETL	COIL	OPTIONS	SAT
BRAIN														
Routine	SAG T1	2D SE	18	400		2	256 × 192	5	1.5	24		Head	POMP	I
	AX FSE	2D FSE	16	2200		1	256 × 192	5	2	21	8	Head	FC, EDR	I
	AX FSE	2D FSE	85	4000		2	256 × 192	5	2	21	8	Head	FC, EDR	I, F
	AX T1	2D SE	16	600		2	256 × 192	5	2	21		Head	CS, EDR	
Post gado	SAG T1	2D SE	18	400		2	256 × 192	5	1.5	24		Head	POMP	I
	AX T1	2D SE	16	600		2	256 × 192	5	2	21		Head	CS, EDR	
R/O MS	SAG T2	2D FSE	85	5000		3	256 × 192	4	1	21	8	Head	FC, EDR	I, F
Epilepsy	COR T2	2D FSE	85	400		2	256 × 192	3	1	21	8	Head	FC, EDR	I, F
	COR or OBL	3D SPGR	min	33	30	1	256 × 192	2		22		Head		
BRAIN MRA														
Circle of Willis	AX	3D SPGR	5.3	50	30	1	512 × 256	1		22 × 16		Head	FC, VBW, MagT	3D TOF
	AX	30 VASC PC		25	20	1	256 × 128	1		18 × 20		Head/Neck	FC	VENC 30
R/O sinus occl.	SAG	2D PC		22	20	8	256 × 192	40		24			FC, SEQ	VENC 20
2D carotids	AX	2D TOF SPGR	0.4	47	60	1.5	256 × 192	2		19 × 21		Neck	FC, SEQ	2D TOF
3D carotids	COR	3D VASC PC	8	25	20	1	256 × 128	1		24		Neck	FC	VENC 30
Sella														
Routine	SAG T1	2D SE	18	400		2	256 × 192	5	1.5	24			POMP, EDR	I
	COR T1	2D SE	17	400		3	256 × 192	3	I	20 × 15			VBW, SqP	S, I
Optional	COR FSE	2D SE	85	3000		3	256 × 192	3	I	20 × 15	8		EDR, SqP	S, I
Post Gado	COR T1	2D SE	17	400		3	256 × 192	3	I	20 × 15			VBW, SqP	S, I
	SAG T1	2D SE	15	400		3	256 × 192	3	I	20			NPW, EDR	S, I
IACs														
Routine	SAG T1	2D SE	18	400		2	256 × 192	5	1.5	24		Head	POMP	I
	AX T1	2D SE	17	400		3	256 × 192	3	I	20 × 15		Head	VBW, SqP	S, I
Post gado	AX T1	2D SE	17	400		3	256 × 192	3	I	20 × 15		Head	VBW, SqP	S, I
	COR T1	2D SE	17	400		3	256 × 192	3	I	20 × 15		Head	VBW, SqP	S, I
Orbits														
Routine	SAG T1	2D SE	18	400		2	256 × 192	5	1.5	24		Head	POMP, EDR	I
	AX T1	2D SE	17	400		3	256 × 192	3	I	18		Head	NPW, EDR, CS, SPF	S, I
	AX FSE	2D SE	76	3600		3	256 × 192	3	I	18		Head	NPW, EDR, SPF	S, I
Post gado	AX T1	2D SE	17	500		3	256 × 192	3	I	18		Head	NPW, EDR, CS, SPF	S, I, F
	COR TI	2D SE	16	6--		3	256 × 192	4	I	20		Head	NPW, EDR, CS	S, I, F
SPINE														
Cervical spine														
Routine	SAG T1	2D SE	15	600		3	256 × 192	3	0.5	28 × 21		PA spine	CS, ED	S, I, A
	SAG FSE	2D FSE	85	3500		3	256 × 192	3	0.5	28 × 28	8	PA spine	EPRNP, SPF	S, I, A
	AX GRE	2D GRE	14	800	25	4	256 × 192	3	1.0	20		PA spine	NPW, SPF, FC/S	S, I

Table A1-3 *(continued)*
MAGNETIC RESONANCE IMAGING PROTOCOLS (GE SIGNA 1.5T/5X)

EXAM	PROJECTION	TECHNIQUE	TE	TR	FLIP	NSA	MATRIX	SLICE THICK	GAP	FOV	ETL	COIL	OPTIONS	SAT
	AX FSE	2D FSE	76	4000		3	256 × 192	4	1	20	8	PA spine	FC/S, NP, ED, SPF	S, I, A
Post gado	SAG T1	Same as precontrast												
	AX T1	Same as precontrast												
Optional	AX T1	2D FSE	17	500	700	2	256 × 192	4	1	20		PA spine	NPW, ED, CS, SPF	S, I, F
Thoracic spine														
Routine	SAG T1	2D SE	15	650		3	512 × 256	3	0.5	48 × 36		PA spine	ED, CS	S, I, A
	SAG FSE	2D FSE	80	4000		3	512 × 256	3	0.5	48 × 48	8	PA spine	NPW, SPF	S, I, A
	AX T1	2D SE	18	800		3	256 × 192	6	1.5	20		PA spine	NPW, CS, ED, SPF	S, I
Optional	AX FSE	2D FSE	76	4000		3	256 × 192	6	1.5	20		PA spine	NPW, SPF, ED, FC/S	S, I, A
Lumbar Spine														
Routine	SAG T1	2D SE	15	650		3	512 × 256	3	0.5	40 × 20		PA spine	CS	S, I, A
	SAG FSE	2D FSE	102	4000		3	512 × 256	3	0.5	40 × 40	8	PA spine	NPW, SPF	S, I, A
	AX T1	2D SE	18	700		3	256 × 192	5	1	18		PA spine	NPW, CS, SPF	S, I
	AX FSE	2D FSE	76	4000		3	256 × 192	5	1	18	8	PA spine	FC/S, NPW, ED, SPF	S, I, A
Trauma	SAG TSE	2D FSE	96	4000		3	512 × 256	3	0.5	40		PA spine	NPW, SPF	S, I, A, F
Post gado	SAG T1	Same as precontrast												
	AX T1	Same as precontrast												
Myelogram	COR FSE	2D FSE	256	6000		2	512 × 256	3	0	40	16	PA spine	NPW	F

Abbreviations: A = anterior saturation band; CS = contiguous slices; ETL = echo train length; F = fat saturation; FC = flow compensation; FC/S = flow compensation/slice direction; FOV = field of view; FSE = fast spin echo; I = inferior saturation band; MagT = magnetization transfer contrast; NPW = no phase wrap; NSA = number of signal averages; PA spine = phased-array spine coil; POMP = phase offset multiplanar; S = superior saturation band; SAT = saturation band; SE = (conventional) spin echo; SPF = swap phase and frequency; SqP = square pixels; VBW = variable bandwidth.

slice or volume. A major disadvantage of TOF MRA is its sensitivity to any area of pronounced T1 shortening.

Methemoglobin in an area of subacute hemorrhage could result in an area of marked T1 shortening and obscure underlying vascular structures. The signal returned from methemoglobin present in a thrombosed vessel or dural venous sinus could also mimic the signal returned from flowing blood in a normal patent vessel, leading to misdiagnosis.

Phase-contrast (PC) methods take advantage of the difference in phase that the spins acquire as they move along a magnetic field gradient. The gradient has no net effect on stationary spins; however, moving spins alter their phase in relation to their direction and velocity of travel. This information can then be manipulated to give both quantitative and directional information. Artifacts related to T1 shortening are not a problem in this technique. Phase-contrast imaging is particularly useful in evaluating the dural venous sinus and other venous structures. A disadvantage of phase-contrast MRA lies in the fact that the sensitivity of the phase-encoding gradients must be set prospectively. An estimate of the velocity of the vessel under study must be made and an encoding velocity (V_{ENC}) set prior to the start of imaging. If the velocity selected is very far off, inadequate visualization of the vessel of interest or artifacts can result. Phase-contrast techniques result in excellent background suppression but suffer from increased imaging time and therefore enhanced sensitivity to motion.

Time-of-flight and phase contrast angiograms can be acquired as **2D or 3D** data sets. Each acquisition mode has its advantages and disadvantages. Typically, 3D acquisitions permit thinner slices to be acquired, whereas 2D acquisitions can be gotten in less time and are less motion-sensitive. Three-dimensional aquisitions tend to have higher signal-to-noise ratios than 2D acquisitions. **Multiple overlapping thin-slab acquisition** (MOTSA) is a strategy that represents an intermediate ground between 2D and 3D acquisitions. Its primary disadvantage is the need to overlap imaging slabs by 20 to 50 percent in order to obtain acceptable images.

GLOSSARY

(Modified from American College of Radiology: *Glossary of MR Terms*, 3d ed.)

1. *Faraday's law of induction* A time-varying magnetic field interacting with a receiver coil will induce a current in that conductor.
2. *FID* (free induction decay) Transient MRI signal that decays with a characteristic time constant after transverse magnetization has resulted from the application of a 90° RF pulse.
3. *Flip angle* The amount of rotation of the macroscopic magnetization vector produced by an RF pulse with respect to the direction of the main magnetic field.
4. *Frequency encoding* Encoding the distribution of sources of MRI signals along a direction by detecting the signal in the presence of a magnetic field gradient along that direction so that there is a corresponding gradient of resonant frequencies along that direction.
5. *Larmor frequency* The frequency at which magnetic resonance can be excited. The frequency of precession is proportional to the magnetic field strength and a constant for a given nucleus called the gyromagnetic ratio.
6. *Magnetic resonance* Resonance phenomenon resulting in the absorption and/or emission of electromagnetic energy by nuclei or electrons in a static magnetic field.
7. *Magnetic susceptibility* Measure of the ability of a substance to become magnetized.
8. *Phase encoding* Encoding the distribution of sources of MRI signals along a direction in space with different phases by applying a pulsed magnetic field gradient along that direction prior to detection of the signal. In general, it is necessary to acquire a set of signals with a suitable set of different phase-encoding gradient pulses in order to reconstruct the distribution of the sources along the encoded direction.
9. *Pulse sequence* A set of RF (and/or gradient) magnetic field pulses and the time spacing between these pulses; used in conjunction with magnetic field gradients and MRI signal reception to produce MR images.
10. *Resonance* A large-amplitude vibration in a mechanical or electrical system caused by a relatively small periodic stimulus with a frequency at or close to the natural frequency of the system.
11. *Saturation* A nonequilibrium state in MRI in which equal numbers of spins are aligned against and with the magnetic field so that there is no net magnetization.
12. *Spin echo* Reappearance of an MRI signal after the FID has apparently died away, as a result of the effective reversal of the dephasing of the spins (refocusing) by techniques such as specific RF pulse sequences.
13. *T1 relaxation* (spin-lattice or longitudinal relaxation time) The time, in milliseconds, required to recover 63 percent of the signal. Regrowth of longitudinal magnetization.
14. *T2 relaxation* (spin-spin or transverse relaxation time) The time, in milliseconds, necessary to lose 63 percent of the signal. Loss of phase coherence.
15. *T2** (T-two-star) The observed time constant of the FID due to loss of phase coherence among spins oriented at an angle to the static magnetic field, commonly due to a combination of magnetic field inhomogeneities, changes in the magnetic field, and spin-spin transverse relaxation.
16. *TE* (echo time) The time between the middle of the excitation pulse and the middle of the echo production.
17. *TR* (repetition time) The time between the beginning of the pulse sequence and the beginning of the succeeding identical pulse sequence.

SUGGESTED READINGS

MRI Physics

1. Newhouse JH, Weiner, JI: *Understanding MRI.* Boston, Little, Brown and Company, 1991.
2. Horowitz AL: *MRI Physics for Radiologists: A Visual Approach.* New York, Springer-Verlag, 1992.
3. Lufkin RB: *The MRI Manual:* Part I. *Basic Principles.* St Louis, Mosby-Year Book, 1990. (Excellent introductions to the physics of magnetic resonance imaging.)

Magnetic Resonance Angiography

1. Anderson CM et al: *Clinical Magnetic Resonance Angiography.* New York, Raven Press, 1993. (Best MRA text.)
2. Listerud J: First principles of magnetic resonance angiography. *Magn Reson Q* 7(2): 136–170, 1991.
3. Magnetic resonance angiography. *Neuro Imaging Clin North Am* 2(4): 623–835, 1992.

APPENDIX 2

Myelography

Scott Agran

Despite the advent of magnetic resonance imaging (MRI), myelography is here to stay. It may not be as frequently used as in the past, but proficiency will still be required to perform useful diagnostic examinations. At least 10 to 20 percent of patients are unable to tolerate MRI. Many patients move, limiting the diagnostic usefulness of the MRI exam; and many scans are nondiagnostic due to other factors such as patient body habitus, severe scoliosis, poor imaging capabilities of the scanner (such as low-field MRI machines), and just plain old diagnostic dilemmas such as findings that do not correlate with the patient's history.

☐ PREPARATION

Prior to beginning a myelogram, personal communication with the referring clinician is imperative to determine the levels of interest (cervical, thoracic, lumbar), symptoms, necessity for CSF collection, and length of stay necessary (see Table A2-1). Certainly, allergic history and any history of prior spinal surgery or myelography (especially using Pantopaque) or other relevant history (such as coagulopathy and medications) is important. Not only should a direct clinical history be derived from the referring clinician but equally important is the patient's own history. Not infrequently, discrepancies between these two sources arise, and it is incumbent upon the neuroradiologist to sort out the truth prior to beginning the myelogram. Prior radiographs, myelograms, CT scans (with or without intrathecal contrast administration), and MRIs should be obtained and reviewed prior to beginning the myelogram.

Table A2-1
RECOMMENDED DOSAGE OF CONTRAST MATERIAL FOR MYELOGRAPHY[a]

	Via Lumbar Puncture	Via C1–C2 puncture
Cervical	10 mL 300 mg I%	10 mL 200 mg I%
Thoracic	15 mL 200 mg I%	15 mL 200 mg I%
Lumbar	10 mL 200 mg I%	10 mL 300 mg I%

[a]For CT/myelography only, the recommended dose may be reduced to half.

Prior to beginning the examination, the procedure should be explained to the patient and a consent form signed. During the explanation, a detailed, step-by-step description of what the patient can expect is necessary to relieve the patient's anxiety. The patient should not receive any unexpected surprises in the middle of the exam, when a dangerous situation could result. Patients often have an unrealistic fear of myelography, and it is easy to assuage these fears with a thorough explanation of the procedure. As the needle enters the spinal canal, most of the nerve roots move away, but occasionally (approximately 5 percent of the time) one is tapped. When that occurs, the patient may feel an electric shock down the leg. I assure patients that if this should happen, I will reposition the needle. Special situations arise with patients who have had prior spinal surgery or Pantopaque myelography. In these situations, there is a high incidence of arachnoiditis. Hence the risk of tapping the nerve root with the needle is much higher (approximately 20 percent).

I also explain to the patient the possibility of complications. Although this is a low-risk procedure, complications can occur. Infection, bleeding, nerve injury, and spinal headache are mentioned. Special note is made in discussion of postmyelogram headache. The patient is told that today, we use smaller needles, and that the incidence of these headaches is lower than it had once been. The risk of headache is directly proportional to the size of the hole made in the dura and hence to the size of the spinal needle. Therefore the smallest needle possible should be used, making sure that the patient remains in bed for at least 4 h postprocedure.

Today, it is possible to do outpatient myelography. The advent of small (25- to 27-gauge) spinal needles has made this a safe procedure. Safeguards are necessary, however. Although I feel that patients can drive themselves home or go home alone, it would certainly be preferable for them to be driven home and supervised for several hours. Inpatient myelograms should be performed with a 22-gauge spinal needle. The smaller-gauge spinal needles are a bit trickier to use at first but soon feel quite natural. Their smaller size allows greater mobility, but they are also more likely to stray from the originally directed line. This can be used to advantage.

☐ PROCEDURE

POSITIONING

Positioning can be performed in the traditional midline approach. However, most neuroradiologists use an oblique paraspinous approach. In this approach, the patient is obliqued to approximately 15 to 20° (although this will vary), such that the side closest to the myelographer is elevated. Under fluoroscopic guidance, the intervertebral foramen (the lucency at the junction of the lamina, the spinous process, and articular facet) is visualized. It is placed into optimal position such that the intervertebral foramen appears as a lucent "keyhole" through which the spinal needle is to be advanced. Once this keyhole appearance is achieved, your metal marker, preferably one with a hole at the end, is placed over the intervertebral foramen and the position marked with indelible ink.

Next, prepare the myelogram tray for the procedure. Before you start the myelogram, be sure that you have everything you will ultimately need. Obtain the spinal needle, contrast, lidocaine, and Betadine. Draw up the contrast into your syringe, attach the extension tubing, remove all air bubbles, and advance the contrast to the end of the extension tubing. Also, draw up the lidocaine into a 3-mL specially marked syringe (tape or a Band-Aid can be affixed for distinction).

THE STERILE FIELD

Next, clean the patient's back with Betadine, in a sterile fashion. This usually entails a circular cleansing technique from the center of the field to the periphery with three different Betadine-soaked sponges. The size of the field should be larger than the size of the hole in the drape. If the drape has no adhesives, then the area should be quite a bit larger, since the drape will usually move slightly during the procedure. After the Betadine has been applied, place the drape over this area and, with a clean 2 × 2, wipe the central area gently to remove the excess Betadine.

NEEDLEWORK

Place a 20-gauge or larger needle at the expected site of entry (usually L2–3 or L3–4) and perform brief fluoroscopy to be certain that landmarks are stable and in the expected location. Since lumbar disk herniations are more common at L4–5 and L5–S1 levels, it is important to remember that lumbar puncture at these sites should be avoided when possible. Administer lidocaine subcutaneously through a 25- or 27-gauge needle and raise a wheal measuring 1 cm. You may add a small amount along the expected needle track as well. Remove the lidocaine syringe to a place well away from all your other equipment so as to never confuse it with any other pieces of equipment. Intrathecal administration of lidocaine can be fatal. If you are certain that you will not be needing it, remove it from the tray setup. At the site of subcutaneous lidocaine administration, place a 20-gauge needle with its tip at your expected entry point and perform brief fluoroscopy to ensure correct positioning. If correct, replace this with your spinal needle (25/27-gauge for outpatient and 22-gauge for inpatient), and advance it along the expected track, with frequent brief fluoroscopic monitoring to ensure proper location. You should have an idea of the depth necessary from having reviewed the scout images previously. With a 22-gauge needle, you will frequently feel a "pop" as you penetrate the thecal sac. This pop marks is a subtle decrease in resistance as you pass through the thecal sac. This is frequently absent with a 25/27-gauge needle; therefore, you will need to have a greater degree of suspicion as to the expected depth of the thecal sac. When you are in the expected location (thecal sac), the technologist should gently elevate the head of the tilt table approximately 30°. This is especially important with the 25/27-gauge needles and in patients with suspected spinal stenosis. It will help to raise the pressure at the needle tip, so that when the stylet is removed, cerebrospinal fluid (CSF) will drain into the needle hub. Prior to removing the stylet, rotate the needle 360° to help eliminate any tenting of the dura at the needle tip and to help keep the tip completely within the thecal sac. After removing the stylet, look down the needle hub to observe CSF flow (good lighting is imperative). If present, note its color, turbidity, and viscosity. If not present, you may tilt the table an additional 15°. If no CSF flows, replace the stylet. If you believe that you have not advanced beyond the anterior margin of the thecal sac or have not reached the thecal sac, advance your needle in 5-mm increments and recheck for CSF flow.

Alternatively, flatten the patient (from the oblique position and from the head-up tilted position) and obtain a cross-table lateral radiograph centered upon the spinal needle (be sure to cone the beam and avoid unnecessary radiation exposure). All you will need to obtain from the radiograph is the location of your needle tip with respect to the thecal sac (whether you are posterior to it, anterior to it, or within the expected location). If posterior, advance under fluoroscopic guidance the expected distance, remove the stylet, and check for CSF flow. If anterior, retract the expected distance and check for CSF flow. If you are within the expected location, try to determine whether you are near one of the edges of the thecal sac and try to position the tip more toward the center. Use any prior imaging studies to guide you.

COLLECTION OF CEREBROSPINAL FLUID

If you have now gained access and CSF is required for laboratory evaluation, carefully attach a short (10-cm) piece of extension tubing to the needle hub. It will behoove you to attach this tubing while you rest your hand, holding the spinal needle on the patient's back for stability. This will prevent you from advancing or retracting the needle during attachment of the extension tube. After this is accomplished, tilt the table (head up) approximately 30 to 45°. Some fine tuning of the angle will be necessary. If CSF collection is requested, do *not* use the 25/27-gauge needle, as this will make it take all day to collect several milliliters.

ADMINISTRATION OF CONTRAST

After collecting the CSF, carefully remove the extension tubing (again, rest your needle hand upon the patient's back to keep the needle stable) and replace it with the long extension tubing connected to the contrast syringe (the connection must be firmly tightened but without changing the needle position). Be certain to eliminate most of the air from the system. Hold the syringe well away from the patient (this is why the extension tubing is long), review how much contrast is in the syringe/extension tubing system, and, under brief intermittent fluoroscopy, administer the contrast into the thecal sac. It will be much harder to administer the contrast through a 25/27-gauge needle than the 22-gauge needle. Just take your time. Too much pressure will dislodge the connection to the needle tip making the contrast squirt in all directions. Try to avoid this, with an even pressure. The rate of contrast administration is not important. After the requisite amount of contrast has been administered (lesser amounts are needed with narrow canals and with high degrees of spinal stenosis), remove the needle and contrast system in a smooth continuous motion and press a 2 × 2 to the puncture site for 10 s. Place a Band-Aid at this site and place the drapes and 2 × 2 into the trash.

LUMBAR IMAGING

If you are performing a lumbar myelogram, place the patient flat (no obliquity) and expose a radiograph in the posteroanterior PA projection if the contrast fills the thecal sac to its most caudal aspect, usually S1 or S2. Cone the field of view significantly, but be certain that a left or right position marker is within this field of view and on the correct side. If the inferior aspect of the thecal sac is not filled with contrast, tilt the table (elevate the head) until it fills. This may require almost vertical positioning. With severe spinal stenosis, the patient may need to flex and extend the lumbar spine while standing; do what it takes. Remove this film and, on two-on-one imaging with a 10 × 10 cassette, expose the patient in shallow obliquity (again, be certain that the marker is visible and cone the exposure). On the same film, expose an oblique view in steep obliquity for good visualization of the exiting nerve roots. Replace this film and repeat shallow and steep oblique radiographs of the opposite obliquity. Next, flatten the patient and obtain a cross-table lateral radiograph centered at approximately L3. Place the patient in lateral position and obtain flexion and extension overhead lateral images again centered at L3. Place the patient supine, and advance the contrast to the conus and expose frontal and cross-table lateral radiographs centered on the conus (usually T12–L1). Again, cone these images somewhat to decrease unnecessary radiation exposure.

THORACIC AND CERVICAL IMAGING

If you are performing a thoracic myelogram, the patient is turned to a supine position and contrast material is manuvered to the thoracic region by tilting the table with patient's head down 15 to 20° while the patient's chin is tugged toward his or her chest. The x-ray table is then moved to a horizontal position, and overhead frontal anteroposterior; cross-table lateral radiographs and a swimmer's view of the cervicothoracic junction is adequate. For performance of a cervical myelogram, after observing the lumbosacral junction and exposing any radiographs that would appear useful, the contrast will have to be advanced to the cervical subarachnoid space. This is accomplished by first connecting small boots to the patient's feet. These boots should be capable of firm connection with a platform at the caudal aspect of the tilt table and should be tied into place in such a way that the patient *cannot conceivably fall* after table tilting. After and only after the contrast has been administered into the thecal sac and the needle removed should the boots be connected to the table. Their firm attachment to the table should be confirmed (confirmation of firm attachment of this platform to the tilt table should be made as well). The patient is placed into a prone position with the chin placed in a head holder or towels placed under the chin such that the patient's neck is as extended as possible. Hand grips will aid stability as well. The technologist should move to a position cranial to the patient's head (just in case support is necessary), and the patient should be tilted head-down. The patient should be tilted slowly, but there is virtually no maximum angle of tilt. Usually, 60° is sufficient; however, in patients with marked accentuation of the thoracic kyphosis, passage of contrast may require a greater angle of tilt. Occasionally, it becomes necessary to choose an alternative means of contrast advancement. If this should occur, place the patient in the lateral position (feet still in boots attached to the table) with towels placed under the ear and the head tilted such that the opposite ear is as close to its ipsilateral shoulder as possible in order to form a depression between the shoulders and head into which contrast will pool. The table is subsequently tilted head down, with fluoroscopic observation of contrast progression from the lumbar to the thoracic and subsequently into the cervical subarachnoid space. When contrast has reached the cervical level, the tilt table can be flattened into a nearly horizontal position. Attempt to maintain the contrast in the cervical region (not into the head and not back down to the lumbar level) while turning the patient into a prone position. When the patient is in the prone position, posteroanterior, lateral views can be obtained. When exposing lateral views, the patient is told to move his or her shoulder as low as possible. A swimmer's view is then obtained. The two oblique views should be obtained last because some contrast dilation can occur while the patient is being moved for oblique positions.

POSTMYELOGRAM COMPUTED TOMOGRAPHY

The required postmyelogram CT images should be individualized to the individual patient and only chosen after review of the myelogram radiographs. As a general rule, cervical spine imaging should be at intervals of 1.5 × 1.5 mm, the thoracic spine at intervals of 10 × 10 mm (with narrower intervals of 3 × 3 or 5 × 5 mm through areas of particular interest) and intervals of 3 × 3 mm at the lumbosacral level. The extent of CT imaging will depend upon clinical and plain-film findings. An L4–5 radiculopathy with solitary thecal sac encroachment at L4–5 on myelogram may require CT imaging solely from the mid-L4 to the mid-L5 levels. Large lesions, such as a large syrinx, may not require such thin slices. Direct communication with the CT technologist is imperative. Drawing the scanning range directly onto the lateral radiograph with slice thickness or making a drawing on paper is recommended. Computed tomography images should be rendered with both bone [W (window width) 4000L (window level) 400] and soft tissue (W40040) images printed. All the disk levels should be numbered with a china marker/wax pencil on both sets of images. Similarly, numbering of the vertebral bodies on the plain-film radiographs should be performed to avoid confusing the radiologist and clinician. Communication will be facilitated.

POSTMYELOGRAM

Before the patient has left for CT, orders should be written in the chart. These should include:

1. Bed rest for 4 h.
2. Diet—as tolerated. Encourage oral fluid.
3. Acetaminophen or ibuprofen for pain or headache.
4. Other medications the patient uses.
5. No phenothiazines for 24 h.
6. Pager number or other number at which you can be reached in an emergency.
7. Vital signs on arrival and every hour for 2 h.

The patient may be monitored in any appropriate environment. A recovery room is probably overkill and unnecessary. Prior to discharge, the patient should demonstrate appropriate ambulatory skills. Any patient who experiences severe discomfort, pain, numbness and tingling, or worsening of symptoms should be reevaluated, with consideration of orthopedic or neurosurgical consultation. Appropriate pain medication as well as overnight stay should be considered

☐ COMPLICATIONS

HEADACHE

Headache is the most frequent complication/complaint related to myelography. There are numerous theories concerning the cause; however, suffice it to say that the larger the hole, the higher the percentage of patients with postmyelogram headaches. As radiologists, we do not realize the frequency of these headaches, but talk with your orthopedic surgeon, neurologist, or neurosurgeon for enlightenment. The use of 22-gauge needles results in approximately 40 percent postmyelogram headaches, while 25/27-gauge needles cause headaches in approximately 5 percent of cases.

Postmyelogram headaches are less likely if the patient maintains bed rest following the myelogram—overnight for a 22-gauge and 4 h for a 25/27-gauge needle.

One procedure for the relief of a post LP (lumbar puncture)/postmyelogram headache is the blood patch. This should *not* be used prophylactically but only on patients with intractable headaches. It should rarely be necessary when 25/27-gauge needles are being used, and this is one reason that I recommend the use of these needles for myelography.

A blood patch is performed by placing an intravenous line into a peripheral vein (usually the antecubital fossa), and then performing an LP at approximately the level of the prior LP/myelogram. After CSF is demonstrated,

5 mL of autologous blood is withdrawn from the intravenous line into a syringe. The spinal needle is retracted until CSF flow ceases. At this point, the stylet is removed and the autologous blood is administered through the spinal needle into the extradural space while the spinal needle is slowly removed. The concept involves blood clotting around the prior LP site and closing the CSF leak responsible for the headache. Sterile technique is of vital concern, as blood is a great medium for bacterial growth, and the spinal canal and extradural spaces are terrible sites for infection.

INFECTION

Other common complications include infection (very uncommon, and eliminated with good sterile technique).

PAIN

Severe and unrelenting pain, with or without numbness, tingling, and other sensory or motor findings, is occasionally encountered, especially in patients with severe spinal stenosis. In patients with demonstrated severe spinal stenosis, a smaller dose of contrast should be administered. The pain and other symptoms usually subside after 30 to 60 min but can occasionally persist for hours or days. If some relief is not demonstrated after 30 to 60 min, direct examination and consideration of orthopedic or neurosurgical consultation should be considered. Analgesics should be given sparingly, because an acute block or compression may necessitate intervention and should not be obscured due to analgesia.

SUBDURAL INJECTION

A subdural injection is an infrequent complication that will be encountered by every physician who does enough myelograms. This should not cause major anxiety. At the very worst, the patient will require a repeat myelogram, which is very unlikely to result in patient harm. However, you may be able to salvage information. Sometimes, especially if the contrast is anterior to the thecal sac, extradural defects such as disk bulges and herniations can be well demonstrated on radiographs and especially on CT.

ADVERSE REACTION RELATED TO CONTRAST MATERIAL

The most frequently reported adverse reactions following intrathecal administration of nonionic contrast materials are headache, nausea, vomiting, and musculoskeletal pain. Major motor seizures, facial neuralgia, and tinnitus have rarely been reported. Hypotension, tachycardia, and chest pain have been reported. Allergy, CNS irritation, cardiac arrhythmias, and apnea may also occur. Detailed information is available in the package insrt for each contrast agent.

□ THE CERVICAL PUNCTURE

In the event of a complete block or possibly when one cannot obtain lumbar access due to severe degenerative changes, scoliosis, or infection, it may become necessary to perform a cervical spinal tap. This carries a much higher risk of complication (though still quite low at 0.17 percent) than the lumbar route, owing to the presence of the spinal cord and the vertebral arteries. Hence, special care must be taken. Begin by placing the patient in a lateral position. Find the inferior aspect of the mastoid process, and place a marker (a 20-gauge needle is ideal) 1 cm posteriorly and 1 cm caudally. Observe under fluoroscopy, and adjust it such that the tip lies between the spinous processes of C1 and C2, approximately two-thirds of the way posteriorly along a line between the posterior aspect of the dens and the spinal lamina line. Mark the spot with indelible ink and, using Betadine, sterilize the area and place a sterile drape with a hole in it over the area of interest. Anesthetize the skin with 1% lidocaine and advance a 22-gauge spinal needle under intermittent fluoroscopic guidance into the cervical spinal subarachnoid space. Determine approximately how deep you will need to penetrate and slowly advance your needle. Intermittently, remove the stylet and observe for CSF flow. When CSF is demonstrated, the patient is turned into the prone position and contrast material is injected in that position with the patient's chin tilted upward and the neck hyperextended.

APPENDIX 3

Cerebral Angiography

Michael I. Ginsburg
David P. Chason

Despite more recently developed noninvasive vascular imaging techniques such as magnetic resonance angiography (MRA) and computed tomography angiography (CTA), catheter angiography remains the "gold standard" for the evaluation of cerebrovascular disease. However, because of the risk of stroke, catheter angiography should not be performed in cases where equivalent information may be obtained in a noninvasive manner. The purpose of this guide is to provide the reader with a brief review of the basic issues required to perform catheter angiography safely.

☐ RADIOGRAPHIC FACILITIES

Cerebral angiography may be accomplished in any standard angiographic facility with either cut film or ideally biplane digital capabilities. The spatial resolution presently available on digital subtraction angiography (DSA) allows for excellent examination of the arch branches and intracerebral vessels, obviating the need for cut film studies even for aneurysm and the evaluation of arteriovenous malformation (AVM). The overall procedure time and contrast dose to the patient are decreased by DSA. Furthermore, each injection can be evaluated almost instantaneously and in real time. This allows the exam to be tailored more easily and may permit more subtle diagnosis.

Mechanical pressure injectors should be used routinely, as these ensure precise injection volumes, injection pressures, and pressure rise times.

Medical support systems such as monitoring equipment and anesthetic/resuscitative equipment should be readily available in the angiography suite.

☐ PREPROCEDURAL ASSESSMENT OF THE PATIENT

The preprocedure visit should be used to clarify the indication(s) for the specific examination and to provide information about the patient's current clinical condition and past medical history. Current medications, drug allergies, laboratory values (blood urea nitrogen, creatinine, prothrombin time, partial thromboplastin time, and platelets), and heparin status should be noted. Pertinent CT and MRI studies should be reviewed and are often valuable in the planning and interpretation of the angiogram.

☐ COMMONLY USED MEDICATIONS DURING ANGIOGRAPHY

The reader is referred to the *Physician's Desk Reference* for further and more complete information.

SEDATION

1. Midazolam (Versed) IV is a short-acting benzodiazepine. The starting dose ranges from 0.25 mg to 1 mg depending on the patient's status. A total dose of 4 to 6 mg (0.07 mg/kg) should not be exceeded.
2. Lorazepam (Ativan) 1 to 3 mg IV.
3. Diazepam (Valium) 5 to 10 mg IV.

ANALGESICS

1. Fentanyl (Sublimaze) IV is a synthetic opioid. In young adults, dose increments are between 50 and 100 μg; in elderly or frail patients, 25 μg increments

may be used. Its onset of action is almost immediate with the effect lasting 0.5 to 1 h.
2. Meperidine (Demerol) IV or IM is usually given in a dose of 25 to 50 mg.

ANTINAUSEANTS

1. Prochlorperazine IV (Compazine) in a dose of 2.5 to 5 mg (contraindicated for myelography).
2. Metoclopramide (Reglan) 10 mg PO.

ANTIHYPERTENSIVES

1. Nifedipine (Procardia) 10 mg sublingually is useful in the treatment of hypertension and can also be used for treatment of arterial spasm. The patient's blood pressure should be closely monitored, as this drug may lead to precipitous falls in blood pressure, concomitantly reducing cerebral perfusion pressure.
2. Labetalol (Normadyne) IV may be titrated against blood pressure, making it a useful choice for patients in whom only a mild antihypertensive effect is desired.
3. Hydralazine (Apresoline) may be given in a dose of 5 mg IV as an antihypertensive agent.

ANTICOAGULANTS

1. Heparin is often given to patients undergoing interventional procedures; however, its use in diagnostic angiography is controversial. On occasion, heparin is given at the onset of a diagnostic angiogram in older individuals or in those with aortoiliac grafts to be used for vascular access. Heparin is contraindicated by the presence of active bleeding, hemorrhagic stroke, intracranial tumor, recent surgery, trauma, or a history of heparin hypersensitivity. At our institution, a loading dose of approximately 5000 U is administered intravenously and followed by an infusion at the rate of 400 to 1000 U/h. The half-life of heparin is approximately 45 min.

REVERSAL AGENTS

1. Reversal of benzodiazepines—flumazenil (Romazicon). This is a benzodiazepine antagonist with a half-life of 40 to 80 min. Increments of 0.2 mg are given up to a maximum dosage of approximately 3 mg IV. The drug may be used to reverse the effects of Versed, Valium, or Ativan.
2. Reversal of anticoagulants—protamine. The dosage is 1 mg for every 100 U of heparin remaining (calculate using a half-life of approximately 45 min) and is administered over 15 to 20 min. Overdosage should be avoided, as unopposed protamine also has an anticoagulant effect.
3. Reversal of narcotic analgesics—naloxone (Narcan). This is given intravenously in dosages of 0.4 mg at 2- to 3-min. intervals up to a total of 2 mg.

☐ SELECTION OF NEEDLES, GUIDE WIRES, AND CATHETERS

GENERAL CONSIDERATIONS

1. The number of needles required to fill a space 1 inch wide is equal to the gauge number of that needle. Therefore, the smaller the needle, the larger its gauge number.
2. The French size of a catheter or sheath is defined as the circumference of the outer wall in millimeters for a catheter and the circumference of the inner wall in millimeters for a sheath.
3. The wall of an arterial needle is generally thinner than that of a venous needle of the same gauge. For example, an 18-gauge arterial needle will permit passage of up to a 0.038-in. wire, whereas an 18-gauge venous needle will only permit the passage of a 0.025-in. wire or smaller.

☐ SELECTION OF NEEDLES

Vascular access in the femoral, brachial, or axillary arteries is usually initiated with an 18-gauge Seldinger needle. This permits the passage of a 0.035- to 0.038-in. guide wire. The Seldinger needle has a sharp stylet, a blunt cannula, and a funnel-shaped hub (see Fig. A3-1).

If a 4 French catheter is to be used, a 19-gauge needle may be substituted. In cases of difficult vascular access or for pediatric work, micropuncture sets are available that utilize a 21-gauge needle, a 0.018-in. wire and a 4 or 5 French sheath.

Single-wall needles (Potts needle) are also available, which consist of a Seldinger-style hub and a sharp beveled needle tip with no stylet (see Fig. A3-1). Some angiographers perform single-wall punctures routinely, while others do so in selective cases only. Relative indications for performing a single-wall puncture include (1) an axillary puncture, (2) prosthetic graft puncture, (3) uncontrolled hypertension, (4) coagulopathy, and (5) a high femoral puncture. It is felt by some that the use of a single-wall technique diminishes the chances of arterial hemorrhage, while others insist that the risk of intimal dissection is increased.

☐ SELECTION OF GUIDE WIRES

Guide wires are used for initial vascular access and selective catheterization of branch vessels and may be subdivided according to a number of criteria including

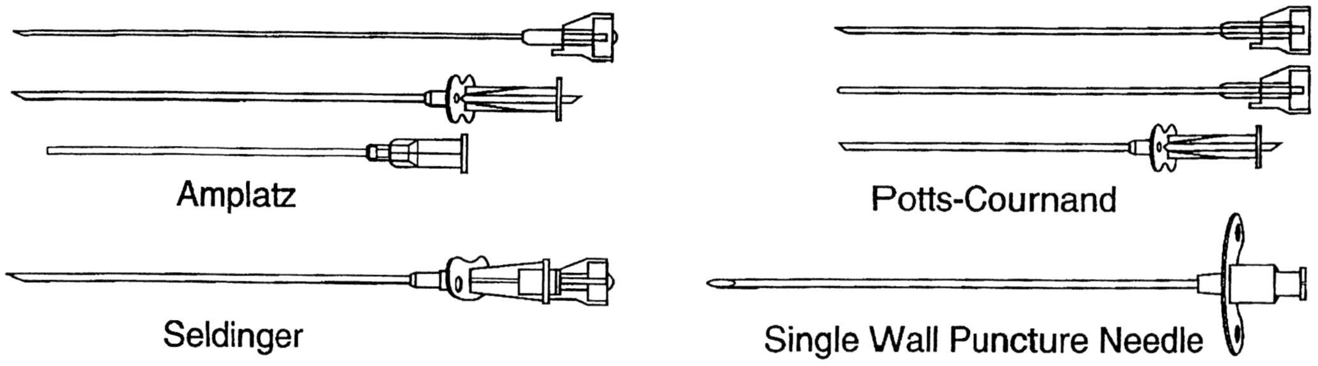

Figure A3-1 Arterial access needles. Note the presence of an occlusive stylet in double-wall needles (Amplatz, Seldinger). Single-wall needles have no central stylet. Pulsatile arterial backflow is therefore evident immediately after penetration of the anterior wall with single-wall needles.

length, stiffness, surface coating/slipperiness, and tip configuration. With the exception of hydrophilic guide wires, the basic construction includes an inner-coil mandril, an outer coil spring, and a safety wire. The hydrophilic wires have a surface coating of hydrophilic material that becomes extremely slippery upon hydration. Standard guide wire length is 145 cm. Exchange wires are 225 to 300 cm long.

INITIAL ACCESS WIRES (SEE FIG. A3-2)

In our institution we have found the Bentson wire (0.035 or 0.038) or less commonly a J wire (3 or 15 mm) to be useful as a safe initial access wire. Hydrophilic wires are used by some; however, they probably should not be used for initial vascular access by the inexperienced for several reasons. Hydrophilic wires are extremely slippery, may be more difficult to manage, and can also result in dissection with little resistance felt by the angiographer.

SELECTIVE CATHETERIZATION OF BRANCH VESSELS

In selecting a wire for selective branch vessel catheterization, the tip configuration and the stiffness of the distal portion of the wire are of particular importance. In general, the stiffer wires provide greater torquability and steerability but pose a greater hazard to the intima than floppier wires (e.g., Bentson). The hydrophilic wires are particularly useful for catheterizing extremely tortuous or small vessels. Furthermore, they are unsurpassed in allowing the catheter to follow over the wire because of their stiffness and decreased resistance between the catheter and wire. The tips of hydrophilic wires may be straight, slightly angled, or adjustable (Naviguide). All these wires should be used with extreme caution as they may dissect into the subintimal space without apparent feel of resistance. The Bentson wire may be difficult to use in patients with tortuous vessels because catheters may not follow its floppy tip unless it is well secured in the vessel.

☐ CATHETER CHOICE

Features to consider in the selection of a catheter include steerability, torquability, visibility, friction, stability, and flow rate. Smaller catheters (5 French or smaller) track more easily over wires but may be limited in flow rate, torquability, and visibility. Larger catheters (6 French or greater) allow greater flow rates, torquability, and visibility but may increase the likelihood of vascular injury.

In selecting the shape of a catheter tip, the anatomy and configuration of the vessels is of great importance (Fig. A3-3). In younger patients, the arch branches tend to arise at a more perpendicular angle from the arch, with less tortuosity. In older patients, the arch branches arise at an increasingly acute angle. Younger patients (less than 40 years of age) may be examined routinely with a JB1, H1, or H1H catheter. Older patients may require an HN4, JB2, Simmons 2, or Newton catheter, as these catheters allow engagement of vessels arising at acute angles. These latter catheters also may be used routinely with younger patients.

☐ NEEDLE PUNCTURE AND SHEATH PLACEMENT

After standard groin preparation, the common femoral artery should be palpated between two fingers as it passes over the femoral head. Fluoroscopic observation of the femoral head may be of value, particularly in the obese patient. Recommended anesthesia is 1 percent lidocaine without epinephrine. The skin incision should be made slightly below the level of the femoral head, ideally at the groin crease just below the inguinal ligament, to allow for the cephalad angulation of the needle. Attention should be paid to the planned angle of puncture (approximately 45°). Retracting the skin with the index finger and thumb, a #11 scalpel blade held flat is used to make a small incision. This helps to ensure that

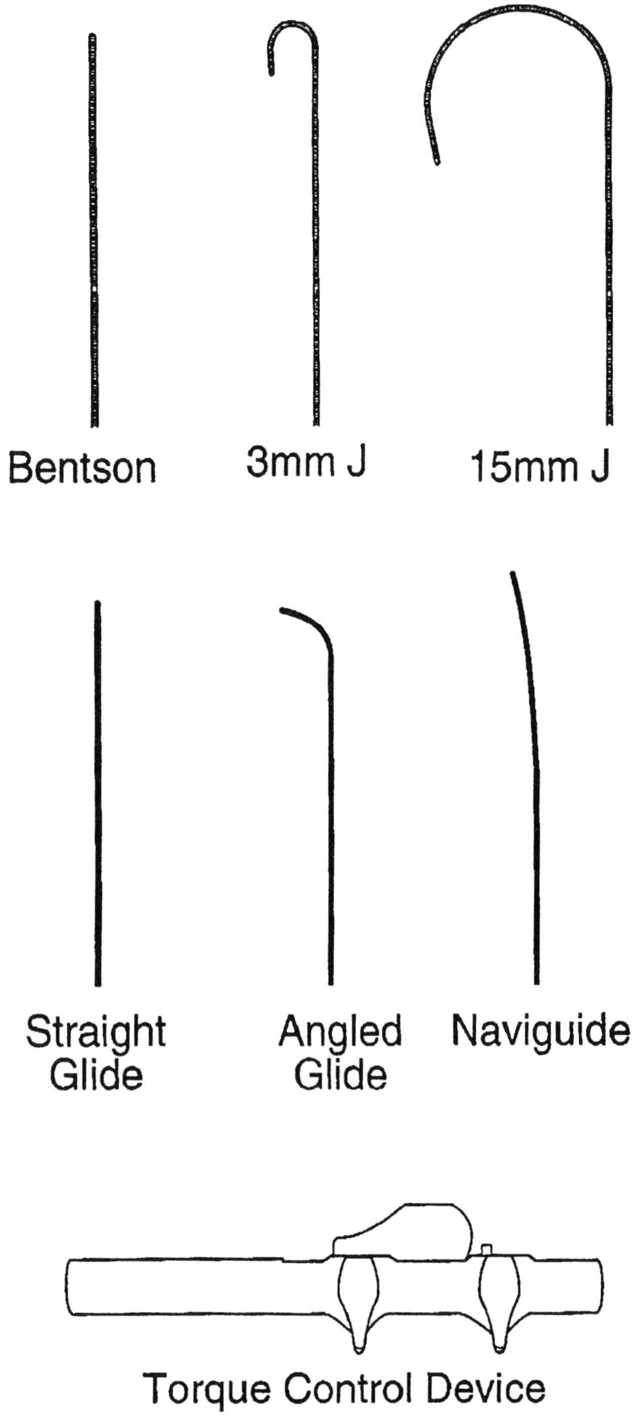

Figure A3-2 Configuration of the distal tips of various neuroangiography guide wires. The straight glide, angled glide, and Naviguide are hydrophilic wires and may be used with the torque-control device to facilitate wire rotation (*bottom*). The tip of the Bentson is floppy and atraumatic, making it a safe wire for general use. The J-tipped wires are useful in minimizing intimal damage.

the scalpel blade does not injure the femoral artery. The dermatotomy may then be widened with a hemostat as needed.

Needle punctures are performed using the standard Seldinger technique. The puncture needle is held with the index and third fingers resting in front of the hub shield, with the thumb on the hub. The needle is slowly advanced through the incision and subcutaneous tissue until a transmitted pulse is felt along the needle to the thumb. The needle is then firmly advanced in a single motion to pierce both the anterior and posterior walls of the common femoral artery. A nodding "yes" motion (up-and-down) of the needle usually indicates adequate central placement, while a side-to-side "no" motion may indicate that the needle is adjacent to the artery or in its side wall. The stylet of the needle is then withdrawn. The hub of the needle is then tilted to lie more parallel to the skin. The needle is then withdrawn and, as the tip enters the arterial lumen, arterial spurting of blood will occur and the guide wire can be introduced. The near parallel position of the needle facilitates passage of the guide wire into the central portion of the artery. Slow venous-type backflow should not be mistaken for the arterial pulsation of blood. If venous return is obtained, the needle should be withdrawn further, as in approximately 8 percent of patients the femoral vein lies directly posterior to the femoral artery. The guide wire is then passed through the needle and advanced into the lower abdominal aorta. The wire should not be advanced if any resistance is felt. If so, fluoroscopy should be utilized to determine the nature of the problem. Often the hub of the needle may only need to be reangled to allow smooth passage of the wire initially. With the wire in place, either a catheter or sheath may be introduced into the common femoral artery. A sheath allows multiple catheter exchanges, especially when catheters are of different sizes, and facilitates catheter manipulation in patients with severe aortoiliac disease. Furthermore, a sheath is used in most interventional cases or when vascular access is needed for long periods of time (Fig. A3-4).

☐ GRAFT PUNCTURE

The risk of graft infection from graft puncture is controversial; however, the morbidity from a graft infection can be extremely high. Consequently, many consider giving a prophylactic dose of antibiotics intravenously 1 h prior to the procedure. Furthermore, heparinization may be considered, as the risk of thrombosis may be greater in grafts than in native femoral vessels. Contraindications to graft puncture include placement of the graft within the last 6 months, graft infection, anastomotic pseudoaneurysm, and active skin infection overlying the graft site.

☐ ALTERNATIVE ROUTES OF ARTERIAL ACCESS

The transaxillary approach is an occasionally employed alternative to femoral catheterization. The Seldinger

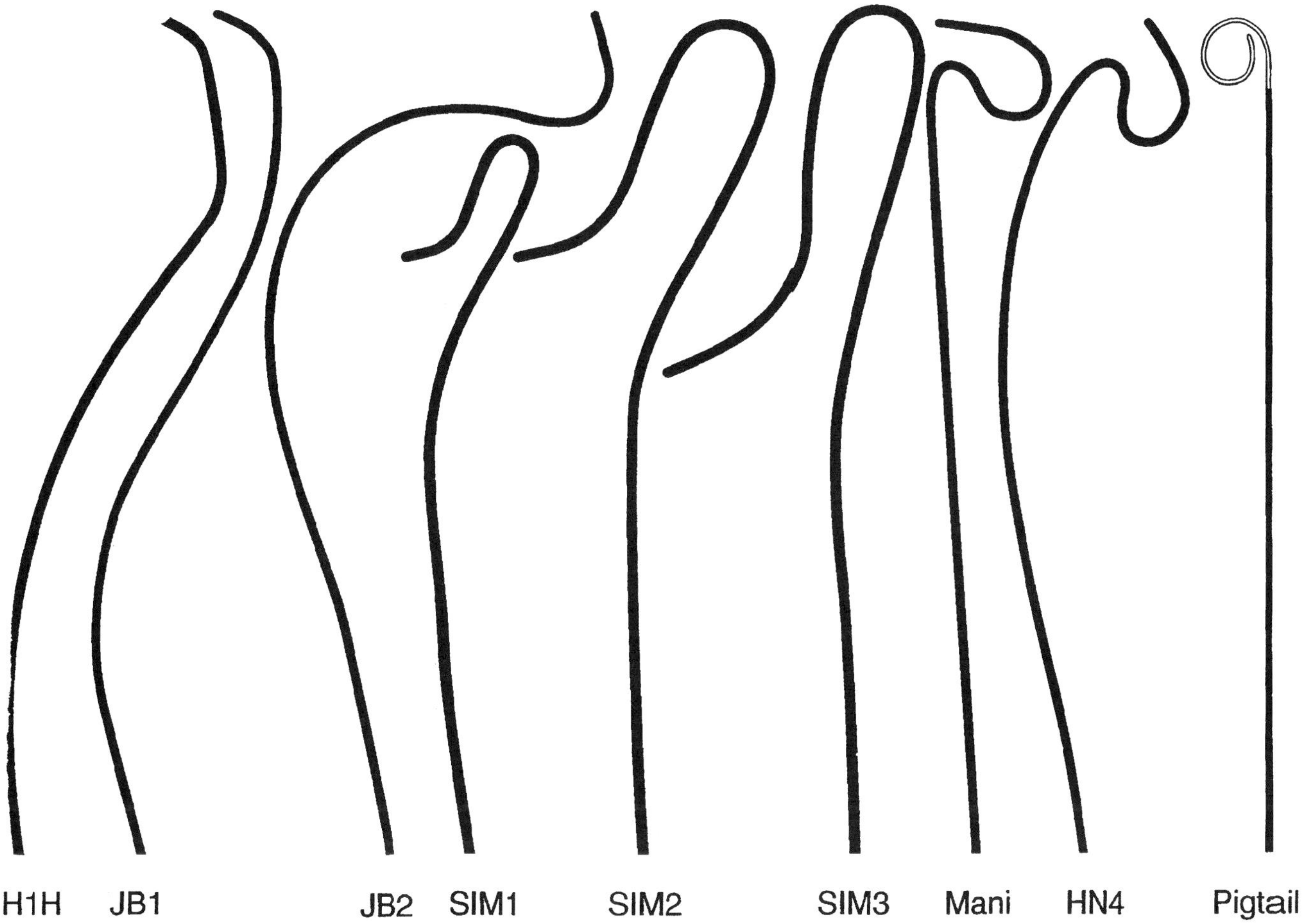

Figure A3-3 Configuration of the distal tips of commonly used neuroangiography catheters. Note the obtusely angled, gentle curvature of the catheter tip in catheters designed for younger patients (H1H, JB1) and the relatively acute angled distal bends in catheters designed for use in older patients (JB2, HN4).

technique is used, preferably from the right, with a 4 or 5 French catheter. Potential complications of this approach include hematoma formation, axillary thrombosis, and brachial plexopathy.

The transbrachial approach is felt by some to be safer than the transaxillary, with regard to arterial hemostasis and nerve injury. The brachial artery is punctured two to three fingers above the elbow crease using the Seldinger technique. A 4 French catheter is recommended or alternatively a 4 French catheter can be used with a 4 French sheath.

☐ STANDARD FILMING TECHNIQUE

Routine filming technique using cut film for cerebral angiography is two films per second for 3 s and one film per second for 6 s. If filming is done digitally, three to six frames per second is standard throughout the arterial and venous phase of the injection. Some digital units are capable of 15 to 30 frames per second, which is invaluable for evaluating extremely rapid circulation [i.e., AVM, arteriovenous fistula (AVF), and carotid-cavernous fistula (CCF)]. Refer to Table A3-1 for standard filming techniques.

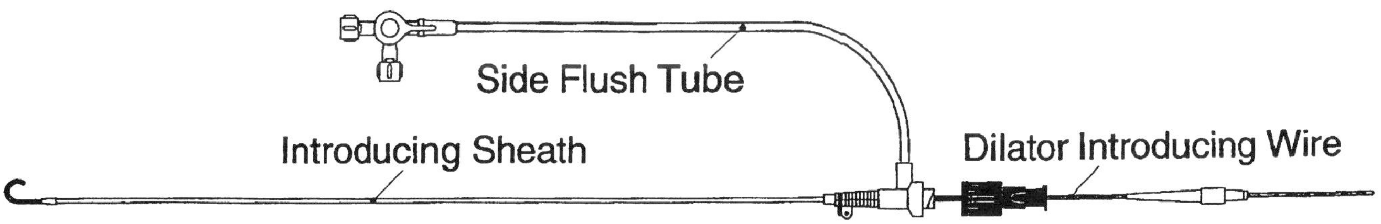

Figure A3-4 Introducing set. The set consists of a 3-mm J wire over which the dilator and sheath are inserted as a unit. The dilator is then withdrawn and heparinized saline allowed to flow through the side-port tubing.

Table A3-1
GUIDELINES FOR SELECTION OF TECHNICAL VARIABLES

		Arch	Common Carotid	Internal Carotid	External Carotid	Vertebral
Catheter choice		5F pigtail		JB1 and Hinck, for younger patients JB2, Simmons 2, Simmons 3, HN4, Mani, for older patients		
Catheter tip position		Ascending arch (1–2 cm proximal to innominate)	Below the bifurcation	C2–3	C3–4	C5–6 or at orifice of vertebral off the subclavian
Injection pressures and rise time		1050 psi 0.3 s		900 psi; 0.3–0.9 s rise time depending on stability of catheter tip position		
Injection volumes	Cut film	25 mL/s for a total of 50 mL	8 mL/s for a total of 12 mL	6 mL/s for a total of 8 mL	4 mL/s for a total of 6 mL	6 mL/s for a total of 8 mL
	Digital	20 mL/s for a total of 40 mL	6 mL/s for a total of 8 mL	4 mL/s for a total of 6 mL	3 mL/s for a total of 5 mL	4 mL/s for a total of 7 mL
Film rates	Digital	6 frames per second		6 frames per second for ± 10 s		
	Cut film	2:2:2:1:0:1:0:1		2:2:2:1:1:1:1:1:1		
Projections		1. AP: a transfacial to show circle of Willis plus distal cervical vessels 2. LAO (45–60°) over arch and arch branches	1. AP: standard angiographic angle 2. Lateral 3. Obliques over common carotid bifurcation	1. AP: standard angio angle 2. Lateral 3. Transorbital oblique with contralateral compression 4. SMV	1. AP: off-centered 2. Lateral	1. AP a. Townes' b. Transfacial 2. Lateral 3. Stenver's 4. Alcock's maneuver

☐ INJECTION VOLUMES

It is necessary to replace approximately one-third of the normal blood flow in the target vessel for contrast opacification to be adequate. For digital opacification, this estimation may be reduced by 25 to 33 percent. Hand test injections may help predict the actual flow rate when needed. The hand injection is important for assessing vessel size and flow rate, establishing catheter tip position, and assessing the course and status of the vessel. Common injection rates and volumes are listed in Table A3-1.

☐ ARTERIOVENOUS CIRCULATION TIME

The period of time from the peak concentration of contrast material in the carotid siphon to the maximum concentration in the parietal veins is called the arteriovenous circulation time and is approximately 4.2 s in normal adults and is normally more rapid in children. A circulation time greater than 6 s is prolonged.

☐ COMMONLY PERFORMED NEUROANGIOGRAPHIC PROCEDURES

The aim of neuroangiography is to demonstrate the arch branches and intracranial circulation. The examination should be tailored to the clinical situation. For routine exam paradigms, refer to Table A3-2.

The workup for transient ischemic attack (TIA) is usually begun with an arch aortogram in order to demonstrate the anatomic configuration of the arch and its branches as well as to determine regions of stenosis, ulceration, or occlusion prior to more selective catheterization. Catheterization of the common carotid arteries is then performed to evaluate the extra and intracranial circulation. The decision to perform routine vertebral angiography in TIA/stroke studies without posterior circulation symptomatology varies from institution to institution. The entire cerebral circulation, circle of Willis, and other collateral blood flow, however, cannot be completely assessed without this information.

In performing common carotid artery injections, oblique filming over the neck may be needed to best demonstrate the carotid bifurcation, with anteroposterior (AP) and lateral filming to display the intracranial circulation. The AP projection utilizes the standard angiographic angle (petrous ridges superimposed over the orbital roofs), and the lateral is centered over the sella. For vertebral angiography in the TIA/stroke setting, the AP projection is a Towne's projection in order to best demonstrate the posterior cerebral, superior cerebellar, anterior inferior cerebellar artery (AICA), and posterior inferior cerebellar artery (PICA) arteries.

In the setting of subarachnoid or intracerebral hemorrhage, the angiogram is tailored to demonstrate the intracranial vessels and the circle of Willis for exclusion of aneurysm or AVM. Fifteen to 20 percent of intracranial

Table A3-2
DIAGNOSTIC APPROACHES TO VARIOUS CLINICAL SITUATIONS

I. STROKE/TIA
  A. Arch aortogram
    1. LAO over arch—arch anatomy and origins of great vessels.
    2. Transfacial—distal cervical vessels and circle of Willis.
  B. Right and left common carotid artery (CCA)
    1. Oblique projections or AP and lateral over the bifurcations.
    2. Standard angiographic angle AP and lateral over intracranial circulation.
  C. Vertebrobasilar
    1. Towne's (frontooccipital – 30°).
    2. Lateral.

II. ANEURYSM EVALUATION
  A. Carotid circulation
    1. Selective *catheterization of internal carotid artery*, if possible, after fluoroscopic observation of bifurcation to exlcude significant plaque, stenosis, or vasospasm.
    2. *Projections*
      AP—standard angiographic angle
      Lateral—centered over sella
      Transorbital oblique—with cross compression to demonstrate anterior communicating (ACom) artery and the posterior carotid wall
      ± *Submentovertical view*—to better delineate the orientation of an ACom artery aneurysm
      ± *Houghton's view*—zygomaticoparietal projection to better delineate the middle cerebral artery bifurcation
  B. Vertebral
    1. If ipsilateral injection refluxes the contralateral vertebral to the level of PICA, it may not be necessary to catheterize both vertebral arteries.
    2. *Projections*
      AP—transfacial (petrous ridge overlaps floor of orbit) or *Towne's*.
      Stenvers—to demonstrate basilar tip and the angles between the basilar, superior cerebellar arteries (SCAs) and posterior cerebral arteries (PCAs). Origin of PICA also well seen.
      Lateral—centered over posterior fossa ± utilization of Alcock's maneuver to retrogradely opacify the PCom A.

III. VASCULITIS
  A. Essentially same as the TIA/stroke approach.
  B. Magnification views may be useful.
  C. A selective external carotid study may be useful in evaluating subtle changes of early temporal arteritis.

IV. AVM EVALUATION
  A. Essentially same as II, above, with the addition of external carotid artery sequences in AP and lateral projections.
  B. Filming or framing rate may need to be increased.
  C. Attention should also be paid to the venous circulation.
  D. Associated aneurysms should be carefully excluded, both proximally and within the arteriovenous malformation.

V. TRAUMA
  A. Survey study with arch aortogram.
  B. Selective CCA and vertebral catheterization after exclusion of injury more proximally.
  C. AP, lateral, ± oblique filming as necessary, preferably with magnification.

VI. DIRECT CAROTID CAVERNOUS FISTULAS
  A. AP and lateral projections of a selective internal carotid artery injection are performed.
  B. Flow may be too rapid to delineate exact site of fistula; therefore maximum filming rate is necessary.
  C. An Alcock's maneuver may be a useful adjunct in this regard.

VII. INDIRECT CAROTID-CAVERNOUS FISTULA (CCF)
  A. Separate selective external carotid artery injections in AP plus lateral projections.

VIII. VENOUS SINUS THROMBOSIS
  A. Filming in lateral and off axis (20°) AP projections (venous phase).

aneurysms are multiple; therefore a complete aneurysm workup is necessary in any case where a single aneurysm is found. Furthermore, arteriovenous malformations may be associated with aneurysms, and often a complete study is necessary.

Aneurysm studies may be performed with a selective internal carotid injection if the vessel is safe to enter. In addition to standard AP and lateral views, bilateral transorbital oblique (optic canal in the inferolateral quadrant of the orbit) projections with cross compression of the contralateral carotid artery are used to demonstrate the anterior communicating artery. Visualization of the anterior and posterior communicating arteries is essential, and every safe effort should be made to demonstrate these vessels. If the posterior communicators fail to fill from the carotid injections, a vertebral injection can be performed while doing an Alcock's maneuver (i.e., compression of the ipsilateral carotid artery to induce forward filling through the posterior communicator) if necessary. The submentovertical view is occasionally helpful to see the anterior and posterior communicators. A transfacial view may be useful to demonstrate the vertebrobasilar system in the AP projection (rather than a Towne's projection) when searching for basilar tip and posterior fossa aneurysms. The Stenver's view (oblique transfacial) can aid in demonstrating aneurysms in the basilar tip, those partially obscured in the angle between the origins of the PCAs and SCAs, and to better visualize the PICAs. Both vertebral arteries may need to be evaluated unless the injected vertebral artery refluxes the contralateral distal vertebral artery and demonstrates the PICA origin.

SUGGESTED READINGS

1. Chapman S, Nakielny R: *A Guide to Radiological Procedures*. London, Baillière Tindall, 1981, pp 107–117.
2. Earnest F IV et al: Complications of cerebral angiography: Prospective assessment of risk. *AJR* 142:247–253, 1984.
3. Grzyska U et al: Selective cerebral intra-arterial DSA. *Neuroradiology* 32:296–299, 1990.
4. Hankey GJ et al: Cerebral angiographic risk in mild cerebrovascular disease. *Stroke* 21:209–222, 1990.
5. Hansen M et al: *Angiography, Interventional Radiology and Neuroradiology Resident Handbook*. Dallas, TX, Parkland Memorial Hospital, 1994.
6. Heiserman JE et al: Neurologic complications of cerebral angiography. *AJNR* 15:1401–1407, 1994.
7. Osborn AG: *Introduction to Cerebral Angiography*. Philadelphia, Harper & Row, 1980, pp 1–31.
8. Osborn AG: *Diagnostic Neuroradiology*. St Louis, Mosby-Year Book, 1994, pp 117–153.
9. Polak JF et al: Carotid endarterectomy: Preoperative evaluation of candidates with combined Doppler sonography and MR angiography. *Radiology* 186:333–338, 1993.
10. Ramsey RG: *Neuroradiology*, 3d ed. Philadelphia, Saunders, 1994, pp 34–74.

Index

Page numbers in **boldface** indicate tables or illustrations.

ISBN 0-07-057128-7

90000>
9 780070 571280